# THE HUMAN ENDOMETRIUM

ANNALS OF THE NEW YORK ACADEMY OF SCIENCES
Volume 734

# THE HUMAN ENDOMETRIUM

*Edited by Carlo Bulletti, Erlio Gurpide, and Carlo Flamigni*

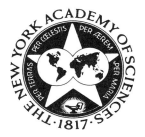

*The New York Academy of Sciences*
*New York, New York*
*1994*

Copyright © 1994 by the New York Academy of Sciences. All rights reserved. Under the provisions of the United States Copyright Act of 1976, individual readers of the Annals are permitted to make fair use of the material in them for teaching or research. Permission is granted to quote from the Annals provided that the customary acknowledgment is made of the source. Material in the Annals may be republished only by permission of the Academy. Address inquiries to the Executive Editor at the New York Academy of Sciences.

Copying fees: For each copy of an article made beyond the free copying permitted under Section 107 or 108 of the 1976 Copyright Act, a fee should be paid through the Copyright Clearance Center, Inc., 222 Rosewood Drive, Danvers, MA 01923. For articles of more than 3 pages the copying fee is $1.75.

∞ The paper used in this publication meets the minimum requirements of American National Standard for Information Sciences—Permanence of Paper for Printed Library Materials, ANSI Z39.48-1984.

Cover: *Implantation of the embryo on the endometrium.*

### Library of Congress Cataloging-in-Publication Data

The human endometrium / edited by Carlo Bulletti, Erlio Gurpide, and Carlo Flamigni.
    p.  cm. — (Annals of the New York Academy of Sciences, ISSN 0077-8923 ; v. 734)
    Papers from the Second Conference on the Endometrium, held in Bologna, Italy, September 20–22, 1993.
    Includes bibliographical references and index.
    ISBN 0-89766-871-5 (pbk. : alk. paper). — ISBN 0-89766-870-7 (cloth : alk. paper)
    1. Endometrium—Congresses.  2. Endometrium—Diseases—Congresses. I. Bulletti, Carlo.  II. Gurpide, Erlio, 1927–   . III. Flamigni, C.  IV. Conference on the Endometrium (2nd : 1993 : Bologna, Italy) V. Series.
    [DNLM: 1. Endometrium—congresses.  W1 AN626gg v.734s 1994 / WP 400 H918 1994]
Q11.N5  vol. 734
[QP262]
500 s—dc20
[612.6′2]
DNLM/DLC
for Library of Congress
                                                94-28726
                                                  CIP

BiComp/PCP
*Printed in the United States of America*
**ISBN 0-89766-870-7** (cloth)
**ISBN 0-89766-871-5** (paper)
**ISSN 0077-8923**

ANNALS OF THE NEW YORK ACADEMY OF SCIENCES
Volume 734
September 30, 1994

# THE HUMAN ENDOMETRIUM[a]

*Editors and Conference Chairs*
Carlo Bulletti, Erlio Gurpide, and Carlo Flamigni

## CONTENTS

| | |
|---|---|
| Preface. *By* the Editors | xi |

**Part I. Endometrial Cell Proliferation, Decidualization, and Decidual Products**

| | |
|---|---|
| Regulatory Roles of IFN-Gamma in Human Endometrium. *By* S. Tabibzadeh | 1 |
| Growth Factors and Decidualization *in Vitro*. *By* Juan C. Irwin, Lisa De Las Fuentes, and Linda C. Giudice | 7 |
| Mechanism of Human Endometrial Stromal Cells Decidualization. *By* Baiqing Tang, Seth Guller, and Erlio Gurpide | 19 |
| Decidual Progesterone and Estrogen Receptors in the First Trimester of Pregnancy. *By* Ivo Noci, Patrizia Borri, Enrico Periti, Francesco Branconi, Gianni Messeri, Paola Tozzi, Francesca Torricelli, Lucia Nutini, Milena Paglierani, Gianni Taddei, and Gianfranco Scarselli | 26 |
| Protease and Protease Inhibitor Expression during *in Vitro* Decidualization of Human Endometrial Stromal Cells. *By* Frederick Schatz, Csaba Papp, Erno Toth-Pal, Vito Cudemo, Virginia Hausknecht, Graciela Krikun, Leszek Markiewicz, Beni Gavi, En-Yu Wang, Naum Feygin, Zoltan Papp, and Charles J. Lockwood | 33 |
| The Adhesion Molecules on Human Endometrial Stromal Cells: Immunological Implications. *By* Mauro Busacca, Paola Viganò, Barbara Magri, and Mario Vignali | 43 |

---

[a] This volume contains papers from a conference entitled *Second Conference on the Endometrium*, which was held by the University of Bologna and the Mount Sinai School of Medicine of New York in Bologna, Italy on September 20–22, 1993.

## Part II. Endometrial Vascularization, Hemostasis, and Dysfunctional Uterine Bleeding (DUB)

Vascularization of Human Endometrium: Uterine Blood Flow in Healthy Condition and in Primary Dysmenorrhoea. *By* MATS ÅKERLUND .... 47

The Role of Progestationally Regulated Stromal Cell Tissue Factor and Type-1 Plasminogen Activator Inhibitor (PAI-1) in Endometrial Hemostasis and Menstruation. *By* CHARLES J. LOCKWOOD, GRACIELA KRIKUN, CSABA PAPP, ERNO TOTH-PAL, LESZEK MARKIEWICZ, EN-YU WANG, THOMAS KERENYI, XIAODONG ZHOU, VIRGINIA HAUSKNECHT, ZOLTAN PAPP, and FREDERICK SCHATZ .... 57

Dysfunctional Uterine Bleeding (DUB). *By* C. BULLETTI, C. FLAMIGNI, R. A. PREFETTO, V. POLLI, and E. GIACOMUCCI .............. 80

## Part III. Uterine Receptivity and Human Blastocyst Implantation: Basic

Potential Roles for the Low Density Lipoprotein Receptor Family of Proteins in Implantation and Placentation. *By* GEORGE COUKOS, MATS E. GÅFVELS, FRANK WITTMAACK, HIROYA MATSUO, DUDLEY K. STRICKLAND, CHRISTOS COUTIFARIS, and JEROME F. STRAUSS III ................................... 91

The Endometrial Cell Surface and Implantation: Expression of the Polymorphic Mucin MUC-1 and Adhesion Molecules during the Endometrial Cycle. *By* J. D. APLIN, M. W. SEIF, R. A. GRAHAM, N. A. HEY, F. BEHZAD, and S. CAMPBELL .................... 103

Human Trophoblast Invasion: Autocrine Control and Paracrine Modulation. *By* MICHAEL T. MCMASTER, KATHRYN E. BASS, and SUSAN J. FISHER............................................ 122

Negative Regulation and Placental Fibronectin Expression by Glucocorticoids and Cyclic Adenosine 3',5'-Monophosphate. *By* SETH GULLER, ROBERT WOZNIAK, MATTHEW I. LEIBMAN, and CHARLES J. LOCKWOOD ....................................... 132

Hormone Regulation and Hormone Antagonist Effects on Protein Patterns of Human Endometrial Secretion during Receptivity. *By* KARIN BEIER-HELLWIG, KARL STERZIK, BARBARA BONN, ULRIKE HILMES, MARC BYGDEMAN, KRISTINA GEMZELL-DANIELSSON, and HENNING M. BEIER ......................... 143

The Role of Leukemia Inhibitory Factor (LIF) and Other Cytokines in Regulating Implantation in Mammals. *By* COLIN L. STEWART....... 157

Formation of the Chorio-Decidual Interface of Human Fetal Membranes: Is It Analogous to Anchoring Villi Development in the Placenta? *By* S. C. BELL and T. M. MALAK ............................. 166

## Part IV. Uterine Receptivity and Human Blastocyst Implantation: Clinical

Morphology of the Human Endometrium in the Peri-Implantation Period. *By* T. C. LI, M. A. WARREN, C. J. HILL, and H. SARAVELOS....... 169

Human Endometrial Lymphocytes in Normal Pregnancy and Pregnancy
  Loss. *By* JUDITH N. BULMER ............................... 185

Is Controlled Ovarian Stimulation Associated with Adverse Endometrial
  Effects? *By* ARIE BIRKENFELD ............................. 193

The Use of the Donor Oocyte Program to Evaluate Embryo
  Implantation. *By* JEROME H. CHECK ........................ 198

Hormonal Control of Endometrial Receptivity: the Egg Donation Model
  and Controlled Ovarian Hyperstimulation. *By* DOMINIQUE DE
  ZIEGLER, RENATO FANCHIN, MARC MASSONNEAU, CHRISTINE
  BERGERON, RENÉ FRYDMAN, and PHILIPPE BOUCHARD ........... 209

Endometrial and Embryonic Factors Involved in Successful Implantation.
  *By* C. BULLETTI, V. POLLI, F. LICASTRO, and R. PARMEGGIANI .... 221

Intravenous Immunoglobulin (IVIG) in the Prevention of Implantation
  Failures. *By* G. DE PLACIDO, F. ZULLO, A. MOLLO, F. CAPPIELLO,
  A. NAZZARO, N. COLACURCI, and G. PALUMBO................. 232

Immunologically Mediated Abortion (IMA): a Minireview.
  *By* E. GIACOMUCCI, C. BULLETTI, V. POLLI, and C. FLAMIGNI ..... 235

## Part V. The Endometrium under Contraception

Regulation of Endometrial Differentiation by Synthetic Steroids *in Vitro*.
  *By* L. KIESEL and M. MAPPES .............................. 237

Interaction between Steroid Hormones and Endometrial Opioids.
  *By* ACHILLE GRAVANIS, ANTONIS MAKRIGIANNAKIS, CHRISTOS
  STOURNARAS, and ANDREW N. MARGIORIS .................... 245

Hormonal Contraception: Current Status and Future Perspectives.
  *By* CHRISTIAN F. HOLINKA ................................. 257

## Part VI. The Endometrium under Hormone Replacement Therapy

Morphological Aspects of Human Endometrium during Hormone
  Replacement Therapy. *By* LUIGI DE CECCO, DANIELA GERBALDO,
  PAOLO CRISTOFORONI, ANTONELLA FERRAIOLO, VALENTINO
  REMORGIDA, PATRIZIA BARACCHINI, and EZIO PULCHERI ........ 263

Aspects of Hormone Replacement Therapy. *By* CHRISTIAN F. HOLINKA.. 271

*In Vitro* Bioassays for Drugs with Dual Estrogenic and Progestagenic
  Activities. *By* LESZEK MARKIEWICZ and ERLIO GURPIDE .......... 285

## Part VII. Endometrial Cancer

Epidermal Growth Factor Receptor Expression and Endometrial Cancer
  Histotypes. *By* VALERIO M. JASONNI, DONATELLA SANTINI,
  ANDREA AMADORI, CLAUDIO CECCARELLI, and SILVIA NALDI...... 298

Clinical Response of Abnormal Endometrial Growth to Hormonal
  Treatment. *By* E. LÓPEZ DE LA OSA GONZÁLEZ................. 306

Tamoxifen and Endometrial Cancer. *By* P. SISMONDI, N. BIGLIA, E. VOLPI, M. GIAI, and T. DE GRANDIS ..................... 310

## Part VIII. Endometriosis

Cytokine Regulation of Cellular Proliferation in Endometriosis. *By* NANCY A. KLEIN, GABRIELA M. PÉRGOLA, RAJESHWAR RAO TEKMAL, IRIS A. MONTOYA, TAMMY D. DEY, and ROBERT S. SCHENKEN ..................... 322

Deeply Infiltrating Endometriosis Is a Disease Whereas Mild Endometriosis Could Be Considered a Non-Disease. *By* PHILIPPE R. KONINCKX, DIDIER OOSTERLYNCK, THOMAS D'HOOGHE, and CHRISTEL MEULEMAN ..................... 333

Peritoneal Endometriosis: Two-Dimensional and Three-Dimensional Evaluation of Typical and Subtle Lesions. *By* JACQUES DONNEZ, MICHELLE NISOLLE, and FRANÇOISE CASANAS-ROUX ..................... 342

Epidemiology and Diagnosis of Endometriosis. *By* G. B. MELIS, S. AJOSSA, S. GUERRIERO, A. M. PAOLETTI, M. ANGIOLUCCI, B. PIRAS, A. CAFFIERO, and V. MAIS ..................... 352

The Recurrence of Endometriosis. *By* LUIGI FEDELE, STEFANO BIANCHI, GIULIANA DI NOLA, MASSIMO CANDIANI, MAURO BUSACCA, and MARIO VIGNALI ..................... 358

## Part IX. Parturition

Parathyroid Hormone and Parathyroid Hormone-Related Protein Stimulate Adenylate Cyclase in Human Endometrial Stromal Cells. *By* M. LINETTE CASEY, AHMET ERK, and PAUL C. MACDONALD.... 365

Is Vasopressin Involved as a Local Mediator in the Mechanism of Parturition? *By* ALESSANDRO MAURI, CARLO TICCONI, ANNIBALE VOLPE, and EMILIO PICCIONE ..................... 372

Secretion and Putative Role of Activin and CRF in Human Parturition. *By* FELICE PETRAGLIA, PASQUALE FLORIO, ANDREA GALLINELLI, ANTONELLO A. DE MICHEROUX, ALLESANDRO FERRARI, DAVIDE DE VITA, LORENZO AGUZZOLI, ALESSANDRO D. GENAZZANI, and COSTANTINO DI CARLO ..................... 380

Antiprogestins in the Induction of Labor. *By* KRISTOF CHWALISZ and ROBERT E. GARFIELD ..................... 387

The Preterm Labor Syndrome. *By* ROBERTO ROMERO, MOSHE MAZOR, HERNAN MUNOZ, RICARDO GOMEZ, MAURIZIO GALASSO, and DAVID M. SHERER ..................... 414

Morphometric Characteristics of the Decidua, Cytotrophoblast, and Connective Tissue of the Prelabor Ruptured Fetal Membranes. *By* T. M. MALAK, G. MULHOLLAND, and S. C. BELL ..................... 430

## Part X. Gynecologic Endoscopy

Operative Laparoscopy: Videolaparoscopy and Videolaseroscopy.
By CAMRAN NEZHAT, FARR NEZHAT, and CEANA NEZHAT . . . . . . . . . .   433

The Rationale for Use of Medical Suppressive Therapy Prior to
Endoscopic Surgery. By VEASY C. BUTTRAM, JR. . . . . . . . . . . . . . . .   445

Laparoscopic Myomectomy: Operative Procedure and Results. By JEAN-
BERNARD DUBUISSON and CHARLES CHAPRON . . . . . . . . . . . . . . . . . .   450

Endoscopic Treatment of Dermoid Cyst. By MAURIZIO ROSATI . . . . . . . . .   455

Therapeutic Strategy in Tubal Infertility. By FRANÇOIS AUDIBERT . . . . . . .   460

Operative Hysteroscopy: Ten Years' Experience. By A. PERINO,
P. CRISTOFORONI, and N. CHIANCHIANO . . . . . . . . . . . . . . . . . . . . . . .   469

Ultrasound, Hysteroscopy, and Histological Assessment of the
Endometrium in Postmenopausal Women. By G. POSSATI, V. M.
JASONNI, S. NALDI, S. MAZZONE, S. GABRIELLI, M. BEVINI,
G. MUSERRA, A. PARESCHI, and C. FLAMIGNI . . . . . . . . . . . . . . . . . . .   479

Can Hysteroscopic Evaluation of Endometrial Carcinoma Influence
Therapeutic Treatment? By G. L. TADDEI, D. MONCINI,
G. SCARSELLI, C. TANTINI, and G. BARGELLI . . . . . . . . . . . . . . . . . . .   482

Hysteroscopic Metroplasty. By ALBERTO MARABINI, GIAMPIETRO
GUBBINI, ROBERTA STAGNOZZI, MARCO STEFANETTI, MANUELA
FILONI, and ALESSANDRO BOVICELLI . . . . . . . . . . . . . . . . . . . . . . . . .   488

Subject Index . . . . . . . . . . . . . . . . . . . . . . . . . . . . . . . . . . . . . . . . . . . . . .   493

Index of Contributors . . . . . . . . . . . . . . . . . . . . . . . . . . . . . . . . . . . . . . .   499

**Financial assistance was received from:**

*Major funder*
- ZENECA SpA

*Supporter*
- SANOFY WINTHROP SpA

*Contributors*
- A.C.R. ANGELINI FRANCESCO SpA
- ASTA MEDICA SpA
- ORGANON ITALIA SpA
- BRACCO SpA
- CIBA GEIGY SpA
- WYETH SpA
- SCS INTERNATIONAL Srl

---

The New York Academy of Sciences believes it has a responsibility to provide an open forum for discussion of scientific questions. The positions taken by the participants in the reported conferences are their own and not necessarily those of the Academy. The Academy has no intent to influence legislation by providing such forums.

# Preface

This volume of the *Annals of the New York Academy of Sciences* includes communications presented at the Second Conference on the Endometrium held under the auspices of the University of Bologna on September 20–22, 1993 with truly international participation.

The proceedings of the First Conference on the Primate Endometrium were published as Volume 622 of these *Annals* in 1991. The Introduction to that volume emphasized the clinical, endocrine, and biochemical relevance of studies on the endometrium. It also called attention to the wide variety of possibilities that the human endometrium offers for research, including *in vitro* studies with tissue fragments, homogeneous preparations of cells of different types, which could also be mixed to observe their paracrine interactions.

This second conference, in addition to reporting new results on these subjects, covered topics of increasing current interest in endometrial research including proliferation and differentiation of endometrial cells, vascularization and hemostasis, contraception and hormonal replacement, embryo receptivity, implantation, pregnancy, and parturition.

The rich mine for biochemical and hormonal research provided by human endometrial tissue, available at various phases of the menstrual cycle, continues to yield novel findings of potential clinical significance on topics as important as assisted human reproduction, pregnancy maintenance, and contraception. Furthermore, the special characteristics of cells isolated from the endometrium and the cell lines derived from human endometrial adenocarcinomas are helping in studies of the biology of these tumors and of the susceptibility of endometrial cancer to anticancer drugs.

We extend thanks to all those whose efforts made this conference possible, beginning with the members of the Program Committee, Drs. H. M. Beier, J. N. Bulmer, V. M. Jasonni, R. Romero, R. S. Schenken, J. F. Strauss, and D. de Ziegler. The various sessions were chaired by Drs. D. Amadori, F. Audibert, H. M. Beier, G. Benagiano, A. Birkenfeld, L. Bovicelli, J. N. Bulmer, J. H. Check, L. Fedele, A. R. Genazzani, A. G. Gravanis, C. F. Holinka, C. J. Lockwood, E. López de la Osa Gonzalez, C. Melega, C. Nezhat, M. Nisolle, R. Romero, G. Scarselli, and J. F. Strauss. The Department of Obstetrics, Gynecology, and Reproductive Science of the Mount Sinai School of Medicine in New York and the Reproductive Medicine Unit of the Department of Obstetrics and Gynecology of the University of Bologna provided helpful support. The staff of our organizing secretariat, O.S.C. Bologna, particularly Ms. Maria Antonietta Dioli and Ms. Lilia De Santis, in collaboration with Ms. Ann Rogers of the Mount Sinai School of Medicine, contributed importantly to the arrangements for the conference. Finally, Ms. Sheila Kane and Dr. Cook Kimball of the Editorial Department of the New York Academy of Sciences efficiently edited and directed the production of this volume.

*Carlo Bulletti*
*Erlio Gurpide*
*Carlo Flamigni*

# Regulatory Roles of IFN-Gamma in Human Endometrium[a]

S. TABIBZADEH[b]

*Department of Pathology*
*University of South Florida Health Sciences Center*
*and*
*Moffitt Cancer Center*
*12902 Magnolia Drive*
*Tampa, Florida 33612*

## Microenvironments in Human Endometrium: Contribution of Cytokines to Their Development

Human endometrium is composed of glandular structures invested with endometrial stroma. The structure of endometrium after birth is quite simple and is composed of a surface epithelium, and short simple glands surrounded by stroma. The complex structure of endometrium exhibiting the development of several microenvironments is not attained until puberty.[1] This includes the well-known basalis and functionalis microenvironments. The stromal cells around the spiral arteries delineate a different microenvironment where predecidua associated with the expression of VLA-1 and $\alpha_1$ PEG first appears.[2-3] Stromal cells that reside around glands and underneath surface epithelium and that express Ber-EP4 and those that surround lymphoid cells and express HLA-DR molecules exemplify other distinct microenvironments within the endometrial tissue.[4] Concomitant with the development of this complex and distinct tissue architecture, endometrium begins to undergo characteristic phases of proliferation, and secretion followed by menstrual shedding. The role of systemic steroids, estradiol-17$\beta$ (E2) and progesterone (P) as signals paramount in driving the endometrial cells through these cycles is well studied. Since receptors for E2 and P are present in all endometrial epithelial cells, development of microenvironments peculiar to the endometrial tissue may not simply be explained based on the effects of these factors.[5-7] This includes regional specific attributes that may be well delineated by characterizing proliferation, and expression of diverse proteins in the endometrial cells.[4,8-12] It is more likely that effects of sex steroid hormones are mediated by paracrine modulators of cell function. For example it was suggested that the proliferative effect of E2 in the mouse endometrium is mediated through epidermal growth factor (EGF)/transforming growth factor (TGF)-$\alpha$.[13-14] Recognizing the paracrine driving forces behind the unique local features of this tissue is extremely important in view of the role of endometrium in conception and the high incidence of morbidity that results from its aberrant development. For example, it is suggested that certain cytokines including tumor necrosis factor (TNF)-$\alpha$, interleukin (IL)-1, IL-8, colony stimulating factor (CSF)-1, granulocyte-macrophage (GM)-

---

[a] This work is supported by Public Health Research Grant CA46866.
[b] Address for correspondence: S. Tabibzadeh, MD, Department of Pathology, Moffitt Cancer Center, 12902 Magnolia Drive, Tampa, FL 33612.

CSF and TGF-α may be involved in parturition.[14–19] We demonstrated expression of protein and mRNA of TNF-α, IL-1α, IL-1β, interleukin receptor antagonist protein (IRAP), IL-6, TGF-α, TNF-α and CSF-1 in human endometrium.[20–23] Despite the species differences, expression of various cytokines including IL-1, IL-6, TNF-α and CSF-1 have also been shown in the mouse uterus.[24–25] On the surface, the function of such large array of endometrial cytokines may seem alarmingly too complex to dissect. However, undoubtedly a delicate balance in regulation of their function is attained by their active interactive network and by the regulatory control of steroid hormones.[26–41]

Based on the mitotic rate in the primate uterus, it was suggested that a quadripartite zonation exists in endometrium.[42] However, our work has allowed us, based on the expression of various proteins and proliferative activity, to show that division of endometrium into such distinct compartments is not warranted.[8–10,12] Proliferation is a characteristic feature of endometrial epithelium during the proliferative phase. Autoradiographic studies in explant cultures support the view that proliferation is observed until the third postovulatory day.[11] We demonstrated that the proliferative activity is marked in the upper functionalis epithelium and gradually diminishes towards the basalis.[10] Expression of various proteins gradually rather than abruptly changes from the basalis towards the surface.[8,12] Such gradual changes argue against the presence of distinct regions separated by sharp, demarcating boundaries. In contrast, such data provide support for the existence of a polarized gradient likely to be produced by paracrine factors. This concept does not represent a radical departure from the traditional view that steroids are the primary and essential regulators of endometrial function. Demonstration of steroid hormone receptors in lymphoid cells, positive regulation of IFN-gamma promoter by E2, modulation of release of IL-1 and TNF-α from leukocytes and modulation of cytokine actions by E2 all show the tight interaction of steroid hormones and the cytokine network.[7,26–41]

Based on the concept that the development of a polarized environment is dependent on local rather than systemic factors, we postulated the existence of paracrine factors that are potentially responsible for creation of these microenvironments in human endometrium.[8] The distribution of the lymphoid aggregates in the basalis is the only anatomically impressive difference that one can observe between the functionalis and basalis regions.[1,8,43–47] Lymphoid aggregates exhibit a predominant population of T cells.[7–8,43–47] Expression of HLA-DR, HLA-DP, HLA-DQ and VLA-1 in endometrial T cells suggested that they are activated and are potentially capable of cytokine secretion.[48] The major theme of our hypothesis rests on the premise that the development of a polarized microenvironment identifiable by growth characteristics and HLA-DR expression of endometrial epithelium are T cell/IFN-gamma driven. Confirmatory evidence for the validity of this hypothesis has been provided as IFN-gamma has been localized to these aggregates as well as a scattering of other cells in the stroma.[49] We reported that HLA-DR expression and proliferation in human endometrium are differentially regulated.[2,8–10] Differential protein expression was not exclusive of HLA-DR and was also observed for some members of the integrin family of molecules.[12] The differential regulation of endometrial epithelial function could not be based on the disparate expression of IFN-gamma receptor in the basalis versus functionalis epithelium.[48] Furthermore, addition of the endometrial T cells to autologous epithelial cells focally induced expression of HLA-DR molecules in epithelial cells to which the leukocytes were bound. Supernatants of endometrial T cells also induced HLA-DR molecules in the endometrial epithelial cells. Finally, the HLA-DR-inducing activity of the supernatant was inhibited with an antiserum to IFN-gamma.[50] We also demonstrated that IFN-gamma induces HLA-DR expression and inhibits proliferation of endometrial epithelial cells.[51-52] We recently devised an *in vitro* model that allowed determination of the impact of a cytokine gradient on diverse epithelial cell attributes. Our experimentation with this model system clearly showed that at a given time, growth and HLA-DR expression in epithelial cells are uniquely dictated by the amount of IFN-gamma and the distances of the epithelial cells from the source of the cytokine.[53] We showed that endometrial epithelial cells are extremely sensitive to IFN-gamma and IL-1$\alpha$.[41,51-52,54] The class II molecules (HLA-DR, HLA-DP and HLA-DQ) were differentially induced by IFN-gamma treatment of endometrial epithelial cell lines with HLA-DR being the predominant induced molecule.[9] This finding was in accord with the expression of class II molecules in human endometrium.[9] Taken together, these findings concur with the view that the differential regulation of proliferation and HLA-DR expression within endometrial epithelium is under the regulatory role of T cells activated within lymphoid aggregates.

## SUMMARY

Available data suggest that several microenvironments exist within the complex structure of human endometrium. Predecidual reaction which is associated with the expression of VLA-1 and $\alpha_1$ PEG first appears in the stromal cells around the spiral arteries. Expression of Ber-EP4 is limited to a distinct group of stromal cells that reside around glands and underneath surface epithelium. A distinctly different group of stromal cells that surround lymphoid cells express HLA-DR molecules. The proliferative activity of endometrial epithelium is markedly higher in the upper functionalis and is gradually diminished towards the basalis. In addition, several proteins, including HLA-DR and some members of the integrin family of molecules are strongly expressed in the basalis epithelium. The expression of these proteins in endometrial epithelium is gradually diminished towards the surface. The gradual rather than abrupt changes in the expression of proteins and proliferative activity across the length of endometrial epithelium argues against separation of endometrium into the distinct regions of basalis and functionalis. Rather, such distribution is in favor of existence of a polarized microenvironment in human endometrium. Emerging evidence suggests that the development of this microenvironment is mediated by T cells activated within lymphoid aggregates with consequent secretion of IFN-gamma. IFN-gamma regulates HLA-DR expression and proliferation of endometrial epithelium. Maximal impact of the cytokine is exerted in regions close to the source of cytokine with a gradual dissipation of the effect distant from this source. Therefore, this cytokine may be the prototype of a group of paracrine factors that induce a polarized microenvironment in human endometrium.

## REFERENCES

1. BLAUSTEIN, A. 1982. Pathology of the Female Genital Tract. Second Edit. A. Blaustein, Ed. Springer-Verlag. New York.
2. TABIBZADEH, S. 1990. Immunoreactivity of human endometrium: correlation with endometrial dating. Fertil. Steril. **54:** 624–631.
3. WAITES, G. T., R. F. L. JAMES & S. C. BELL. 1988. Immunohistological localization of the human endometrial secretory protein pregnancy-associated endometrial

$\alpha_1$-globulin, an insulin-like growth factor-binding protein, during the menstrual cycle. J. Endocrinol. Metab. **67:** 1100.
4. TABIBZADEH, S. 1991. Distinct subsets of stromal cells confined to unique microenvironments in human endometrium throughout the menstrual cycle. Am. J. Reprod. Immunol. **26:** 5-10.
5. PRESS, M. F. & G. L. GREENE. 1984. Method in laboratory investigation. An immunocytochemical method for demonstrating estrogen receptor in human uterus using monoclonal antibodies to human estrophilin. Lab. Invest. **50:** 480-486.
6. PRESS, M. F., N. A. NOUSEK-GOEBL, M. BUR & G. L. GREENE. 1986. Estrogen receptor localization in the female genital tract. Am. J. Pathol. **123:** 280-292.
7. TABIBZADEH, S. S. & P. G. SATYASWAROOP. 1989. Sex steroid receptors in lymphoid cells of human endometrium. Am. J. Clin. Pathol. **91:** 656-663.
8. TABIBZADEH, S. S., A. BETTICA & M. A. GERBER. 1986. Variable expression of Ia antigens in human endometrium and in chronic endometritis. Am. J. Clin. Pathol. **86:** 153-160.
9. TABIBZADEH, S. S. & P. G. SATYASWAROOP. 1989. Differential expression of HLA-DR, HLA-DP and HLA-DQ antigenic determinants of the major histocompatibility complex in human endometrium. Am. J. Reprod. Immunol. Microbiol. **18:** 124-130.
10. TABIBZADEH, S. S. 1990. Proliferative activity of lymphoid cells in human endometrium throughout the menstrual cycle. J. Endocrinol. Metab. **70:** 437-443.
11. FERENCZY, A., G. BERTRAND & M. M. GELFAND. 1979. Proliferation kinetics of human endometrium during the normal menstrual cycle. Am. J. Obstet. Gynecol. **133:** 859-867.
12. TABIBZADEH, S. 1992. Patterns of expression of integrin molecules in human endometrium throughout the menstrual cycle. Hum. Reprod. **7:** 876-882.
13. NELSON, K. G., T. TAKAHASHI, D. C. LEE, N. C. LUETTEKE, N. L. BOSSERT, K. ROSS, B. E. EITZMAN & J. A. MCLACHLAN. 1992. Transforming growth factor-$\alpha$ is a potential mediator of estrogen action in the mouse uterus. Endocrinology **131:** 1657-1664.
14. MCLACHLAN, J. A., K. G. NELSON, T. TAKAHASHI, N. L. BOSSERT, R. R. NEWBOLD & K. S. KORACH. 1991. Do growth factors mediate estrogen action in the uterus? *In* The New Biology of Steroid Hormones. R. B. Hochberg & F. Naftolin, Eds. Vol. 74: 337-344. Raven Press. New York.
15. ROMERO, R., M. MAZOR & B. TARTAKOVSKY. 1991. Systemic administration of interleukin-1 induces preterm parturition in mice. Am. J. Obstet. Gynecol. **165:** 969-971.
16. ROMERO, R., K. R. MANOGUE, D. M. MURRAY, Y. K. WU, E. OYARZUN, J. C. HOBBINS & A. CERAMI. 1989. Infection and labor. IV. Cachectin-tumor necrosis factor in the amniotic fluid of women with intraamniotic infection and preterm labor. Am. J. Obstet. Gynecol. **161:** 336-341.
17. ROMERO, R., Y. K. WU, E. OYARZUN, J. C. HOBBINS & M. D. MITCHELL. 1989. A potential role of epidermal growth factor/$\alpha$ transforming growth factor in human parturition. Eur. J. Obstet. Gynecol. Reprod. Biol. **33:** 55-60.
18. DUDLEY, D. J., M. S. TRAUTMAN & M. D. MITCHELL. 1993. Inflammatory mediators regulate interleukin-8 production by cultured gestational tissues: evidence for a cytokine network at the chorio-decidual interface. J. Endocrinol. Metab. **76:** 404-410.
19. HILL, J. A. 1992. Cytokines considered critical in pregnancy. Am. J. Reprod. Immunol. **28:** 123-126.
20. TABIBZADEH, S. & X. Z. SUN. 1992. Cytokine expression in human endometrium throughout the menstrual cycle. Hum. Reprod. **7:** 1214-1221.
21. TABIBZADEH, S. 1991. Ubiquitous expression of TNF-$\alpha$/cachectin in human endometrium. Am. J. Rep. Immunol. **26:** 1-5.
22. HUNT, J. S., H.-L. CHEN, X.-L. HU & S. TABIBZADEH. 1992. Tumor necrosis factor-$\alpha$ mRNA and protein in human endometrium. Hum. Reprod. **47:** 141-147.
23. PAMPFER, S., S. TABIBZADEH, F.-C. CHUAN & J. W. POLLARD. 1991. Molecular cloning of a novel transcript for colony stimulating factor-1 from human endometrial glands. Production of a transmembrane form of the protein. J. Mol. Endocrinol. **5:** 1931-1938.

24. SANFORD, M. D. T. R. & G. W. WOOD. 1993. Expression of interleukin 1, interleukin 6 and tumour necrosis factor $\alpha$ in mouse uterus during the peri-implantation period of pregnancy. J. Reprod. Fertil. **97:** 83–89.
25. ARCECI, R. J., F. SHANHAN, E. R. STANLEY & J. W. POLLARD. 1989. Temporal expression and location of colony-stimulating factor 1 (CSF-1) and its receptor in the female reproductive tract are consistent with CSF-1-regulated placental development. Proc. Natl. Acad. Sci. USA **86:** 8818–8822.
26. TABIBZADEH, S. 1991. Human endometrium: an active site of cytokine production and action. Endocr. Rev. **12:** 272–290.
27. BRIGSTOCK, D. R. 1991. Growth factors in the uterus: steroidal regulation and biological actions. Baillier's Clin. Endocrinol. Metab. **5:** 791–808.
28. ININNS, E. K., M. GATANAGA, F. CAPPUCCINI, C. A. DETT, R. S. YAMAMOTO, G. A. GRANGER & T. GATANAGA. 1992. Growth of the endometrial adenocarcinoma cell line AN3 CA is modulated by tumor necrosis factor and its receptor is upregulated by estrogen *in vitro*. Endocrinology **130:** 1852–1856.
29. LOY, R. A., J. A. LOUKIDES & M. L. POLAN. 1992. Ovarian steroids modulate human monocyte tumor necrosis factor alpha messenger ribonucleic acid levels in cultured human peripheral monocytes. Fertil. Steril. **58:** 733–739.
30. FUKUOKA, M., K. YASUDA, H. FUJIWARA, H. KANZAKI & T. MORI. 1992. Interactions between interferon $\gamma$, tumour necrosis factor $\alpha$, and interleukin-1 in modulating progesterone and oestradiol production by human luteinized granulosa cells in culture. Hum. Reprod. **7:** 1361–1364.
31. POLLARD, J. W., A. BARTOCCI, R. ARCECI, A. ORLOFSKY, M. B. LANDER & E. R. STANLEY. 1987. Apparent role of the macrophage growth factor, CSF-1, in placental development. Nature **330:** 484–486.
32. GONZALEZ, F., J. LAKSHAMANN, S. HOATH & D. A. FISHER. 1984. Effect of oestradiol-17$\beta$ on uterine epidermal growth factor concentration in immature mice. Acta Endocrinol. **105:** 425–428.
33. MUKKU, V. R. & G. M. STANCEL. 1985. Regulation of epidermal growth factor receptor by estrogen. J. Biol. Chem. **260:** 9820–9824.
34. FOX, H., B. L. BOND & T. G. PARSLOW. 1991. Estrogen regulates the IFN-$\gamma$ promoter. J. Immunol. **146:** 4362–4367.
35. MORI, H., M. NAKAGAWA, N. ITOH, K. WADA & T. TAMAYA. 1990. Danazol suppresses the production of interleukin-1$\beta$ and tumor necrosis factor by human monocytes. Am. J. Reprod. Immunol. **24:** 45–50.
36. POLAN, M. L., A. DANIELE & A. KUO. 1988. Gonadal steroids modulate human monocyte interleukin-1 (IL-1) activity. Fertil. Steril. **49:** 964–968.
37. PACIFICI, R., C. BROWN, E. PUSCHECK, E. FRIEDRICH, E. SLATOPOLOSKY, D. MAGGIO, R. MCCRACKEN & L. V. AVIOLI. 1991. Effect of surgical menopause and estrogen replacement on cytokine release from human blood mononuclear cells. Proc. Natl. Acad. Sci. USA **88:** 5134–5138.
38. DANFORTH, D. N., JR. & M. K. SGAGIAS. 1991. Interleukin 1$\alpha$ blocks estradiol-stimulated growth and down-regulates the estrogen receptor in MCF-7 breast cancer cells *in vitro*. Cancer Res. **51:** 1488–1493.
39. WANG, Y., H. D. CAMPBELL & I. G. YOUNG. 1993. Sex hormones and dexamethasone modulate interleukin-5 gene expression in T lymphocytes. J. Steroid Biochem. Mol. Biol. **44:** 203–210.
40. TABIBZADEH, S. S., U. SANTHANAM, P. B. SEHGAL & L. MAY. 1989. Cytokine-induced production of interferon $\beta_2$/interleukin-6 by freshly explanted human endometrial stromal cells. Modulation by estradiol-17$\beta$. J. Immunol. **142:** 3134–3139.
41. TABIBZADEH, S. S., A. SIVARAJAH, D. CARPENTER, B. M. OHLSSON-WILHELM & P. G. SATYASWAROOP. 1990. Modulation of HLA-DR expression in epithelial cells by interleukin 1 and estradiol-17$\beta$. J. Endocrinol. Metab. **71:** 740–747.
42. PADYKULA, H. A., L. G. COLES, J. A. MCCRACKEN, N. W. KING, JR., C. LONGCOPE & I. R. KAISERMAN-ABRAMOF. 1984. A zonal pattern of cell proliferation and differentiation in the Rhesus endometrium during the estrogen surge. Biol. Reprod. **31:** 1103–1118.

43. KLENTZERIS, L. D., J. N. BULMER, A. WARREN, L. MORRISON, T.-C. LI & I. D. COOKE. 1992. Endometrial lymphoid tissue in the timed endometrial biopsy: morphometric and immunohistochemical aspects. Am. J. Obstet. Gynecol. **167:** 667–674.
44. SEN, D. K. & H. FOX. 1967. The lymphoid tissue of the endometrium. Gynaecologia **163:** 371–378.
45. MARSHAL, R. J. & D. B. JONES. 1988. An immunohistochemical study of lymphoid tissue in human endometrium. Int. J. Gynecol. Pathol. **7:** 225–235.
46. KAMAT, B. R. & D. M. ISAACSON. 1987. The immunocytochemical distribution of leukocytic subpopulations in human endometrium. Am. J. Pathol. **127:** 66–73.
47. MORRIS, H., J. EDWARDS, A. TILTMAN & E. MALCOLM. 1985. Endometrial lymphoid tissue: an immunohistological study. J. Clin. Pathol. **38:** 644–652.
48. TABIBZADEH, S. S. 1990. Evidence of T cell activation and potential cytokine action in human endometrium. J. Endocrinol. Metab. **71:** 645–649.
49. STEWART, C. J. R., A. FARQUAHARSON & A. K. FOULIS. 1992. The distribution and possible function of gamma interferon-immunoreactive cells in normal endometrium and myometrium. Virchows Archiv A Pathol. Anat. **420:** 419–424.
50. TABIBZADEH, S. 1991. Induction of HLA-DR expression in endometrial epithelial cells by endometrial T cells: potential regulatory role of endometrial T cells *in vivo.* J. Endocrinol. Metab. **73:** 1352–1359.
51. TABIBZADEH, S. S., M. A. GERBER & P. G. SATYASWAROOP. 1986. Induction of HLA-DR antigen expression in human endometrial epithelial cells *in vitro* by recombinant gamma-interferon. Am. J. Pathol. **125:** 90–96.
52. TABIBZADEH, S. S., P. G. SATYASWAROOP & P. N. RAO. 1988. Antiproliferative effect of interferon gamma in human endometrial epithelial cells *in vitro:* potential local growth modulatory role in endometrium. J. Endocrinol. Metab. **67:** 131–138.
53. TABIBZADEH, S., X. Z. SUN, Q. F. KONG, G. KASNIC, J. MILLER & P. G. SATYASWAROOP. 1993. *In vitro* induction of a polarized micro-environment by T cells and IFN-gamma in three dimensional spheroid cultures of endometrial epithelial cells. Hum. Reprod. **8:** 182–192.
54. TABIBZADEH, S. S., K. L. KAFFKA, P. G. SATYASWAROOP & P. L. KILIAN. 1990. IL-1 regulation of human endometrial function: presence of IL-1 receptor correlates with IL-1 stimulated $PGE_2$ production. J. Endocrinol. Metab. **70:** 1000–1006.

# Growth Factors and Decidualization in Vitro[a]

JUAN C. IRWIN, LISA DE LAS FUENTES,
AND LINDA C. GIUDICE

*Department of Gynecology and Obstetrics*
*Stanford University Medical Center*
*Stanford, California 94305*

## INTRODUCTION

The success of the human reproductive process is dependent on the synchronous development of endometrial changes during the ovulatory cycle.[1] In the postovulatory phase, under the influence of progesterone (P), glandular secretion and stromal decidualization become the dominant features of the endometrium.[2] In fertile cycles the implanting embryo breaches the epithelial barrier and invades the underlying stroma, to lie in intimate contact with the decidualized cells during the early stages of gestation. Throughout pregnancy, decidual cells are believed to fulfill paracrine,[3] nutritional,[4] immunoregulatory,[5,6] and embryoregulatory[7,8] functions. The decidualization of the endometrium involves the differentiation of the stromal cells which acquire distinct morphological and functional features. Morphological decidualization is expressed histologically by a change to a polyhedral cell shape with an increase in cell size,[2] and ultrastructurally by an extensive development of the organelles involved in protein synthesis (rough endoplasmic reticulum) and secretion (Golgi apparatus), and by the appearance of specialized intercellular contacts (gap junctions).[9] Functionally, decidualization is associated with increased cell proliferation in a P-dominated environment,[2,10] and with the onset of prolactin (PRL)[11] and insulin-like growth factor binding protein-1 (IGFBP-1)[12,13] secretion. Decidualized stromal cells produce a basement membrane-like extracellular matrix (rich in laminin, fibronectin, collagen type IV, and heparan sulfate proteoglycan),[14] and express increased levels of tissue factor.[15]

Growth factors have been implicated as autocrine/paracrine regulators of endometrial function. Several growth factors including epidermal growth factor (EGF), the insulin-like growth factors (IGF-I and IGF-II), transforming growth factor-$\alpha$ (TGF-$\alpha$), platelet-derived growth factor (PDGF), fibroblast growth factor (FGF), transforming growth factor-$\beta$ (TGF-$\beta$), and colony-stimulating factor-1 (CSF-1) have been identified in the endometrium.[16] Both EGF and IGF-I have been shown to be regulated by sex steroids in rodent uterus, and are believed to be mediators of steroid hormone action in uterine tissues.[17–20] In human endometrium, the immunolocalization of EGF peptide and levels of IGF-I and IGF-II mRNAs have been shown to vary throughout the menstrual cycle,[21,22] suggesting the involvement of these growth factors in endometrial cyclic activity. The decidualization of the human endometrial stroma is known to occur during the secretory phase under the influence of P,[2] but knowledge of the regulation of decidual differentiation and function by growth factors is still limited. IGF-II mRNA is abundantly expressed

---

[a] Supported by National Institutes of Health Grant HD-25220 (to L.C.G.).

in mid to late secretory endometrium[22] where intense EGF immunostaining is localized around the spiral arteries of the stroma[21] (the areas of early decidualization), suggesting these two growth factors may play a role in decidual differentiation and function *in vivo*. Our previous studies with an *in vitro* model system for human endometrial stromal cell decidualization[23] have shown that stromal cell responsiveness to growth factors *in vitro* is P-dependent,[24] and although EGF, FGF and PDGF were equally effective in stimulating cell proliferation, decidual differentiation markers were induced *in vitro* specifically by EGF.[23-25] The present study examines the interaction of the IGFs with EGF in the decidualization of human endometrial stromal cells in culture, as measured by a P-dependent growth response, and by the production of the decidual secreted proteins IGFBP-1 and PRL.

## MATERIALS AND METHODS

### Cell Cultures

Endometrial samples were obtained at the time of endometrial biopsy or hysterectomy for benign reasons at various stages of the menstrual cycle. Informed consent was obtained from patients in accordance with the guidelines of *The Declaration of Helsinki,* and the study was approved by the Stanford University Human Subjects Committee. Tissue samples were collected in DMEM (GIBCO, Grand Island, NY) and transported to the laboratory. Stromal cells were separated from epithelium after collagenase digestion of endometrial tissue, and subsequently cultured and passaged as previously described.[24] For experiments, stromal cells (passages 1–4) were grown in 24-well trays (Costar, Cambridge, MA), in DMEM supplemented with 5 $\mu$g/ml bovine insulin (Sigma, St. Louis, MO) and 10% charcoal-stripped fetal bovine serum (GIBCO). Confluent cultures were rinsed and maintained thereafter in serum-free medium [75% DMEM (GIBCO), 25% MCDB-104, 50 $\mu$g/ml ascorbic acid, 1 mg/ml RIA grade bovine serum albumin, 10 $\mu$g/ml human transferrin (all from Sigma)]. Where indicated, 20 ng/ml EGF (Collaborative Research, Bedford, MA), 1 $\mu$M progesterone (Sigma), and 0.1–1000 ng/ml insulin (Sigma), IGF-I and IGF-II (Bachem, Torrance, CA) were included in the culture medium. The culture medium was renewed every 2–3 days and the conditioned medium collected, clarified by centrifugation, and stored at $-70°C$ for further analysis. Cell counts were obtained after trypsinization of stromal cultures using a Coulter counter.

### Analysis of Conditioned Media

*Western Ligand Blots and Densitometry*

Conditioned media of human endometrial stromal cells were analyzed by ligand blotting as described previously,[26] according to the method of Hossenlop *et al.*[27] Briefly, nonreduced samples of serum (2 $\mu$l), or conditioned medium (90 $\mu$l) were electrophoresed on 12% SDS nonreducing acrylamide gels without boiling, and electrotransferred to nitrocellulose membrane. The blots were incubated with 1 million cpm $^{125}$I IGF-I overnight at 4°C, washed, air-dried and exposed to XAR film (Eastman Kodak, Rochester, NY). Autoradiographs were scanned on a laser

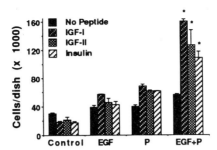

**FIGURE 1.** Steroid and growth factor interactions in the stimulation of human endometrial stromal cell proliferation. Stromal cells were cultured for 14 days in serum-free medium without steroids or growth factors (Control), or containing 20 ng/ml EGF, 1 μM P, or EGF+P; without added peptides, or with 100 ng/ml of IGF-I or IGF-II, or 1 μg/ml insulin. After the treatment period, cultures were trypsinized for cell counts. The values represent the mean ± SEM (*bars*) of duplicate or triplicate cultures. $p < 0.01$ (*) compared to the no-peptide control group.

densitometer (LKB, Bromma, Sweden), the integrated areas under the absorbance curves for each band being expressed in arbitrary units × mm.

*Immunoassays*

Conditioned media from duplicate or triplicate cultures of each experimental group were assayed in duplicate. The immunoenzymometric assay (IEMA) that measured IGFBP-1 levels used an IGFBP-1 IEMA kit from Medix Biochemica (Kauniainen, Finland). The sensitivity was 0.4 ng/ml, and intraassay and interassay coefficients of variation were 3.4% and 7.4% respectively. A Tandem-R PRL kit from Hybritech Inc. (San Diego, CA) was used for PRL radioimmunoassay, with sensitivity of 4.7 ng/ml, and intraassay and interassay coefficients of variation of 3.1% and 4.2% respectively.

*Statistics*

The experimental variables were tested in duplicate or triplicate cultures. Statistical analysis of the data was carried out using analysis of variance, and significance of the differences between treatment groups determined by Dunnett's or Scheffe's test as appropriate.

## RESULTS

Initial studies investigated the effects of IGF-I and IGF-II on the proliferation of human endometrial stromal cells cultured without other growth factors or steroid hormones, or receiving concurrently EGF, or EGF+P. In the absence of IGFs, no significant growth stimulation was observed in stromal cells cultured in the presence of EGF, P, or EGF+P (FIG. 1). Addition of physiological doses (100

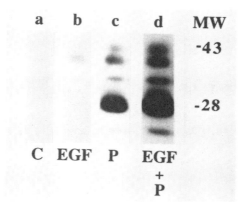

**FIGURE 2.** Autoradiograph of Western ligand blot of conditioned media from endometrial stromal cells cultured for 10 days without steroids or growth factors (C, *lane* a), or in the presence of 20 ng/ml EGF, (*lane* b), 1 μM P (*lane* c), or EGF+P (*lane* d). Position of the molecular weight markers is indicated on the *right margin*, expressed in kilodaltons. Autoradiographs were exposed for 10 days.

ng/ml) of IGF-I or IGF-II stimulated cell proliferation in stromal cultures receiving combined treatment with EGF and P, but neither one of the IGFs was found to elicit a significant growth response when used alone or in combination with either EGF or P. Suprahysiological concentrations of insulin (1 μg/ml) could substitute for the IGFs in supporting P-dependent growth stimulation by EGF.

In contrast to the strict requirement of IGFs for P-dependent growth stimulation, treatment of stromal cells with EGF+P induced IGFBP-1 and PRL secretion in the absence of exogenous IGFs. The secretion of IGFBP-1 by human endometrial stromal cells was examined by Western ligand blot analysis of conditioned media from stromal cells cultured for 10 days in medium without steroids or growth factors (control cultures), or containing EGF, P, or EGF+P (FIG. 2). In the absence of growth factors and steroid hormones (FIG. 2, lane a) confluent stromal cultures secreted minimal amounts of IGFBPs, and EGF (FIG. 2, lane b) did not affect this basic profile. The conditioned medium of cultures receiving P alone contained a major IGFBP band of 28 kDa (FIG. 2, lane c) that previous studies have shown to represent predominantly IGFBP-1 with a small amount of glycosylated IGFBP-4.[25] Combined treatment with EGF and P increased the levels of the 28-kDa band (FIG. 2, lane d), which was shown by densitometry to be 60% higher than in cultures receiving P alone (data not shown). Measurement of the levels of immunoreactive IGFBP-1 in stromal cultures using an immunoenzymometric assay (IEMA) confirmed that the 28-kDa band shown by Western ligand blot analysis represents predominantly IGFBP-1. Consistent with the results of the Western ligand blot analysis, this quantitative assay showed undetectable levels of IGFBP-1 in the conditioned medium of both control and EGF-treated cultures (FIG. 3A). Stromal cells treated with P secreted 27 ± 9 μg (mean + SEM) of immunoreactive IGFBP-1/day/$10^6$ cells,

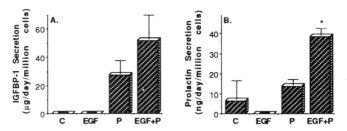

**FIGURE 3.** Growth factor and steroid hormone regulation of **(A)** IGFBP-1 and **(B)** PRL secretion by human endometrial stromal cells. Stromal cells were cultured for 12 days in serum-free medium without steroids or growth factors (C), or containing 20 ng/ml EGF, 1 μM P, or EGF+P. IGFBP-1 and PRL were assayed in 2-day conditioned medium, and the values represent the mean ± SEM (*bars*) of triplicate cultures assayed in duplicate. $p < 0.01$ (*) compared to the no-steroid and growth factor group (C).

while cultures receiving combined treatment with EGF and P secreted IGFBP-1 levels twofold higher than those obtained with P alone. Optimal induction of PRL secretion in stromal cultures also required combined treatment with EGF and P (FIG. 3B). PRL levels were low and variable in control cultures (ranging from 0–4 ng/ml) and undetectable in cultures treated with EGF. P caused a modest and not significant increase in PRL levels, whereas treatment with EGF+P increased PRL secretion sixfold compared to control ($p < 0.01$), and threefold compared to P alone ($p < 0.05$).

In sharp contrast to their synergism in stimulating stromal cell proliferation, the IGFs antagonized the stimulation of IGFBP-1 secretion by EGF+P in stromal cultures. FIGURE 4 shows the Western ligand blot analysis of conditioned media

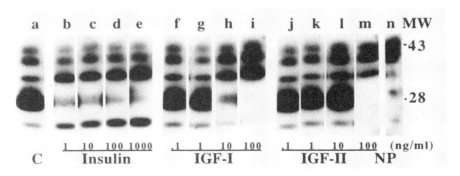

**FIGURE 4.** Autoradiograph of a Western ligand blot of conditioned media from endometrial stromal cells cultured for 10 days with EGF (20 ng/ml) + P (1 μM), with no further additions (C, *lane* a), or in the presence of insulin (*lanes* b–e), IGF-I (*lanes* f–i), or IGF-II (*lanes* j–m), at various concentrations (ng/ml) as indicated; nonpregnant female serum (NS) was run as a control (*lane* n). Position of the molecular weight markers is indicated on the *right margin*, expressed in kilodaltons. Autoradiograph was exposed for 10 days.

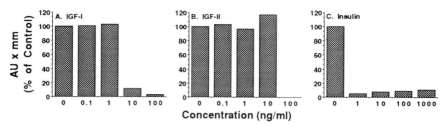

**FIGURE 5.** Densitometric analysis of the 28-kDa IGFBP secreted by endometrial stromal cells cultured for 10 days with EGF+P and various concentrations of **(A)** IGF-I, **(B)** IGF-II, or **(C)** insulin. Integrative densitometry measured in arbitrary units (AU) per mm is expressed as a percentage of the value in conditioned medium of control cultures (EGF+P without peptides). The analyses were performed on a 10-day exposure of an autoradiograph of the Western ligand blot shown in FIGURE 4.

from stromal cells cultured for 10 days in medium containing EGF+P with no further additions or with various concentrations of IGF-I, IGF-II, or insulin. The densitometry of the 28-kDa band in the autoradiogram shown in FIGURE 4 is presented in FIGURE 5. IGF-I (FIG. 4, lanes f–i; FIG. 5A) had no effect on the 28-kDa band at the lowest concentrations tested (0.1 and 1 ng/ml), but treatment with 10 and 100 ng/ml of IGF-I reduced the intensity of this band by 88% and 97% respectively. IGF-II (FIG. 4, lanes j–m; FIG. 5B) which was also without effect at 0.1 or 1 ng/ml, increased the 28-kDa IGFBP by 17% at 10 ng/ml, and reduced it to undetectable levels at 100 ng/ml. Insulin (FIG. 4, lanes b–e; FIG. 5C) induced a marked decrease of the 28-kDa band (over 90% reduction) at all concentrations tested (1–1000 ng/ml).

Quantitative assessment of the regulation of IGFBP-1 levels in stromal cultures using IEMA, revealed biphasic concentration-dependent effects of the IGFs that were not evident on Western ligand blot analysis, probably due to the lower sensitivity of this technique compared to the IEMA. Stromal cells treated with EGF+P for 10 days in the absence of peptides (control values) produced $25.5 \pm 3.2$ $\mu$g of immunoreactive IGFBP-1/day/$10^6$ cells (FIG. 6). IGF-I concentrations from 0.1 to 1 ng/ml increased IGFBP-1 levels by a maximum of 200%, while higher concentrations caused a reduction of IGFBP-1, with a half-maximal effect at 3 ng/ml (FIG. 6A). IGF-II was approximately tenfold less potent than IGFI in suppressing IGFBP-1 secretion. It had a stimulatory effect up to a concentration of 10 ng/ml (250% of control), followed by inhibition to 2% of control values at 100 ng/ml (FIG. 6B). Insulin induced a dose-dependent reduction of IGFBP-1 levels, with half-maximal effect at a concentration <1 ng/ml, and a maximal reduction to 1% of control values (FIG. 6C).

PRL secretion was also regulated in stromal cultures by IGFs. Both IGF-I and IGF-II had concentration-dependent effects on PRL secretion that paralleled the changes of IGFBP-1 levels (compare FIG. 6 to FIG. 7). Stromal cells cultured with EGF+P in the absence of peptides secreted basal PRL levels of $38.3 \pm 3.5$ ng/day/$10^6$ cells (FIG. 7). IGF-I increased PRL levels by a maximum of 243% at 1 ng/ml, and induced a dose-dependent inhibition at higher concentrations, to reach 8% of basal levels at 100 ng/ml (FIG. 7A). IGF-II stimulated PRL secretion

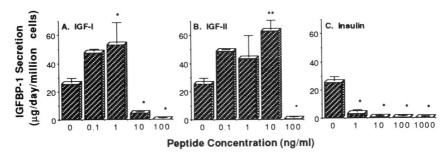

**FIGURE 6.** Dose-dependent regulation of IGFBP-1 secretion in endometrial stromal cultures by **(A)** IGF-I, **(B)** IGF-II, and **(C)** insulin. Stromal cells were cultured with EGF (20 ng/ml) + P (1 μM) for 12 days, with the indicated concentrations of IGF-I, IGF-II, or insulin. IGFBP-1 was assayed in 2-day conditioned medium, and the values represent the mean ± SEM (*bars*) of duplicate or triplicate cultures, assayed in duplicate. $p < 0.05$ (*), $p < 0.01$ (**) compared to 0 peptide.

by more than threefold at 10 ng/ml, but reduced PRL levels to 22% of the basal output at 100 ng/ml (FIG. 7B). With increasing insulin concentrations (FIG. 7C), an overall trend to lower PRL levels was observed in stromal cultures ($p > 0.05$).

In view of the known regulatory effects of IGFBPs on IGF action, it was of interest to determine whether the changes in endogenous IGFBP-1 levels in stromal cultures were associated with changes in the biological effects of the IGFs on stromal cells. Since our initial experiments showed that IGFs were required in combination with EGF and P to stimulate stromal cell proliferation (see FIG. 1), the mitogenic response in the presence of EGF+P provided an indicator of IGF bioactivity in stromal cultures. IGF-induced mitogenesis was inversely correlated with the endogenous IGFBP-1 levels in stromal cultures receiving EGF+P (com-

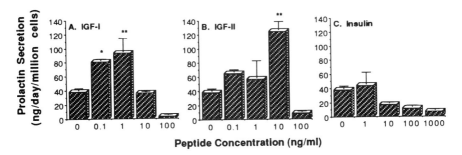

**FIGURE 7.** Dose-dependent regulation of PRL secretion in endometrial stromal cultures by **(A)** IGF-I, **(B)** IGF-II, and **(C)** insulin. Stromal cells were cultured with EGF (20 ng/ml) + P (1 μM) for 12 days, with the indicated concentrations of IGF-I, IGF-II, or insulin. PRL was assayed in 2-day conditioned medium, and the values represent the mean ± SEM (*bars*) of duplicate or triplicate cultures, assayed in duplicate. $p < 0.05$ (*), $p < 0.01$ (**) compared to 0 peptide.

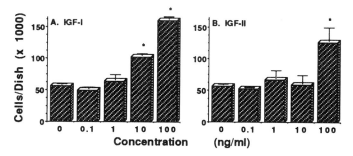

**FIGURE 8.** Dose-dependent stimulation of cell proliferation in endometrial stromal cultures by **(A)** IGF-I and **(B)** IGF-II. Stromal cells were cultured in serum-free medium containing EGF (20 ng/ml) + P (1 μM), with the indicated concentrations of IGF-I, or IGF-II. After 14 days of treatment cells were trypsinized and counted, and the values represent the mean ± SEM (*bars*) of duplicate or triplicate cultures. $p < 0.01$ (*) compared to 0 peptide.

pare FIG. 6 to FIG. 8). IGF-1 induced a dose-dependent stimulation of cell proliferation with half-maximal effect at 10 ng/ml (FIG. 8A), while IGF-II stimulated growth only at 100 ng/ml (FIG. 8B), the concentration that also caused suppression of IGFBP-1 (see FIG. 6B).

## DISCUSSION

A growing body of evidence implicates growth factors as autocrine/paracrine regulators of endometrial function.[16] Considerably less information exists regarding the precise cellular targets and the specific functions regulated by growth factors in this tissue. In particular, knowledge of the role of growth factors in decidualization is still limited. In the present study, we have used an *in vitro* model system to provide experimental evidence of the involvement of growth factors in the regulation of decidual differentiation and function. The data presented herein show that in the presence of EGF and P, factors known to effect decidualization *in vitro*,[23-25] the IGFs not only are mitogenic for human endometrial stromal cells, but also regulate their secretion of IGFBP-1 and PRL, two products of decidualized endometrium. Our studies thus define a set of endocrine (P), and autocrine/paracrine (EGF and IGFs) effectors that interact to regulate endometrial cell differentiation and function *in vitro*, and suggest that decidual differentiation and function *in vivo* may be regulated by the interplay between locally produced growth factors and ovarian steroid hormones.

A variety of biochemical changes associated with the morphological decidualization of the endometrium *in vivo*[10-15] serve as indicators of decidualization *in vitro*.[15,23-25,28] Our previous studies have shown that human endometrial stromal cell responsiveness to growth factors *in vitro* is P-dependent,[24] and although EGF, FGF, and PDGF were equally effective in stimulating cell proliferation, decidual differentiation markers were induced *in vitro* specifically by EGF.[23-25] These *in vitro* findings[23,24] are consistent with recent studies by Hofmann *et al.*[21] showing intense EGF immunostaining in late secretory endometrium, localized around the spiral arteries (the areas of early decidualization), and taken together suggest a role for EGF in decidualization *in vivo*. The IGFs act in concert with other growth factors to control cell proliferation[29] and differentiation,[30] and in uterine tissues, the IGFs may interact with other steroid-inducible growth factors such as EGF,[17,18] to regulate the growth and differentiation of endometrial cells. The results of the present study are consistent with this hypothesis, as they show that IGFs act in conjunction with EGF and P to regulate the secretion of two decidual proteins (IGFBP-1 and PRL) by human endometrial stromal cells *in vitro*. Both IGF-I and IGF-II had concentration-dependent biphasic effects on IGFBP-1 levels in stromal cultures, and this regulatory pattern was unique for IGFBP-1 and not evident in the other IGFBPs secreted by decidualized endometrial stromal cells (see FIG. 3). IGF concentrations within the physiological range regulated IGFBP-1 and PRL secretion in stromal cultures, and these IGF effects were clearly distinct from the changes induced by the structurally related peptide hormone insulin. Therefore, the effects of the IGFs are likely to be mediated via IGF receptors and not through binding to the insulin receptor with which the IGFs are known to crossreact.[31]

In the cycling human endometrium the proliferation of stromal cells is observed in the areas of early decidualization,[2,32] and in rodents, hormonally induced cell proliferation is believed to be a prerequisite for decidual differentiation.[33] Recent studies from our laboratory have shown that IGF-II mRNA is abundantly expressed in mid to late secretory endometrium and early pregnancy decidua, suggesting a role for IGF-II in decidual differentiation and function. The data presented herein show that IGFs are strictly required to stimulate the proliferation of human endometrial stromal cells, in the presence of EGF and P, known to induce decidualization *in vitro*.[24,25] Therefore the EGF+P-dependent stimulation of stromal cell proliferation by the IGFs *in vitro* may represent the mitogenic activation associated with the decidual differentiation program.[33] In addition, IGFI and IGF-II were not only mitogenic for stromal cells, but also regulated their secretion of the decidual proteins IGFBP-1 and PRL. Taken together, our findings suggest that IGF-II may be involved in the control of stromal cell proliferation during decidualization, and may also act as a local regulator of decidual cell function throughout the early stages of gestation.

IGFBP-1 is the major secreted protein of the decidualized endometrium during the late secretory phase and pregnancy.[34] IGFBP-1 is known to compete with endometrial membrane receptors for the binding of IGF-I,[35] suggesting it is an inhibitory regulator of IGF action in this tissue. Thus IGFBP-1, in addition to being an indicator of decidualization, is a potential modulator of growth factor action in the endometrium. Our *in vitro* studies showed an inverse correlation between endogenous IGFBP-1 levels and IGF-induced mitogenesis in stromal cultures, suggestive of an inhibitory role for IGFBP-1 in this system. Consistent with this interpretation, recent studies by Frost *et al.*[36] have shown that the mitogenic effects of IGF-I and IGF-II in endometrial stromal cultures can be inhibited by exogenously added IGFBP-1. Both the inhibitory effects of IGFBP-1 *in vitro*, and the increased expression of IGF-II mRNA in mid-to-late secretory endometrium *in vivo*,[22] are consistent with the hypothesis that endometrial IGFBP-1 may provide a physiological mechanism to limit IGF-II induced mitogenesis during the proliferation/differentiation program of decidualization.

At present we speculate that the regulatory actions of IGF-II on decidualized stromal cell function may represent a physiological mechanism whereby the implanting embryo can interact with the maternal endometrium. Consistent with this hypothesis is the widespread expression of IGF-II mRNA in fetal tissues[37] and in preimplantation stage embryos.[38] Thus locally produced IGF-II[22] may stimulate the secretory activity of the decidualized stromal cells throughout the endometrium, while embryo-derived IGF-II[39] may generate high levels of this peptide at the implantation site to induce suppression of IGFBP-1 secretion. This paracrine network would enable the implanting embryo to modify the surrounding maternal environment and ensure the bioavailability of IGFs to regulate the differentiation[30] and function[37] of the invading trophoblast. Recent studies by Andoh et al.[40] showing a delay of the decidual reaction in endometrial biopsies of conception cycles are consistent with the regulation of decidualization by embryo-derived factors.

In the current study we have challenged a specific endometrial cell type with individual growth factors and assessed discrete cellular responses *in vitro*. Taken together our results suggest that complex autocrine/paracrine interactions involving growth factors and their binding proteins differentially regulate the proliferation/differentiation program of decidualization, and may also be involved in the regulation of decidual function in early pregnancy.

## SUMMARY

Growth factors are believed to act as local regulators of endometrial cyclic activity, but there is limited information on their regulation of decidual differentiation and function. Cell cultures of human endometrial stroma treated with progesterone (P) undergo morphologic, proliferative and secretory changes characteristic of decidualizing endometrium. In the presence of P, different growth factors can stimulate cell proliferation, but decidual differentiation is induced specifically by EGF, as shown by the production of prolactin (PRL), fibronectin, laminin, and insulin-like growth factor binding protein 1 (IGFBP-1). The present study investigates the effects of the insulin-like growth factors (IGF-I, IGF-II) on decidualization *in vitro*, as indicated by a P-dependent growth response and by the secretion of PRL and IGFBP-1. IGFs were required together with EGF and P to stimulate stromal cell proliferation. In contrast, PRL ($38 \pm 4$ ng/day/$10^6$ cells) and IGFBP-1 ($26 \pm 3$ μg/day/$10^6$ cells) were secreted by *in vitro* decidualized cells in the absence of exogenous IGFs. However, IGFs regulated both IGFBP-1 and PRL secretion in a dose-dependent biphasic manner. Stimulation of IGFBP-1 (200–250%) and PRL (243–324%) peaked at 1 ng/ml for IGF-I, and 10 ng/ml for IGF-II, followed by inhibition at higher peptide concentrations ($ED_{50}$s 3 and 30 ng/ml, respectively). Maximal physiological doses (100 ng/ml) of IGF-I and IGF-II virtually abolished IGFBP-1 secretion (1% and 2% of basal levels, respectively), but did not cause total suppression of PRL secretion (8% and 22% of basal levels). IGF-induced mitogenesis was inversely correlated with endogenous IGFBP-1 levels in *in vitro* decidualized stromal cultures. Our studies show that growth factor interactions regulate decidual function, and that specific cellular functions associated with the decidual response are differentially regulated by growth factor interactions. Our findings support a role for the IGF system in autocrine/paracrine interactions during decidualization and early pregnancy. It is speculated that IGF-II may constitute one of the embryonic signaling mechanisms during early postimplantation stages.

## ACKNOWLEDGMENTS

We wish to thank Dr. Y. Chandrasaker for her critical review of the manuscript, and Dr. T-F. Wu for conducting the prolactin assays.

## REFERENCES

1. WEITLAUF, H. M. 1988. Biology of implantation. *In* The Physiology of Reproduction. E. Knobil, J. Neil, L. L. Ewing, G. S. Greenwald, C. L. Markert & D. W. Pfaff, Eds. Vol. 1: 231–262. Raven Press Ltd. New York.
2. NOYES, R. W., A. T. HERTIG & J. ROCK. 1950. Dating the endometrial biopsy. Fertil Steril. **1:** 3–25.
3. MASLAR, I. A., B. M. KAPLAN, A. A. LUCIANO & D. H. RIDDICK. 1980. Prolactin production by the endometrium of early human pregnancy. J. Clin. Endocrinol. Metab. **51:** 78–83.
4. KEARNS, M. & P. K. LALA. 1983. Life history of decidual cells: a review. Am. J. Reprod. Immunol. Microbiol. **3:** 78–82.
5. GOLANDER, A., V. ZAKUTH, Y. SHECHTER & Z. SPIRER. 1981. Suppression of lymphocyte reactivity *in vitro* by a soluble factor secreted by explants of human decidua. Eur. J. Immunol. **11:** 849–851.
6. MCKAY, D. B., M. A. VAZQUEZ, R. W. REDLINE & C. Y. LU. 1992. Macrophage functions are regulated by murine decidual and tumor extracellular matrices. J. Clin. Invest. **89:** 134–142.
7. PIJNENBORG, R., G. DIXON, W. B. ROBERTSON & I. BROSENS. 1980. Trophoblastic invasion of human decidual from 8 to 128 weeks of pregnancy. Placenta **1:** 3–19.
8. REN, S.-G. & G. D. BRAUNSTEIN. 1991. Decidua produces a protein that inhibits choriogonadotropin release from human trophoblasts. J. Clin. Invest. **87:** 325–330.
9. WYNN, R. M. 1974. Ultrastructural development of the human decidua. Am. J. Obstet. Gynecol. **118:** 652–670.
10. FERENCZY, A., G. BERTRAND & M. M. GELFAND. 1979. Proliferation kinetics of human endometrium during the normal menstrual cycle. Am. J. Obstet. Gynecol. **133:** 859–867.
11. MASLAR, I. A. & D. H. RIDDICK. 1979. Prolactin production by human endometrium during the normal menstrual cycle. Am. J. Obstet. Gynecol. **135:** 751–754.
12. JULKUNEN, M., R. KOISTINEN, A.-M. SUIKKARI, M. SEPPÄLÄ & O. A. JANNE. 1990. Identification by hybridization histochemistry of human endometrial cells expressing mRNAs encoding a uterine $\beta$-lactoglobulin homologue and insulin-like growth factor binding protein-1. Mol. Endocrinol. **4:** 700–707.
13. BELL, S. C. 1991. The insulin-like growth factor binding proteins—the endometrium and decidua, Ann. N.Y. Acad. Sci. **622:** 120–137.
14. WEWER, U. M., M. FABER, L. A. LIOTTA & R. ALBRECHTSEN. 1985. Immunocytochemical and ultrastructural assessment of the nature of the pericellular basement membrane of human decidual cells. Lab Invest. **53:** 624–633.
15. LOCKWOOD, C. J., Y. NEMERSON, S. GULLER, G. KRIKUN, M. ALVAREZ, V. HAUSKNECHT, E. GURPIDE & F. SCHATZ. 1993. J. Clin. Endocrinol. Metab. **76:** 231–236.
16. GIUDICE, L. C. 1994. Growth factors and growth modulators in human uterine endometrium: their potential relevance to reproductive medicine. Fertil. Steril. **61:** 1–17.
17. HUET-HUDSON, Y. M., C. CHAKRABORTY, S. K. DE, Y. SUZUKY, G. K. ANDREWS & S. K. DEY. 1990. Estrogen regulates the synthesis of epidermal growth factor in mouse uterine epithelial cells. Mol. Endocrinol. **4:** 510–523.
18. NELSON, K. G., T. TAKAHASHI, N. L. BOSSERT, D. K. WALMER & J. A. MCLACHLAN. 1991. Epidermal growth factor replaces estrogen in the stimulation of female genital-tract growth and differentiation. Proc. Natl. Acad. Sci. USA **88:** 21–25.
19. MURPHY, L. J., L. C. MURPHY & H. G. FRIESEN. 1987. Estrogen induces insulin-like growth factor-I expression in the rat uterus. Mol. Endo. **1:** 445–450.
20. KAPUR, S., H. TAMADA, S. K. DEY & G. K. ANDREWS. 1992. Expression of insulin-like growth factor-I (IGF-I) and its receptor in the peri-implantation mouse uterus, and cell-specific regulation of IGF-I gene expression by estradiol and progesterone. Biol. Reprod. **46:** 208–219.
21. HOFMANN, G. E., R. T. SCOTT, P. A. BERGH & L. DELIGDISCH. 1991. Immunohistochemical localization of epidermal growth factor in human endometrium, decidua, and placenta. J. Clin. Endocrinol. Metab. **73:** 882–887.

22. GIUDICE, L. C., B. A. DSUPIN, I. H. JIN, T. H. VU & A. R. HOFFMAN. 1993. Differential expression of messenger ribonucleic acids encoding insulin-like growth factors and their receptors in human uterine endometrium and decidua. J. Clin. Endocrinol. Metab. **76:** 1115–1122.
23. IRWIN, J. C., W. H. UTIAN & R. L. ECKERT. 1991. Sex steroids and growth factors differentially regulate the growth and differentiation of cultured human endometrial stromal cells. Endocrinology **129:** 2385–2392.
24. IRWIN, J. C., D. KIRK, R. J. B. KING, M. M. QUIGLEY & R. B. L. GWATKIN. 1989. Hormonal regulation of human endometrial stromal cells in culture: an *in vitro* model for decidualization. Fertil. Steril. **52:** 761–768.
25. GIUDICE, L. C., B. A. DSUPIN & J. C. IRWIN. 1992. Steroid and peptide regulation of insulin-like growth factor-binding proteins secreted by human endometrial stromal cells is dependent on stromal differentiation. J. Clin. Endocrinol. Metab. **75:** 1235–1241.
26. GIUDICE, L. C., D. A. MILKOWSKI, G. LAMSON, R. G. ROSENFELD & J. C. IRWIN. 1991. Insulin-like growth factor binding proteins in human endometrium: steroid-dependent messenger ribonucleic acid expression and protein synthesis. J. Clin. Endocrinol. Metab. **72:** 779–787.
27. HOSSENLOPP, P., D. SEURIN, B. SEGOVIA-QUINSON, S. HARDOUIN & M. BINOUX. 1986. Analysis of serum insulin-like growth factor binding proteins using Western blotting: use of the method for titration of the binding proteins and competitive binding studies. Anal. Biochem. **154:** 138–143.
28. TABANELLI, S., B. TANG & E. GURPIDE. 1992. *In vitro* decidualization of human endometrial stromal cells. J. Steroid Biochem. Mol. Biol. **42:** 337–344.
29. LEOF, E. B., W. WHARTON, J. J. VAN WYK & W. J. PLEDGER. 1982. Epidermal growth factor (EGF) and somatomedin C regulate $G_1$ progression in competent Balb/c-3T3 cells. Exp. Cell Res. **141:** 107–115.
30. BHAUMICK, F., D. GEORGE & R. M. BALA. 1992. Potentiation of epidermal growth factor-induced differentiation of cultured human placental cells by insulin-like growth factor-I. J. Clin. Endocrinol. Metab. **74:** 1005–1011.
31. NAGAMANI, M., C. A. STUART, P. A. DUNHARDT & M. G. DOHERTY. 1991. Specific binding sites for insulin and insulin-like growth factor I in human endometrial cancer. Am. J. Obstet. Gynecol. **165:** 1865–1871.
32. FERENCZY, A., G. BERTRAND & M. M. GELFAND. 1979. Proliferation kinetics of human endometrium during the normal menstrual cycle. Am. J. Obstet. Gynecol. **133:** 859–867.
33. BELL, S. C. 1983. Decidualization: regional differentiation and associated function. Oxf. Rev. Reprod. Biol. **5:** 220–271.
34. BELL, S. C. 1991. The insulin-like growth factor binding proteins—the endometrium and decidua. Ann. N.Y. Acad. Sci. **622:** 120–137.
35. RUTANEN, E.-M., F. PEKONEN & T. MAKINEN. 1988. Soluble 34K binding protein inhibits the binding of insulin-like growth factor I to its receptors in human secretory phase endometrium: evidence for autocrine/paracrine regulation of growth factor action. J. Clin. Endocrinol. Metab. **66:** 173–180.
36. FROST, R. A., J. MAZELLA & L. TSENG. 1993. Insulin-like growth factor binding protein-1 inhibits the mitogenic effect of insulin-like growth factors and progestins in human endometrial stromal cells. Biol. Reprod. **49:** 104–111.
37. BRICE, A. L., J. E. CHEETHAM, V. N. BOLTON, N. C. W. HILL & P. N. SCHOFIELD. 1989. Temporal changes in the expression in the insulin-like growth factor II gene associated with tissue maturation in the human fetus. Development **106:** 543–554.
38. RAPPOLEE, D. A., K. S. STURM, G. A. SCHULTZ, C. A. BASILICO, D. BOWEN-POPE, R. A. PEDERSEN & Z. WERB. 1991. Expression and function of growth factor ligands and receptors in preimplantation mouse embryos. *In* Growth Factors in Reproduction. D. W. Schomberg, Ed. 207–218. Springer-Verlag. New York.
39. HEMMINGS, R., J. LANGLAIS, T. FALCONE, L. GRANGER, P. MIRON & H. GUYDA. 1992. Human embryos produce transforming growth factor $\alpha$ activity and insulin-like growth factor II. Fertil. Steril. **58:** 101–104.
40. ANDOH, K., H. MIZUNUMA, Y. NAKAZATO, K. YAMADA, M. MICHISHITA & Y. IBUKI. 1992. Endometrial dating in the conception cycle. Fertil. Steril. **58:** 1127–1130.

# Mechanism of Human Endometrial Stromal Cells Decidualization

BAIQING TANG,[a] SETH GULLER, AND ERLIO GURPIDE[b]

*Departments of Obstetrics, Gynecology
and Reproductive Science
and
Department of Biochemistry
Mount Sinai School of Medicine (CUNY)
One Gustave L. Levy Place
New York, New York 10029-6574*

## INTRODUCTION

As described by Noyes *et al.* in their classic article of 1950 on the histologic dating of the endometrium,[1] one of the characteristic events in the morphologic changes that this tissue undergoes during the menstrual cycle is the differentiation of the stromal cells to the decidual phenotype. On day 23 of the regular 28-day cycle, the elongated, fibroblast-like stromal cells of the proliferative tissue begin to differentiate around the endometrial blood vessels into larger, rounder and often binucleated decidual cells.[2] Since many of the endometrial changes are clearly linked to ovarian cyclic events (*e.g.*, secretory changes in the glandular epithelium after ovulation) decidualization has been traditionally associated with the production of progesterone (P) by the ovarian luteal cells. Since the placenta secretes large amounts of P, such hormonal connection was consistent with the massive decidualization of the endometrium of pregnancy (*viz* the decidua). Early *in vitro* experiments supported this view, since addition of P to fragments of human proliferative endometrium in culture resulted in detectable changes of the stromal component to the decidual phenotype, both morphologically and by the appearance of prolactin (PRL), a characteristic secretory product of decidual cells.[3] However, the belief that P, with or without estradiol ($E_2$), was solely responsible for decidualization of human endometrial stromal cells was not supported by a series of *in vitro* studies reported by Tseng and co-workers.[4-6] They showed that medroxyprogesterone acetate (MPA), a metabolically stable progestin, had only slow and moderate effects on PRL production, even in the presence of $E_2$, while a faster and much larger effect on PRL output was elicited in the same system by a mixture of MPA and relaxin (RLX), a hormone that is also secreted by the corpus luteum. Also casting doubts on the role of P as the single factor affecting decidualization is a recent report[7] on pregnancies in women with serum levels of P at 4 weeks

---

[a] Present address: Department of Medicine, Memorial Sloan-Kettering Cancer Center, New York, NY 10021.
[b] Corresponding author.

**TABLE 1.** Products Induced or Affected by Decidualization of Human Endometrial Stromal cells[a]

| Type of Product | Product |
|---|---|
| Cytokines | CSF-1 |
|  | TNF-$\alpha$ |
|  | IL-1$\beta$ |
|  | IL-6 |
|  | TGF-$\beta$ |
| ECM components | laminin |
|  | fibronectin |
|  | collagen IV |
|  | heparan sulfate proteoglycan |
| Hypophyseal hormones, neuropeptides | prolactin |
|  | oxytocin |
|  | somatostatin |
|  | inhibin, activin |
|  | CRF |
| Ovarian hormones | relaxin |
| Enzymes | diamine oxidase |
|  | aromatase |
|  | steroid sulfatases |
|  | proteases (PAs, collagenases) |
|  | protease inhibitors (PAIs, TIMPs) |
|  | 25-OH-$D_3$-1$\alpha$ hydrolase |
|  | prorenin, renin |
| Miscellaneous | platelet-activating factor (PAF) |
|  | desmin |
|  | IGF-I binding protein (IGFBP-1, PP12) |
|  | 24K protein (hsp27) |
|  | tissue factor |
|  | endothelin-1 |

[a] Modified from Gurpide et al.[12]

gestation which were as low as 1.9 nM (0.6 ng/ml), even lower than the mean concentration of P at the time of endometrial decidualization during the normal menstrual cycle (about 10 ng/ml). These observations suggest that other physiologic effectors play a role in the process of decidualization.

Since it had been reported that RLX generates cAMP in a variety of systems,[8-10] we tested for and demonstrated a direct inductive action of the cyclic nucleotide on the expression of PRL and other products of decidualization by stromal cells isolated from proliferative endometrium.[11] Results from a series of studies based on this observation allowed us to propose other mechanisms for the differentiation of fibroblast-like stromal cells to the decidual phenotype.

In addition to PRL, decidualized cells acquire the capability of expressing a large number of bioactive compounds, including cytokines, extracellular matrix components, hypophyseal hormones, neuropeptides, ovarian hormones and enzymes not detectable in stromal cells of proliferative endometrium. Some of these products are listed in TABLE 1, modified from previous publications,[12] and used as markers of decidualization in these studies.

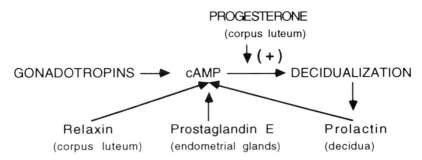

**FIGURE 1.** Schema showing a proposed mechanism by which endometrial stromal cells are decidualized during the luteal phase of the menstrual cycle and during pregnancy.

## MECHANISMS RELEVANT TO HUMAN ENDOMETRIAL DECIDUALIZATION

FIGURE 1 is based on our experimental observations concerning the mechanism by which human endometrial stromal cells are decidualized and on results published by other investigators.

This model postulates that gonadotropins of pituitary or chorionic origin act on endometrial stromal cells to generate cAMP, which acts as the autocrine inducer of PRL expression. Prolactin is depicted as a product of decidualization as well as a cAMP generator. Other reported generators of cAMP in the endometrium, *i.e.*, $PGE_2$ and RLX, are also shown in FIGURE 1. Progesterone or synthetic progestins are shown in the schema as participating in the decidualization process by enhancing the effect of cAMP on PRL expression.

What follows is an account of the experimental evidence justifying each of the connections in FIGURE 1 and a discussion of their physiologic relevance.

### *Gonadotropins Induce cAMP in Human Endometrial Stromal Cells*

Fragments of proliferative endometrium, collected as biopsies or scraped from excised uteri, were used to isolate stromal cells as published.[14] These procedures involve digestion of the tissue with collagenase, separation of glands by filtration through a 30-$\mu$m pore size sieve and collection of the filtrate in plastic dishes, allowing 15–30 min for attachment of the dispersed stromal cells to the plastic surface of culture dishes before changing medium, thus removing erythrocytes and nonrapidly attaching cells. The near homogeneous stromal cell preparations were allowed to reach confluency in RPMI 1640 medium containing 0.2 U/ml insulin and 10% charcoal-treated fetal bovine serum (RPMI/2% ctFBS) and were further incubated with RPMI 1640 medium containing 0.1 U/ml insulin and 2%

charcoal-treated fetal bovine serum (RPMI/2% ctFBS) in the presence or absence of the following gonadotropins:

- FSH, extracted from urine of postmenopausal women (Metrodin,$^R$ Serono Laboratories, Randolph, MA), used at 0.1 IU/ml concentration in the *in vitro* experiments to be described;
- FSH + LH, extracted from urine of postmenopausal women (Pergonal,$^R$ Serono Laboratories, Randolph, MA), used at 0.1 IU/ml FSH + 0.1 IU/ml LH concentrations; or
- hCG extracted from urine of pregnant women (Schein Pharm, Inc., Port Washington, NY), used at 5 USP unit/ml concentration.

Confluent stromal cells were cultured in the presence or absence of these gonadotropin preparations for a 6-day period, replacing the medium every 24 h. At the end of the culture period the cells in the 6-cm Petri dishes were washed, covered with 1.5 ml of 0.1 N HCl and incubated for 45 min at room temperature to extract intracellular cAMP and to measure its concentration by using a cAMP-competitive enzyme immunoassay (EIA) kit (Advanced Magnetics, Inc., Cambridge, MA).

In a series of 3 separate experiments carried out in duplicate, each of the gonadotropin preparations tested (FSH, FSH + LH, or hCG) significantly increased intracellular cAMP concentrations, as reported in a previous publication.[13]

As implied in the schema in FIGURE 1, the same gonadotropin preparations were found to induce morphologic changes to the decidual phenotype, *viz* to larger and rounder cells, and the expression of PRL, demonstrated immunocytochemically, by Western blotting technique, and by measuring the accumulation of PRL in the culture medium.[13] At the concentrations used, the PRL outputs induced by each of the 3 gonadotropin preparations tested were similar.

### *Cyclic AMP Induces Prolactin Production by Human Endometrial Stromal Cells*

Stromal cells isolated from human proliferative endometrium were cultured in the presence of dibutyryl-cyclic AMP (db-cAMP, 0.5 mM), 8-Br-cAMP (0.5 mM) or forskolin (15 $\mu$M), a stimulator of adenylate cyclase, for different periods of time (up to 12 days) changing medium every 2 days. The effects of each of these compounds on PRL expression, as well as other products of decidualization, was ascertained by different methods, as follows.

*Immunocytochemistry*

Induction of PRL expression by db-cAMP, was demonstrated by culturing stromal cells on Lab-Tek slides for 8 days and subjecting them to immunocytochemical analysis using rabbit polyclonal anti-hPRL antibody and the avidin-biotin immunoperoxidase method (Vectastain ABC kit). Application of the same immunocytochemical procedures, utilizing the appropriate antibodies, revealed effects of db-cAMP on other products of decidualization, such as IGFBP-1, hsp-27, desmin and laminin.[11] Morphologic changes to the decidual phenotype induced by treatment of the stromal cells with db-cAMP were also obtained during these experiments.

*[$^{35}$S]-Methionine Incorporation and Immunoprecipitation*

Stromal cells were cultured with db-cAMP for 5 days in RMI/2% ctFBS medium and then exposed for 3–6 h to high specific activity [$^{35}$S]-methionine in serum- and methionine-free medium. [$^{35}$S]-labeled PRL released to the culture medium was determined by precipitation with rabbit anti-hPRL antibody and Protein A sepharose followed by solubilization of the labeled PRL and radioautographic measurement of [$^{35}$S]-PRL and SDS-PAGE performed under reducing conditions.[11] No PRL was detected in control preparations.

*PRL Output into the Culture Medium*

Prolactin output by stromal cells exposed to db-cAMP was demonstrated by RIA, using rabbit anti-hPRL antibody (supplied by S. Raiti, National Hormone and Pituitary Program), and by ELISA procedures, as previously described.[11] This method was also used to demonstrate time and concentration dependence of the effects of db-cAMP on PRL production.[11]

*Western Blotting*

Samples of media collected after exposure of stromal cells isolated from proliferative endometrium to db-cAMP (0.5 mM) for 3, 7 or 11 days were subjected to SDS-PAGE, running PRL standards in parallel. After transfer to a nitrocellulose membrane, PRL on the membrane was detected by incubation with rabbit polyclonal anti-PRL antibody followed by labeling with [$^{125}$I]-Protein A to allow the localization and quantitative evaluation of PRL expression based on densitometric values obtained with samples and appropriate PRL standards.[11]

*Northern Blotting*

RNA extracted from stromal cells treated or untreated with db-cAMP (0.5 mM) for 2, 6 and 10 days was denatured and subjected to 1% agarose-formaldehyde gel electrophoresis, transferred to a nylon membrane and hybridized with a [$^{32}$P]-labeled probe of pituitary hPRL cDNA to localize and estimate the levels of PRL message by using X ray film. In order to normalize for the amount of RNA loaded, the PRL blots were rehybridized to a [$^{32}$P]-labeled cyclophilin DNA probe.[11]

These procedures demonstrated the presence of an approximative 1.1 kb PRL mRNA in cells exposed to db-cAMP for 6 and 10 days but not in cells untreated with db-cAMP or exposed to the cyclic nucleotide for only 2 days.

### *Progestins Enhance the Effect of cAMP on Prolactin Expression by Endometrial Stromal Cells*

The inductive effects of db-cAMP, 8-Br-cAMP and forskolin on PRL production by endometrial stromal cells in culture were enhanced by MPA (1 $\mu$M), as demonstrated by measuring PRL output into the medium and by Western blotting procedures,[11] even though MPA was by itself incapable of eliciting detectable PRL production under the same experimental conditions.

### *Prolactin Induces Differentiation of Endometrial Stromal Cells to the Decidual Phenotype*

Prolactin, one of the products characteristic of decidualization, was found to be by itself capable of inducing differentiation of stromal cells isolated from proliferative endometrium,[15] likely by generating cAMP.

Decidualization, (morphologic changes, immunocytochemical determination of IGFBP-1, desmin and hsp-27, and elevation of estrone sulfate sulfatase activity) was observed when hPRL [received from Dr. S. Raiti through the National Hormone and Pituitary Program (NIADDK)] was added at a concentration of 500 ng/ml to cultures of human endometrial stromal cells and maintained in RPMI 1640 medium containing 10% charcoal-treated fetal bovine serum and 7 $\mu$g/ml insulin.[15,16]

### *Participation of RLX and $PGE_2$ in the Decidualization Process*

Since RLX has been shown to generate cAMP in endometrial epithelial[8] and stromal[9] cells, it can be expected to play a role in decidualization, as reported by Tseng et al.[4-6] Similarly, Houserman et al.[17] have shown that $PGE_2$ can induce cAMP synthesis in cultured human endometrial stromal cells and, as predictable by the model presented in FIGURE 1, Frank et al. found decidualizing effects of $PGE_2$ in the same stromal cell system.[18]

## DISCUSSION

The presence of LH/hCG receptors in human endometrial stromal and epithelial cells[19] enhances the physiologic relevance of the unexpected finding of direct effects of gonadotropins on this tissue. Moreover, endometrial biopsies obtained from women undergoing ovarian stimulation with gonadotropins in preparation for *in vitro* fertilization procedures showed out-of-phase epithelial and stromal events consistent with stromal decidualization.[20,21] For instance, it was found during histologic and immunocytochemical studies of such biopsies that subnuclear glycogen accumulation in the glandular epithelium, characteristic of the first days of the secretory phase, coexisted with positive staining for PRL in the stroma, which in untreated subjects only appears several days later during the menstrual cycle, when glycogen accumulation is no longer histologically detectable.

The physiological and clinical implications of the findings that gonadotropins, in addition to their steroidogenic actions in the ovary, can exert direct effects on the endometrium are of considerable interest since decidualization of the stromal cells affects implantation and development of the embryo.

### REFERENCES

1. NOYES, R. W., A. T. HERTING & J. ROCK. 1950. Dating the endometrial biopsy. Fertil. Steril. **1:** 3–25.

2. DALLENBACH-HELLWEG, G. 1987. Histopathology of the Endometrium. Fourth Edit. 25–93. Springer-Verlag. Berlin, Heidelberg, New York.
3. DALY, D. H., I. A. MASLAR & D. H. RIDDICK. 1982. Prolactin production during *in vitro* decidualization of proliferative endometrium. Am. J. Obstet. Gynecol. **145:** 672–678.
4. HUANG, J. R., L. TSENG, P. BISCHOFF & O. A. JANNE. 1987. Regulation of prolactin production by progestin, estrogen and relaxin in human endometrial stromal cells. Endocrinology **121:** 2011–2017.
5. ZHU, H. H., J. R. HUANG, J. MAZELLA, M. ROSENBERG & L. TSENG. 1990. Differential effects of progestin and relaxin on the synthesis and secretion of immunoreactive prolactin in long term culture of human endometrial stromal cells. J. Clin. Endocrinol. Metab. **71:** 889–899.
6. TSENG, L., J-G. GAO, R. CHEN, H. H. ZHU, J. MAZELLA & D. R. POWELL. 1992. Effect of progestin, antiprogestin, and relaxin on the accumulation of prolactin and insulin-like growth factor-binding protein-1 mesenger ribonucleic acid in human endometrial stromal cells. Biol. Reprod. **47:** 441–450.
7. AZUMA, K., I. CALDERON, M. BESANKO, V. MACLACHLAN & D. L. HEALY. 1993. Is the luteal-placental shift a myth? Analysis of low progesterone levels in successful art pregnancies. J. Clin. Endocrinol. Metab. **77:** 195–198.
8. CHEN, G., J. R. HUANG & L. TSENG. 1988. The effects of relaxin on cAMP concentrations in human endometrial glandular epithelial cells. Biol. Reprod. **39:** 519–525.
9. FEI, D. T. W., M. C. GROSS, J. L. LOFGREN, M. MORA-WORMS & A. B. CHEN. 1990. Cyclic AMP response to recombinant human relaxin by cultured human endometrial cells: a specific and high throughput *in vitro* bioassay. Biochem. Biophys. Res. Commun. **170:** 214–222.
10. KRAMER, S. M., U. E. M. GIBSON, B. M. FENDLY, M. A. MOHLER, D. W. DRLER & P. D. JOHNSTON. 1990. Increase in cAMP levels by relaxin in new born rhesus monkey uterus cell culture. In vitro Cell Dev. Biol. **26:** 647–656.
11. TANG, B., S. GULLER & E. GURPIDE. 1993. Cyclic adenosine 3′,5′-monophosphate induces prolactin expression in stromal cells isolated from human proliferative endometrium. Endocrinology. **133:** 2197–2203.
12. GURPIDE, E., S. TABANELLI & B. TANG. 1992. Human endometrial stromal cells. *In* Hormones in Gynecological Endocrinology. A. R. Genazzani & F. Petraglia, Eds. 717–724. Partenon Press. Casterton Hall. Carnforth, Lancs, UK.
13. TANG, B. & E. GURPIDE. 1993. Direct effects of gonadotropins on decidualization of human endometrial stromal cells. J. Steroid Biochem. Mol. Biol. **47:** 115–121.
14. FLEMING, H. & E. GURPIDE. 1982. Growth characteristics of primary cultures of stromal cells from human endometrium. J. Steroid Biochem. **16:** 717–720.
15. TABANELLI, S., B. TANG & E. GURPIDE. 1992. *In vitro* decidualization of human endometrial stromal cells. J. Steroid Biochem. Mol. Biol. **42:** 337–344.
16. BENEDETTO, M. T., S. TABANELLI & E. GURPIDE. 1990. Estrone sulfate sulfatase activity is increased during *in vitro* decidualization of stromal cells from human endometrium. J. Clin. Endocrinol. Metab. **70:** 342–345.
17. HOUSSERMAN, V. L., H. TODD & F. HERTELENDY. 1989. Progesterone treatment *in vitro* enhances prostaglandin E and forskolin-promoted cyclic AMP production in human endometrial stromal cells. J. Reprod. Fertil. **85:** 195–202.
18. FRANK, G. R., A. BRAR, M. CEDARS & S. HANDWERGER. 1993. Prostaglandin $E_2$ dramatically enhances endometrial stromal cell differentiation. Program and Abstracts of the 75th Annual Meeting of The Endocrine Society, Las Vegas, NV, p. 350 (Abstract #1197).
19. RESHEF, E., Z. M. LEI, CH. V. RAO, D. D. PRIDHAM, N. CHEGINI & J. L. LUBORSKY. 1990. The presence of gonadotropin receptors in nonpregnant human uterus, human placenta, fetal membranes, and decidua. J. Clin. Endocrinol. Metab. **70:** 421–430.
20. TABANELLI, S., A. BIRKENFELD, D. NAVOT, C. BULLETTI, C. FLAMIGNI & E. GURPIDE. 1993. Insulin-like growth factor-I binding protein and stress responsive protein 27; expression in the endometrium of women undergoing IVF and correlation with pregnancy. Program and Abstracts of the 75th Annual Meeting of The Endocrine Society, Las Vegas, NV, p. 899 (Abstract #1340).
21. DELIGDISH, L. 1993. Effects of hormone therapy on the endometrium. Mod. Pathol. **6:** 94–106.

# Decidual Progesterone and Estrogen Receptors in the First Trimester of Pregnancy

IVO NOCI,[a,e] PATRIZIA BORRI,[a] ENRICO PERITI,[a]
FRANCESCO BRANCONI,[a] GIANNI MESSERI,[c]
PAOLA TOZZI,[c] FRANCESCA TORRICELLI,[d]
LUCIA NUTINI,[d] MILENA PAGLIERANI,[b]
GIANNI TADDEI,[b] AND GIANFRANCO SCARSELLI[a]

[a]*Department of Obstetrics and Gynecology*
[b]*Department of Pathology*
*University of Florence*
*Florence, Italy*

*and*

[c]*Endocrinology Laboratory*
[d]*Cytogenetics Laboratory*
*Careggi Hospital*
*Florence, Italy*

## INTRODUCTION

Concentrations of progesterone and estrogens in maternal blood increase from the beginning of pregnancy progressively. These hormones, synthetized first in the rescue corpus luteum and later on in the placenta (luteoplacental shift),[1] play an important role in the maintenance of pregnancy due to the activity they exercise on many target tissues.

Hormone action on myometrium has long been studied and is the best known. Surgical ablation of the corpus luteum before the luteoplacental shift, providing a sudden decrease in progesterone, causes increased contractile activity in the uterus following abortion; this effect is antagonized by the administration of exogenous progesterone.[2] Such studies yielded the model, still accepted at this time,[3] showing that the uterus is an intrinsically active organ which is suppressed by progesterone. On the contrary, the administration of exogenous estrogens to luteoctomized women does not prevent the abortive evolution of a pregnancy.[2]

Another important function of progesterone and estrogens is the preparation of the mammary glands for lactation.[4] Moreover, local modifications of the immune response have been recently attributed to progesterone.[5]

Progesterone and estrogens have a key function in the preparation of the endometrium for implantation whereas their functional role regarding the decidua is uncertain. Administration during early pregnancy of the antiprogesterone RU 486 is followed by the increase of myometrium contractile activity[6] as well as by other decidual alterations[7] resulting in abortion. This is the reason why

---

[e] Corresponding author: Dr. Ivo Noci, I. Clinica Ginecologica e Ostetrica, Università di Firenze, viale Morgagni, 85, 50 139 Florence, Italy.

progesterone is thought to have a protective function on the decidua. On the other hand, the effect of antiestrogen on the decidua during early pregnancy is not understood.

The prerequisite for hormonal influence on a tissue is, up to now, the presence of specific intracellular receptor proteins. The few studies that have been done on the state of decidual receptors for progesterone (PR) and estrogens (ER) have yielded conflicting results.[8–10]

The aim of our study was to investigate PR and ER in the decidua of physiological pregnancies in the first trimester. The study was carried out by using both biochemical ligand techniques and immunocytochemical methods in order to integrate quantitative data of the binding capacity of receptors to their localization.

## MATERIALS AND METHODS

### Patients

The study was carried out on 59 women between January and December 1992 at the Department of Gynecology and Obstetrics of the University of Florence. All women voluntarily decided to undergo abortion and each patient gave her informed consent to the study. The mean female age was 24.3 years, ranging from 19 to 38. Gestational age ranged from 6 to 12 weeks. At the moment of the operation, each woman had a blood sample drawn for blood progesterone and estrogen assay. The gestational age was always confirmed by ultrasonography. Decidua samples, obtained by aspiration, were sent on ice to the laboratory within a few minutes. The decidual tissue homogeneity was soon assessed microscopically ($\times$ 2.5, Zeiss, Germany). The tissue was then divided in two equivalent portions (200 to 400 mg), which were frozen and stored in liquid nitrogen separately. These were later used for the two different determinations of PR and ER within 6 months.

### Methodology

Progesterone and estrogen serum assay was performed using a commercial kit (ES-700, Boehringer-Mannheim, Tutzing, Germany).

The measurement of PR and ER was carried out using both biochemical ligand techniques (LBA) and immunohistochemical (IH) methods.

LBA was performed as previously described.[11] Briefly, the tissue was mechanically homogenized and the resulting suspension centrifuged at 105,000 $\times$ g. The cytosol was then incubated, in triplicate, with a single concentration (1 nmol/L) of high specific activity tritiated steroids, 3H-E2 and 3H-ORG 2058, respectively. A parallel series of tubes contained, in addition, a saturating concentration of the nonradioactive steroid (100 nmol/L) to measure nonspecific (not saturable) binding. After removing the unbound steroids by dextran coated charcoal, the soluble fraction-associated radioactivity was measured and the amount of bound steroids computed. The protein content of the cytosol was measured by Comassie Blue staining and the receptor content expressed as fmol/mg protein. We defined those cases with values higher than 10 fmol/mg protein as positive, while receptors were considered to be undetectable in the presence of concentrations of less than 3 fmol/mg protein. Those cases with receptor concentrations of between 3 and 10 fmol/mg protein were considered to be borderline. Six cases (three from the ninth and three from the tenth week of pregnancy) were eliminated due to the scanty biological sample. Therefore, there were 53 evaluable cases.

The ER and PR immunostaining was performed in accordance with the manufacturer's instructions using anti-ER and anti-PR monoclonal antibodies that are commercially available in kit form (Abbott GmbH, Germany). Cryostat sections were cut at 6 micro-m and immediately fixed in phosphate buffered saline (PBS) 0.01M pH 7.4 containing 10 formaldehyde solution for 15 minutes. Sections were washed in PBS for at least 5 minutes and then soaked in cold methanol at $-20°C$ for 4 minutes and subsequently in cold acetone at $-20°C$ for 2 minutes. After being rinsed in PBS they were treated differently according to whether ER or PR were to be detected. In both cases, however, sections were incubated with normal goat serum for 15 minutes to reduce nonspecific binding of subsequent reagents. The tissue sections were then incubated separately with the monoclonal (rat) antibody to human ER or PR (0.1 micro-g/ml) or normal rat IgG (0.1 fg/ml), goat antibody to rat IgG, and rat peroxidase-antiperoxidase (PAP) for 30 minutes each at room temperature in a moist chamber. Each incubation was followed by a 5-minute washing in PBS. After a final PBS rinse, sections were incubated in the chromogen substrate solution containing substrate reagent (hydrogen peroxide) and DAB (diaminobenzidine 4HCl) for 6 minutes, rinsed in tap water and weakly counterstained with Harris hematoxylin. A negative control established by replacing the primary antibody with normal rat IgG in the same dilution was performed on each specimen. A positive check was performed using a frozen piece of carcinomatous mammary tissue in which there was the presence of PR and ER. With every run, a known ER- and PR-positive and ER- and PR-negative specimen was incubated in parallel with the unknown specimens. Results were evaluated as the percentage of positive cells. Values greater than 10% were considered positive for ER and PR. In addition, one piece of tissue was colored with hematoxylin and eosin to verify purity of the decidual tissue and perform histological evaluation.

### Statistical Analysis

The variation in serum concentration of progesterone and estrogen in comparison to gestational age was evaluated with regression analysis of the median values for each complete week of pregnancy.

Any variation in decidual PR and/or ER from the various weeks of the first trimester was analyzed using the Kruskall-Wallis analysis of variance for ranges.

A $p$ value $<0.05$ was considered significant.

## RESULTS

### Serum Progesterone and Estrogen Concentration

Progesterone and estrogen levels in peripheral blood fell within a physiological range.

Median progesterone values were calculated for each gestational week by weighted linear regression of the log median. The regression equation was described as follows: $\text{Log P} = 2.285 - 3.471/\text{wk}$ ($r = -0.90$); wk is gestational age

TABLE 1. Serum Progesterone and Estradiol Values (Expressed as Regressed Median) in the First Trimester of Pregnancy

| Pregnancy Week | No. of Women | Progesterone (nmol/L) | Estradiol (nmol/L) |
|---|---|---|---|
| 6 | 7 | 50.87 | 2.61 |
| 7 | 9 | 61.54 | 3.79 |
| 8 | 6 | 70.98 | 5.02 |
| 9 | 6 | 79.31 | 6.23 |
| 10 | 5 | 86.68 | 7.42 |
| 11 | 11 | 93.21 | 8.55 |
| 12 | 9 | 99.03 | 9.63 |

expressed as weeks. The regressed median of progesterone was 50.87 nmol/L at the 6th week and progressively rose to 99.03 nmol/L in the 12th week (TABLE 1).

Blood estradiol behaved in an analogous manner (TABLE 1), with a regression equation: $\text{Log E} = 1.55 - 6.797/\text{wk}$ ($r = 0.99$).

### Progesterone Receptors

When using LBA, PR were undetectable in three decidua samples and borderline in six cases. In the remaining 44 cases the PR concentration was >10 fmol/mg protein, (median 32.7 fmol/mg protein, range 10–234 fmol/mg protein). Analysis of variance showed no significant differences among the various weeks (Kruskal-Wallis $H = 9.0608$, two-tailed $p = 0.1702$) (TABLE 2).

No correlation was apparent between decidual PR and serum progesterone levels ($r = 0.18$).

IH, besides confirming the presence of decidual tissue, showed a marked positivity of PR in the nucleus of stromal and epithelial cells in all the 53 samples.

### Estrogen Receptors

ER were undetectable by LBA in 36 decidual samples, borderline in 15 and slightly positive in the remaining two.

IH did not detect any ER in all the samples.

## DISCUSSION

The few studies performed on decidual ER and PR used only binding techniques.[8-10] The only exception was Padayachi's report[12] in which decidua from four extrauterine pregnancies was studied by an immunoenzymatic technique. Before our study, no other paper reported the simultaneous detection of decidual ER and PR by using both LBA and IH.

LBA measures the capacity of receptor molecules to recognize and bind their respective steroids, thus furnishing quantitative results but primarily of unbound receptors.

In contrast, IH seems to be capable of recognizing both free and bound receptors as well as their location (nucleus, cytoplasm).

The use of both methods allows a better understanding of the results.

Both methods detected PR in 44 cases out of 53 (83% of cases). LBA showed wide fluctuations of PR values, ranging from 10 to 234 fmol/mg protein (median of 32.7 fmol/mg protein). The analysis of variance showed the absence of significant differences in the distribution of PR values among the different gestational weeks. We found no correlation between blood progesterone levels and decidual PR. IH showed an intense and constant positivity of PR localized in the nuclei of epithelial and stromal cells of the decidua.

Our results on PR in decidua are not easily compared with previous data from the literature[8-9] since the methods used are different. Tamaya,[8] using only the LBA, found constant PR concentration values in 26 cases between the 6th and 12th weeks of pregnancy. Padayachi,[9] on the other hand, reported a constant reduction of PR with the progress of the pregnancy. The lowering was more evident when comparing secretive endometrium and early pregnancy than when comparing decidua of different gestation weeks.

As far as ER are concerned, 36 samples were negative by both methods, 15 samples were negative by IH and borderline by LBA, and only 2 samples were positive for LBA and negative for IH: the two methods are in agreement in the 96.2% of cases.

We can hypothesize that the progressive increase of progesterone in the course of the first trimester of pregnancy reduces decidual ER.

However, a reduction of decidual ER, even if expected, is difficult to explain, since the presence of PR always required the presence of even lower amounts of functional ER.[13]

A variation of the ER affinity, as suggested by Padayachi[9] might explain the phenomenon. As a matter of fact, the LBA measures only high affinity and low capacity receptors. A variation in the affinity characteristics of the receptor might make them undetectable to the radiometric method. IH, on the other hand, detects the receptor protein independently from the binding to the steroid, but the available methods are not sufficiently sensitive.

In addition, it may be suggested that the receptor modifications responsible for the binder affinity variation make the molecule epitopes undetectable by the antibody used in available kits.

In any case, some of the clinical and experimental data reported in the literature is in agreement with our observations concerning the presence of a minimal amount, if any, of decidual ER. The use of the antiestrogen tamoxifen (TMX) in

TABLE 2. Decidual Progesterone Receptor (PR) Concentrations (fmol/mg Protein, Expressed as Median and Range) in the First Trimester of Pregnancy

| Pregnancy Week | No. of Women | PR (fmol/mg protein)[a] | |
|---|---|---|---|
| | | Median | Range |
| 6 | 7 | 44.6 | 220.5 |
| 7 | 9 | 17.9 | 74.5 |
| 8 | 6 | 12.7 | 44.2 |
| 9 | 6 | 41.6 | 51.1 |
| 10 | 5 | 22.3 | 80.7 |
| 11 | 11 | 62.3 | 107.7 |
| 12 | 9 | 33.1 | 101.7 |

[a] Kruskal-Wallis $H = 9.0608$; two-tailed $p = 0.1702$.

the luteal phase in primates is able to block implantation without interfering with luteal function,[14] but probably blocking the decidual reaction of the endometrial stroma;[15] this confirms the importance of estrogen in preparation of the endometrium for implantation. On the contrary, unplanned taking of TMX in early unrecognized pregnancy has been followed by ordinary continuation of pregnancy (ICI Italia, personal communication). The only report of an abortive effect of TMX refers to its combination with prostaglandin.[16]

As stated before about PR, our data is not easily comparable with that of the literature. Padayachi[9] and Kreitmann,[10] using the radiometric method alone, detected very low amounts of ER, but not having IH confirmation considered them positive. On the other hand, Tamaya[8] reported that ER, nuclear and cytoplasmic, increase from the 6th to the 12th week; this conflicting result may be due to the small number of cases considered.

In conclusion, our results seem to prove that the decidua in the first trimester of pregnancy has consistent and constant levels of PR, whereas ER are nearly absent. The adequacy of current techniques in revealing very low amounts of receptors needs to be further confirmed.

## SUMMARY

Receptor content of human decidua in early pregnancy (weeks 6–12) was investigated. Fifty-three tissue samples were obtained from voluntary patients undergoing abortion and whose gestational age range from 6 to 12 weeks. Blood samples were drawn at the time of operation in order to mesure circulating estradiol (E) and progesterone (P) concentrations. Tissue samples underwent first histological confirmation and then were analyzed for receptor content by immunohistochemistry (IH) and by the conventional ligand binding technique (LBA). Estrogen receptors (ER) appeared to be always undetectable by IH (53 samples). LBA measured a significant amount of ER ($>10$ fmol/mg) in two samples, borderline levels (3–10 fmol/mg) in 15, and no binding ($<3$ fmol/mg) in the other 36. Progesterone receptors were always revealed by IH as a strong nuclear staining. LBA measured PR amounts ranging from 10 up to 280 fmol/mg in 44 samples, borderline values (3–10 fmol/mg) in 6 and no binding in the other three. No relation was apparent between PR levels and either gestational age or blood P concentration. ER were possibly downregulated by the high E levels, and their synthesis inhibited by the high P levels.

## REFERENCES

1. SCOTT, R., D. NAVOT, H.-C. LIU & Z. ROSENWAKS. 1991. A human *in vivo* model for the luteoplacental shift. Fertil. Steril. **56:** 481–484.
2. CSAPO, A. I., M. O. PULKKINEN & W. G. WIEST. 1973. Effects of luteoctomy and progesterone replacement therapy in early pregnant patients. Am. J. Obstet. Gynecol. **115:** 759–765.
3. BYDGEMAN, M. & M. L. SWAHN. 1990. Uterine contractility during pregnancy and the effect of abortifacient drugs. Baillihre's Clin. Obstet. Gynaecol. **4:** 249–261.
4. MCNEILLY, A. S. 1977. Physiology of lactation. J. Biosoc. Sci. **4:** 5–21.
5. HANSEN, K. A., M. S. OPSAHL, L. K. NIEMAN, J. R. BAKER & T. A. KLEIN. 1992. Natural killer cell activity from pregnant subjects is modulated by RU 486. Am. J. Obstet. Gynecol. **166:** 87–90.
6. SWAHN, M. L. & M. BYDGEMAN. 1988. The effect of the antiprogestin RU-486 on

uterine contractility and sensitivity to prostaglandin and oxytocin. Br. J. Obstet. Gynecol. **95:** 126–134.
7. AVRECH, O. M., A. GOLAN, Z. WEINRAUB, I. BUKOVSKY & E. CSAPI. 1991. Mifepristone (RU-486) alone or in combination with a prostaglandin analogue for termination of early pregnancy: a review. Fertil. Steril. **56:** 385–393.
8. TAMAYA, T., K. ARABORI & H. OKADA. 1985. Relation between steroid receptor levels and prolactin levels in the decidua of early human pregnancy. Fertil. Steril. **43:** 761–765.
9. PADAYACHI, T., R. J. PEGORARO, J. HOFMEYR, S. M. JOUBERT & R. J. NORMAN. 1987. Decreased concentrations and affinities of oestrogen and progesterone receptors of intrauterine tissue in human pregnancy. J. Steroid Biochem. **26:** 473–479.
10. KREITMANN, B. & F. BAYARD. 1979. Oestrogen and progesterone receptor concentrations in human endometrium during gestation. Acta Endocrinol. **92:** 547–552.
11. GION, M., R. DITTADI & A. E. LEON. 1991. Comparison between single saturating dose ligand binding assay and enzyme immunoassay for low salt extractable estrogen and progesterone receptors in breast cancer: a multicenter study. Eur. J. Cancer **27:** 996–1002.
12. PADAYACHI, T., R. J. PEGORARO, L. ROM & S. M. JOUBERT. 1990. Enzyme immunoassay of oestrogen and progesterone receptors in uterine and intrauterine tissue during human pregnancy and labour. J. Steroid. Biochem. Mol. Biol. **37:** 509–511.
13. MARSIGLIANTE, S., J. R. PUDDEFOOT, S. BARKER, J. GLEDHILL & G. P. VINSON. 1990. Discrepancies between antibody (EIA) and saturation analysis of estrogen receptor content in breast tumor samples. J. Steroid Biochem. Mol. Biol. **37:** 643–648.
14. RAVINDRANATH, N. & N. R. MOUDGAL. 1987. Use of tamoxifen, an antioestrogen, in establishing a need for oestrogen in early pregnancy in the bonnet monkey (*Macaca radiata*). J. Reprod. Fertil. **81:** 327–336.
15. BARKAI, U., T. KIDRON & P. F. KRAICER. 1992. Inhibition of decidual induction in rats by clomiphene and tamoxifen. Biol. Reprod. **46:** 733–739.
16. LINAN, C., Z. YUFENG, C. YUNHONG, J. ZHAOYING, W. KUIQING & L. QUAN. 1990. Combined use of tamoxifen and dl-15-methylprostaglandin F2alpha for termination of early pregnancy. Acta Acad. Med. Shangai **17:** 378–391.

# Protease and Protease Inhibitor Expression during *in Vitro* Decidualization of Human Endometrial Stromal Cells

FREDERICK SCHATZ, CSABA PAPP,[a] ERNO TOTH-PAL,[a]
VITO CUDEMO, VIRGINIA HAUSKNECHT,
GRACIELA KRIKUN, LESZEK MARKIEWICZ,
BENI GAVI, EN-YU WANG, NAUM FEYGIN,
ZOLTAN PAPP,[a] AND CHARLES J. LOCKWOOD

*Department of Obstetrics, Gynecology
and Reproductive Science
Mount Sinai Medical Center
One Gustave L. Levy Place
New York, New York 10029-6574*

and

[a]*Department of Obstetrics and Gynecology
Semmelweis University Medical School
Baross utca 27
1088 Budapest, Hungary*

## INTRODUCTION AND BACKGROUND

### *The Integral Role of Extracellular Matrix Turnover in Decidualization*

Decidualization involves hormone-mediated growth, differentiation and transformation of the endometrial stromal cell to the decidual cell. It occurs in species in which the trophoblast successively penetrates the luminal epithelial barrier, the extracellular matrix (ECM) of the stromal compartment, and the ECM of decidual cell-enveloped blood vessels. While this process provides the embryo direct access to maternal blood prior to the onset of placentation, it risks pregnancy-ending local hemorrhage.[1] Since they are concentrated at perivascular sites, decidual cells are strategically positioned to counteract this threat of hemorrhage. Recent evidence from this laboratory suggests that they may accomplish this in part via the expression of tissue factor, the potent procoagulant mediator of hemostasis.[2,3] In species with a hemochorial placenta, the extent of trophoblast invasiveness is positively correlated with the degree of decidualization.[4] Across species lines, the human trophoblast is the most invasive, and human endometrium displays the most extensive decidualization reaction.[4]

During decidualization in women, the interstitial-type ECM surrounding the stromal cells, in which collagen types I, III, V and VI predominate, is converted to a basal laminar type ECM surrounding the decidual cells, which contains characteristically high levels of laminin, fibronectin, heparin sulfate proteoglycan, collagen type IV and osteonectin.[5-8] This ECM subserves the decidual cell function of limiting trophoblast invasion of the endometrium.[1] The turnover of the ECM surrounding decidual cells therefore plays a key role in implantation. A large body of evidence indicates that efficient ECM degradation depends on the concerted actions of two classes of proteases; the plasminogen activators (PAs) and the matrix metalloproteinases (MMPs).

### The PA/Plasmin System and ECM Degradation

The PAs are highly substrate-specific serine proteases that cleave a unique Arg-Val peptide bond to convert plasminogen to plasmin, a serine protease with broad substrate specificity. The catalytic activity of tissue type PA (tPA) depends on high affinity binding of its structural domain to fibrin, which enables tPA to mediate fibrinolysis by the local generation of plasmin.[9] The urokinase-type PA (uPA) is secreted in its predominantly inactive, single chain form. Its "growth factor"-like structural domain binds to membrane receptors concentrated at the "leading edge" of tumor cell invasion *in situ*[10] and of migration *in vitro*.[11] Similarly, human trophoblast cells, secrete uPA,[12] display saturated cell surface receptors,[13] and are highly invasive *in vitro*.[14] Surface receptor-bound single chain uPA is readily converted to the active double chain form, which resists endocytosis and degradation.[15] Since plasminogen also binds to cell surface receptors, it can be utilized efficiently by active uPA at focal cell surface sites. Binding to specific cell surface receptors protects newly generated plasmin against inhibition by plasma-derived alpha-2-macroglobulin and alpha-2-antiplasmin.[16] While plasmin can utilize such ECM components as fibronectin, laminin, and proteoglycans as substrates,[17] its prime impact on ECM degradation results from activation of MMP zymogens.[18-21]

### The MMPs and ECM Degradation

Based on molecular weight and substrate specificity, the MMPs can be divided into *collagenases,* which preferentially degrade interstitial ECM components; *gelatinases,* which preferentially degrade basement membrane components; and *stromelysins,* which effectively degrade both. The MMPs are released as zymogens that are activated by hydrolytic decoupling of a cysteine in the 10,000-$M_r$ propeptide amino terminus.[22] Since plasmin can activate the MMPs, and the active form of at least one member, stomelysin-1 can, in turn, activate other MMPs,[22] the combined effects of uPA, plasmin and the MMPs generate a proteolytic cascade directed at ECM degradation.

### Specific PA and MMP Inhibitors

Recent attention has been directed at two members of the SERPIN family of inhibitors, the endothelial-type inhibitor $PAI_1$ and the placental-type inhibitor $PAI_2$, which bind to and inactivate both PAs with particularly high affinity.[23] PAI-1 is secreted as an active PA inhibitor, but rapidly undergoes a unique conformational change to its latent form. Stabilization of PAI-1 in its active form, by binding to circulating vitronectin[23] and to ECM-sequestered vitronectin,[24] is integral to the regulation of fibrinolysis and of proteolysis of ECM components respectively.

The MMPs can be inhibited by tissue inhibitors of metalloproteinases (TIMPs).[22,25] $TIMP_1$ is a 28,500-MW glycoprotein which forms a 1 : 1 stoichiometric complex with the active form of a number of MMP subfamilies including the interstitial collagenases and stromelysins. $TIMP_2$ is a 20,000-MW protein, which can bind to and block the activation of gelatinase zymogens. The MMPs are inhibited in plasma by alpha-2-macroglobulin.[22]

### *The Requirement for Human Cells in Studying Human Decidualization* in Vitro

*In vitro* studies permit evaluation of protease and protease inhibitor expression during hormone-induced decidualization of endometrial stromal cells, while eliminating complications from hormonal effects on extraneous cell types. Fundamental differences in the decidualization reaction in humans compared with species generally available for study emphasize the importance of using human cells to study human decidualization. Thus in women, the sequential effects of E2 and progesterone induce stromal cells to decidualize during each normal menstrual cycle.[1] In contrast, the occurrence of decidualization in nonprimates depends firstly on progesterone priming of the uterus for the actions of E2 (*i.e.*, the reverse steroid conditioning sequence of the human),[26,27] and secondly on physical and/or chemical implantational signal(s) (reviewed in Kennedy[28]). Increased endometrial vascular permeability (EVP) and EVP-dependent decidualization of the underlying stroma are among the earliest events of implantation. These changes remain localized at the sites of implantation in the rodent uterus, and are generally constrained in nonhuman primates.[4] However, increased EVP and the decidualization reaction occurs in waves throughout the luteal phase human endometrium.[26,28]

Consistent with ovarian steroid dependence of decidualization *in vivo*, cultured stromal cells derived from specimens of predecidualized cycling human endometrium manifest many decidualization-related changes in response to progestins. These include elevated production of prolactin[29,30] and of IGF-BP;[31,32] increased accumulation of the decidual cell ECM-associated proteins, laminin and fibronectin;[30,33] and enhanced expression of enkephalinase,[34] and tissue factor,[2,3] which are important regulators of hemostasis. Despite a lack of response to E2 alone, E2 generally augments the progestin-mediated effects in the stromal cell monolayers. This synergy *in vitro* is thought to reflect E2 enhancement of progesterone receptor levels *in vivo*, which primes the endometrial stromal cells for the differentiating actions of progesterone.[35]

## OVARIAN STEROID-REGULATED PROTEASE AND PROTEASE INHIBITOR EXPRESSION IN CULTURED HUMAN ENDOMETRIAL STROMAL CELLS

We have evaluated the effects of ovarian steroids on the expression of PAs and PA inhibitors, and of MMPs in primary monolayers of stromal cells derived from specimens of predecidualized human endometrium. The results obtained are included in three recent manuscripts, which are referenced under the appropriate heading below. Following a brief description of the culturing technique used, the results are summarized and discussed.

## Primary Culture of Stromal Cells

Stromal cells were isolated from specimens of predecidualized cycling endometrium following hysterectomy, purified to homogeneity and grown to confluence ($3-5 \times 10^4$ cells/cm$^2$) on polystyrene dishes in a culture medium with 10% charcoal-stripped calf serum.[2] Experimental incubations were initiated in a defined medium[3] containing either 0.1% ethanol vehicle, or E2, or the synthetic progestin medroxyprogesterone acetate (MPA), or E2 + MPA, then placing the dishes in a 37°C : 95% air : 5% CO2 incubator. At three-day intervals: 1) the conditioned media were collected, centrifuged and the supernatants stored frozen; 2) the media were replenished with the corresponding fresh media; and 3) the cells were harvested and analyzed for DNA and protein content. Parallel stromal cell cultures were washed with HBSS and frozen at −80°C for RNA extraction and Northern analysis.

## PA Expression in the Stromal Cell Cultures[a]

As a consequence of their concentration at perivascular sites and abundance, human decidual cells are well situated to both control bleeding as trophoblastic cells breech endometrial blood vessels, and to exert paracrine control against overinvasion of the pregnant endometrium. Therefore, we investigated whether: 1) cultured stromal cells synthesize and release tPA, the primary fibrinolytic agent, and/or uPA, the initiator of an ECM-degrading proteolytic cascade mediating invasion of tissues; and 2) the expression of either PA was altered during steroid-induced decidualization *in vitro*. Previously, explants[36] and stromal cell monolayers[37] derived from human endometrium were shown to secrete both uPA and tPA, with E2 elevating and progesterone lowering the output of uPA.

Use of specific ELISAs enabled us to confirm and extend the latter report. Thus, both uPA and tPA were detected in the conditioned medium of confluent stromal cell cultures under control conditions. Moreover, $10^{-6}-10^{-8}$ M MPA depressed the output of both tPA and uPA. Despite the lack of inhibition by $10^{-8}$ M E2 alone, the progestin-mediated inhibition was sharply augmented in response to E2 + MPA. Similar results were seen with SDS-PAGE separation of stromal cell secreted $^{35}$S-labelled proteins after immunoprecipitation with monoclonal antibodies to tPA (major band at 67 kd) and uPA (major band at 55 kd), indicating that at least part of these steroid effects reflects changes in newly synthesized PAs. To determine whether stromal secreted uPA and tPA were catalytically active, aliquots of the stromal cell conditioned medium were subjected to substrate gel zymography (SDS gels polymerized with small amounts of plasminogen and large amounts of the plasmin substrate casein). As expected, medium from control incubations contained major lytic zones at 67 kd and 55 kd, which were reduced by MPA and further reduced by E2 + MPA. A chromogenic assay that utilizes fibrin binding to discriminate between tPA and uPA activity in the same test sample[38,39] revealed that the progestin selectively inhibited levels of secreted tPA activity compared with the tPA antigen, and that this differential inhibition was even greater in response to E2 + MPA.

---

[a] More details are provided in a recently submitted manuscript: Schatz, F., S. Aigner, C. Papp, V. Hausknecht & C. J. Lockwood. Steroid regulation of plasminogen activators and plasminogen activator inhibitor (PAI-1) during *in vitro* decidualization of human endometrial stromal cells.

## PAI Expression in the Stromal Cell Cultures[b]

Effects of hormones, cytokines and drugs on *in vitro* PA production are frequently associated with opposite effects on the expression of specific PA inhibitors.[41,42] Littlefield and colleagues suggested that the greater inhibition by dexamethasone of secreted tPA verus uPA activity in an ovarian cancer cell line reflected preferential inactivation of the tPA protein by PAI-1.[43] As described above, the progestin MPA selectively inhibited stromal cell secreted tPA activity versus tPA antigen. Therefore, we questioned whether the stromal cell monolayers produced either PAI-1 or PAI-2, and whether the progestin exerted an effect on the expression of either or both PAI moieties that correlated with preferential reduction of tPA activity.

Aliquots of the conditioned medium from confluent stromal cell cultures incubated as described in the previous section were analyzed for PAI-1 and PAI-2 content by sensitive ELISAs. After 3 days of experimental incubation, MPA, but not E2, significantly elevated PAI-1 levels. Despite the refractoriness to E2 alone, an additional doubling of the MPA effect was seen in response to E2 + MPA. Immunoblot analysis confirmed that the secreted PAI-1 conformed to its established molecular weight (50,000). Northern analysis showed that the stromal cells contained a major band at 3.2 kb, and a minor band at 2.2 kb, which conforms to the known species of PAI-1 mRNA.[44] Furthermore, exogenous steroids elicited changes in the expression of PAI-1 message that corresponded to those of the PAI-1 protein (*i.e.*, MPA, but not E2, elevated PAI-1 mRNA levels, with further enhancement of the progestin-mediated effect evident with E2 + MPA).

The cultured stromal cells secreted about one fifth as much PAI-2 as PAI-1. Moreover, unlike PAI-1, PAI-2 levels in the stromal cell conditioned medium were unaffected by exogenous steroids. The preferential production of PAI-1 during *in vitro* decidualization has important implications when extrapolated to decidual cell involvement in regulating periimplantational trophoblast invasion. Thus, PAI-1, but not PAI-2, binds to plasma-derived vitronectin sequestered in ECM, and is maintained in the biologically active form as a result of this binding.[45,46] Such decidual cell-derived PAI-1 could act as a barrier to invasion of the endometrial ECM by trophoblastic cells.

## MMP Expression in the Stromal Cell Cultures[c]

In view of the well documented role of PA-MMP interactions in mediating efficient ECM degradation[9,15,17-19,21,22] we sought to determine whether the ovarian steroid-elicited effects on the production of the PAs and PAI-1 in primary cultures of human endometrial stromal cells as described above, were paralleled by effects on the expression of specific MMPs. Thus, aliquots of conditioned medium obtained from confluent stromal cell cultures in control and steroid-supplemented medium were subjected to substrate gel zymography utilizing gels polymerized in the presence of gelatin. Those gelatin-lysing zones that are abolished by developing the gel in the chelating agent, 1,10-phenanthroline, but not by serine protease inhibitor, PMSF, are considered to reflect MMP activity.[47,48] Accordingly, several

---

[b] See Schatz, F. & C. J. Lockwood[40] for details.

[c] Presented in greater detail in a recently submitted article: Schatz, F., C. Papp, E. Toth-Pal & C. L. Lockwood. Ovarian steroid modulated stromelysin-1 expression in human endometrial stromal and decidual cells.

zones of MMP activity were evident in lanes loaded with conditioned media from control incubations. Of these, three lytic zones proved to be steroid-regulated: 1) a zone of extensive lysis inclusive of both 72-kD type IV/V collagenase and stromelysin-1; 2) a zone showing much less lysis that would be consistent with 92-kD type IV/V collagenase; and 3) a more prominent zone at 135 kD. Incubation with $10^{-6}$ M MPA produced a time-dependent reduction in the magnitude of these zones (*i.e.*, barely seen at 0–3 days, but clearly evident at 3–6 days). While the stromal cells failed to respond to $10^{-8}$ M E2 alone, progestin-mediated inhibition was enhanced by E2 + MPA at both 0–3 days and 3–6 days of experimental incubation.

Stromelysin-1 appears to be pivotal in regulating an ECM-degradating proteolytic cascade. Among the MMPs, it degrades the broadest spectrum of ECM components, and is uniquely capable of activating the zymogenic (*i.e.*, secreted) forms of other MMPs.[22,49,50] Therefore, our efforts were directed at identification of stromelysin-1 as a secreted product of the stromal cells. Immunoblot analysis of five separate experiments indicated the presence of a single band in the stromal cell conditioned medium with the apparent molecular weight of stromelysin-1 (50,000). Moreover, the magnitude of this band was predictably affected by exogenous steroids (*i.e.*, compared with the corresponding controls, no response to $10^{-8}$ M E2 at 0–3 days and 0–6 days; 37% inhibition by $10^{-6}$ M MPA at 3–6 days; and 56% and 64% inhibition at 0–3 days and 0–6 days respectively by E2 + MPA.

We sought to determine whether alterations in levels of secreted stromelysin-1 reflected steady state levels of stromelysin-1 mRNA. Thus, Northern analysis was carried out on RNA extracted from stromal cell monolayers after 3 days of experimental incubation using a cDNA probe generously made available by Dr. N. Hutchinson (Merck Research Laboratories, Rahway, NJ). The stromal cell stromelysin-1 mRNA of approximately 2.1 kb is similar in size to that reported for cultured synovial fibroblasts.[51] Furthermore, as was the case with secreted stromelysin-1 protein, $10^{-8}$ M E2 failed to affect, whereas E2 + MPA markedly reduced stromelysin-1 mRNA expression. Interestingly, E2 added with MPA at $10^{-8}$–$10^{-6}$ M to simulate the physiological range of progesterone concentrations from luteal phase through pregnancy, reduced steady state levels of stromelysin-1 mRNA about 66%.

## DISCUSSION AND CONCLUSIONS

In species with a hemochorial placenta, decidualized endometrial stromal cells control invasion of implanting trophoblast cells. During decidualization, the interstitial ECM surrounding precursor stromal cells is converted to the basal laminar-type ECM around the decidual cells, which forms a barrier against invading trophoblasts.[1,5–8] This transformation requires the synthesis of ECM components, and would be augmented by the simultaneous inhibition of enzymes that degrade the new proteins. Our results indicate that exogenous steroids effect changes in protease expression in human endometrial stromal cells that are consistent with the latter. Accordingly, we observed that a synthetic progestin enhanced the expression of the potent PA inhibitor PAI-1, while reducing that of uPA, and stromelysin-1. Moreover, these effects were increased by mimicking the steroidal milieu of the luteal phase by adding the progestin together with E2. Since uPA-generated plasmin mediates the dissolution of ECM components that are rapidly remodelled, whereas the MMPs tend to degrade the more slowly turning over scaffolding proteins,[50] inhibiting both classes of proteases during decidualization would be expected to help maintain the integrity of the decidual cell ECM.

Results obtained during *in vitro* decidualization can also be extrapolated to decidual cell-trophoblast cell interactions involved in the maintenance of hemostasis during early pregnancy. Consistent with the threat to pregnancy by local hemorrhage posed by trophoblast invasion of the decidual cell-enveloped spiral arterioles, we observed that the expression of the primary fibrinolytic agent tPA was inhibited, while that of its inhibitor PAI-1 were elevated, during steroid-induced decidualization of human endometrial stromal cells. These results, taken together with the parallel increase in expression of the potent procoagulant tissue factor during *in vitro* decidualization of the stromal cells,[2,3] suggest that prevention of hemorrhage during trophoblast invasion is an acute function of the decidual cell.

Finally, simultaneous progestion-elevation of PAI-1 and inhibition of uPA and stromelysin-1 outputs by the cultured stromal cells suggests mechanisms whereby the decidual cell could control ECM degradation mediated by the trophoblast, and hence limit its invasion. Thus, enhanced expression of decidual cell PAI-1 and reduced release of uPA could respectively inhibit the activity of uPA bound to receptors on the trophoblast cell surface, and limit the paracrine supply of uPA to such receptors.[13] Moreover, there is strong evidence linking invasiveness of first trimester trophoblast cells to their expression of the 92-kD gelatinase/type IV collagenase.[48] Since the zymogenic form of this enzyme is activated by stromelysin-1,[52] progestin-mediated suppression of stromelysin-1 expression by decidual cells could serve as a restraint against trophoblast invasion.

In summary, ovarian steroid-induced decidualization of human endometrial stromal cells is accompanied by a reduction in their potential to mediate proteolysis. This phenotypic change is reflected in reduced expression of MMPs such as stromelysin-1, as well as that of the PAs, uPA and tPA, and by enhanced production of the potent PA inhibitor PAI-1. Alterations in the production of these proteins during and following decidualization are postulated to play important roles in: 1) the conversion of the interstitial-type ECM of stromal cells to the basal laminar-type ECM surrounding decidual cells; 2) preventing local hemorrhage during the invasion of the endometrial vasculature by implanting trophoblasts; and 3) limiting the invasion of implanting trophoblasts.

## REFERENCES

1. BELL, S. C. 1990. Decidualization and relevance to menstruation. *In* Contraception and Mechanisms of Endometrial Bleeding. C. d'Arcangues, I. S. Fraser & J. R. Newton, Eds. 187–212. Cambridge: Cambridge University Press.
2. LOCKWOOD, C. J., Y. NEMERSON, S. GULLER, G. KRIKUN, M. ALVAREZ, V. HAUSKNECHT, E. GURPIDE & F. SCHATZ. 1993. Progestational regulation of human endometrial stromal cell tissue factor expression during decidualization. J. Clin. Endocrinol. Metab. **76:** 231–236.
3. LOCKWOOD, C. J., Y. NEMERSON, G. KRIKUN, V. HAUSKNECHT, L. MARKIEWICZ, M. ALVAREZ, S. GULLER & F. SCHATZ. 1993. Steroid-modulated stromal cell tissue factor expression: a model for the regulation of endometrial hemostasis and menstruation. J. Clin. Endocrinol. Metab. **77:** 1014–1019.
4. RAMSEY, E. M., M. L. HOUSTON & J. W. HARRIS. 1976. Interactions of the trophoblast and maternal tissues in three closely related primate species. Am. J. Obstet. Gynecol. **124:** 647–652.
5. WEWER, U. M., M. FABER, L. A. LIOTTA & R. ALBRECHTSEN. 1985. Immunochemical and ultrastructural assessment of the nature of the pericellular basement membrane of human decidual cells. Lab. Invest. **53:** 624–633.
6. KISLAUS, L. L., J. C. HERR & C. D. LITTLE. 1987a. Immunolocalization of extracellular

matrix proteins and collagen synthesis in first trimester human decidua. Anat. Rec. **218:** 402–415.
7. KISLAUS, L. L., E. C. NUNLEY & J. C. HERR. 1987b. Protein synthesis and secretion in human decidua of early pregnancy. Biol. Reprod. **36:** 785–798.
8. WEWER, U. M., R. ALBRECHTSEN, L. W. FISHER, M. F. YOUNG & J. D. TERMINE. 1988. Osteonectin/SPARC/BM-40 in human decidual and carcinoma tissues characterized *de novo* formation of basement membrane. Am. J. Pathol. **132:** 345–355.
9. VASSELLI, J. D., A. P. SAPPINO & D. BELIN. 1991. The plasminogen activator/plasmin system. J. Clin. Invest. **88:** 1067–1072.
10. KWAAN, H. C., H. N. KEER, J. A. RADOSEVICH, J. F. CAJOT & R. ERNST. 1991. Components of the plasminogen-plasmin system in human tumor cell lines. Semin. Thromb. Hemostasis **17:** 175–182.
11. ESTREICHER, A., J. MUHLHAUSER, J. L. CARPIENTIER, L. ORCI & J. D. VASSALLI. 1990. The receptor for urokinase type plasminogen activator polarizes expression of the protease to the leading edge of migrating monocytes and promotes degradation of enzyme inhibitor complexes. J. Cell Biol. **111:** 783–792.
12. QUEENAN, J. T., JR., L. C. KAO, C. E. ARBOLEDA *et al.* 1987. Regulation of urokinase-type plasminogen activator production by cultured human cytotrophoblasts. J. Biol. Chem. **262:** 10903–10906.
13. ZINI, J. M., S. C. MURRAY, C. H. GRAHAM *et al.* 1992. Characterization of urokinase receptor expression by human placental trophoblasts. Blood **79:** 2917–2929.
14. YAGEL, S., R. S. PARHAR, J. J. JEFFREY & P. K. LALA. 1988. Normal nonmetastatic human trophoblast cells share *in vitro* invasive properties of malignant cells. J. Cell. Physiol. **136:** 455–462.
15. KIRCHHEIMER, J. C. & B. R. BINDER. 1991. Function of receptor-bound urokinase. Semin. Thromb. Hemostasis **17:** 246–250.
16. STEPHENS, R. W., J. POLLANEN, H. TAPIOVAARA *et al.* 1989. Activation of pro-urokinase and plasminogen on human sarcoma cells: a proteolytic system with surface-bound reactants. J. Cell Biol. **108:** 1987–1995.
17. LACK, C. H. & H. J. ROGERS. 1958. Action of plasmin on cartilage. Nature **182:** 948–949.
18. MULLIN, D. E. & S. T. RORLICH. 1983. The role of proteinases in cellular invasiveness. Biochim. Biophys. Acta **695:** 177–214.
19. O'GRADY, R. L., L. I. UPFOLD & R. W. STEPHENS. 1981. Rat mammary carcinoma cells secrete active collagenase and active latent enzymes in the stroma via plasminogen activator. Int. J. Cancer **28:** 509–515.
20. TRYGGVASON, K., M. HOYHTYA & T. SALO. 1987. Proteolytic degradation of extracellular matrix in tumor invasion. Biochim. Biophys. Acta **907:** 191–217.
21. WERB, A., C. L. MAIARDIL, C. A. VATER & E. D. HARRIS, JR. 1977. Endogenous activation of latent collagenases by rheumatoid synovial cells: evidence for a role of plasminogen activator. N. Engl. J. Med. **296:** 1017–1023.
22. WOESSNER, J. F., JR. 1991. Metalloproteinases and their inhibitors in connective tissue remodeling. FASEB J. **5:** 2145–2154.
23. LOSKUTOFF, T., M. SAWDEY & J. MIMURO. 1989. Type 1 plasminogen activator. Prog. Hemostasis Thromb. **9:** 87–115.
24. SALONEN, E., M. A. VAHERI, J. POLLANEN *et al.* 1989. Interaction of plasminogen activator inhibitor (PAI-1) with vitronectin. J. Biol. Chem. **264:** 6339–6343.
25. KHOKHA, R. & D. T. DENHARDT. 1989. Matrix metalloproteinases and tissue inhibitor of metalloproteinases: a review of their role in tumorigenesis and tissue invasion. Invasion Metastasis **9:** 391–405.
26. PSYCHOYOS, A. Endocrine control of egg implantation. *In* Handbook of Physiology Section 7, Vol. 2, Part 2. R. O. Greep, E. B. Asstwood & S. R. Geiger, Eds. 187–215. American Physiological Society. Bethesda, MD.
27. CASTRACANE, V. D. & V. C. JORDAN. 1975. The effect of estrogen and progesterone on uterine prostaglandin biosynthesis in the ovariectomized rat. Biol. Reprod. **34:** 327–335.
28. KENNEDY, T. G. 1987. Interactions of eicosanoids and other factors in blastocyst implantation. *In* Eicosanoids and Reproduction. K. Hillier, Ed. 73–88. MTP Press. Lancaster.

29. HUANG, J. R., L. TSENG, P. BISCHOFF & O. A. JANNE. 1987. Regulation of prolactin production by progestin, estrogen, and relaxin in human endometrial stromal cells. Endocrinology **121:** 2011–2017.
30. IRWIN, J. C., D. KIRK, R. J. B. KING, M. M. QUIGLEY & R. B. GWATKIN. 1989. Hormonal regulation of human endometrial stromal cells in culture: an *in vitro* model for decidualization. Fertil. Steril. **52:** 761–768.
31. BELL, S. C., J. A. JACKSON, J. ASHMORE, H. H. ZHU & L. TSENG. 1991. Regulation of insulin-like growth factor binding protein-1 synthesis and secretion by progestin and relaxin in long term cultures of human endometrial stromal cells. J. Clin. Endocrinol. Metab. **72:** 1014–1024.
32. GIUDICE, L. K., D. A. MILKOWSKI, G. LAMSON, R. G. ROSENFELD & J. C. IRWIN. 1991. Insulin-like growth factor binding proteins in human endometrium: steroid-dependent messenger ribonucleic acid expression and protein synthesis. Endocrinology **72:** 779–787.
33. ZHU, H. H., J. R. HUANG, J. MAZELLA, J. ELIAS & L. TSENG. 1992. Progestin stimulates the biosynthesis of fibronectin and accumulation of fibronectin mRNA into human endometrial stromal cells. Hum. Reprod. **7:** 141–146.
34. CASEY, M. L., J. W. SMITH, K. NAGAI, L. B. HERSH & P. C. MACDONALD. 1991. Progesterone-regulated modulation of membrane metallopeptidase (enkephalinase) in human endometrium. J. Biol. Chem. **266:** 23041–23047.
35. TSENG, L., J. MAZELLA & B. L. SUN. 1986. Modulation of aromatase in human endometrial stromal cells by steroids, tamoxifen and RU486. Endocrinology **118:** 1312–1318.
36. CASSLEN, B., A. ANDERSON, D. M. NILSSON & B. ASTEDT. 1986. Hormonal regulation of the release of plasminogen activators and of a specific activator inhibitor from endometrial tissue in culture. Proc. Soc. Exp. Biol. Med. **182:** 419–424.
37. CASSLEN, B., S. URANO, I. LECANDER & T. NY. 1992. Plasminogen activators in the human endometrium, cellular origin and hormonal regulation. Blood Coag. Fibrinolysis **3:** 133–138.
38. KARLAN, B. Y., A. S. CLARK & B. A. LITTLEFIELD. 1987. A highly sensitive chromogenic microtiter plate assay for plasminogen activators in cultured human lymphocytes. Biochem. Biophys. Res. Commun. **142:** 147–154.
39. KARLAN, B. Y., W. AMIN, V. BAND, V. R. ZURAWSKI & B. A. LITTLEFIELD. 1988. Plasminogen activator secretion by established cell lines of human ovarian carcinoma cells *in vitro*. Gynecol. Oncol. **31:** 103–112.
40. SCHATZ, F. & C. L. LOCKWOOD. 1993. Progestin regulation of plasminogen activator inhibitor type 1 in primary cultures of endometrial stromal and decidual cells. J. Clin. Endocrinol. Metab. **77:** 621–625.
41. DANO, K., P. A. ANDERSEN, J. GRONDAHL-HANSEN *et al*. 1985. Plasminogen activators, tissue degradation and cancer. Adv. Cancer Res. **44:** 139–266.
42. LOSKUTOFF, D., M. SAWDEY & J. MIMURO. 1989. Type I plasminogen activator inhibitor. Prog. Hemostasis Thromb. **9:** 87–115.
43. KARLAN, B. Y., J. A. RIVERO, M. E. CRABTREE & B. A. LITTLEFIELD. 1989. Different mechanisms contribute to simultaneous inhibition of urokinase and tissue-type plasminogen activators by glucocorticoids in human ovarian carcinoma cells. Mol. Endocrinol. **3:** 1006–1013.
44. FATTAL, P. G., D. J. SCHNEIDER, B. E. SOBEL & J. J. BILLADELLO. 1992. Posttranscriptional regulation of expression of plasminogen activator inhibitor type I mRNA by insulin and insulin-like growth factor. J. Biol. Chem. **267:** 12412–12415.
45. SEIFFERT, D., J. MIMURO, R. R. SCHLEFF & D. J. LOSKUTOFF. 1990. Interactions between type I plasminogen activator inhibitor, extracellular matrix and vitronectin. Cell Differ. Dev. **32:** 287–292.
46. PREISSNER, K. T. & D. JENNE. 1991. Structure of vitronectin and its biological role in hemostasis. Thromb. Haemostasis **66:** 123–132.
47. FISHER, S. J., T. Y. CUI, L. ZHANG *et al*. 1989. Adhesive and degradative properties of human placental cytotrophoblast cells *in vitro*. J. Cell Biol. **109:** 891–902.
48. LIBRACH, C. L., Z. WERB, M. L. FITZGERALD *et al*. 1991. 92-kD type IV collagenase mediates invasion of human cytotrophoblasts. J. Cell Biol. **113:** 437–449.

49. MATRISIAN, L. M. 1990. Metalloproteinases and their inhibitors in matrix remodelling. Trends Genet. **6:** 121–125.
50. BIRKEDAL-HANSEN, H., E. G. I. MOORE, M. K. BODDEN, L. J. WINDSOR, B. BIRKEDAL-HANSEN, A. DECARLO & J. A. ENGLER. 1993. Matrix metalloproteinases: a review. Crit. Rev. Oral Biol. Med. **4:** 197–250.
51. MACNAULT, K. L., N. CHARTRAIN, M. LARK, M. J. TOCCI & N. I. HUTCHINSON. 1990. Discoordinate expression of stromelysin, collagenase, and tissue inhibitor of metalloproteinase-1 in rheumatoid human synovial fibroblasts. J. Biol. Chem. **265:** 17238–17245.
52. OGATA, Y., J. J. ENGHILD & H. NAGASE. 1992. Matrix metalloproteinase 3 (stromelysin) activates the precursor for human metalloproteinase 9. J. Biol. Chem. **267:** 3581–3584.

# The Adhesion Molecules on Human Endometrial Stromal Cells

## Immunological Implications

MAURO BUSACCA, PAOLA VIGANÒ, BARBARA MAGRI,
AND MARIO VIGNALI

*II Department of Obstetrics and Gynecology*
*University of Milan*
*Clinica Ostetrico-Ginecologica "L. Mangiagalli"*
*Via Commenda 12*
*20122 Milan, Italy*

Currently available data seem to indicate that retrograde menstruation and altered cellular immunity are both important aetiological factors in the development of endometriosis. According to these findings, endometriosis may develop when the peritoneal immune surveillance is defective and permits the outgrowth of endometrial cells in ectopic sites. In particular, recently both Oosterlynck's and our study demonstrate, in these patients, a significantly decreased natural killer-mediated cytotoxicity to autologous endometrial antigens.[1-2] An impaired natural killer response may result in the inability to remove refluxed menstrual debris, thereby increasing the possibility of endometriosis. This decrease in natural killer activity strongly correlated with the severity of the disease.[1]

Furthermore, when endometrial cells were separated in their stromal and epithelial components, the altered cell-mediated immunity was observed toward both cell populations, but was significantly decreased only in presence of stromal cell antigens.[2] Thus, in endometriosis patients, only the stromal compartment seems to be significantly less susceptible to lymphocyte lysis when compared to controls.

Natural killing and interactions of leukocyte to endothelial cells and fibroblasts requires cell-cell contact and adhesion. The recent identification and characterization of a family of glycoproteins, known as integrins, that mediate such interactions have dramatically altered earlier speculations about the nature of cell signaling and cell adhesion molecules.[3-4] These adhesion receptors mediate cell adhesion to a wide variety of extracellular matrix components and potentiate cell-cell interactions.[5]

At a molecular level, one possible explanation for our results is that the stromal cells of the endometrium might present an impairment of these surface molecules involved in the cell-to-cell adhesion mechanism. As a consequence, the lack of a lytic effect towards the stroma could allow ectopic development of endometrial fragments. The expression of these glycoproteins on endometrial stromal cell surface and their role in endometrial metabolism and functions have not yet been extensively investigated. Thus, the aim of this study was to assess the surface expression of two of these molecules, known as intercellular adhesion molecule-1 (ICAM-1) and lymphocyte function-related antigen-3 (LFA-3), on resting and activated human endometrial stromal cells. To this end endometrial biopsies were obtained from 11 regularly cycling women who had undergone diagnostic laparoscopy for unexplained infertility or pelvic pain. Stromal cells were isolated and

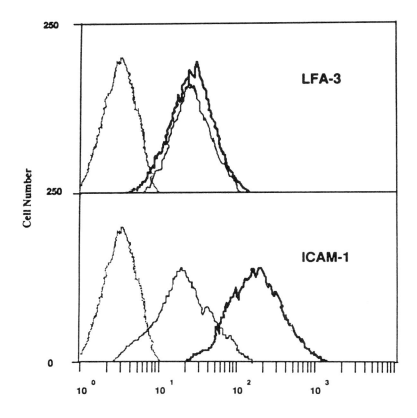

**FIGURE 1.** Representative experiment of LFA-3 and ICAM-1 expression on human dermal fibroblasts measured by immunofluorescence flow cytometry. Cells were treated with medium (*solid line*) or with 40 units/ml IL-1β (*bold line*). *Dotted line* represents nonbinding control.

cultured in Ham's F-10 with 10% fetal calf serum in presence and absence of recombinant human interleukin (IL)-1β. Dermal fibroblasts were used as control cells. To perform flow cytometric analysis, cells were labelled with marker specific monoclonal antibodies (mAbs). The expression of LFA-3 and ICAM-1 was defined as flow cytometry mean fluorescence values and peak fluorescence values.

FIGURE 1 shows the cytometry pattern of ICAM-1 and LFA-3 expression on dermal cells and FIGURE 2 on endometrial stroma. The dotted line represents nonbinding control. Dermal fibroblasts have moderate expression of LFA-3 and ICAM-1. The bold line shows that exposure of this cell type to 40 units/ml of recombinant IL-1β resulted in a 5–10-fold increase in ICAM-1 expression but had no effect on LFA-3 expression. Endometrial stromal cells express LFA-3 at approximately the same level as dermal fibroblasts while ICAM-1 seems to be more expressed on endometrial stromal cells. Furthermore, IL-1$\beta$ is able to enhance ICAM-1 expression while LFA-3 is not upregulated upon exposure to the cytokine.

TABLE 1 confirms the results since ICAM-1 mean fluorescence values and peak fluorescence values are higher on endometrial stromal cells than on dermal fibroblasts. This finding suggests that ICAM-1 might be constitutively more expressed on endometrial stromal cells. In conclusion, our results indicate that LFA-3 has a uniform distribution on dermal fibroblasts as well as on endometrial stromal cells. Its expression does not appear to be modulated by IL-1$\beta$. On the contrary, ICAM-1 expression on cultured endometrial cells seems to be constitutively higher than that found on dermal fibroblasts. Thus, cultured endometrial

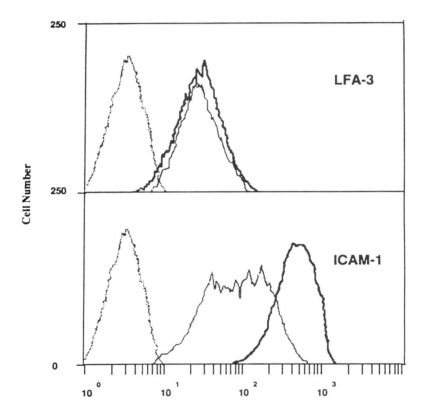

**FIGURE 2.** Representative experiment of LFA-3 and ICAM-1 expression on human endometrial stromal cells measured by immunofluorescence flow cytometry. Cells were treated with medium (*solid line*) or with 40 units/ml IL-1$\beta$ (*bold line*). Dotted line represents nonbinding control.

**TABLE 1.** Constitutive Expression of LFA-3 and ICAM-1 on Endometrial versus Dermal Cells

| Cell Type | Antigen | No. Samples | Mean Channel Fluorescence Values | Peak Channel Fluorescence Values |
|---|---|---|---|---|
| Endometrial | ICAM-1 | 11 | 353 ± 160 | 120 ± 97 |
| | LFA-3 | 11 | 96.5 ± 34 | 21 ± 12 |
| Dermal | ICAM-1 | 3 | 130 ± 43.5 | 55 ± 43.3 |
| | LFA-3 | 3 | 105 ± 3.5 | 25 ± 2.7 |

stromal cells appear to be in an intermediate state of activation. ICAM-1 upregulation might be important in regulating both the natural non-antigen-dependent infiltration of human endometrium by leukocytes and the lymphocyte response at the site of inflammation in the peritoneal cavity.

Furthermore, our results indicate that IL-1$\beta$ has a regulatory action on ICAM-1 expression. This finding could have a physiological relevance, as cells capable of producing lymphokines are commonly present both in the endometrium and in the peritoneum. We are now investigating their functional activity and their possible involvement in conjugate formation and NK-mediated cytotoxicity and shall therefore clarify if any antigenic differences exist between the endometrium of women with endometriosis and that of normal women.

## REFERENCES

1. OOSTERLYNCK, D. J., F. J. CORNILLIE, M. WAER, M. VANDEPUTTE & P. R. KONINCKX. 1991. Women with endometriosis show a defect in natural killer activity resulting in a decreased cytotoxicity to autologous endometrium. Fertil. Steril. **56:** 45–51.
2. VIGANÒ, P., P. VERCELLINI, A. M. DI BLASIO, A. COLOMBO, G. B. CANDIANI & M. VIGNALI. 1991. Deficient antiendometrium lymphocyte-mediated cytotoxicity in patients with endometriosis. Fertil. Steril. **56:** 894–899.
3. HYNES, R. O. 1987. Integrins: a family of cell surface receptors. Cell **48:** 549–554.
4. RUOSLAHTI, E. & M. D. PIERSCHBACHER. 1987. New perspectives in cell adhesion-RGD and integrins. Science **238:** 491–497.
5. SPRINGER, T. A. 1990. Adhesion receptors of the immune system. Nature **346:** 425–434.

# Vascularization of Human Endometrium

## Uterine Blood Flow in Healthy Condition and in Primary Dysmenorrhoea[a]

MATS ÅKERLUND

*Department of Obstetrics and Gynecology*
*University Hospital*
*S-221 85 Lund, Sweden*

## INTRODUCTION

In order to provide for nutrition of a newly nidated ovum the anatomy of the human uterine vascular tree changes repeatedly in a specific and complex way with the normal variations in hormonal state during the menstrual cycle. The innervation of arteries is also under the influence of hormonal changes. Furthermore, hormonal factors influence the spontaneous contractile activity of the smooth muscle of vessel walls as well as the motor responses to different vasoactive substances. Vascular compression can also be due to increased myometrial activity.

In this overview present knowledge about the circulation of the human uterus in healthy condition will be discussed. Menstrual disturbances with respect to blood flow will also be covered to some extent, in particular primary dysmenorrhoea.

*Morphology*

The main blood supply to the human uterus, as well as to the foetoplacental unit during pregnancy is provided by the uterine arteries (FIG. 1). They reach the uterus at the upper cervix where a descending ramification, the vaginal artery, is given off. An ascending branch follows the lateral part of the uterus between the folds of the broad uterine ligament and numerous branches are given off to the myometrium. After further ramification the vessels eventually reach the endometrium. They connect with the coiled arterioles, which are well developed at the time of ovulation and finally ramify into capillaries. At the lateral upper part of the uterus below the istmic part of the fallopian tube, the uterine artery splits into the ovarian and tubal branches, both of which anastomose with branches of the ovarian artery, which also contributes to the uterine circulation. The venous circulation follows a corresponding pattern.

The anatomy of endometrial blood vessels changes in a typical way during the menstrual cycle. Microhysteroscopic studies[1] allowed a definition of five different

---

[a] This study was supported by the Swedish Medical Research Council (B94-17X-06571-12) and the University of Lund, Sweden.

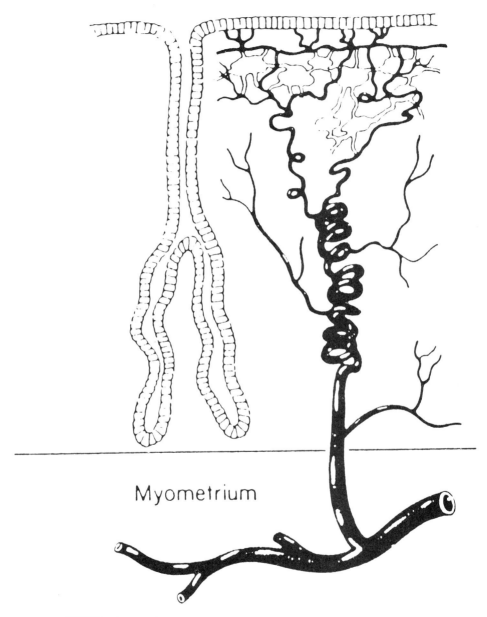

**FIGURE 1.** Arterial and capillary vasculature of the human uterus.

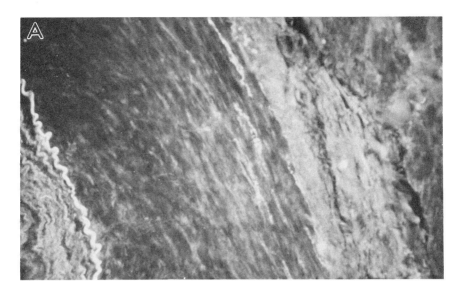

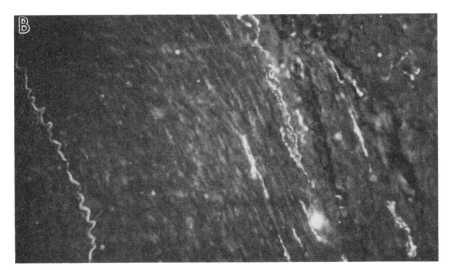

**FIGURE 2.** Immunohistochemical demonstration of separate nerve fibers containing thyroxin hydroxylase as a marker for **(A)** noradrenaline and **(B)** neuropeptide (NP) Y in a branch of the human uterine artery, and **(C)** NPY and **(D)** vasoactive intestinal peptide in the same fibers of the smooth muscle of the uterine arterial wall.

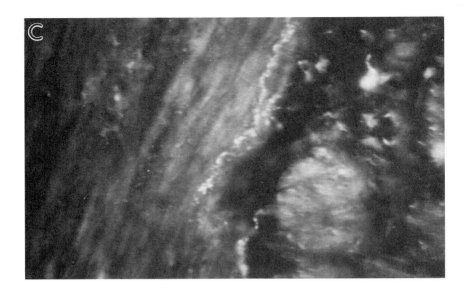

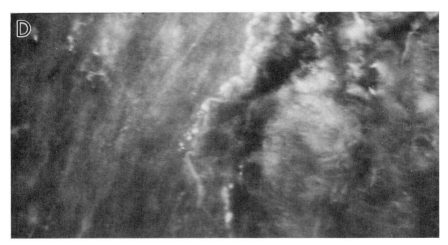

**FIGURE 2** (*Continued*).

and typical phases of the menstrual cycle in humans, *i.e.*, early proliferative, late proliferative, early secretory, late secretory and premenstrual phases. The postovulatory period of the menstrual cycle is characterized by rapid growth of the coiled arteries and development of capillaries and venules.[2] Definite coiled arterioles consist of interlinked endothelial smooth muscle cells which provide flexibility for rapid changes in shape. Progressive differentiation continues up to the premenstrual stage. This abundant angiogenesis may reflect preparation and maintenance of a suitable uterine environment for possible implantation and pregnancy during each menstrual cycle.

## *Innervation of Uterine Arteries*

The basic and abundant adrenergic and cholinergic nerve supply to the human uterine arteries, mediating both contraction and relaxation, has been well described previously.[3] The postjunctional contractile adrenoceptors are primarily of the alfa-1 type.[4] Correspondingly, studies in the guinea pig demonstrated that relaxant adrenoceptor effects and extraneuronal uptake are of minor importance in the main branch of the uterine artery.[5]

The smooth muscle of the vascular walls of human uterine arteries contains peptidergic nerves, which also mediate both contraction and relaxation. Immunohistochemical studies (FIG. 2) demonstrated separate fibers containing vasoactive intestinal peptide, peptide histidine methionine, neuropeptide Y and, to some extent, leuenkephaline.[6] Some nerve fibers contain more than one transmitter peptide (FIG. 2). The density of peptide-containing nerves increases with a decreased diameter of arteries, the greatest concentration being seen around resistance vessels.[7]

## *Endometrial Circulation during the Menstrual Cycle: Influence of Ovarian Steroids*

Apart from causing cyclical changes in vascular anatomy, ovarian steroids have direct effects on endometrial circulation. During the menstrual cycle there are variations in endometrial blood flow, which were described already in the classic reports by Markee[8] and Prill and Götz.[9] Markee studied endometrial transplants in the eye chamber of monkeys and Prill and Götz, although studying humans, used a primitive thermodilution technique. In more recent quantitative estimations by Frazer *et al.*[10] using the 123-Xe-technique similar but not identical results were obtained, probably due to discrepancies in the methods employed. The latter author showed blood flows in the endometrium varying from 10–70 ml/100 g tissue/min in healthy women of fertile age. When results obtained at different days of the menstrual cycle were compared a significant correlation between plasma estradiol levels and endometrial blood flow was seen in the follicular phase with an elevation of flow in the days preceding ovulation.[10] This is in agreement with the well-established potent vasodilatory effect of estrogens on uterine arteries.[11] A morphometric study of endometrial capillaries during the normal menstrual cycle[12] also demonstrated dynamic changes during the normal menstrual cycle with a significant dilatation of the vessels during the postovulatory phase.

In the luteal phase there seems to be no correlation between blood flow and estradiol levels, but a gradual increase until the onset of menstruation when a

TABLE 1. Concentrations (mol/L) of Agonists Giving 50% of Maximal Response of Different-Sized Branches of the Isolated Human Uterine Artery[a]

| Agonist (Bath Conc. Factor) | Type of Artery | | |
|---|---|---|---|
| | Main Stem ($EC_{50}$) | Medium-Sized ($EC_{50}$) | Small-Sized ($EC_{50}$) |
| Arginine vasopressin ($\times 10^{-10}$) | 10 | 7 | 3 |
| Endothelin ($\times 10^{-9}$) | 43 | 32 | 8 |
| Oxytocin ($\times 10^{-8}$) | 17 | 10 | 6 |
| Noradrenaline ($\times 10^{-7}$) | 32 | 26 | 8 |
| $PGF_{2\alpha}$ ($\times 10^{-6}$) | 2 | 5 | 6 |
| Dopamine ($\times 10^{-6}$) | 82 | 160 | 7 |

[a] Small-sized artery preparations gave significantly more pronounced responses to arginine vasopressin, endothelin, oxytocin and noradrenaline than the main stem of the uterine artery.

fall is observed.[10] Women with dysfunctional bleeding due to unovulation have exceedingly variable flow rates.[10]

A direct effect of estradiol with reduced vascular resistance and corresponding increase in uterine blood flow was demonstrated by transvaginal Doppler-sonography.[13] Progesterone seemed to counteract this effect of estradiol.[13] The effect is probably mediated by specific estrogen and progesterone receptors in human uterine vessel walls.[14,15]

### Effects of Some Peptides and Other Vasoactive Substances on Human Uterine Blood Flow

In Vitro *Data*

The contractile potencies *in vitro* of some neutropeptides and other important humoral factors on human uterine arteries are shown in TABLE 1. The most potent of the studied substances was arginine vasopressin, followed in order by endothelin, oxytocin, noradrenaline and dopamine.[6,16] Vasopressin, endothelin, oxytocin and noradrenaline also had the most pronounced effects on the smaller arteries, the so called resistant vessels.[16] Acetylcholine and tyrosine had only a small effect on uterine arteries and VIP caused relaxation of contractile activity induced by prostaglandin (PG)$F_{2\alpha}$.[6,16]

The important role of different PGs in the regulation of menstrual bleeding has been known for some time and has been extensively reviewed.[17,18] Laudanski et al.[19] found that the effect of PGs on human uterine arteries are limited with $PGF_{2\alpha}$ causing contraction and $PGE_2$ to some extent inducing relaxation. Meigaard et al. (1985)[18] demonstrated a difference between extra- and intramyometrial arteries with these PGs and recorded relaxation only in the latter type of vessels.

## In Vivo *Findings*

Vasopressin has a potent effect *in vivo* on human endometrial blood flow, particularly during early menstruation.[21,22] When the effect of vasopressin is inhibited by a newly developed oxytocin and type V1 vasopressin receptor blocking agent, 1-deamino-2-D-(OEt)-4-Thr-8-Orn-oxytocin the blood flow rises markedly and the uterus relaxes (FIG. 3).

There is little *in vivo* data on the effect on endometrial blood flow of other physiological and pharmacological factors, with the exception of the $\beta_2$-adrenoceptor-stimulating agent terbutaline. This drug causes a rise in flow, which varies in magnitude during the menstrual cycle and is most pronounced at the onset of menstruation.[23]

### *Spontaneous Blood Flow in Healthy Condition and in Primary Dysmenorrhoea*

During spontaneous, well-demarked uterine contractions in healthy women, which occur around the onset of menstruation, blood flow generally decreases (FIG. 3). This is due to an effect of the increased intrauterine pressure on uterine vessels.[21–23] In primary dysmenorrhoea myometrial hyperactivity causes uterine ischemia and pain by an even more pronounced compression of uterine vessels, but blood flow recordings also indicate the presence of vasoconstrictive agents acting directly on the vessel walls.[24] One such factor which has been shown to have an important role in dysmenorrhoea is vasopressin.[25,26] Oxytocin may also play a role in view of the recent demonstration of both oxytocin and type V1 vasopressin receptors in the myometrium and pronounced *in vivo* and *in vitro* effects of this substance at certain stages of the menstrual cycle.[27] The variation in effects of vasopressin and oxytocin during different hormonal states may reflect differences in oxytocin receptor concentrations.[27] The involvement of both oxytocin and vasopressin in the aetiology of dysmenorrhoea is in agreement with demonstrated therapeutic effect of 1-deamino-2-D-(OEt)-4-Thr-8-Orn-oxytocin.[28]

## CONCLUSION

The regulation of endometrial blood flow is complex, involving adrenergic and peptidergic nerves and humoral factors. A considerable amount of *in vitro* data on these factors is available, but the importance in the *in vivo* situation in physiological and pathophysiological conditions still largely remains to be determined. Furthermore, when considering endometrial circulatory effects of different agents, the effect of myometrial activity also needs to be taken into account. Ovarian steroids have both a tropic effect on the endometrial vessels, which are repeatedly changing each menstrual cycle and also direct effects on the vessel walls via specific receptors. Disturbances of any of these factors probably influence mechanisms of menstrual bleeding, and this is an area of important future research.

## SUMMARY

The anatomy of the human uterine vascular tree changes repeatedly with the variations in hormonal state during each menstrual cycle, with progressive

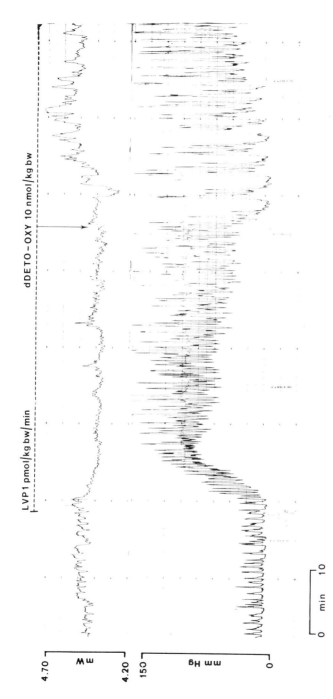

**FIGURE 3.** Recording of intrauterine pressure and added power reflecting uterine blood flow in a nonpregnant woman at the onset of menstruation. Infusion of lysine vasopressin (LVP) induced hyperactivity, reduction of blood flow and dysmenorrhoea-like pain, which was counteracted by injection of the competitive type V1 vasopresin and oxytocin receptor antagonist, 1-deamino-2-D-Tyr(OEt)-4-Thr-8-Orn-oxyto-cin (dDETO-OXY).

differentiation of arterioles up to the premenstrual state. Hormonal factors also influence the innervation of uterine arteries, both cholinergic, adrenergic and peptidergic, and regulate the spontaneous contractile activity of the smooth muscle of vessel walls as well as the motor responses of these tissues to different vasoactive substances. The smaller branches of uterine arteries, *i.e.*, the resistance arteries appear to be of particular importance in the regulation of uterine blood flow, since they are most densely innervated. Furthermore, the most effective uterine vasoconstrictors *in vitro*, vasopressin, endothelin, oxytocin and noradrenaline have a more pronounced effect on these vessels than on the main branches of the uterine artery. Vascular compression may also result from changes in the myometrial activity.

A hormonal disturbance may cause dysfunctional bleeding by changing vessel growth as well as the uterine smooth muscle activity of both vessels and myometrium. An example of the latter phenomenon is primary dysmenorrhoea, women with this condition having an increased secretion of vasopressin. By an action on type V1 vasopressin receptors of the uterus, this peptide causes myometrial hyperactivity and vasoconstriction, with resultant uterine ischemia and pain. Further support for a pathophysiological role of vasopressin and also of oxytocin in dysmenorrhoea is the therapeutic effect of a competitive type V1 vasopressin and oxytocin receptor antagonist in the condition.

## REFERENCES

1. VAN HERENDAEL, B. J., M. J. STEVENS, A. FLAKIEWICZ-KULA & C. H. HANSCH. 1987. Dating of the endometrium by microhysteroscopy. Gynecol. Obstet. Invest. **24:** 114–118.
2. KAISERMAN-ABRAMOF, I. R. & H. A. PADYKULA. 1989. Angiogenesis in the postovulatory primate endometrium: the coiled arteriolar system. Anat. Res. **224:** 479–489.
3. OWMAN, CH. & M. STJERNQUIST. 1988. Origin, distribution, and functional aspects of aminergic and peptidergic nerves in the male and female reproductive tracts. *In* Handbook of Chemical Neuroanatomy, Vol. 6. The Peripheral Nervous System. A. Björklund, T. Hökfelt & Ch. Owman, Eds. 445–544. Elsevier. Amsterdam.
4. STJERNQUIST, M. & CH. OWMAN. 1990. Adrenoceptors mediating contraction in the human uterine artery. Hum. Reprod. **5:** 19–24.
5. FALLGREN, B. & L. EDVINSSON. 1986. Characterisation of adrenoceptor mechanisms in isolated guinea-pig uterine arteries. Eur. J. Pharmacol. **131:** 163–170.
6. EKESBO, R., P. ALM, P. EKSTRÖM, L.-M. LUNDBERG & M. ÅKERLUND. 1991. Innervation of the human uterine artery and motor responses to neuropeptides. Gynecol. Obstet. Invest. **31:** 30–36.
7. ALM, P., M. ÅKERLUND & T. BOSSMAR. 1993. Differences in innervation between main stem and smaller branches of the human uterine artery. In manuscript.
8. MARKEE, J. E. 1950. The relation of blood flow to endometrial growth and the inception of menstruation. *In* Menstruation and Its Disorders. E. T. Engle, Ed. 165–185. C. C. Thomas. Springfield, IL.
9. PRILL, H. J. & F. GÖTZ. 1961. Blood flow in the myometrium and endometrium of the uterus. Am. J. Obstet. Gynecol. **82:** 102–108.
10. FRASER, I. S., G. MCCARRON, B. HUTTON & D. MACEY. 1987. Endometrial blood flow measured by xenon-133 clearance in women with normal menstruation cycles and dysfunctional uterine bleeding. Am. J. Obstet. Gynecol. **156:** 158–166.
11. MAKOWSKI, E. L. 1977. Vascular physiology. *In* Biology of the Uterus. R. M. Wynn, Ed. 77–100. Plenum Press. New York.
12. PEEK, M., B. M. LANDGREN & E. JOHANNISSON. 1992. The endometrial capillaries during the normal menstrual cycle: a morphometric study. Hum. Reprod. **7:** 906–911.
13. DE ZIEGLER, D., R. BESSIS & R. FRYDMAN. 1991. Vascular resistance of uterine

arteries: physiological effects of oestradiol and progesterone. Fertil. Steril. **55:** 775–779.
14. BATRA, S. & S. IOSIF. 1987. Nuclear oestrogen receptors in human uterine arteries. Gynecol. Obstet. Invest. **24:** 250–255.
15. BERGQVIST, A., D. BERGQVIST & O. M. FERN. 1993. Oestrogen and progesterone receptors in vessel walls. Biochemical and immunochemical assays. Acta Obstet. Gynecol. Scand. **72:** 10–16.
16. EKSTRÖM, P., M. L. FORSLING, H. KINDAHL, T. LAUDANSKI & M. ÅKERLUND. 1992. Stimulation of vasopressin release in women with primary dysmenorrhoea and after oral contraceptive treatment effect on uterine contractility. Br. J. Obstet. Gynaecol. **98:** 680–684.
17. CHRISTIAENS, G. C. M. L., J. J. SIXMA & A. A. HASPELS. 1981. Haemostasis in menstrual endometrium in the presence of an intrauterine device. Br. J. Obstet. Gynaecol. **88:** 825–837.
18. GRANSTRÖM, E., M.-L. SWANN & V. LUNDSTRÖM. 1983. The possible roles of prostaglandins and related compounds in endometrial bleeding. A mini-review. Acta Obstet. Gynecol. Scand. **113:** 91–99.
19. LAUDANSKI, T., A. KOSTRZEWSKA & M. ÅKERLUND. 1984. Interaction of vasopressin and prostaglandins in the nonpregnant human uterus. Prostaglandins **27:** 441–452.
20. MAIGAARD, S., A. FORMAN & K.-E. ANDERSSON. 1985. Differences in contractile activation between human extra- and intramyometrial arteries. Acta Physiol. Scand. **124:** 371–379.
21. ÅKERLUND, M. & K.-E. ANDERSSON. 1976. Vasopressin response and terabutaline inhibition of the uterus. Obstet. Gynecol. **47:** 529–535.
22. HAUKSSON, A., M. ÅKERLUND & P. MELIN. 1988. Uterine blood flow and myometrial activity at menstruation, and the action of vasopressin and a synthetic antagonist. Br. J. Obstet. Gynaecol. **95:** 898–904.
23. ÅKERLUND, M. & K.-E. ANDERSSON. 1976. Effects of terbutaline on myometrial activity and endometrial blood flow during the menstrual cycle. Obstet. Gynecol. **47:** 529–536.
24. ÅKERLUND, M., K.-E. ANDERSSON & I. INGEMARSSON. 1976. Effects of terbutaline on myometrial activity, endometrial blood flow, and lower abdominal pain in women with primary dysmenorrhoea. Br. J. Obstet. Gynaecol. **83:** 673–678.
25. ÅKERLUND, M., P. STRÖMBERG & M. L. FORSLING. 1979. Primary dysmenorrhoea and vasopressin. Br. J. Obstet. Gynaecol. **86:** 484–487.
26. STRÖMBERG, P., M. ÅKERLUND, M. L. FORSLING, E. GRANSTROM & H. KINDAHL. 1984. Vasopressin and prostaglandin in premenstrual pain and primary dysmenorrhoea. Acta Obstet. Gynecol. Scand. **63:** 533–538.
27. BOSSMAR, T., M. ÅKERLUND, G. FANTONI, M. MAGGI, J. SZAMATOWICZ & T. LAUDANSKI. 1993. Uterine response to oxytocin and vasopressin in non-pregnant women—receptor mediated effects. Br. J. Obstet. Gynecol. In manuscript.
28. ÅKERLUND, M. 1987. Can primary dysmenorrhoea be alleviated by a vasopressin antagonist? Acta Obstet. Gynecol. Scand. **66:** 459–461.

# The Role of Progestationally Regulated Stromal Cell Tissue Factor and Type-1 Plasminogen Activator Inhibitor (PAI-1) in Endometrial Hemostasis and Menstruation

CHARLES J. LOCKWOOD,[a] GRACIELA KRIKUN,
CSABA PAPP, ERNO TOTH-PAL, LESZEK MARKIEWICZ,
EN-YU WANG, THOMAS KERENYI, XIAODONG ZHOU,
VIRGINIA HAUSKNECHT, ZOLTAN PAPP,
AND FREDERICK SCHATZ

*Department of Obstetrics, Gynecology and
Reproductive Science
Mount Sinai School of Medicine
1 Gustave L. Levy Place
New York, New York 10029*

## INTRODUCTION

The maintenance of endometrial *hemostasis* is crucial to the success of implantation and placentation. Survival of the implanting human blastocyst requires that syncytiotrophoblasts breach the endometrial vasculature to establish the primordial uteroplacental circulation.[1] Subsequently, extravillous cytotrophoblasts penetrate the uterine spiral arteries to mediate extensive morphological changes.[2] Both invasive processes involve profound vascular perturbations which must occur in the absence of hemorrhage. In contrast, the absence of implantation leads to menstrual *hemorrhage* which is accompanied by diffuse disruption of endometrial vessels.

The mechanisms by which the endometrium can paradoxically prevent focal hemorrhage during implantation and permit diffuse bleeding during menstruation, are poorly understood.[3] This lack of knowledge has hampered efforts to treat a number of serious obstetrical and gynecological disorders. Derangements in endometrial hemostasis are a potential source of miscarriage, abruptio placenta and preterm delivery. In nonpregnant women, disorders of endometrial bleeding are a primary indication for hysterectomy.[4] Furthermore, endometrial "breakthrough-bleeding" is a major cause for the discontinuation of hormonal contraception leading to unplanned pregnancy.[5]

---

[a] Address for correspondence: Charles J. Lockwood, MD, The Mount Sinai School of Medicine, Department of Obstetrics, Gynecology and Reproductive Medicine, Division of Maternal Fetal Medicine, 1 Gustave L. Levy Place, New York, NY 10029-6574.

## Decidual Cells as Regulators of Hemostasis and Menstruation

Progesterone acts on the estrogen-primed human endometrium to transform stromal cells to decidual cells. In humans, histologically identifiable decidual cells first appear at perivascular sites at about day 23 of the menstrual cycle and spread wave-like throughout the endometrium.[6] During implantation, perivascular decidualized stromal cells are strategically positioned to promote endometrial hemostasis during trophoblast penetration and subsequent remodeling of endometrial vessels. That decidual cells participate in periimplantational and placental hemostasis is suggested by the close correlation between the extent of trophoblast invasion and decidualization in species with a hemochorial placenta;[7] both processes reaching their fullest expression in women.[8] Since endometrial blood vessels are enveloped by decidual cells by the end of the luteal phase, they are also well positioned to promote and control "hemorrhage" during menstruation. Further support for the participation of decidualized endometrial stromal cells in implantational hemostasis and menstrual hemorrhage is suggested by: 1) the association of ectopic pregnancy, a condition marked by an absence of decidua, with hemorrhage; and 2) the limitation of spontaneously occurring decidualization to species exhibiting menstruation.[9]

## Tissue Factor as a Decidual Mediator of Endometrial Hemostasis

As the initiator of the extrinsic pathway of coagulation, tissue factor (TF) is primarily responsible for the maintenance of hemostasis *in vivo*[10] and, thus, a likely mediator of decidual hemostasis. Tissue factor is a cell membrane-bound glycoprotein comprised of 263 amino acids including a hydrophilic extracellular domain of 219 residues, a 23-residue membrane spanning hydrophobic domain and a cytoplasmic tail of 21 residues.[10] The mature protein displays an apparent molecular mass of 46 kDa on SDS-PAGE.[11] The TF gene maps to the short arm of chromosome 1,[12-15] is 9.4 kb in length with at least two introns and a 2.5-kb message, which has been cloned.[12]

The extrinsic coagulation pathway is poised to initiate hemostasis following vascular disruption. Tissue factor is not normally expressed by endothelial cells, and, therefore, is not in contact with the intact circulation. However, once exposed to blood, TF avidly binds to plasma factor VII, a 406-amino acid vitamin K-dependent serine protease, and the TF-factor VII complex converts factor X to factor Xa either directly or indirectly via the initial activation of factor IX to factor IXa.[10] In turn, factor Xa converts prothrombin to thrombin to initiate clotting.[10]

As a co-factor, TF does not require proteolytic modification to exert its procoagulant function. Moreover, factor VII is unique among coagulation factor zymogens, in that it exerts its procoagulant activity immediately upon binding to TF without need for an initial proteolytic modification.[16,17] This zymogenic activity obviates a crucial objection to the intrinsic pathway paradigm of coagulation, namely that an endless series of clotting factor zymogen activations is theoretically required to initiate clotting. However, the initial stage of factor VII-mediated clotting is exponentially enhanced by the subsequent cleavage of factor VII to VIIa by either thrombin, factor IXa, Xa, or XIIa which results in a 120-fold increase in factor VII activity.[10,18]

As noted, TF is not normally in contact with the circulation. However, such contact would follow focal trophoblast-mediated disruption of the uterine vasculature, where TF expression by perivascular decidual cells would serve to prevent hemorrhage. Alternatively, a premenstrual reduction in perivascular decidual cell TF expression might contribute to the diffuse uterine bleeding of menstruation.

### *Plasminogen Activator Inhibitor and Endometrial Hemostasis*

The maintenance of hemostasis depends not only on the initiation of coagulation but on the maintenance of vascular stability and the prevention of fibrinolysis. The latter two functions are opposed by urokinase-type and tissue-type plasminogen activators, uPA and tPA, respectively. These substrate-specific serine proteases cleave an Arg-Val peptide bond in plasminogen to convert it to plasmin.[19] Plasmin, in turn, mediates fibrinolysis and degrades extracellular matrix (ECM) components to promote hemorrhage. High levels of plasminogen are present in plasma and tissues.[19]

The stability of the decidual vasculature is crucially dependent on the integrity of its ECM. By binding to cell membrane receptors, uPA can directly degrade this ECM,[20,21] but its major role in ECM degradation is via the generation of plasmin. As a consequence of wider substrate specificity, plasmin can degrade several decidual ECM components directly (*e.g.*, fibronectin, laminin, proteoglycans) and activate metalloproteinase zymogens.[22-26] Thus, the generation of endometrial uPA could initiate the degradation of the decidual vascular ECM leading to vessel instability. Endometrial hemostasis can also be adversely affected by fibrinolysis mediated by tPA which binds to the fibrin clot to generate plasmin and acts as the primary initiator of fibrinolysis.[27]

The activities of the PAs are controlled by specific inhibitors. Two of these, $PAI_1$ and $PAI_2$, bind the PAs with particularly high affinity.[27] As a primary inhibitor of both ECM degradation and fibrinolysis, PAI-1[27] is a likely mediator of these activities in the decidua. The mature PAI-1 glycoprotein is a single polypeptide chain containing 379 amino acids with a Mr of 50,000.[27] Its Ka for both tPA and uPA is in the order of $10^7$ $M^{-1}$ $sec^{-1}$. The PAI-1 gene maps to the long arm of chromosome 7, is 12.2 kB in length and contains 9 exons and 8 introns.[27-29] Two distinct PAI-1 mRNAs are transcribed, 3.2 and 2.3 kB. They appear to differ only in the length of their 3′ untranslated region and both contain an identical 1.2 kB codogenic region.[27]

Recently, attention has been focused on the sequestration of PAI-1 in the ECM via its binding to vitronectin.[30] This binding results in a conformational change which greatly augments its inhibitory activity. Enhanced deposition of PAI-1 in the perivascular decidual ECM could modulate trophoblast invasion, promote vascular stability and enhance hemostasis. Conversely, a reduction in perivascular decidual PAI-1 expression could promote vascular ECM degradation and enhance fibrinolysis to facilitate menstruation.

### *Hypothesis: Decidualization is Associated with Enhanced Stromal Cell Tissue Factor and PAI-1 Expression*

Based on the above information we postulated that progesterone-induced decidualization of endometrial stromal cells was likely to be associated with enhanced expression of TF and PAI-1, which would serve to promote hemostasis during trophoblast implantation and endovascular invasion. Conversely, we hypothesized that withdrawal of progesterone would likely be associated with reduced decidual cell TF and PAI-1 expression creating an environment conducive to menstrual-associated vascular and tissue disruption and hemorrhage. The following is a review of prior work from our laboratory as well as recent unpublished findings which strongly support this hypothesis.

## MATERIALS AND METHODS

### Collection of Tissues

Endometrial specimens were obtained from premenopausal women undergoing hysterectomies for reasons other than neoplasia. A portion was formalin fixed, stained with hematoxylin-eosin and dated according to the criteria of Noyes and associates.[6] Decidua was obtained following first trimester elective terminations. Endometrial stromal cells were isolated by the method of Satyaswaroop et al.[31] as modified by Schatz and colleagues.[32] Decidual cells were isolated according to the method of Braverman et al.[33] The >98% purity of these preparations was confirmed by selective immunocytochemical staining for cytokeratin and vimentin.

### Experimental Culture Conditions

*Stromal Cell Cultures*

Stromal cells were grown to confluence ($3-5 \times 10^4$ cells/cm$^2$) in a 37°C 95% air:5% $CO_2$ incubator in basal medium (BM), a phenol red-free 1:1 v/v mixture of Dulbecco's MEM (Gibco) and Ham's F-12 (Flow Labs), with 100 $\mu$/ml penicillin, 100 $\mu$g/ml streptomycin, 0.25 $\mu$g/ml fungizone and 10% charcoal-treated calf serum (10% SCS). At confluence, the cells were either maintained in BM or washed twice with a defined medium (DM) [BM + ITS$^+$ (Collaborative Research) + 5 $\mu$M $FeSO_4$, 50 $\mu$M $ZnSO_4$, 1 nM $CuSO_4$, trace elements (Gibco), with 50 ng/ml EGF and 50 $\mu$g/ml ascorbic acid (Sigma)]. The experimental period was initiated by adding either BM + 10% SCS or DM containing either $10^{-8}$ M E2, $10^{-8}$ to $10^{-6}$ M MPA, E2 + MPA, or 0.1% ethanol, as a vehicle control. After 2–24 days, the incubations were terminated after collecting the medium which was centrifuged and stored at $-70$°C, and harvesting the cells by washing with HBSS, scraping with a rubber spatula and transferring to cold HBSS containing a mixture of protease inhibitors [10 $\mu$g/ml each of PMSF, soybean trypsin inhibitor, aprotinin, pepstatin A and leupeptin (Sigma)]. The cells were then pelleted and frozen at $-70$°C until assayed. Parallel cultures were washed with HBSS and frozen at $-70$°C for Northern analysis.

The effects of steroid withdrawal were also assessed. Confluent stromal cell cultures were incubated in BM + 10% SCS with $10^{-8}$ M E2 + $10^{-7}$ M MPA, replacing the media every two days. After 10 days, the cultures were washed twice with BM + 10% SCS and parallel cultures exposed to either the same steroidal regimen or vehicle control for 4 or 7 days, since a minimum of three days incubation with control media is required to clear steroids from their receptors.[34]

*Decidual Cell Cultures on Type I Collagen Gels*

Isolated decidual cells were suspended in BM + 2% SCS + ITS$^+$ containing vehicle control or steroids and 500,000 cells seeded on Millicell CM inserts (Millipore) coated with a collagen gel as described.[35] After the cells had adhered to the collagen surface for 48 hours in a 37°C 95% air : 5% $CO_2$ incubator, the medium was exchanged for DM containing the corresponding control and steroid treatments. Cultures were maintained for another 4 days, and the medium was then collected, centrifuged and stored at −70°C and decidual cells were harvested by digesting with 0.25% collagenase (Worthington).

## Immunohistochemistry

Specimens were fixed in 10% formalin × 3 hr, then dehydrated, infiltrated and embedded in paraffin. Five micron sections were placed on 1% poly-D-lysine (Sigma) coated glass slides. After deparaffinization and rehydration, select sections were exposed to 1% $H_2O_2$ and preincubated with 0.1% pepsin (Sigma) in 0.01 N HCl for 20 min at 37°C. The latter step is required for visualization of TF- and PAI-1 antigen in formalin-fixed tissues. Immunoperoxidase staining was then carried out with an avidin-biotin peroxidase complex (Vector Labs, Burlingame, CA). The TF studies utilized 300 ng/ml of an anti-human TF rabbit IgG polyclonal antibody, raised and purified as described.[19] The PAI-1 studies utilized a specific anti-PAI-1 monoclonal antibody as per the manufacturer's recommendation (American Diagnostica). Controls were routinely performed by replacing the primary antibody with appropriate nonimmune serum, or by using antibody preadsorbed with excess immunopurified human brain TF prepared as described[39] or immunopurified PAI-1 (American Diagnostica).

## Biochemical Assay

### Tissue Factor Assays

Cell pellets were solubilized with Triton X-100 and TF content measured by a previously described enzyme linked immunoassay (ELISA).[36,37] The slope of optical absorbance vs TF concentration was linear between 0 to 220 pM with R > 0.99. A previously detailed[36,37] two-stage TF clotting assay was employed to measure functionally active TF. The linear range of the assay's standard curve of TF content vs the log of clot time was 0.1 to 8 pM.

### PAI-1 and PAI-2 Immunoassay

Concentrations of PAI-1 and PAI-2 in the medium were measured by ELISA (American Diagnostica) employing either a specific anti-PAI-1 or anti-PAI-2 monoclonal antibody in the solid phase and a second peroxidase conjugated goat anti-human PAI-1 or PAI-2 IgG to amplify the PAI signal. The inter- and intra-assay errors were <7% and the detection limits for PAI-1 and PAI-2 were 1 and 6 ng/ml, respectively. The PAI-1 assay detects both active and inactive forms, and PAI-1 complexed with PA. The PAI-2 assay detects both the 46.6-kD (placental) and 60-kD (plasma) MW forms of the molecule.

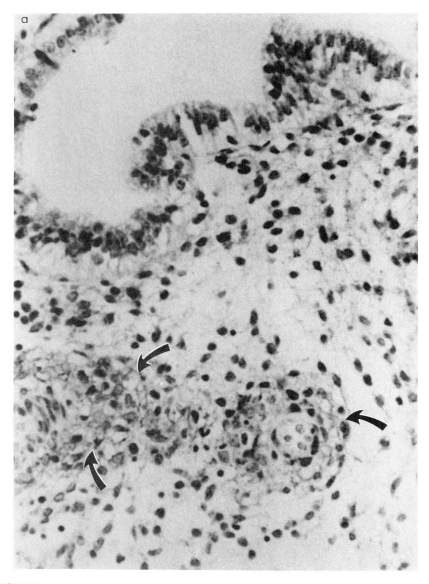

**FIGURE 1.** Immunohistochemical staining for tissue factor in late secretory endometrium and plasminogen activator inhibitor (PAI-1) in gestational endometrial tissue. **(a)** Late secretory endometrium displaying staining for TF in the cytoplasm and cell membranes of perivascular decidualized stromal cells (*arrows*). The glandular epithelium failed to display detectable TF antigen. **(b)** Decidual cells from gestational endometrium obtained in the first trimester displaying cytoplasmic staining for PAI-1 (*arrows*).

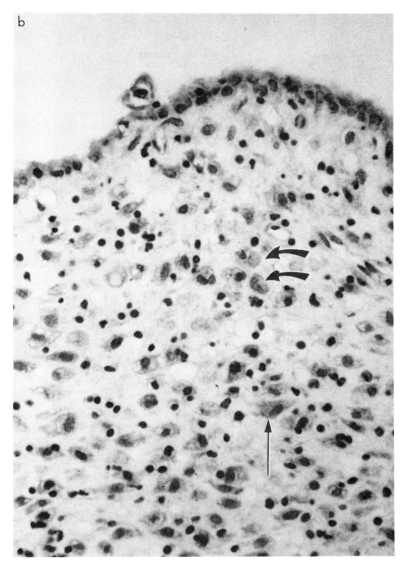

**FIGURE 1** (*Continued*).

*Prolactin Assay*

Immunoreactive prolactin (irPRL) levels in the medium were measured as described[37] using a double antibody kit according to the manufacturer's specifications (Amersham, Arlington Heights, IL).

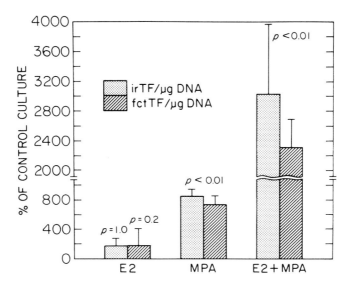

**FIGURE 2.** Progestin-enhanced tissue factor expression. Confluent endometrial stromal cell cultures were incubated in media containing serum with either vehicle control, $10^{-8}$ M E2, $10^{-6}$ M MPA, or E2 + MPA for 20 days. Immunoreactive (ir) and functionally active (fct) tissue factor (TF) content is normalized to culture DNA and expressed as percent of control cultures (mean and SEM for cultures from 5 patient specimens; $p$ values for comparison with control cultures).

## Protein and DNA Assays

Concentrations of total protein were measured with a modified Bradford assay (Bio-Rad), while total DNA content was assayed by the method of Hinegardner.[38]

## *Immunoblot Studies*

Immunopurified human brain TF (2.5 ng) or 10 μg of cultured cell protein was suspended in an appropriate volume of Laemmli sample buffer with 5% 2-mercaptoethanol, and subjected to 10% SDS-PAGE. The gel was then electrotransferred overnight onto nitrocellulose (Bio-Rad) and nonspecific protein binding sites blocked with 3% powdered low-fat milk. The blot was then incubated overnight with 1 μg/ml of the anti-TF polyclonal antibody described above, treated with a 1:2000 dilution of goat-anti-rabbit IgG conjugated to alkaline phosphatase (Bio-Rad) and developed for 10–20 min with BCIP/NBT according to the manufacturer's specifications (Bio-Rad).

Immunopurified PAI-1 standards (American Diagnostica) or unconcentrated conditioned medium from 6-day stromal cell cultures in DM were subjected to 10% SDS-PAGE under reducing conditions, electrotransferred overnight onto nitrocellulose (Bio-Rad), blocked and incubated with anti-PAI-1 monoclonal antibody (1:500) (American Diagnostica). The filters were then washed, treated with goat-anti-mouse antibody (1:500) (Sigma) for 90 min, exposed to [$^{125}$I]-protein A

(200,000 cpm/ml) for 30 min (New England Nuclear), then washed and autoradiographed for one week.

### Northern Analyses of Tissue Factor and PAI-1 mRNA

Approximately 15 μg of RNA extracted from each culture with RNAzol-B (Cinna Biotecx Labs), as well as ethidium bromide stained RNA standards were separated on a 1% agarose gel containing 2.2 M formaldehyde and transferred to a Zeta Probe membrane (Bio-Rad). Levels of TF mRNA were detected using a TF probe consisting of a 1.2-kb Hind III/Sma I fragment corresponding to base pairs 148–1354 of TF cDNA, isolated from the plasmid, pLB4TF.[12] Levels of PAI-1 mRNA were detected using a 5.2-kb PAI-1 insert derived from a 7.9-kb plasmid obtained from ATCC (Rockville, MD). All plasmids were grown and purified using a CIRCLEPREP Kit (Bio 101 Inc., La Jolla, CA). Probes/inserts were labeled with $^{32}$P-dCTP to high specific activity by random priming.[39] Hybridization was performed by standard methods[39] and the washed filters exposed to Kodak XAR film and hybridization signals quantitated by densitometric scanning.

Probes were then stripped from the filters by soaking in a solution composed of 5 mM (pH 8.0), 0.2 mM EDTA, 0.05% sodium pyrophosphate, 0.02% polyvinylpyrolidone, 0.02% BSA, and 0.02% Ficoll at 70°C for 30–60 min. Removal of probe was confirmed by X-ray autoradiography before filters were reused. Additional

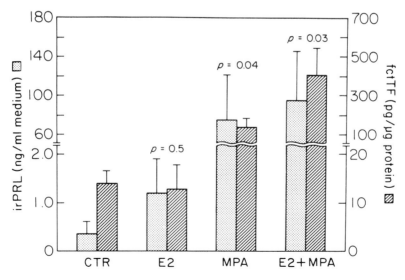

**FIGURE 3.** Concordant expression of endometrial stromal cell tissue factor activity and prolactin in response to progestin treatment. Confluent stromal cell cultures were incubated in media with either vehicle control, $10^{-8}$ M E2, $10^{-6}$ M MPA, or E2 + MPA for 20 days. Data are derived from 5 experiments and expressed as the mean ± SEM for cell-associated functionally active tissue factor (fctTF) in pg/μg of culture protein (*hatched bars*) and the mean ± SEM for immunoreactive prolactin (irPRL) released into the medium and expressed in ng/ml of medium (*stippled bars*) (p values for comparison with controls).

**TABLE 1.** Expression of Immunoreactive (ir) and Functionally Active (fct) Tissue Factor (TF) by Endometrial Stromal Cells Cultured in Serum-Containing Medium with Vehicle Control (Ctr), $10^{-8}$ M Estradiol (E2), $10^{-6}$ M Medroxyprogesterone Acetate (MPA) or E2 + MPA[a]

| Days in Culture | Mean/(SEM); pmoles TF/mg Culture Protein | | | | | |
|---|---|---|---|---|---|---|
| | Ctr | E2 | MPA | $p^b$ | E2 + MPA | $p^c$ |
| 2–4 days | | | | | | |
| irTF | 3.80 | 5.07 | 6.24 | NS | 5.90 | NS |
| | (1.27) | (1.90) | (2.18) | | (1.76) | |
| fctTF | 3.29 | 3.84 | 4.84 | NS | 4.76 | NS |
| | (0.94) | (1.00) | (1.17) | | (1.17) | |
| 8–12 days | | | | | | |
| irTF | 1.29 | 1.42 | 9.10 | 0.02 | 18.95 | 0.02 |
| | (0.57) | (0.50) | (2.68) | | (5.96) | |
| fctTF | 1.22 | 1.29 | 8.17 | 0.001 | 15.48 | 0.0005 |
| | (0.28) | (0.32) | (2.78) | | (3.33) | |
| 20–24 days | | | | | | |
| irTF | 0.84 | 1.00 | 6.15 | 0.04 | 25.31 | 0.02 |
| | (0.28) | (0.22) | (3.20) | | (15.76) | |
| fctTF | 1.79 | 0.94 | 5.83 | 0.1 | 16.78 | 0.09 |
| | (1.00) | (0.52) | (2.55) | | (6.92) | |

[a] Confluent endometrial stromal cells were incubated in a basal medium containing 10% SCS plus either vehicle control, $10^{-8}$ M E2, $10^{-6}$ M MPA, or E2 + MPA for 2–24 days (see Methods). Each result represents an average of 4–8 cultures derived from separate patient specimens. Levels of immunoreactive and functionally active TF are normalized to stromal cell protein.
[b] Comparison of cultures exposed to vehicle control vs MPA.
[c] Comparison of cultures exposed to vehicle control vs E2 + MPA.

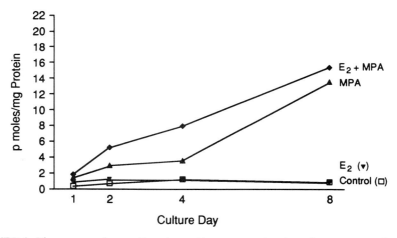

**FIGURE 4.** Time course of progestin-enhanced immunoreactive tissue factor content. Stromal cells were cultured in a serum-free defined medium with either vehicle control; $10^{-8}$ M E2; $10^{-6}$ M MPA; and E2 + MPA (each data point represents the average of 2 specimens; tissue factor levels expressed in pM/mg culture protein). Similar results were obtained for tissue factor activity.

TABLE 2. Release of PAI-1 by Endometrial Stromal Cells Cultured in a Serum-Free Defined Medium with Vehicle Control (Ctr), $10^{-8}$ M Estradiol (E2), $10^{-6}$ M Medroxyprogesterone Acetate (MPA) or E2 + MPA[a]

| Days in Culture | Mean/(SEM); ng PAI-1/$\mu$g Culture Protein | | | | | |
|---|---|---|---|---|---|---|
| | Ctr | E2 | MPA | $p^b$ | E2 + MPA | $p^c$ |
| 3 | 0.68 (0.10) | 0.78 (0.08) | 4.0 (0.7) | 0.03 | 8.46 (1.98) | 0.02 |
| 6 | 0.47 (0.08) | 0.33 (0.10) | 14.65 (6.78) | 0.01 | 34.79 (14.03) | 0.01 |

[a] Confluent endometrial stromal cells were incubated in a DM containing either vehicle control, $10^{-8}$ M E2, $10^{-6}$ M MPA, or E2 + MPA for 3 or 6 days (see Methods). Levels of immunoreactive PAI-1 in the conditioned medium were normalized to stromal cell protein.
[b] Comparison of cultures exposed to vehicle control vs MPA.
[c] Comparison of cultures exposed to vehicle control vs E2 + MPA.

sequential hybridizations were then carried out with the labeled PAI-1 insert and a cloned cDNA probe for cyclophilin.[40]

## RESULTS

To evaluate whether TF and PAI-1 were indicators of the state of endometrial hemostatic, proteolytic and fibrinolytic potential across the menstrual cycle and in pregnancy we: 1) determined the distinct cell types expressing TF and PAI-1 by immunohistochemical examination of human cycling and gestational endometrium; and 2) evaluated the hormonal regulation of TF and PAI-1 in primary cultures of isolated endometrial stromal and decidual cells.

### Immunohistochemical Localization of Tissue Factor and PAI-1

Immunohistochemical examination of endometrial specimens from multiple proliferative, and early to late secretory phases of the menstrual cycle and uterine curettings from first trimester terminations, revealed that TF and PAI-1 expression correlated with stromal cell decidualization (FIG. 1). While minimal staining for TF was noted in stromal cells from proliferative and early secretory phase endometrium, prominent staining for TF was observed in decidualized stromal cells from late secretory phase tissues (FIG. 1a). Staining for TF was most intense in decidual cells from gestational endometrium.[37] Detectable immunostaining for PAI-1 was present in the stromal cells of secretory phase specimens but pronounced staining was present only in the decidual cells of gestational endometrium (FIG. 1b). As expected, controls performed with nonimmune serum or antibody preadsorbed with excess TF and PAI-1 failed to stain.

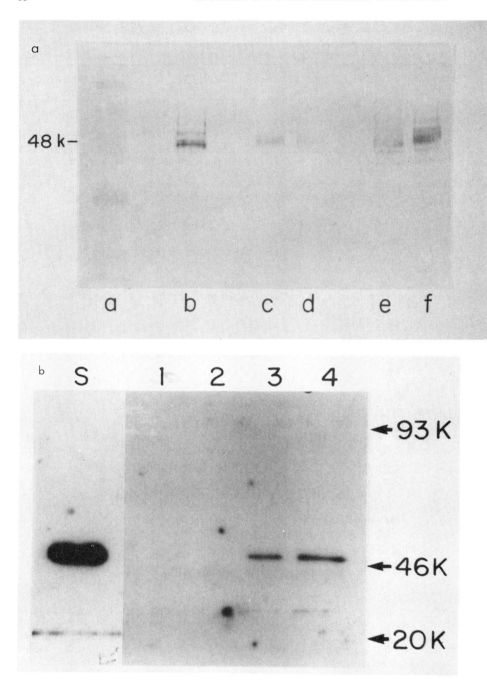

## Tissue Factor and PAI-1 Expression in Stromal Cell Cultures

*Dose Response and Time Course of Tissue Factor Protein Expression*

Given these immunohistochemical results we sought to determine whether there was an enhancement of TF expression during *in vitro* decidualization of endometrial stromal cells.[41] Thus, confluent stromal cell cultures in BM with 10% SCS or DM were exposed to either vehicle control (0.1% ethanol), $10^{-8}$ M estradiol (E2), $10^{-8}$ to $10^{-6}$ M medroxyprogesterone acetate (MPA), or E2 + MPA. The medium was replenished every 2–4 days with the appropriate control or steroid-supplemented media. FIGURE 2, which presents stromal cell TF content following 20 days of culture in BM + 10% SCS, indicates that despite a lack of response to E2 relative to control cultures, addition of MPA significantly elevated the content of both irTF and fctTF (about 10-fold), and that the addition of E2 + MPA further increased in the content of irTF and fctTF (20 to 30-fold). Comparable progestin effects on stromal cell TF expression were observed at concentrations of $10^{-7}$ and $10^{-8}$ M MPA ± E2.[42] FIGURE 3 demonstrates that the progestin-elevated expression of TF paralleled enhanced secretion of irPRL, confirming that increased TF expression accompanies decidualization.

Time course studies demonstrated that maximal TF expression was achieved following 10 days' exposure to E2 + MPA in serum-containing medium and that TF expression continued to increase through 20 to 24 days of culture (TABLE 1). Interestingly, during exposure to progestin alone TF expression peaked at 10 days, declining thereafter. This observation is consistent with downregulation of progesterone receptor levels in response to progestin exposure in the absence of E2. FIGURE 4 presents the time course of a typical experiment in serum-free DM. Note a similar pattern of steroid responsiveness, although progestin-induction of TF expression occurs earlier in DM.

*Dose Response and Time Course Studies of PAI-1 Protein Expression*

TABLE 2 compares the effects of $10^{-8}$ M E2, $10^{-6}$ M MPA and E2 + MPA on levels of PAI-1 measured by ELISA in the conditioned medium of stromal cells derived from 5 specimens.[43] After 3 days of treatment, E2 had no effect, whereas MPA significantly enhanced and E2 + MPA synergistically enhanced levels of PAI-1 compared with control cultures. Moreover, in the subsequent 3 days of

---

**FIGURE 5.** Immunoblot of tissue factor present in endometrial stromal cell protein and PAI-1 released into the medium. Standard and samples were loaded under reducing conditions and resolved by SDS-10% PAGE. **(a)** Tissue factor (TF) immunoblot: *lane a*, molecular weight standards (240.6, 117.3, 75.5, 48.0, 28.2, and 19.4 kDa); *lane b*, 2.5 ng human brain tissue factor prepared as described in Methods; *lane c–f*, immunoreactive TF present in 10 μg of cell protein derived from a stromal cell culture exposed to: vehicle control (c); $10^{-8}$ M estradiol (E2) (d); $10^{-6}$ M medroxyprogesterone acetate (MPA) (e); or both E2 + MPA (f). **(b)** PAI-1 immunoblot: *lanes 1–4* contain 28 μl of conditioned medium from 3–6 day confluent stromal cell cultures derived from a single specimen and exposed for 6 days to either: vehicle control (1); $10^{-8}$ M E2 (2); $10^{-8}$ M E2 + $10^{-7}$ M MPA (3); $10^{-8}$ M E2 + $10^{-6}$ M MPA (4); with *lane S* = PAI-1 standard (American Diagnostica), electrophoresed separately. (FIG. 5b from Schatz & Lockwood.[43] Reprinted by permission from the *Journal of Clinical Endocrinology and Metabolism*.)

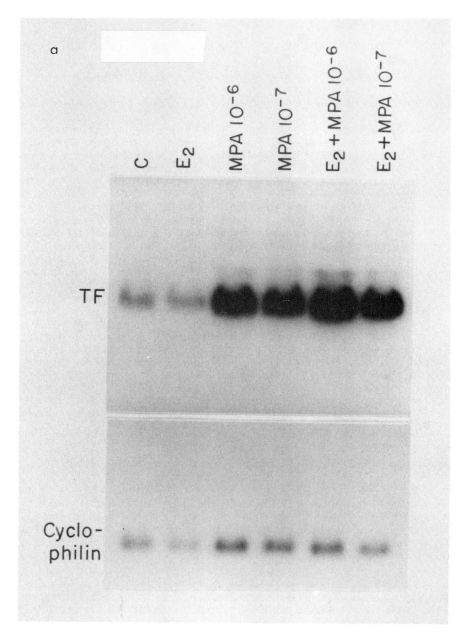

**FIGURE 6.** Northern blots of tissue factor and PAI-1 mRNA levels in confluent endometrial stromal cell cultures derived from a proliferative phase specimen maintained for 8 days in a defined medium with or without steroids. **(a)** Tissue factor Northern blot: vehicle control (C); $10^{-8}$ M E2; $10^{-7}$ or $10^{-6}$ M MPA; or E2 + MPA. (From Lockwood et al.[42] Reprinted by permission from the *Journal of Clinical Endocrinology and Metabolism*.) **(b)** PAI-1 Northern blot: vehicle control (C); $10^{-8}$ M E2; $10^{-7}$ or $10^{-6}$ M MPA; or E2 + MPA. (From Schatz & Lockwood.[43] Reprinted by permission from *Journal of Clinical Endocrinology and Metabolism*.)

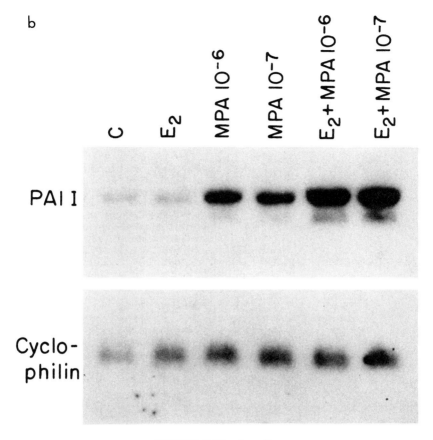

**FIGURE 6** (*Continued*).

culture, despite a significant absolute reduction in the PAI-1 content of the control and E2 exposed cultures ($p < 0.03$ and $0.0003$, respectively), MPA and E2 + MPA produced a substantial further increase in PAI-1 content relative to controls. Additional experiments indicated that concentrations of MPA as low as $10^{-8}$ M MPA with or without $10^{-8}$ M E2 enhanced PAI-1 content 10-fold and 50-fold, respectively, in 6-day cultures derived from 2 specimens.[43] In contrast to the results for PAI-1, negligible quantities of PAI-2 were detected in the conditioned medium and no hormonal effect on PAI-2 release was observed.[43]

*Immunoblot Analysis of Stromal Cell Tissue Factor and PAI-1*

Western blot analyses (FIG. 5) were performed to determine whether the immunoreactive species of TF and PAI-1 measured in stromal cell cultures conformed

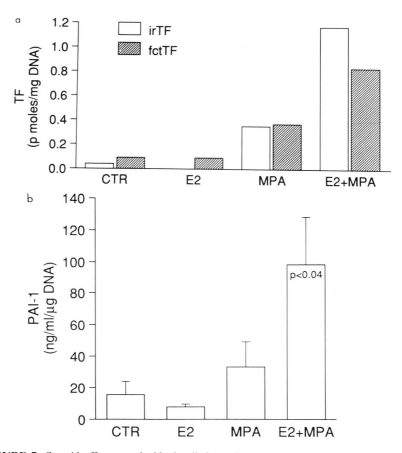

**FIGURE 7.** Steroid effects on decidual cell tissue factor and PAI-1 expression *in vivo*. (a) Representative results for tissue factor content of decidual cells derived from a first trimester endometrium and cultured on collagen I gels in BM + 2% SCS as described in Methods. Cultures were treated with either vehicle control, $10^{-8}$ M E2, $10^{-6}$ M MPA, or E2 + MPA for 5 days. The immunoreactive (ir) and functionally active (fct) TF content is normalized to culture DNA. (b) PAI-1 content in the media of decidual cell cultures treated with either vehicle control, $10^{-8}$ M E2, $10^{-6}$ M MPA, or E2 + MPA for 5 days as described in Methods. Levels of PAI-1 are expressed in ng/ml of medium/$\mu$g culture DNA (mean of 5 separate patient specimens). * = $p < 0.04$ for comparison with control values.

to the electrophoretic mobility of previously characterized human TF[44] and PAI-1.[27] The TF (FIG. 5a) and PAI-1 (FIG. 5b) moieties present in the cultured stromal cells and conditioned medium, respectively, were found to conform to the anticipated MWs of 46–48,000 and 50,000, respectively. Furthermore, the relative intensity of staining for TF and PAI-1 in response to steroids was consistent with the ELISA results (TABLES 1 and 2).

## Northern Analyses of TF and PAI-1 mRNA

Northern analyses were carried out in primary endometrial stromal cell cultures maintained for 6 days in DM with vehicle control, 10 nM E2, $10^{-8}$ M to $10^{-6}$ M MPA or both E2 + MPA. In the control incubations, the size of both the TF (FIG. 6a) and PAI-1 (FIG. 6b) mRNA were 2.5 kb, and 3.2/2.3 kB, respectively, which is consistent with prior reports.[36,45] The steady state levels of mRNA for both endpoints displayed a similar pattern of response to the added steroids. Thus, in contrast to the lack of response to E2 alone, $10^{-7}$ and $10^{-6}$ M MPA increased TF mRNA levels 4- and 5-fold, respectively (FIG. 6a) and PAI-1 mRNA levels 3- and 4-fold, respectively (FIG. 6b); while the combination of E2 + $10^{-7}$ and $10^{-6}$ M MPA caused a synergistic 6- and 7-fold increase, respectively, in both TF and PAI-1 mRNA levels.

## Expression of Tissue Factor and PAI-1 in Decidual Cell Cultures

Decidual cells cultured in collagen I gels were exposed to either vehicle control, E2, MPA, or E2 + MPA. After 5 days of the experimental incubations, the medium was collected and analyzed for PAI-1 while the decidual cells were harvested and analyzed for TF and DNA content. FIGURE 7a, which displays the effects of steroid hormone exposure on decidual TF expression for a representative experiment, indicates that decidual cells retain their responsiveness to progestins and that the combination of E2 + MPA maximizes TF expression FIG. 7b shows the analogous effects of steroid hormones on the PAI-1 content of the decidual cell medium.

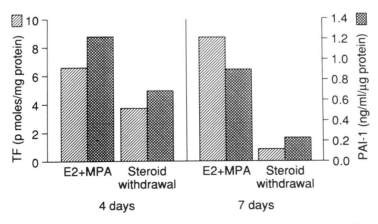

**FIGURE 8.** Steroid withdrawal effects on stromal cell immunoreactive tissue factor (ir) content and medium levels of PAI-1. Confluent stromal cell cultures from a secretory phase specimen were incubated for 10 days with $10^{-8}$ M E2 + $10^{-7}$ M MPA, then washed and exposed to either the steroids (E2 + MPA) or basal media without steroids (steroid withdrawal) for 4 and 7 days. Similar results were obtained from two additional experiments in cultures derived from patients with proliferative phase specimens.

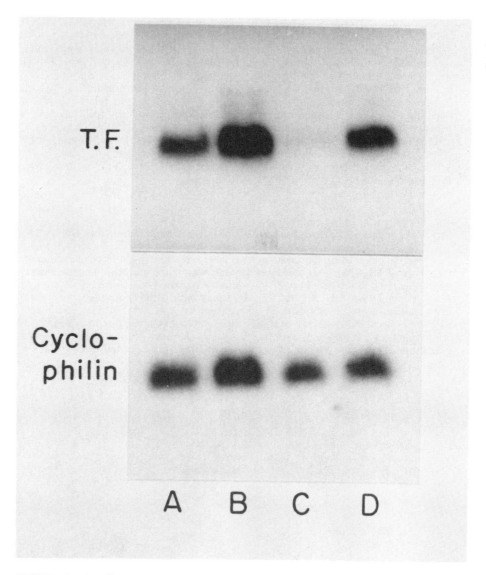

**FIGURE 9.** The effects of steroid withdrawal on stromal cell tissue factor mRNA content. Parallel cultures, derived from the endometrial specimen described in FIGURE 8, were utilized for Northern analysis of tissue factor and PAI-1 mRNA. *Lane A* = culture in which steroids have been withdrawn for 4 days; *lane B* = parallel culture maintained with $10^{-8}$ M E2 + $10^{-7}$ M MPA for the additional 4 days; *lane C* = culture in which steroids have been withdrawn for 7 days; and *lane D* = parallel culture maintained with $10^{-8}$ E2 + $10^{-7}$ M MPA for the additional 7 days. (From Lockwood *et al.*[42] Reprinted by permission from the *Journal of Clinical Endocrinology and Metabolism*.)

## Effects of Progestin Withdrawal on Tissue Factor and PAI-1 Content

Following exposure to $10^{-7}$ M MPA + $10^{-8}$ M E2 for 10 days, confluent stromal cell cultures were divided into a control group maintained in E2 + MPA and an experimental group in which the steroids were withdrawn by exchanging the conditioned media with control BM + 10% SCS. As can be seen from FIG. 8, steroid withdrawal reduced levels of cell-associated irTF as well as PAI-1 released into the medium. Similar results were obtained for fctTF. Northern analysis of similarly treated cultures demonstrated parallel reductions in TF mRNA levels in response to steroidal withdrawal (FIG. 9).

## DISCUSSION

These results indicate that a marked increase in endometrial stromal cell TF and PAI-1 expression accompanies decidualization both *in vivo* and *in vitro*.

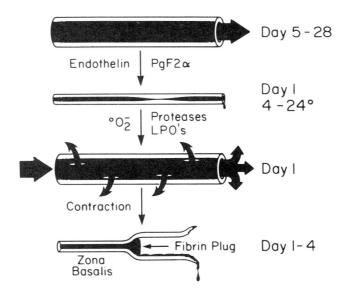

**FIGURE 10.** Schematic depiction of vascular events leading to menstruation. During the initial 5–28 days of the typical menstrual cycle blood flow through those portions of the spiral arteries traversing the hormonally responsive layers of the endometrium is unimpeded (*top figure*). On day one of the cycle these vessels undergo intense vasoconstriction presumably mediated by decidual-derived endothelin and glandular-derived $PgF_{2alpha}$ (*second figure*). The resultant ischemia causes the production of free radicals, lipid peroxides (LPOs) and destabilizes lysozomes in perivascular cells causing protease release damaging vessels to promote hemorrhage (*third figure*). Concomitant reductions in perivascular decidual hemostatic, antiproteolytic and antifibrinolytic proteins potentiate this process leading to extensive hemorrhage and proteolysis, eventual sloughing of the hormonally-responsive portions of the endometrium. Hemostasis is restored by the formation of fibrin clots in the basal aspects of the vessels present in the hormonally unresponsive aspects of the endometrium which presumably retain their full hemostatic potential (*lowest figure*).

The presence of these important regulators of hemostasis in decidualized human stromal cells and decidual cells isolated from gestational endometrium suggests a mechanism to explain the absence of hemorrhage during invasion of the endometrial vasculature by trophoblasts. Decidual cell-derived TF and PAI-1 could also promote the accumulation of fibrin at such trophoblast-decidual interfaces as Nitabuch's layer and the tunica media of trophoblast-transformed spiral arteries.[2]

Conversely, during menstruation, vascular injury is reported to result from ischemia induced by spiral artery vasoconstriction[3,46] (FIG. 10). Interestingly, two potent vasoconstrictors, decidual-derived endothelin[47] and endometrial glandular-derived PgF2-alpha[48] are released in response to progesterone withdrawal.[3,47] Our current observation that progestin withdrawal also results in a profound time-dependent decline in decidualized stromal cell TF and PAI-1 expression suggests a mechanism for the expected reduction in decidual hemostatic potential and enhanced decidual fibrinolytic and proteolytic capacity during menstruation. The latter is supported by the finding of marked fibrinolytic activity in menstrual effluent.[49] Thus, based on our studies, declining progesterone levels at the end of the luteal phase should produce the two requisites for menstrual "hemorrhage," vascular injury and inadequate hemostasis.

This endometrial stromal cell culture model may also prove valuable for investigating the pathophysiologic mechanisms underlying abnormal uterine bleeding. In pregnancy, decidual hemorrhage associated with spontaneous abortion, stillbirth and preterm delivery[50] may reflect abnormalities of decidual TF and PAI-1 expression due to reduced progesterone production or inhibition of progestational effects. Abnormal uterine bleeding accompanying anovulatory cycles is clearly associated with hyperestrogenic-hypoprogestational states which, our model suggests, result in reduced stromal cell TF and PAI-1 content and vascular instability. Finally, breakthrough bleeding, a leading cause for the discontinuation of progesterone-only contraceptives,[5] could result from inadequate E2 stimulation and/or progestin-induced downregulation of stromal cell progesterone receptors,[51] leading to reduced TF and PAI-1 expression and increased expression of vasoactive agents. Therefore, our model should prove useful in studying the effects of aberrant hormonal states and pharmacological manipulations on endometrial hemostatic potential.

## SUMMARY

The physiologic mechanisms whereby the human endometrium maintains hemostasis during endovascular trophoblast invasion, yet permits menstrual hemorrhage, are unknown. This paradoxical relationship was investigated by evaluating endometrial expression of tissue factor (TF), the primary initiator of hemostasis, and plasminogen activator inhibitor-1 (PAI-1), the primary inhibitor of fibrinolysis. We observed increased immunostaining for TF and PAI-1 in sections of decidualized stromal cells from luteal phase and gestational endometrium. To determine whether TF and PAI-1 expression are directly linked to decidualization, both endpoints were monitored in a well described *in vitro* model of decidualization. Thus, confluent stromal cell cultures were exposed to vehicle control, $10^{-8}$ M estradiol (E2), $10^{-8}$ to $10^{-6}$ M medroxyprogesterone acetate (MPA) or both E2 + MPA for 2–24 days in serum-containing or defined media. The progestin enhanced the content of stromal cell-associated immunoreactive and functionally active TF and PAI-1 released into the medium and elevated levels of stromal cell TF and PAI-1 mRNA. While E2 alone was ineffective, it greatly augmented MPA-enhanced TF and PAI-1 protein and mRNA content. Dose-dependent effects on TF and PAI-1 content were observed between $10^{-8}$ to $10^{-6}$ M MPA ± E2. Similar results were observed for decidual cells derived from first trimester endometrium and cultured in type 1 collagen gels. Following optimal induction of TF and PAI-1 expression by E2 + MPA in stromal cell cultures, removal of these steroids greatly reduced levels of both TF and PAI-1 protein and mRNA within 4 days. These studies suggest a mechanism whereby endometrial hemostasis is maintained during trophoblast invasion yet reduced at the end of nonfertile cycles to permit menses.

## REFERENCES

1. MOORE, K. L. 1988. The Developing Human. 4th edit. 40. W. B. Saunders Company. Philadelphia.
2. DE WOLF, F., C. DE WOLF-PEETERS & I. BROSENS. 1973. Ultrastructure of the spiral arteries in the human placental bed at the end of normal pregnancy. Am. J. Obstet. Gynecol. **117:** 833–848.
3. SMITH, S. K. 1990. The physiology of menstruation. In Contraception and Mechanisms of Endometrial Bleeding. C. D'Arcangues, I. S. Fraser, J. R. Newton & V. Odlind, Eds. 41. Cambridge University Press. Cambridge.
4. BURNETT, L. S. 1988. Gynecological history, examination and operation. In Novak's Textbook of Gynecology. 11th edit. H. W. Jones, A. C. Wentz & L. S. Burnett, Eds. 29. Williams and Wilkins. Baltimore.
5. ODLIND, V. & I. S. FRASER. 1990. Contraception and menstrual bleeding disturbances: a clinical overview. In Contraception and Mechanisms of Endometrial Bleeding. C. D'Arcangues, I. S. Fraser, J. R. Newton & V. Odlind, Eds. 5–32. Cambridge University Press. Cambridge.
6. NOYES, R. W., A. T. HERTIG & J. ROCK. 1950. Dating the endometrial biopsy. Fertil. Steril. **1:** 3–25.
7. BELL, S. C. 1990. Decidualization and relevance to menstruation. In Contraception and Mechanisms of Endometrial Bleeding. C. D'Arcangues, I. S. Fraser, J. R. Newton & V. Odlind, Eds. 188. Cambridge University Press. Cambridge.
8. RAMSEY, E. M., M. L. HOUSTON & J. W. HARRIS. 1976. Interactions of the trophoblast and maternal tissues in three closely related primate species. Am. J. Obstet. Gynecol. **124:** 647–652.
9. FINN, C. A. 1987. Why do women and some other primates menstruate? Perspect. Biol. Med. **30:** 566–574.
10. NEMERSON, Y. 1988. Tissue factor and hemostasis. Blood **71:** 1–8.
11. GUHA, A., R. BACH, W. KONIGSBERG & Y. NEMERSON. 1986. Affinity purification of human tissue factor: interaction of factor VII and tissue factor in detergent micelles. Proc. Natl. Acad. Sci. USA **83:** 299–302.
12. SPICER, E. K., R. HORTON, L. BLOEM et al. 1987. Isolation of cDNA clones coding for human tissue factor: primary structure of the protein and cDNA. Proc. Natl. Acad. Sci. USA **84:** 5148–5152.
13. CARSON, S. D., W. M. HENRY, L. HALEY, M. BYERS, & T. SHOWS. 1985. The gene for tissue factor (coagulation factor III) is localized on human chromosome 1pter–1p21, Human Gene Mapping 8. Cytogenet. Cell Genet. **40:** 600.
14. MORRISSEY, J. H., H. FAKHRAI & T. S. EDGINGTON. 1987. Molecular cloning of the cDNA for tissue factor, the cellular receptor for the initiation of the coagulation protease cascade. Cell **50:** 129.
15. SCARPATI, E. M., D. WEN, G. J. BROZE et al. 1987. Human tissue factor: cDNA sequence and chromosome localization of the gene. Biochemistry **26:** 5324.
16. HAGEN, F. S., C. L. GRAY, P. O'HARA et al. 1986. Characterization of a cDNA coding for human factor VII. Proc. Natl. Acad. Sci. USA **83:** 2412.

17. ZUR, M., R. D. RADCLIFFE, J. OBERDICK & Y. NEMERSON. 1982. The dual role of factor VII in blood coagulation. J. Biol. Chem. **257:** 5623-5631.
18. BACH, R. 1988. Initiation of coagulation by tissue factor. CRC Crit. Rev. Biochem. **23:** 339-368.
19. DANO, K., P. A. ANDERSEN, J. GRONDAHL-HANSEN et al. 1985. Plasminogen activators, tissue degradation and cancer. Adv. Cancer Res. **44:** 139.
20. QUIGLEY, J. P., L. I. GOLD, R. SCHWIMMER & L. SULLIVAN. 1987. Limited cleavage of cellular fibronectin by plasminogen activator purified from transformed cells. Proc. Natl. Acad. Sci. USA **84:** 2776-2780.
21. LAIHO, M., O. SAKSELA & J. KESKI-OJA. 1987. Transforming growth factor-beta induction of type-1 plasminogen activator inhibitor. Pericellular deposition and sensitivity to exogenous urokinase. J. Biol. Chem. **262:** 17467-17474.
22. LACK, C. H. & H. J. ROGERS. 1958. Action of plasmin on cartilage. Nature **182:** 948.
23. MULLIN, D. E. & S. T. RORLICH. 1983. The role of proteinases in cellular invasiveness. Biochim. Biophys. Acta **695:** 177-214.
24. O'GRADY, R. L., L. I. UPFOLD & R. W. STEPHENS. 1981. Rat mammary carcinoma cells secrete active collagenase and active latent enzymes in the stroma via plasminogen activator. Int. J. Cancer **28:** 509-515.
25. TRYGGVASON, K., M. HOYHTYA & T. SALO. 1987. Proteolytic degradation of extracellular matrix in tumor invasion. Biochim. Biophys. Acta **907:** 191-217.
26. WERB, A., C. L. MAIARDI, C. A. VATER & E. D. HARRIS, JR. 1977. Endogenous activation of latent collagenases by rheumatoid synovial cells: evidence for a role of plasminogen activator. N. Engl. J. Med. **296:** 1017.
27. LOSKUTOFF, D. J., M. SAWDEY & J. MIMURO. 1989. Type 1 plasminogen activator. Prog. Hemostasis Thromb. **9:** 87-115.
28. GINSBURG, D., R. ZEHEB, A. Y. YANG et al. 1986. cDNA cloning of human plasminogen activator-inhibitor from endothelial cells. J. Clin. Invest. **78:** 1673-1680.
29. LOSKUTOFF, D. J., M. LINDERS, J. KEIJER, H. VEERMAN, H. VAN HEERIKHUIZEN & H. PANNEKOEK. 1987. Structure of the human plasminogen activator inhibitor 1 gene: nonrandom distribution of introns. Biochemistry **26:** 3763-3768.
30. SALONEN, E., M. A. VAHERI, J. POLLANEN et al. 1989. Interaction of plasminogen activator inhibitor (PAI-1) with vitronectin. J. Biol. Chem. **264:** 6339-6343.
31. SATYASWAROOP, P., R. E. BRESSLER, M. M. DE LA PENA & E. GURPIDE. 1979. Isolation and culture of human endometrial glands. J. Clin. Endocrinol. Metab. **38:** 639-641.
32. SCHATZ, F., R. E. GORDON, N. LAUFER & E. GURPIDE. 1990. Culture of human endometrial cells under polarizing conditions. Differentiation **42:** 184-190.
33. BRAVERMAN, M. B., A. BAGNI, D. DE ZIEGLER, T. DEN & E. GURPIDE. 1984. Isolation of prolactin producing cells from first and second trimester decidua. J. Clin. Endocrinol. Metab. **58:** 521.
34. ECKERT, R. L. & B. S. KATZENELLENBOGEN. 1981. Human endometrial cells in primary tissue culture: modulation of the progesterone receptor level by natural and synthetic estrogens *in vitro*. J. Clin. Endocrinol. Metab. **52:** 699-708.
35. SCHATZ, F., V. HAUSKNECHT, R. E. GORDON, D. HELLER, L. MARKIEWICZ, L. DELIGDISCH & E. GURPIDE. 1991. Studies on human endometrial cells in primary culture. Ann. N.Y. Acad. Sci. **622:** 80-88.
36. BLOEM, L. J., L. CHEN, W. H. KONIGSBERG & R. BACH. 1989. Serum stimulation of quiescent human fibroblasts induces the synthesis of tissue factor mRNA followed by the appearance of tissue factor antigen and procoagulant activity. J. Cell. Physiol. **139:** 418-423.
37. LOCKWOOD, C. J., Y. NEMERSON, S. GULLER et al. 1993. Progestational regulation of human endometrial stromal cell tissue factor expression during decidualization. J. Clin. Endocrinol. Metab. **76:** 231-236.
38. HINEGARDNER, R. T. 1971. An improved fluorometric assay for DNA. Annal. Biochem. **39:** 197-201.
39. SAMBROK, J., E. F. FRITSCH & T. MANIATIS. 1989. Molecular Cloning—A Laboratory Manual. 2nd edit. 10.14-10.17. Cold Spring Harbor Laboratory. Cold Spring Harbor, NY.

40. HASEL, K. W. & J. G. SUTCLIFFE. 1990. Nucleotide sequence of a cDNA encoding for mouse cyclophilin. Nucleic Acids Res. **18:** 4019.
41. GURPIDE, E., S. TABANELLI, M. T. B. BENEDETTO & F. SCHATZ. 1989. Secreted endometrial products with a possible role in implantation and maternal tolerance of the embryo. *In* Basic to Clinic. Serono Symposia. G. L. Capitano, L. DeCecco & R. H. Asch, Eds. Vol. 26: 161–174. Raven Press. New York.
42. LOCKWOOD, C. J., Y. NEMERSON, G. KRIKUN *et al.* 1993. Steroid-modulated stromal cell tissue factor expression: a model for the regulation of endometrial hemostasis and menstruation. J. Clin. Endocrinol. Metab. **77.** In press.
43. SCHATZ, F. & C. J. LOCKWOOD. 1993. Progestin regulation of plasminogen activator inhibitor type-1 in primary cultures of endometrial stromal and decidual cells. J. Clin. Endocrinol. Metab. **77:** 621–625.
44. BACH, R., W. H. KONIGSBERG & Y. NEMERSON. 1988. Human tissue factor contains thioester-linked palmitate and stearate on the cytoplasmic half-cysteine. Biochemistry **27:** 4227–4231.
45. FATTAL, P. G., D. J. SCHNEIDER, B. E. SOBEL & J. J. BILLADELLO. 1992. Posttranscriptional regulation of expression of plasminogen activator inhibitor type 1 mRNA by insulin and insulin-like growth factor 1. J. Biol. Chem. **267:** 12412–12415.
46. MARKEE, J. E. 1940. Menstruation in intraocular endometrial transplants in the rhesus monkey. Contributions to Embryology. Carnegie Institution of Washington Publication No. 518, **28**(177): 219–308.
47. ECONOMOS, K., P. C. MACDONALD & M. L. CASEY. 1992. Endothelin-1 gene expression and protein biosynthesis in human endometrium: potential modulator of endometrial blood flow. J. Clin. Endocrinol. Metab. **74:** 14–19.
48. SCHATZ, F., L. MARKIEWICZ & E. GURPIDE. 1987. Differential effects of estradiol, arachidonic acid, and A23187 on prostaglandin F2-alpha output by epithelial and stromal cells on human endometrium. Endocrinology **120:** 1465–1471.
49. LITTLEFIELD, B. A. 1991. Plasminogen activators in endometrial physiology and embryo implantation. Ann. N.Y. Acad. Sci. **622:** 167–175.
50. HARRIS, B. A., H. GORE & C. E. FLOWERS. 1985. Peripheral placental separation: a possible relationship to premature labor. Obstet. Gynecol. **66:** 774–778.
51. READ, L. D., C. E. SNIDER, J. S. MILLER, G. L. GREENE & B. S. KATZENELLENBOGEN. 1988. Ligand-modulated regulation of progesterone receptor messenger ribonucleic acid and protein in human breast cancer cell lines. Mol. Endocrinol. **2:** 263–271.

# Dysfunctional Uterine Bleeding (DUB)[a]

C. BULLETTI, C. FLAMIGNI, R. A. PREFETTO,
V. POLLI, AND E. GIACOMUCCI

*Reproductive Medicine Unit*
*Department of Obstetrics and Gynecology*
*University of Bologna*
*Via Massarenti, 13*
*40138 Bologna, Italy*

## INTRODUCTION

Metrorrhagia is a common disturbance that occurs in perimenopausal women with or without endometrial hyperplasia.[1] The abnormal uterine bleeding is mainly due to an inadequate endogenous estrogen and/or progesterone production[2] or to a disordered estrogen transport from blood into the endometrium.[3,4] The years before menopause represent the period of highest risk for endometrial hyperplasia development, which in turn may result in endometrial cancer in about ten years.[5] Endometrial hyperplasia may be part of a continuum that is ultimately manifested in the histological and biological pattern of the adenocarcinoma.[6] In premenopausal years an increase in estrogen production and/or a deficiency of progesterone plasma levels are often observed.[7] This hormonal production leads to endometrial overstimulation that may be a risk factor for endometrial cancer.

A therapeutical approach with a gonadotrophin-releasing hormone agonist (GnRHa) (Zoladex) in a depot formulation that induces a sustained and reversible hypogonadotropic hypogonadism, was tested.[8,9] Since ovarian suppression is pharmacologically induced with this drug, transdermal of 17-β-estradiol and oral progestin were also administered to obtain adequate endometrial growth and to avoid the potential risk of osteoporosis when low plasma levels of estrogens and hypogonadism are maintained over six months.[10]

## MATERIALS AND METHODS

One hundred and five premenopausal women attended the Reproductive Medicine Unit of the Department of Obstetrics and Gynecology, S. Orsola University Hospital, Bologna for a clinical study (TABLE 1) on the therapeutical association of GnRHa (Zoladex Depot) subcutaneously administered and a sequential therapy with transdermal 17-β-estradiol and oral progestin. The length of the therapy was 6 months plus 6 months of follow-up without any therapy.

Fifty-four women were enrolled in the study but 14 dropped out before the end. All patients gave informed consent; forty women completed the study. They were selected according to the following criteria: 1) age 42–49; 2) metrorrhagia with or without endometrial hyperplasia (without atypia); 3) hemoglobin <11

---

[a] This work was supported by Italian "Consiglio Nazionale delle Ricerche" Grants No. 9300660 and 9202504, and by University of Bologna (Italy) Grant No. 930212100.

TABLE 1. Study Protocol and the Period of Observation[a]

| | Study | Months of Observation Period |
|---|---|---|
| Group A | history | 0, 12 |
| | mammography | |
| | physical examination | 0, 6, 12 |
| | dual photon linear scanner | |
| | endometrial biopsy | |
| | symptoms analysis (by diary) | monthly |
| | hormonal tests | 0, 0.5, 6, 12 |
| | urinary LH peak | 0.5 |
| | blood chemistry tests | 0, 6, 12 |
| Group B | history | 0, 12 |
| | mammography | |
| | physical examination | 0, 6, 12 |
| | dual photon linear scanner | |
| | endometrial biopsy | 0, 3, 6, 9, 12 |
| | symptom analysis (by diary) | monthly |
| | hormonal tests | 0, 6, 12 |
| | blood chemistry tests | |

[a] Group A includes 20 women who received a combined therapy with GnRHa and 17-β-estradiol plus medrogestone administration. Group B includes 20 women who were not treated.

mg/100 ml (anemia was established in close association with metrorrhagia in the last 12–60 months); 4) body weight within 20% of ideal weight;[11] 5) no hormonal therapy received for the last 2 years; 6) they did not show uterine myomata at ultrasonography; 7) no smokers; 8) medical histories did not include carcinomas, hypertension, liver disease, gallbladder disease, diabetes mellitus, cardiovascular diseases, alcoholism or corticosteroid therapy; 9) no osteoporosis, as tested by dual photon computerized linear scanner of distal extremity of left radium (1/10) (Osteoden-P, source I125, A241, NIM srl, Verona, Italy). The women underwent physical examination, electrocardiography, mammography, endometrial biopsy and routine blood and urine chemistry tests, including those to determine the LH surge (Clearplan, Farmades S.p.A. Rome) (TABLE 1). Symptoms and clinical signs were recorded by patients in a diary. Twenty women were considered for the study (group A) and the other 20 were included as controls (group B). The study protocol, for both Groups A and B, during the 12 months of observation period is summarized in TABLE 2. Patients in groups A and B were similar according to criteria based on histologial diagnosis of the endometrium. Endometrial samples

TABLE 2. Study Protocol

| Group | No. Pts. | Treatment |
|---|---|---|
| A | 20 | day 1<br>  GnRHa injection (goserelin, Zoladex) 3.6 mg depot<br>day 15 (day 1 of sequential therapy)<br>  transdermal 17-β-estradiol 50 + 50 μgr/wk (days 1–21)<br>  medrogestone 5 mg/day (days 10–21) |
| B | 20 | no therapy |

were obtained by curettage or under hysteroscopic control at baseline (7th to 8th day of cycle), at LH peak, after 6 months of steroid replacement therapy (7th to 8th day of transdermal 17-$\beta$-estradiol administration), after the beginning of oral progestin administration, and after 12 months, 3 months after the end of treatment. All tissue samples were processed both for routine hematoxylin and eosin (H & E)-stained sections,[12] while endometrial hyperplasia was evaluated using the criteria of DiSaia and Creasman.[13] Immunostaining for laminin was performed on paraffin sections of all specimens as described by Barsky et al.[18] Paraffin sections were attached to slides by 2 components epoxy glue, deparaffinized in xylol, and rehydrated in graded alcohols and distilled water. Monoclonal rabbit antiserum, anti-laminin, was obtained from Furthmayr (Yale University, New Haven, CT); a dilution of 1:500 of this antiserum was used. Laminin was used to establish an adequate differentiation of human endometrium.[3,15,16]

Since the distribution of progesterone of both study groups (A and B) showed a shewness significantly $>0$, and zero values were present in these data, the logarithm of progesterone (log 10 progesterone) was applied. The transformed data and other data of both study groups were normally distributed as assessed by the Kolmogorov-Smirnov test.[17] Statistical analysis was performed by using multivariate (MANOVA) analysis of variance for all factors considered.[18]

## RESULTS

Both study groups (A and B) had similar baseline values. Fifteen days after the first GnRHa injection in Group A there was a reduction in the levels of LH ($p < 0.001$), FSH ($p < 0.001$) and estradiol ($p < 0.001$) with respect to baseline, but no significant change in progesterone ($p$ NS). In Group B there was an increase in LH ($p < 0.001$), FSH ($p < 0.001$), estradiol ($p < 0.001$), and progesterone ($p < 0.001$) (FIG. 1).

After 180 days there was a further significant drop in LH values ($p < 0.001$) in the treated group (A); FSH levels were lower than basal values ($p < 0.001$) but significantly higher than 15 day levels ($p < 0.01$) (FIG. 1). Estradiol levels had increased with respect to baseline and 15 day values following hormone replacement therapy ($p < 0.001$); progesterone levels were similar to baseline ($p$ NS) (FIG. 1). In Group B, LH and FSH values were those of a late proliferative phase and were significantly elevated with respect to baseline ($p < 0.001$). Estradiol and progesterone levels were significantly higher than baseline ($p < 0.001$) but unchanged with respect to the 15-day values ($p$ NS) (FIG. 1).

Three months after the end of treatment, 360 days from the start of the study, LH and FSH values in Group A had increased ($p < 0.05$) to return to levels not significantly different from those observed prior to treatment; estradiol and progesterone had increased ($p < 0.001$) (FIG. 1). In Group B, LH values were the same as those at 180 days but significantly higher than baseline ($p < 0.001$); FSH levels had decreased since 180 days ($p < 0.005$) but were higher than baseline ($p < 0.001$) (FIG. 1).

Hemoglobin levels at 180 days and 360 days (i.e., 6 months after the end of treatment) were much higher than baseline in Group A ($p < 0.001$), whereas values had dropped in a time-dependent fashion (360 versus 180, $p < 0.001$) at 180 days and after suspension ($p < 0.001$) (FIG. 2).

There was a significant difference between 180 days and baseline for bleeding, metrorrhagia and vasomotor symptoms in Group A ($p < 0.001$), but not in Group

B ($p$ NS) (TABLE 3). Comparing values at baseline and 360 days, there was a highly significant difference for bleeding, metrorrhagia and vasomotor symptoms in Group A ($p < 0.001$), but not in Group B ($p$ NS) except for hot flashes which had increased after a year ($p < 0.05$) (TABLE 3).

Comparing 180-day and 360-day values, there was no difference in vaginal bleeding, metrorrhagia and vasomotor symptoms in Group A ($p$ NS) (TABLE 3). Bleeding and metrorrhagia had not changed in Group B ($p$ NS), while vasomotor symptoms changed from 180 to 360 days ($p < 0.05$) (TABLE 3).

The immunohistochemical reaction for laminin was negative for both groups at baseline, whereas Group A showed a 95% positivity at 180 days and 50% at 360 days ($p < 0.001$ with respect to baseline) (TABLE 4). There were no positive reactions in Group B (TABLE 4). Significance of comparison with immunoreaction for laminin to baseline in both groups was $p < 0.001$ at 180 days, $p < 0.002$ at 360 days; significance of comparison with immunoreaction for laminin between 180 and 360 days was $p < 0.003$.

Both groups had the same histological diagnosis at baseline ($p$ NS) (TABLE 5). At 180 days endometrial decidualization was 95% in Group A, adenomatous hyperplasia persisting in only one case ($p < 0.001$) (TABLE 5). At the same time abnormal endometrial hyperproliferation had worsened in Group B: one case went from persistent proliferative to simple glandular hyperplasia (SGH) (total SGH at 180 days, $14 = 70\%$) and another 2 cases developed into adenomatous hyperplasia (AH) (total AH at 180 days, $4 = 20\%$) ($p$ NS) (TABLE 5).

At 360 days, one woman in Group A had AH (5%), 10 had decidualized endometrium (50%) and 9 had proliferative endometrium (45%). In Group B there were 9 cases of SGH (45%) and 11 cases of AH (55%) at 360 days with a marked deterioration in all cases (TABLE 5). Comparison at baseline and at 180 days between Groups A and B showed a significance of $p < 0.001$ for histological diagnosis, as did the comparison between 360 days and baseline, whereas the intergroup comparison at 180 and 360 days was not significant ($p$ NS) (TABLE 5).

## DISCUSSION

One of the most difficult questions for physicians consulted by premenopausal women with metrorrhagia without uterine myomata is how to treat these women. Curettage and/or hysterectomy are often used to stop metrorrhagia and/or to remove endometrial hyperstimulation. The use of progestins has also been proposed for the same purpose.[19] There is no consensus on the elective therapy to be used in these patients,[20] because too many hysterectomies were performed in the past,[19] and progestins may have negative effects on the cardiovascular system, lipoproteins and liver.[22,23]

When metrorrhagia is not associated with the presence of myomata or adenomatous hyperplasia with atypia and endometrial cancer, surgery may be avoided in premenopausal women. Unopposed estrogens cause endometrial hyperstimulation leading to irregular vaginal bleeding, endometrial hyperplasia and cancer,[24] and the cancer risk may persist for as long as 15 years.[5,6] In the premenopausal years endogenous estrogen/progesterone production is inadequate leading to overstimulation of the endometrium.[7] Within the endometrium endogenous or exogenous estrogens stimulate cell mitosis and proliferation and increase DNA synthesis and the concentration of nuclear estradiol receptors. Endogenous progesterone causes morphological changes which include nucleolar channel systems, giant mitochondria, and subnuclear accumulation of glycogen.

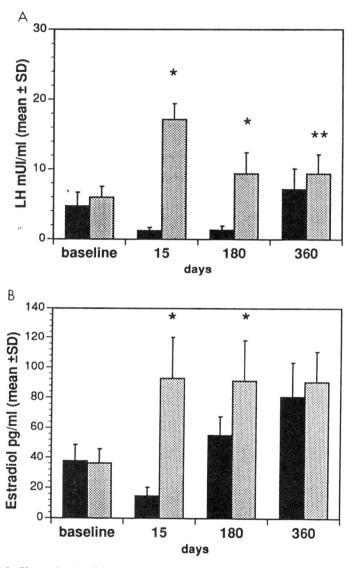

**FIGURE 1.** Plasma levels of **(A)** LH, **(B)** estradiol, **(C)** FSH, and **(D)** the logarithmic of progesterone according to the different steps of the protocol for patients (Group A, *dark columns*) and controls (Group B, *light columns*). * $p < 0.001$; ** $p < 0.05$.

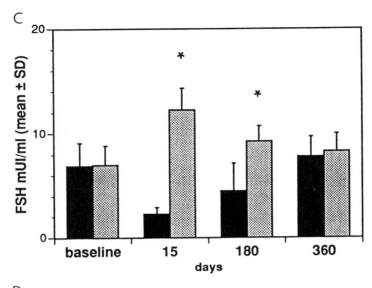
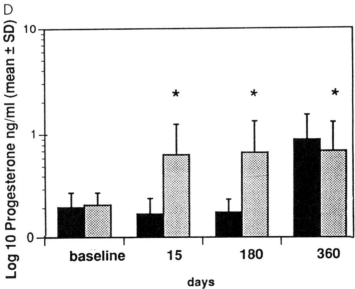

**FIGURE 1** (*Continued*).

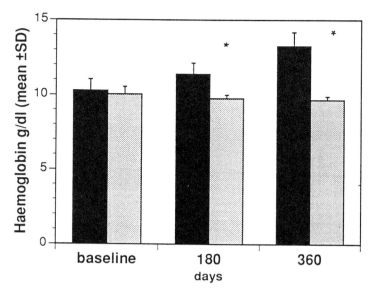

**FIGURE 2.** Hemoglobulin concentration before (baseline) and at the end of (180 days) the administration of the therapy in both patients (Group A, *dark columns*) and controls (Group B, *light columns*); evaluation after 6 months of suspension of the therapy (360 days) was also performed. * $p < 0.001$.

Biochemically, progesterone exposure exerts an antimitotic or antiestrogenic effect in reducing DNA synthesis and nuclear estradiol receptors and exerts a secretory effect by increasing the activity of certain enzymes such as estradiol 17β and isocitric dehydrogenases.[25] Synthetic progestogens reproduce the characteristic morphological and biochemical changes of the secretory phase of the

**TABLE 3.** Variability of Vaginal Bleeding, Metrorrhagia and Vasomotor Symptoms Reported in the Daily Diary and Their Significance

|  | Group A | | Group B | | p Value (Group A versus Group B) |
| --- | --- | --- | --- | --- | --- |
|  | No. | % | No. | % |  |
| Vaginal bleeding |  |  |  |  |  |
| Baseline | 20 | 100% | 20 | 100% | NS |
| 180 days | 1 | 5% | 20 | 100% | <0.001 |
| 360 days | 1 | 5% | 20 | 100% | <0.001 |
| Metrorrhagia |  |  |  |  |  |
| Baseline | 14 | 70% | 14 | 70% | NS |
| 180 days | 0 | 0% | 15 | 75% | <0.001 |
| 360 days | 2 | 10% | 17 | 85% | <0.001 |
| Hot flashes and headache |  |  |  |  |  |
| Baseline | 16 | 80% | 3 | 15% | <0.001 |
| 180 days | 0 | 0% | 3 | 15% | NS |
| 360 days | 6 | 30% | 10 | 50% | NS |

TABLE 4. Positive Immunoreaction for Laminin[a]

| Endometrial Biopsy | Group A | | Group B | |
|---|---|---|---|---|
| | No. | % | No. | % |
| Baseline | 0 | 0% | 0 | 0% |
| 180 days | 19 | 95% | 0 | 0% |
| 360 days | 10 | 50% | 0 | 0% |

[a] Positive immunoreactions of endometrial samples from Group A patients were compared with the positive immunoreactions of endometrial samples collected from Group B patients. The positive immunoreaction represents the predecidualization of the endometrium that in turn corresponds to quiescence of endometrial epithelial cell mitosis.

ovulatory cycle when they are used in combination with exogenous estrogens.[24] The rationale for medication of premenopausal patients with metrorrhagia with or without endometrial hyperplasia (without atypia) is to stop the estrogen production or to add progestins. However there is persuasive evidence that unopposed estrogens reduce the risk of arterial disease, the most common cause of death in postmenopausal women,[26] while oral progestogens oppose favorable estrogen-induced changes in lipid and lipoprotein metabolism.[22] Furthermore the administration of certain progestogens increases the incidence of hypertension and arterial thromboembolic disease in a dose-dependent manner.[27]

The National Institutes of Health in the United States have cautioned against the widespread addition of progestogens to exogenous estrogen treatment.[28] The derivatives of 19-nortestosterone as well as progestins that possess androgenic activity increase plasma insulin concentration (which reflects decreased sensitivity and therefore impaired glucose tolerance), and they lower the concentration of cholesterol in the high density lipoprotein fraction of plasma. This biochemical side effect is inversely related to the incidence of cardiovascular disease in both men and women. Since the beneficial effects of long-term postmenopausal estrogen treatment in possibly reducing mortality from ischemic heart disease[29] may be cancelled by the use of these progestins, a progestin without these biochemical effects was used in our study. Progesterone does not adversely affect plasma high density lipoprotein cholesterol concentrations and causes only minimal changes in carbohydrate metabolism.[29] Medrogestone is a progesterone derivative and its use did not affect plasma high density lipoprotein cholesterol concentration in our study. The suppression of ovarian activity obtained with Zoladex in patients with menstrual disturbances because of unbalanced estrogen/progesterone endogenous production, was effective on the dysfunctional bleeding and reduced the endometrial overstimulation. The beneficial effects of endogenous estrogens were obtained using transdermal estradiol. We did not observe significant changes in lipid or lipoprotein metabolism and the additional use of medrogestone did not have the adverse effect reported with the use of 19-nortestosterone derivative.[29] Patients had a significant increase in hemoglobin concentration and adequate endometrial proliferation and differentiation was restored, thus confirming the potential beneficial role of this therapeutical approach in preventing endometrial hyperplasia and cancer.

TABLE 5. Abnormal Endometrial Growth[a]

| Histological Features | Group A | | | | | | Group B | | | | | |
|---|---|---|---|---|---|---|---|---|---|---|---|---|
| | Baseline | | 180 Days | | 360 Days | | Baseline | | 180 Days | | 360 Days | |
| | No. | % | No. | % | No. | % | No. | % | No. | % | No. | % |
| Persistent proliferative | 6 | 30% | 0 | 0% | 0 | 0% | 5 | 25% | 2 | 10% | 0 | 0% |
| Glandular hyperplasia | 10 | 50% | 0 | 0% | 0 | 0% | 13 | 65% | 14 | 70% | 9 | 45% |
| Adenomatous hyperplasia | 4 | 20% | 1 | 5% | 1 | 5% | 2 | 10% | 4 | 20% | 11 | 55% |
| Decidualized | 0 | 0% | 19 | 95% | 10 | 50% | 0 | 0% | 0 | 0% | 0 | 0% |
| Proliferative | 0 | 0% | 0 | 0% | 9 | 45% | 0 | 0% | 0 | 0% | 0 | 0% |
| Significance | $p$ NS | | $p < 0.001$ | | $p < 0.001$ | | $p$ NS | | $p < 0.001$ | | $p < 0.001$ | |

[a] Abnormal endometrial growth (persistent proliferative, glandular hyperplasia and adenomatous hyperplasia) in the two groups was compared at different times: group A versus group B.

## SUMMARY

Cyclic or irregular uterine bleeding is common in perimenarchal and perimenopausal women with or without endometrial hyperplasia. The disturbance often requires surgical treatment because of its negative effects on both blood loss and abnormal endometrial growth including the development of endometrial cancer. The endometrium is often overstimulated during the perimenopausal period when estrogen/progesterone production is unbalanced. A therapeutical approach with gonadotropin-releasing hormone agonist (GnRHa) was proposed in a depot formulation (Zoladex) that induces a sustained and reversible ovarian suppression. To avoid the risk of osteoporosis and to obtain adequate endometrial proliferation and differentiation during ovarian suppression, transdermal 17-$\beta$-estradiol and oral progestin were administered. Results of 20 cases versus 20 controls showed a reduction of metrorrhagia, a normalization of hemoglobin plasma concentration, and an adequate proliferation and secretory differentiation of the endometrium of patients with abnormal endometrial growth. Abnormal uterine bleeding is mainly due to uterine fibrosis and an inadequate estrogen and/or progesterone production or to a disordered estrogen transport from blood into the endometrium. In premenopausal women, endometrial hyperplasia may be part of a continuum that is ultimately manifested in the histological and biological pattern of endometrial carcinoma. The regression of endometrial hyperplasia obtained by using the therapeutic regimen mentioned above represents a preventive measure for endometrial cancer. Finally the normalization of blood loss offers a good medical alternative to surgery for patients with DUB.

## REFERENCES

1. MERRILL, J. A. 1981. Management of postmenopausal bleeding. Clin. Obstet. Gynecol. **24:** 285–299.
2. GAMBRELL, R. D. 1977. Postmenopausal bleeding. Clin. Obstet. Gynecol. **4:** 129–143.
3. BULLETTI, C., A. GALASSI, V. M. JASONNI, G. MARTINELLI, S. TABANELLI & C. FLAMIGNI. 1988. Basement membrane components in normal, hyperplastic and neoplastic endometrium. Cancer **62**(1): 142–149.
4. BULLETTI, C., V. M. JASONNI, S. TABANELLI, P. M. CIOTTI, F. CAPPUCCINI, A. BORINI & C. FLAMIGNI. 1988. Increased extraction of estrogens in human endometrial hyperplasia and carcinoma. Cancer Detect. Prev. **13:** 123–130.
5. ZIEL, H. K. 1982. Estrogen's role in endometrial cancer. Obstet. Gynecol. **60:** 509–515.
6. KURMAN, R. J. & H. J. NORRIS. 1982. Evaluation of criteria for distinguishing atypical endometrial hyperplasia from well-differentiated adenocarcinoma. Cancer **8:** 2547–2559.
7. GAMBRELL, R. D., JR. 1986. The role of hormones in the etiology and prevention of endometrial cancer. Clin. Obstet. Gynecol. **13**(4): 695–723.
8. WEST, C. P. & D. T. BAIRD. 1987. Suppression of ovarian activity by Zoladex depot (ICI 118630), a long acting luteinizing hormone agonist analogue. Clin. Endocrinol. **26:** 213–220.
9. BIDER, D., Z. BEN-RAFAEL & J. SHALEV. 1989. Pituitary and ovarian suppression rate after high dosage of gonadotropin-releasing hormone agonist. Fertil. Steril. **51**(4): 578–581.
10. MATTA, W. H. & R. W. SHAW. 1987. Hypogonadism induced by luteinizing hormone releasing hormone agonist analogues: effects on bone density in premenopausal women. Br. Med. J. **294:** 1523–1524.
11. THOMAS, A. E., D. A. MCKAY & M. B. CUTLIP. 1976. A monograph method for assessing body weight. Am. J. Clin. Nutr. **29:** 302–304.

12. NOYES, R. W., A. T. HERTIG & J. ROCK. 1950. Dating the endometrial biopsy. Fertil. Steril. **1:** 3–25.
13. DISAIA, P. J. & W. T. CREASMAN. 1984. Clinical Gynecologic Oncology. 2nd edit. 122–133. C. V. Mosby. St. Louis.
14. BARSKY, S. H., N. C. RAO, C. RESTREPO & L. A. LIOTTA. 1984. Immunocytochemical enhancement of basement membrane antigens by pepsin. Applications in diagnostic pathology. Am. J. Clin. Pathol. **82:** 191–194.
15. DALY, D. C., I. A. MASALAR & D. K. RIDDICK. 1983. Prolactin production *in vitro* decidualization of proliferative endometrium. Am. J. Obstet. Gynecol. **145:** 672–678.
16. FABER, M., U. M. WEWER, J. G. BERTHELSEN, L. A. LIOTTA & R. ALBRECHTSEN. 1986. Laminin production by human endometrial stromal cells relates to the cyclic and pathologic state of the endometrium. Am. J. Pathol. **124:** 384–398.
17. SIEGEL, G. 1956. *In* Nonparametric Statistics for the Behavioral Sciences. McGraw-Hill. New York.
18. SPSS Inc. 1985. SPSS/PC+ for IBM PC/XMAT. SPSS Inc. Chicago, IL.
19. WHITEHEAD, M. I., P. T. TOWSEND & J. PRYSE-DAVIES. 1982. Effects of various types and dosage of progestogens on the postmenopausal endometrium. J. Reprod. Med. **27:** 539–548.
20. TRELOAR, A. E. 1981. Menstrual cyclicity and the premenopause. Maturitas **3:** 249–264.
21. Centers for Disease Control Surgical Sterilization Surveillance. Hysterectomy in women aged 15–44. U.S. Department of Health and Human Services, Centers for Disease Control, Center for Health Promotion and Education, Family Planning Evaluation Division, Atlanta.
22. HIRVONEN, E., M. MALKONEN & V. MANNIEN. 1981. Effects of different progestogens on lipoprotein during postmenopausal replacement therapy. N. Engl. J. Med. **304:** 560–563.
23. GORDON, E. M., S. R. WILLIAMS, B. FRENCHEK, C. H. MAZUR & L. SPEROFF. 1988. Dose dependent effects of postmenopausal estrogen/progestin on antithrombin III and factor IX. J. Lab. Clin. Med. **111:** 52–56.
24. WHITEHEAD, M. I. & D. I. FRASER. 1987. The effects of estrogens and progestogens on the endometrium. *In* D. R. Gambrell, Ed. Clinics in Obstetrics and Gynecology of North America, 14(1). The menopause. 299–320. W. B. Saunders. Philadelphia.
25. KING, R. J. B., P. T. TOWSEND, N. C. SIDDLE, M. I. WHITEHEAD & R. W. TAYLOR. 1982. Regulation of estrogen and progesterone receptor levels in epithelium and stroma from pre- and postmenopausal endometria. J. Steroid Biochem. **16:** 21–29.
26. MEADE, T. W., G. GREENBERG & S. G. THOMPSON. 1980. Progestogens and cardiovascular reaction associated with oral contraceptives and a comparison of the safety of 50 and 30 $\mu$gr oestrogen preparations. Br. Med. J. **280:** 1157–1161.
27. National Institutes of Health, National Institute on Aging. 1979. Estrogen use in postmenopausal women. Consensus conference on aging. Bethesda, MD.
28. SPELLACY, W. N., W. C. BUHI & S. A. BURK. 1975. Effects of norethindrone on carbohydrate and lipid metabolism. Obstet. Gynecol. **46:** 560–563.
29. KALKHOFF, R. K. 1982. Metabolic effects of progesterone. Am. J. Obstet. Gynecol. **142:** 735–738.

# Potential Roles for the Low Density Lipoprotein Receptor Family of Proteins in Implantation and Placentation[a]

GEORGE COUKOS,[b] MATS E. GÅFVELS,[b]
FRANK WITTMAACK,[b] HIROYA MATSUO,[b]
DUDLEY K. STRICKLAND,[c] CHRISTOS COUTIFARIS,[c]
AND JEROME F. STRAUSS III[b]

[b]*Department of Obstetrics and Gynecology*
*University of Pennsylvania School of Medicine*
*Philadelphia, Pennsylvania 19104*

*and*

[c]*Biochemistry Laboratory*
*American Red Cross*
*Rockville, Maryland 20855*

## INTRODUCTION

Implantation and placentation encompass complex processes including cell adhesion, cell proliferation, invasion, tissue remodeling and expression of cell specific functions.[1] We have recently come to recognize that the low density lipoprotein (LDL) receptor family of proteins and their ligands could participate in multiple events in the establishment of pregnancy. The state of our knowledge regarding the structure of this family of receptors and their ligands is discussed in this article, emphasizing the potential roles of these molecules in the implantation of the embryo and the development and function of the placenta.

### *The LDL Receptor Family: Structural Similarities and Overlapping Ligand Binding Activities*

The LDL receptor family includes at least five mammalian proteins that share structural features as well as similar ligands. The characteristic structural features of this family are a variable number of cysteine-rich repeats in the ligand-binding domains, multiple tetrapeptide repeats (Tyr-Trp-Thr-Asp), an EGF precursor-like region, a single transmembrane domain and a cytoplasmic domain containing an (Asn-Pro-X-Tyr) (NPXY) consensus sequence that targets the proteins for

---

[a] Work from the authors' laboratories was supported by NIH Grants HD-29946 and GM-42581 and grants from the Mellon Foundation and the American Heart Association.

endocytosis via coated pits (FIG. 1). The mammalian members of this family that have been identified to date, in addition to the LDL receptor, are the $\alpha_2$-macroglobulin receptor/LDL receptor-related protein (LRP), a very low density lipoprotein (VLDL)/apolipoprotein E (apo E) receptor, and two glycoproteins named gp330 and gp280.[2,6] These proteins range in size from about 600 kDa to 100 kDa. Although they are related in structure, the genes that encode them are distributed among several different human chromosomes. Thus, it is likely that they did not arise, at least recently, through a process of gene duplication.

The spectrum of ligands that the members of this family of receptors bind includes lipoprotein particles (LDL, VLDL); protease inhibitors ($\alpha_2$-macroglobulin, pregnancy zone protein, plasminogen activator inhibitor type 1 (PAI-1)); proteases (plasminogen activators); growth factor binding proteins ($\alpha_2$-macroglobulin); metal binding proteins ($\alpha_2$-macroglobulin, lactoferrin); and lipolytic enzymes (lipoprotein lipase). A 39-kDa endogenous inhibitor of ligand binding, called receptor-associated protein (RAP), also binds to at least several members of this family.[7,8] The binding of all the ligands to these receptors is calcium dependent.

The primary ligands have been identified for at least two of these receptors. The most significant ligands for the LDL receptor are the apo B- and apo E-containing lipoproteins, specifically LDL and VLDL. The primary ligand for LRP is $\alpha_2$-macroglobulin, a protease inhibitor, but also a protein that binds certain growth factors including transforming growth factor $\beta$, platelet-derived growth factor, interleukin-1$\beta$, activin and inhibin.[9] The key ligand for the VLDL/apoE receptor is presumably apo E and lipoprotein particles containing apo E, like VLDL.[4] The major ligands for gp280 and gp330 are unknown at present.

While these receptors appear to have primary ligands, they also bind a number of other proteins and consequently have an overlapping repertoire of ligand binding activities.[10–15] For example, apo E-enriched $\beta$-VLDL binds to both LRP and the VLDL/apoE receptor. PAI-1-plasminogen activator complexes bind to LRP and gp330. Lactoferrin binds to both LRP and gp330. Lipoprotein lipase facilitates ligand binding to both LRP and the LDL receptor. RAP, a protein whose carboxyl terminus has 26% homology with apo E, binds to LRP, gp330 and the VLDL/apoE receptor. Since a comprehensive study of all possible ligands has not been carried out with the known members of this family, it is possible that the receptors have an even greater overlap in ligand binding activities than is currently appreciated.

Although the fine structure of the ligand binding domains of the LDL receptor family has not been determined, it is likely that the cysteine-rich repeats in the extracellular domain are the ligand binding sites. The best studied member of this family with respect to identification of the ligand binding sites is LRP. Cross-competition studies carried out with various LRP ligands suggest that there are distinct binding sites for $\alpha_2$-macroglobulin, apo E-enriched VLDL and plasminogen activator, but that these binding sites have similar affinities for RAP.[16] Thus, $\alpha_2$-macroglobulin is not an effective competitor for apo E-enriched $\beta$-VLDL binding and vice versa, but RAP effectively blocks binding of both ligands. Whether there are yet any additional ligand binding sites remains to be determined. The other members of the receptor family presumably have multiple ligand binding domains like LRP.

### *Expression of the LDL Receptor Family in the Trophoblast Lineage*

The members of the LDL receptor family are found in many different tissues, but several of them are highly expressed in placenta, including LRP and the LDL

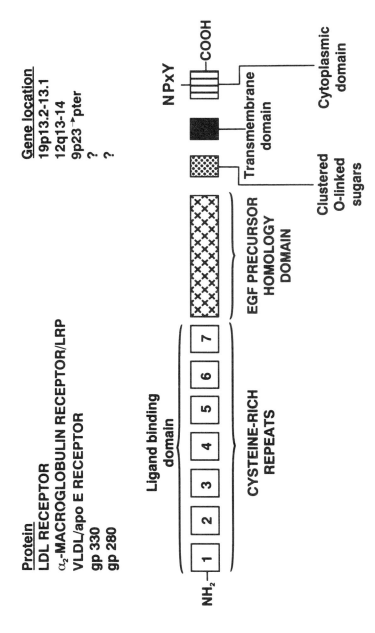

**FIGURE 1.** The mammalian members of the LDL receptor family. The proteins and their genome map positions are indicated. The domains of the receptor family are identified in the *lower panel*.

and VLDL/apoE receptors.[5,17] Detailed studies of the patterns of expression of these proteins in the embryo and placenta have not yet been carried out. However, existing data suggest interesting changes in the expression of these proteins in the trophoblast lineage in space and time. Gp330 has been localized between microvilli in coated pits on the apical surface of trophectoderm of rat pre-implantation blastocysts.[6] Gp330 is apparently lost from trophoblast cells after implantation. LRP has been found on invading cytotrophoblast cells in implantation sites (FIG. 2a,b), in villous cytotrophoblast cells and villous syncytiotrophoblast. As pregnancy advances, LRP becomes localized to the apical surface of syncytiotrophoblast and is lost from villous cytotrophoblast cells.[18] LDL and VLDL/apoE receptor mRNAs have been detected in human placenta and choriocarcinoma cells, but the immunocytochemical localization of these proteins in the various trophoblast forms has not been reported.

The LDL receptor family members expressed by trophoblast cells also appear to be regulated by different mechanisms and in divergent patterns. For example, cAMP increases LDL receptor expression in choriocarcinoma cells while reducing levels of LRP.[18] Collectively, these observations suggest that the different members of the LDL receptor family are expressed in trophoblst cells in distinctive patterns.

### *Trophoblast Cells Produce Ligands for the LDL Receptor Family*

Trophoblast cells synthesize several of the ligands that bind to the LDL receptor family including apo E, PAI-1, urokinase, and RAP.[18,21] Apo E synthesis has been demonstrated in human choriocarcinoma cells and perfused placental cotyledons.[19] It has also been detected by immunocytochemistry in murine trophoblast cells.[22] Recognized by both the LDL and VLDL/apoE receptors and LRP, this protein associates with lipoprotein particles and is believed to have a key function in determining the binding of these particles to lipoprotein receptors. However, apo E may have other roles in addition to lipoprotein metabolism. The addition of apo E to cultures of neurites affects their outgrowth.[23] Apo E also associates with proteoglycans and could, therefore, have a role in extracellular matrix metabolism. Alternatively, the binding of apo E to its receptor might generate a cascade of second messengers, resulting in a change in cell function.

PAI-1, an inhibitor of plasminogen activators, also associates with components of the extracellular matrix. Invading trophoblast cells elaborate both urokinase and PAI-1 and it is probable that these proteins control, in part, trophoblast invasion during the implantation process.[20,21]

The elaboration of both apo E and PAI-1 by trophoblast cells and the presence of receptors capable of binding these proteins once they have complexed with other particles (*e.g.*, lipoproteins) or molecules (*e.g.*, urokinase) has suggested a model of secretion-recapture wherein the trophoblast cells secrete a receptor ligand that associates locally with other molecules and then is reclaimed by the trophoblast cells by receptor-mediated endocytosis.[10] Such a mechanism might facilitate uptake of lipoprotein-carried cholesterol and fatty acids to support placental steroidogenesis, membrane synthesis and fetal nutrition (FIG. 3), as well as removal of inactivated proteases (FIG. 4) and remodeling of the extracellular matrix (FIG. 5), processes that are likely to be critical during implantation. Since LRP has recently been shown to mediate internalization of prourokinase and two-chain (active) urokinase, this receptor may regulate levels of active enzyme on the cell

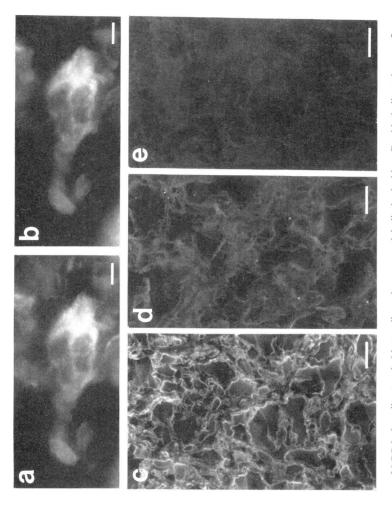

**FIGURE 2.** Presence of LRP in invading trophoblast cells and $\alpha_2$-macroglobulin in decidua. Double indirect immunofluorescence staining of a multinucleated giant trophoblast cell deep within maternal decidua stained for LRP (**a**) and cytokeratin (**b**) in a representative section from a first trimester human implantation site. Human decidua was also stained for $\alpha_2$-macroglobulin (**c**) and pregnancy zone protein (**d**). Note the presence and distribution of $\alpha_2$-macroglobulin in the decidual extracellular matrix and the absence of PZP. Control (**e**). *Bars:* (a,b) = 10 $\mu$; (c–e) = 100 $\mu$.

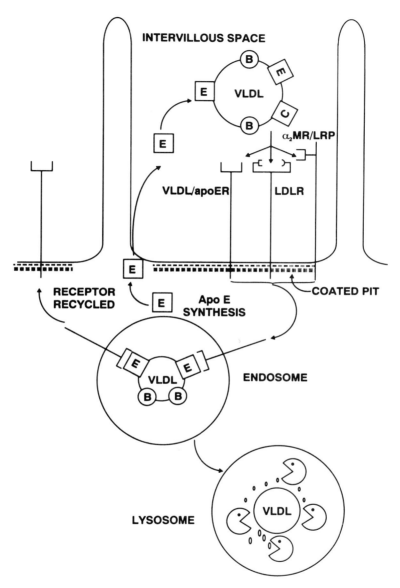

**FIGURE 3.** Model for the secretion-recapture of apo E by trophoblast cells. Apo E is secreted into the intervillous space where it associates with VLDL particles. These particles bind to either the VLDL/apoE or LDL receptors or LRP, which mediate endocytosis of the receptor-ligand complexes with subsequent degradation of the lipoprotein particles in lysosomes and recycling of the receptors to the plasma membrane.

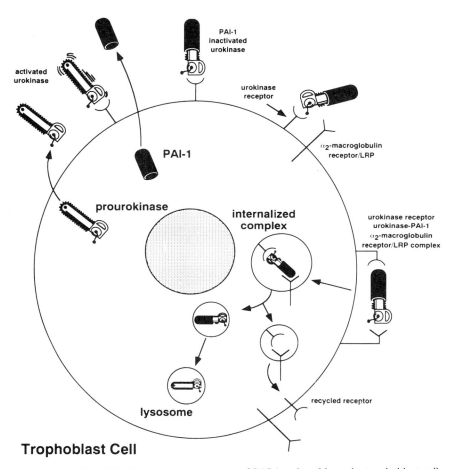

**FIGURE 4.** Model for the secretion-recapture of PAI-1 and urokinase by trophoblast cells. Trophoblast cells invading into the endometrium produce prourokinase which, once activated, binds to specific cell surface receptors that fix the active enzyme at the leading edge of moving cells. The active enzyme can be inactivated by PAI-1, also secreted by the trophoblast cells. The inactivated enzyme is internalized via the LRP, which binds PAI-1. The inactivated enzyme is degraded in lysosomes while the urokinase receptor and LRP are recycled back to the plasma membrane.

surface through a secretion-recapture mechanism functioning independently of PAI-1.[24]

RAP is a 39-kDa heparin-binding protein that was co-purified with LRP. It binds to LRP, the VLDL/apoE receptor and gp330 with high affinity and is able to block the binding of all known ligands for these receptors.[16] Hence, RAP has been proposed to be an endogenous modulator of receptor function. RAP and LRP are frequently co-expressed and double indirect immunofluorescence studies

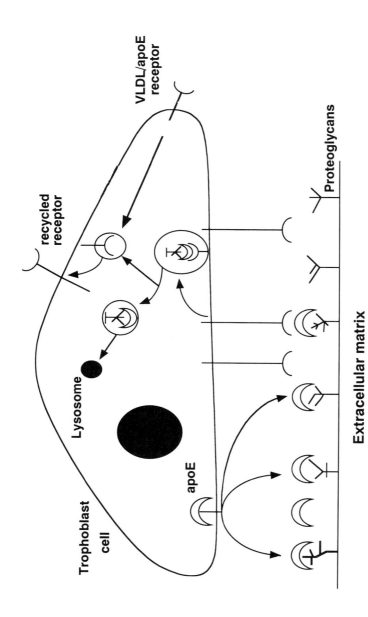

**FIGURE 5.** Secretion-recapture mechanism for apo E and of the extracellular matrix (ECM). Trophoblast cells secrete apo E which binds to ECM proteoglycans. The apo E–proteoglycan complex is then bound by VLDL/apoE receptors, subsequently internalized, and degraded in lysosomes while the VLDL/apoE receptor is recycled to the plasma membrane.

reveal co-localization in certain cells.[18] Interestingly, expression of LRP and RAP is spatially dissociated in some invading trophoblast columns in placental bed biopsies, suggesting LRP expression in the relative absence of RAP in the leading edge of invading trophoblasts.[18] The relative lack of RAP may make the LRP system more efficient in binding and internalization of ligands.

RAP is apparently not secreted by cells. It associates with receptors (LRP) soon after the receptor protein is made and then travels with the receptor to the cell membrane. Hence, nascent receptors may be initially inserted into the plasma membrane in a "blocked" form. RAP may dissociate from the receptor when receptor ligands are presented to the cell and then be reclaimed by unoccupied receptors that recycle back to the cell surface. Alternatively, RAP may dissociate from the receptors prior to insertion into the plasma membrane.

## *Ligands for the LDL Receptor Family Are Produced by Uterine Tissue*

The trophoblast LDL receptor family of proteins are also exposed to ligands generated by uterine tissues with which the trophoblast cells have intimate contact. Lactoferrin, a ligand for gp330 and LRP, is produced in the endometrial glandular epithelium.[25] Lactoferrin could promote the transfer of iron or other molecules into the preimplantation blastocyst via gp330 expressed by the trophectoderm and after implantation by LRP.

The rat decidua beneath the trophoblast elaborates large quantities of $\alpha_2$-macroglobulin.[26,27] $\alpha_2$-Macroglobulin is also detected by immunocytochemistry in human decidua (FIG. 2c). During human pregnancy, a protein that is structurally related to $\alpha_2$-macroglobulin, called pregnancy zone protein (PZP), is also found in plasma in high concentrations. The source of this protein is presumed to be the liver. It is apparently not produced by the decidua since it is not detectable in this tissue by immunocytochemical methods (FIG. 2d). Both $\alpha_2$-macroglobulin and PZP inactivate serine proteases as well as collagenases (metalloproteinases). The inhibiting mechanism of $\alpha_2$-macroglobulin involves trapping of the protease as a large molecular weight complex, effectively shielding the enzyme from high molecular weight substrates (FIG. 6). As noted above, $\alpha_2$-macroglobulin also binds growth factors including transforming growth factor $\beta$, platelet-derived growth factor, interleukin-$1\beta$, basic fibroblast growth factor, activin and inhibin.[9] The binding of growth factors/cytokines to $\alpha_2$-macroglobulin is presumably part of a mechanism to inactivate and remove the biologically active factors from the extracellular space. It is possible, however, that binding to $\alpha_2$-macroglobulin and/or subsequent uptake into cells via the LRP represents a novel mechanism by which $\alpha_2$-macroglobulin delivers active growth factor to trophoblast cells (FIG. 6).[9]

## *Roles for the LDL Receptor Family in Implantation and Placentation*

The LDL receptor family of proteins may have several different roles in trophoblast biology because of the functions of their specific ligands. These roles include the clearance of proteases and growth factors and the delivery of lipids to trophoblast cells. Although it remains to be determined if specific members of the LDL family have essential functions in trophoblast cells, experiments of nature and targeted gene disruption have provided important information regarding the indispensability or lack thereof of certain of these receptors in fetal development.

The absence of LDL receptors does not impair implantation, placentation or

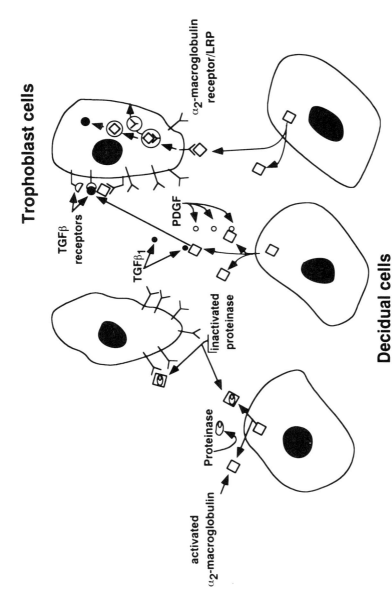

**FIGURE 6.** Interactions between decidual and trophoblast cells via the LRP. Decidual cells secrete $\alpha_2$-macroglobulin, which can serve as a protease inhibitor or growth factor binding protein. The inactivated proteases are internalized by trophoblast cells via LRP and degraded. The receptors are recycled to the plasma membrane of trophoblast cells. Growth factors bound by $\alpha_2$-macroglobulin may also be cleared by this mechanism. Alternatively, the $\alpha_2$-macroglobulin-growth factor complex may bind to LRP and thus present the growth factor to its specific receptor, resulting in a biological response by the trophoblast cells.

fetal growth and development, as humans with homozygous familial hypercholesterolemia, who lack LDL receptors, are born with no known abnormalities in gestation, as are Watanabe rabbits homozygous for mutant LDL receptors and mice whose LDL receptor genes have been disrupted by homologous recombination.[28] Thus, trophoblast cells can function in the absence of LDL receptors. The transport of sufficient levels of maternal lipids to support gestation and fetal development appears to be mediated by other receptors in the absence of active LDL receptors. The VLDL/apoE receptor and LRP may serve as back-ups to the LDL receptor in lipid transport and account for the successful pregnancies in the absence of placental LDL receptors. On the other hand, disruption of the LRP gene in mice is lethal with the fetuses undergoing demise by day 13.5 of pregnancy.[22] These observations suggest that the initial events of implantation can occur in the absence of LRP, but that some subsequent events in placentation or fetal development are abnormal. Homozygous mutations or disruption of the VLDL/apoE receptor and gp330 genes have yet to be reported.

## CONCLUSIONS

Trophoblast cells express several members of the LDL receptor family of proteins. These receptors may have multiple functions during implantation, placentation and maintenance of pregnancy including clearance of inactivated proteases, removal of growth factors and the accumulation of lipids. The overlapping spectrum of ligands may provide redundancy, so that these important roles are maintained in the absence of one of the proteins.

## ACKNOWLEDGMENTS

We thank Ms. Barbara McKenna and Ms. Marianne Winberg for help in preparation of the manuscript.

## REFERENCES

1. APLIN, J. D. 1991. J. Cell Sci. **99**: 681–692.
2. RUSSELL, D. W., W. J. SCHNEIDER, T. YAMAMOTO, K. L. LUSKEY, M. S. BROWN & J. L. GOLDSTEIN. 1984. Cell **37**: 577–585.
3. STRICKLAND, D. K., J. D. ASHCOM, S. WILLIAMS, W. H. BURGESS, M. MIGLIORINI & W. S. ARGRAVES. 1990. J. Biol. Chem. **265**: 17401–17404.
4. HERZ, J., R. C. KOWAL, J. L. GOLDSTEIN & M. S. BROWN. 1990. EMBO J. **9**: 1569–1576.
5. GÅFVELS, M. E., M. CAIRD, D. BRITT, C. L. JACKSON, D. PATTERSON & J. F. STRAUSS, III. 1993. Somatic Cell Mol. Genet. **19**: 557–569.
6. SAHALI, D., N. MULLIEZ, F. CHATELET, C. LAURENT-WINTER, D. CITADELLE, J-C. SABOURIN, C. ROUX, P. RONCO & P. VERROUST. 1993. Am. J. Pathol. **142**: 1654–1667.
7. KOUNNAS, M. Z., J. HENKIN, W. S. ARGRAVES & D. K. STRICKLAND. 1993. J. Biol. Chem. **268**: 21862–21867.
8. STRICKLAND, D. K., J. D. ASCHOM, S. WILLIAMS, F. BATTEY, E. BEHRE, K. MCTIQUE, J. F. BATTEY & W. S. ARGRAVES. 1991. J. Biol. Chem. **266**: 13364–13369.
9. BORTH, W. 1992. FASEB J. **6**: 3345–3353.
10. BROWN, M., J. HERZ, R. C. KOWAL & J. L. GOLDSTEIN. 1991. Curr. Opin. Lipidol. **2**: 65–72.

11. Kowal, R. C., J. Herz, J. L. Goldstein, V. Esser & M. S. Brown. 1989. Proc. Natl. Acad. Sci. USA **86:** 5810–5814.
12. Nykjaer, A., C. M. Peterson, B. Moller, P. A. Jensen, S. K. Moestrup, T. L. Holfet, M. Etzerodt, H. C. Thogersen, M. Munch, P. A. Andreasen & J. Gliemann. 1992. J. Biol. Chem. **267:** 14543–14546.
13. Willnow, T. E., J. L. Goldstein, K. Orth, M. S. Brown & J. Herz. 1992. J. Biol. Chem. **267:** 26180.
14. Bu, G., S. Williams, D. K. Strickland & A. L. Schwartz. 1992. Proc. Natl. Acad. Sci. USA **89:** 7427–7431.
15. Beisiegel, U., W. Weber & G. Bengtsson-Olivecrona. 1991. Proc. Natl. Acad. Sci. USA **88:** 8342–8346.
16. Williams, S. E., J. D. Ashcom, W. S. Argraves & D. K. Strickland. 1992. J. Biol. Chem. **267:** 9035–9040.
17. Gåfvels, M. E., G. Coukos, R. Sayegh, C. Coutifaris, D. K. Strickland & J. F. Strauss III. 1992. J. Biol. Chem. **267:** 21230–21234.
18. Coukos, G., M. E. Gåfvels, S. Wisel, E. A. Ruelaz, D. K. Strickland, J. F. Strauss III & C. Coutifaris. 1994. Am. J. Pathol. **144:** 383–392.
19. Rindler, J. F., M. G. Traber, A. L. Esterman, N. A. Bersinger & J. Dancis. 1991. Placenta **12:** 615–624.
20. Feinberg, R. F., L.-C. Kao, J. E. Haimowitz, J. E. Queenan, T.-C. Wun, J. F. Strauss III & H. J. Kliman. 1989. Lab. Invest. **61:** 20–26.
21. Queenan, J. T., L.-C. Kao, C. E. Arboleda, A. Ulloa-Aguirre, T. G. Golos, B. D. Cines & J. F. Strauss III. 1987. J. Biol. Chem. **262:** 10903–10906.
22. Herz, J., D. E. Clouthier & R. E. Hammer. 1993. Cell **71:** 411–421. Correction. 1993. Cell **73:** 428.
23. Handelmann, G. E., J. K. Boyles, K. H. Weisgraber, R. W. Mahley & R. E. Pitas. 1992. J. Lipid Res. **33:** 1677–1688.
24. Kounnas, M. Z., J. Henkin, W. S. Argraves & D. K. Strickland. 1993. J. Biol. Chem. **268:** 21862–21867.
25. Pentecost, B. T. & C. T. Teng. 1987. J. Biol. Chem. **262:** 10134–10139.
26. Gu, Y., P. G. Jayatilak, J. Fauldie, G. H. Frey & G. Gibori. 1992. Endocrinology **131:** 1321–1328.
27. Thomas, T. 1993. Placenta **14:** 417–428.
28. Ishibashi, S., M. S. Brown, J. L. Goldstein, R. D. Gerard, R. E. Hammer & J. Herz. 1993. J. Clin. Invest. **92:** 883–893.

# The Endometrial Cell Surface and Implantation

## Expression of the Polymorphic Mucin MUC-1 and Adhesion Molecules during the Endometrial Cycle

J. D. APLIN,[a] M. W. SEIF, R. A. GRAHAM, N. A. HEY, F. BEHZAD, AND S. CAMPBELL

*Department of Obstetrics and Gynaecology*
*and*
*School of Biological Sciences*
*University of Manchester*
*Manchester, U.K.*

### Cell Surface and Secretory Mucins in Epithelial Cells

Mucins are high molecular weight glycoproteins bearing relatively high levels of glycan in O-linkage with serine or threonine residues in the core protein. They are associated with secretory epithelial cells in numerous tissues and are thought to play a role in protecting the cell surface against environmental insult.[1,2] Several mammalian mucin genes have been cloned[1-7] and it has become apparent that the corresponding glycoproteins fall into two categories: cell surface-associated and true secretory mucins. The same cells can produce more than one mucin.[8,9] The true secretory mucins (MUC-2,3,4,5,6) self-associate, usually by disulphide bonding, to form large oligomers.[10,11] Highly O-glycosylated and hydrated domains lie between the disulphide knots and display extended conformations,[1,11] which in turn give rise to the specific rheological properties that these molecules exhibit.

A feature of the O-glycosylated, serine and threonine-rich domains of mucins is the presence of repeat sequences whose length varies from 11 to 81 residues.[1,2] High molecular weight secretory mucin has long been known to be produced by cervical tissue and to exhibit menstrual cycle stage-specific physical properties.[11] It is likely that endometrium also produces one or more large secretory mucins[12] but this has not yet been studied in detail.

The cell surface-associated mucins include MUC-1,[4-6] ASGP-1 (ascites sialoglycoprotein 1)[7] and epiglycanin.[13] MUC-1 was first recognised in association with breast cancer cells[14] and it has since been shown to be present at the surface of many different carcinomas, where expression often appears to be higher than in the corresponding normal cells. In normal epithelial tissues including breast, intestine, pancreas, placental villi and others, MUC-1 is specific to the apical cell surface, while in carcinoma cells this polarisation of expression is lost.[15] MUC-1

---

[a] Address for correspondence: Dr. John Aplin, Research Floor, St. Mary's Hospital, Manchester M13 0JH, U.K.

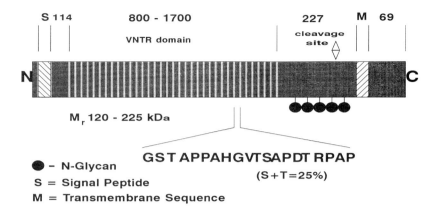

**FIGURE 1.** Diagrammatic representation of the MUC-1 glycoprotein. Numbers above represent amino acids. (Based on data reported in Refs. 4–6 and 21.)

has also been observed in certain bone marrow-derived cells including the large granulated lymphocytes of the mouse uterus.[16] The properties of epiglycanin suggest that it may be related to MUC-1.[13]

ASGP-1 is also a tumour-associated mucin, having been characterised as a product of an ascites tumour subline of the 13762 rat mammary adenocarcinoma.[7,17] Like MUC-1 (see next section), ASGP-1 is cleaved during biosynthesis into two components, a transmembrane polypeptide with a short C-terminal cytoplasmic domain and a larger extracellular domain rich in serine and threonine.

### The Structure of MUC-1

The cDNA for MUC-1 has been independently isolated and sequenced by several groups.[4–6,18,19] FIGURE 1 shows the salient features of the deduced peptide. It contains a short C-terminal cytoplasmic domain of 69 amino acids, a transmembrane domain and a large N-terminal extracellular domain dominated by a 20 amino acid repeat motif which may occur between 21 and 125 times, the most common allelic variants being 41 and 85. The region of the molecule containing these repeats is known as the variable number tandem repeat (VNTR) domain. Sequences flanking the VNTR contain degenerate repeats, so that this sequence dominates the extracellular part of the molecule. At the N-terminus two alternatively spliced forms have been described,[6] and there is unconfirmed evidence for another alternative form that lacks the transmembrane domain.[20] There is also a proteolytic cleavage site reported in the membrane proximal extracellular domain (FIG. 1).[21] The secreted form of MUC-1 lacks the cytoplasmic tail,[22] but it is not clear whether this is the result of alternative splicing or of proteolysis and release of the free extracellular domain.

### MUC-1 Polypeptide in Endometrium

Arklie et al.[14] first reported immunoreactivity in human endometrial epithelium using monoclonal antibodies HMFG1 and HMFG2, reagents produced using a milk fat globule membrane antigen preparation. These antibodies were later shown to bind the pentapeptide PDTRP that occurs in the tandem repeat of MUC-1 (FIG. 1).[23,24] We have used Western blotting and immunohistochemistry with HMFG1, HMFG2 and three other monoclonal antibodies, SM3,[23] BC2 and BC3,[15] all of which recognise sequences that overlap the PDTRP motif, to investigate the expression of MUC-1 in endometrium.

The antibodies bind to glycoprotein products of molecular mass in the range 220–400,000 in extracts of secretory phase endometrium; the molecular mass varies between individuals and sometimes more than one immunoreactive band can be detected (see FIG. 5).[25,26] There is a fraction of MUC-1 that is soluble in aqueous buffer as well as one that requires detergent for its solubilisation (see FIG. 5).[25] The binding of antibody HMFG1 is significantly enhanced after treatment of the extract with sialidase, presumably because of steric hindrance by short oligosaccharides of the NeuNAc-GalNAc (sialyl-Tn) type attached either to the threonine residue in the peptide epitope or at an adjacent serine or threonine.[26] There is evidence that GalNAc alone at these sites does not hinder the binding of the antibody (A. Singhal, personal communication). Binding of antibodies BC2, HMFG2 and SM3 is also inhibited to a greater or lesser extent by glycosylation.[26-28]

Inhibition by TR-associated glycan is also demonstrable in endometrium by immunohistochemistry; antibody SM3 fails to bind to secretory MUC-1, localising only a fraction associated with cytoplasmic sites (not shown). This fraction presumably reflects nascent mucin that has not yet been fully glycosylated. HMFG1 recognises secreted MUC-1 in gland lumens, but enhanced reactivity is observed after desialylation.[26]

Taking into account these considerations, we have used immunohistochemistry and blotting to investigate the cyclic pattern of expression of MUC-1 in normal endometrium. All reactivity is associated with the epithelium, both glandular and luminal. Immunoreactive mucin is present in the proliferative phase, but many cells and a significant fraction of whole gland profiles are negative. Reactivity is either cytoplasmic or associated with the apical cell surface. In early secretory phase, basal immunoreactive deposits appear in the gland cells. This material is later translocated to the apical cytoplasm and cell surface and then released into gland lumens, where maximal reactivity is found in the mid secretory phase coinciding with the predicted time of implantation. FIGURE 2 shows immunostaining of mid secretory phase endometrium with antibody HMFG1.

We have also used explant cultures of secretory phase endometrium pulse-labelled with [35]S-sulphate[29] to demonstrate by immunoprecipitation that endogenous synthesis of MUC-1 is occurring in the tissue and that the product is sulphated.

In primary endometrial epithelial cell cultures, intercellular heterogeneity is evident of both polypeptide and glycan expression (FIG. 3).[30] MUC-1 has been demonstrated at the cell surface as well as intracellularly. Secreted MUC-1 has been detected in culture medium conditioned by epithelial cell monolayers.

### *Transcriptional Regulation of MUC-1 in Endometrium*

Evidence has been obtained for transcriptional regulation of MUC-1 expression in breast cancer cells.[31] Given the variation in core protein production observed during the endometrial cycle, it was important to establish whether transcriptional or post-transcriptional mechanisms were responsible in this tissue. Using a Northern blotting approach with a cDNA to the tandem repeat domain we have investigated the relative abundance of the MUC-1 mRNA in tissue obtained from various phases of the endometrial cycle (FIG. 4).[26] Blots containing total endometrial RNA were probed sequentially for MUC-1 and then two control species, 28S rRNA and β-actin. Signals from the control probes did not vary significantly during the cycle. The data indicate that detectable levels of transcript are present in the proliferative phase. There is approximately a 6-fold increase from proliferative to early secretory phase. Approximately the same high level of transcript is maintained in the mid secretory phase, followed by a decrease in the late secretory phase. The observations suggest that transcriptional regulation does occur and that progesterone may play a role in stimulating increased transcription.

In mouse uterine epithelium, transcriptional regulation of homologous Muc-1 mRNA has also been demonstrated using a quantitative PCR approach.[16] In this species, however, the pattern of expression is quite distinct from human; higher levels of mRNA were observed in proestrus and estrus than at other stages of the cycle, coinciding with high plasma estrogen. In metestrus and diestrus, approximately 2-fold lower Muc-1 levels were observed, and levels were also lower in the implantation phase of pregnancy. Uteri of ovariectomised mice expressed Muc-1 mRNA, and this could be reduced to about 40% of the control value by administration of progesterone. The data suggest the possibility that constitutive expression of Muc-1 occurs (independent of estrogen) and that progesterone may cause down-regulation.

In mouse mammary gland a different pattern of regulation occurs, with low levels of mRNA in virgin animals and increases in pregnancy to a maximum at

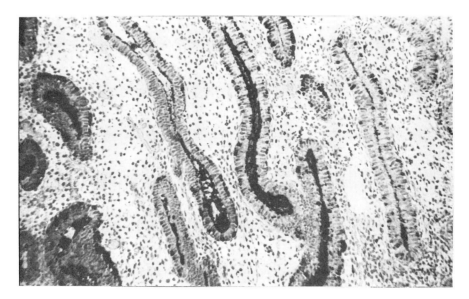

**FIGURE 2.** Immunoperoxidase localisation of MUC-1 core protein using monoclonal antibody HMFG1 in endometrial tissue 5 days after the LH peak. Tissue was fixed in glutaraldehyde and embedded in JB4. Semithin sections were immunostained as described previously.[46] Light nuclear counterstaining (toluidine blue) is visible particularly in the stroma. Immunostaining is seen in the base of some gland cells and is abundant in the gland lumens.

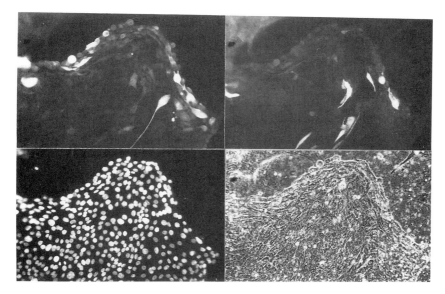

**FIGURE 3.** Mosaicism of MUC-1 core protein and glycan expression in a primary culture of proliferative phase epithelial cells cultured for 8 days on a matrigel-coated filter in the presence of 100 ng/ml progestin R5029. *Top left:* indirect immunofluorescence of MUC-1 core protein (antibody HMFG-1) shows that some cells in this epithelial island, particularly those at the edge, stain intensely while others are either more weakly stained or not at all. *Top right:* staining of the same cell island with the lectin Dolichos biflorus shows that some cells which express MUC-1 also have cell surface oligosaccharides containing terminal N-acetyl-galactosamine. However, the two markers are not co-distributed and the mosaic is complex. *Bottom left:* nuclear staining (bis-benzimide). *Bottom right:* phase microscopy of the same island showing that it is a densely packed confluent sheet characteristic of polarised cultures.

day 14–15.[32] In mammary epithelial cell cultures, the combination of insulin, prolactin and hydrocortisone stimulated increased expression and a further increase could be obtained by culturing the cells on a basement membrane-like substrate.[32]

## *Glycosylation of MUC-1*

In the tandem repeat unit of the MUC-1 polypeptide, 5 of the 20 amino acid residues are serine or threonine and it is clear that some of these are O-glycosylated (see above). In addition, sequences flanking the VNTR are rich in hydroxy amino acids. In the membrane-proximal region there are also 5 potential N-glycosylation sites, and evidence exists to suggest some of these may be used.[33] Based on estimates of its Mr from SDS-PAGE, the endometrial product is probably about 40–50% by weight carbohydrate. There is evidence that tissue-specific glycosylation occurs in MUC-1. Thus, for example, the pancreatic form of the molecule is considerably larger than the breast or endometrial product despite having an

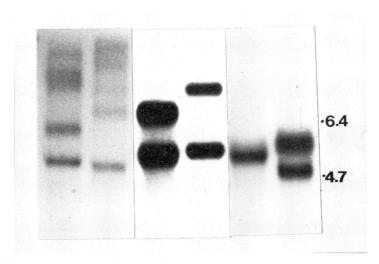

**FIGURE 4.** Representative Northern blot of total endometrial RNA probed with cDNA for MUC-1. Pairs of lanes (15 μg RNA) are shown from proliferative (*left*), mid secretory (*centre*) and menstrual phase (*right*). Note the transcript is most abundant in the mid secretory phase specimens. The two bands correspond to different alleles. Size markers shown at *right* are given in kb.

essentially identical transcript.[5] The suggestion that neoplastic transformation is associated with an increased preponderance of shorter O-glycans in the VNTR is based primarily on the observation that steric hindrance to the binding of anti-core protein antibodies is reduced. So far, relatively little direct structure determination has been carried out on MUC-1-associated glycan, but Hanisch and co-workers[34] have reported that the mucin isolated from human milk carries branched O-linked lactosaminoglycans (LAGs).

The presence of LAGs on MUC-1 is of interest since they have been demonstrated to be produced by endometrial epithelium in other species.[35] Rat uterine explants from immature animals secrete sulphated LAG (keratan sulphate; KS) in glycoprotein or proteoglycan and production could be elevated more than 10-fold by adding estradiol.[36] Polarised rat uterine epithelial cells in culture also produce sulphated LAG (keratan sulphate, KS) as a secretory product at the apical cell surface, although its abundance (expressed per cell) was not affected by estrogen.[36,37] In mice, uterine strips in culture produce LAGs, and the levels are elevated about 3–4-fold in the presence of estradiol or estradiol and progesterone. These glycans are N-linked to protein as well as being sialylated.[38,39] Babiarz and Hathaway[40] have studied various epitopes associated with chain capping modifications of LAG-type glycans in ovariectomised mouse uterus and shown that specific sialic acid and fucose substituents are produced in response to estrogen or progesterone. Kimber and Lindenberg[41–43] have shown that a blood group H type 1 structure, which has a core N-acetyl lactosamine disaccharide, is hormonally regulated and is present in the implantation phase. They have also demonstrated that the initial attachment of mouse embryos to cultured epithelial monolayers can be inhibited to the extent of about 40% by a soluble oligosaccharide analogue.[43]

We initiated a screen for human implantation phase-specific components by immunising mice with endometrial glandular epithelial cells isolated by collagenase digestion from secretory phase tissue. One antibody, D9B1, recognised a secretory and cell-surface-associated component[44,45] that was shown to bind a sialoglycan epitope associated with high molecular weight glycoprotein.[25] Western blotting (FIG. 5) suggested strongly that this glycan is present on a glycoprotein with the electrophoretic characteristics of MUC-1. Further evidence that this is the case has been obtained and will be presented elsewhere. Study of the behaviour of the epitope during the cycle indicated that it is absent in the normal proliferative phase, and produced and secreted in epithelial cells in the secretory phase, achieving maximal levels in secretions 6–7 days after the LH peak (FIG. 6).[45] Production of the epitope was shown to depend on progesterone.[46]

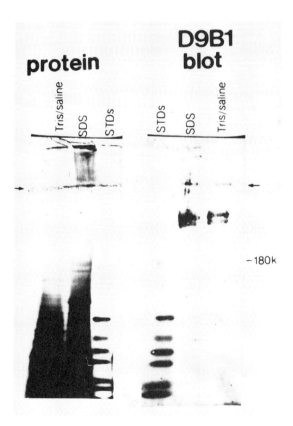

FIGURE 5. Electrophoretic analysis of the D9B1 epitope in endometrium. Secretory phase endometrial tissue was homogenised into Tris-buffered isotonic saline and the supernatant prepared for SDS-PAGE. The tissue pellet was solubilised in SDS sample buffer. The *left lanes* show a coomassie-stained gel, while the *right lanes* show a Western blot of duplicate lanes probed with D9B1. An immunoreactive doublet of Mr > 250,000 is present in both buffer and denaturing detergent extracts. *Arrows* indicate the top of the resolving gel. (From Hoadley *et al.*[25] Reprinted by permission from *Biochemical Journal*.)

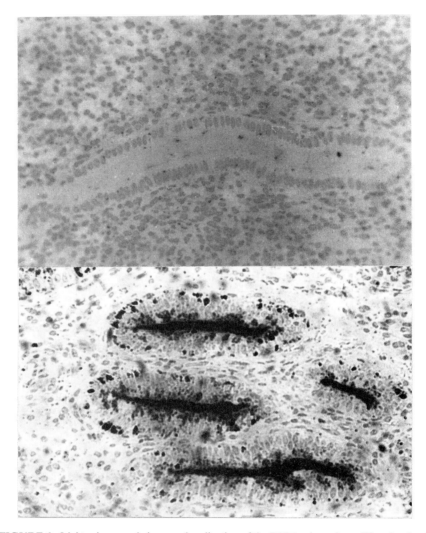

**FIGURE 6.** Light microscopic immunolocalisation of the D9B1 epitope in proliferative (*top*) and early secretory phase endometrium (6 days after the LH peak; *bottom*). No reactivity is observed in the proliferative phase. In mid secretory phase there is abundant immunopositive secretory material in gland lumens, and some residual intracellular reactivity.

Electron microscopic immunolocalisation studies of the D9B1 epitope were carried out in secretory phase endometrium (FIG. 7)[29] and demonstrated the association of the epitope with golgi and post-golgi secretory apparatus in the epithelial cells, as well as with apical glycocalyx on both microvillous and ciliated cells.

In situ characterisation of the glycan was carried out using immunohistochemistry of tissue sections pretreated with specific glycosidases. In addition to being abolished by sialiase pretreatment, binding of D9B1 was also abolished or significantly reduced using endo-$\beta$-galactosidase or keratanase.[25] Based on this we hypothesise that the D9B1 epitope is a terminal nonreducing sialic acid residue on a keratan sulphate-type glycan. Not all the residues on the LAG backbone carry sulphate residues since both keratanase and endo-$\beta$-galactosidase cleave at unsulphated galactose residues. Support for this interpretation came from the observation that the D9B1 epitope is present as a minor component of proteoglycan from articular cartilage (Seif, unpublished); this molecule is rich in keratan sulphate chains, some of which are sialylated. There is preliminary evidence (Nieduszynski, unpublished) that the sialic acid residue is in $\alpha$2–3 linkage with the penultimate sugar in the chain. We assume the D9B1 epitope includes this sialic acid as well as adjacent sugar residues.

Further investigations were then carried out to obtain independent evidence that keratan sulphate is present in human endometrium. Immunohistochemistry using antibody 5D4 to keratan sulphate (FIG. 8) indicated not only that KS is present as a cell surface-associated and secretory product of endometrium, but also that it shows a hormonal pattern of regulation that resembles closely that of the D9B1 sialoepitope.[47] Keratan sulphate is detectable in association with a fraction of the gland cells in proliferative phase tissue, but a very significant increase in production occurs beginning 2–3 days after the luteinising hormone (LH) peak.

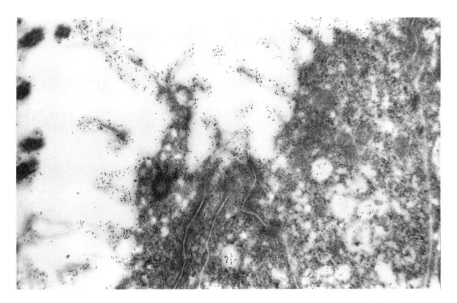

**FIGURE 7.** Electron microscopic immunolocalisation of the D9B1 epitope in mid secretory phase endometrium (6 days after the LH peak). The micrograph demonstrates the association of the epitope with glycocalyx at the apical cell surface of gland cells, including microvilli. Tissue was glutaraldehyde-fixed, epon-embedded and etched before immunolabelling with antibody-conjugated 10 nm gold particles. Method according to Reference 29.

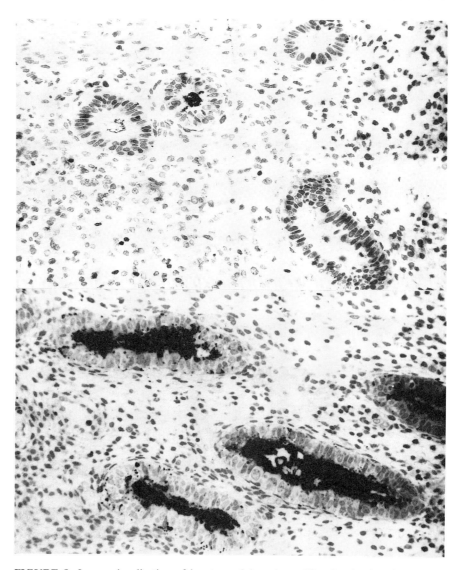

**FIGURE 8.** Immunolocalisation of keratan sulphate in proliferative (*top*) and secretory phase endometrium (5 days after the LH peak; *bottom*). A few proliferative phase glands are immunoreactive in cells and secretions, but a great increase in production occurs after ovulation, with intracellular deposits in gland cells visible in early secretory phase and increasing secretions thereafter. Semithin sections counterstained with toluidine blue.

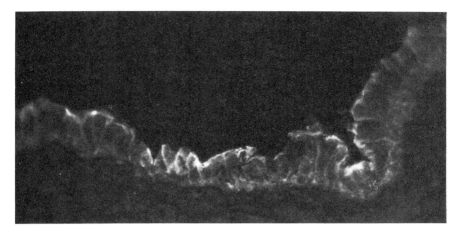

**FIGURE 9.** Immunofluorescence localisation of integrin $\beta 5$ in endometrial luminal epithelial cells. Note the obvious apical staining.

During the period from 3–5 days after the LH peak, intracellular immunoreactivity is preponderant in the gland cells. This appears at the cell base but is subsequently mobilised through the apical cytoplasm and into gland secretions. Maximal immunoreactivity in the secretions occurs in the period from 6–8 days after the LH peak, coinciding with the expected time of implantation.

### Adhesion Molecules in the Maternal Epithelium

The presence of molecules of the integrin family at the maternal epithelial cell surface has been demonstrated by Lessey et al.,[48] Tabibzadeh[49] and Klentzeris et al.[50] These authors report the presence of integrin subunits $\alpha v$, $\alpha 1$, $\alpha 2$, $\alpha 3$, $\alpha 4$, $\alpha 6$, $\beta 3$ and $\beta 4$ at the epithelial cell surface. The light microscopic data is consistent with the presence of $\alpha v$, $\alpha 1$, $\alpha 2$, $\alpha 3$, $\alpha 4$, and $\beta 3$ in the apical domain, though confirmatory evidence is required. We have also demonstrated the presence of integrin $\beta 5$ subunit in the apical epithelium (FIG. 9). Subunits $\alpha 6$ and $\beta 4$ are basally distributed and presumably play a role as the complex $\alpha 6\beta 4$ in cell anchorage to basement membrane.[51] The distribution of integrin $\beta 1$ has not been reported.

Based on the known patterns of association of these subunits, this raises the possibility that integrin heterodimers $\alpha v\beta 1$, $\alpha v\beta 3$, $\alpha v\beta 5$, $\alpha 1\beta 1$, $\alpha 2\beta 1$, $\alpha 3\beta 1$ and $\alpha 4\beta 1$ (TABLE 1)[52] could all be present in the apical cell surface domain, though further work is required to complete the dimerisation analysis.

We have examined sections of endometrium for expression of molecules of the CD44 family. CD44 (FIG. 10) is a transmembrane glycoprotein with a short C-terminal cytoplasmic tail and larger N-terminal extracellular domain containing a region of alternative splicing. It is glycosylated and can contain sulphated glycosaminoglycan chains.[53] The shortest form of the molecule, known as CD44H because it was first detected in hematopoietic cells, acts as a surface receptor for hyaluronic acid.[54] This isoform lacks the whole of the E region shown in FIGURE

10. CD44 is also involved in the cell-cell interaction required to attach lymphocytes to specialised endothelial cells during homing to lymph nodes.[55] Other forms of CD44 known as CD44E may contain some or all of the additional 5 domains shown in FIGURE 10. Analysis of the structure of the CD44 gene indicates that there is also an alternative cytoplasmic domain not shown in FIGURE 10.[56] CD44E has been detected in epithelial cells but does not appear to retain the affinity for hyaluronate shown by the CD44H form of the molecule.[57] The function of CD44E is unknown, but its presence at the cell surface is associated with alteration in the migratory properties of tumour cells.[58]

We have detected CD44 in endometrium by immunofluorescence with antibodies that recognise epitopes common to all the isoforms of the molecule (FIG. 11). CD44 is present in both epithelial and stromal compartments and is usually evident in all epithelial plasma membrane domains. We have not detected any cyclical variation in its apparent abundance using this technique. Further work will be needed to characterise the CD44 spliceoforms and glycoforms present.

## *Molecular Interactions between the Implanting Embryo and the Maternal Epithelium: Models*

One model of implantation in human involves as a first stage the receptor-mediated attachment of trophectoderm to the apical surface of luminal epithelial cells.[59] Although the simple presence of a molecule at the cell surface by no means guarantees its involvement in implantation, it is interesting to speculate as to how MUC-1 and adhesion receptors might function individually or in concert to regulate and/or mediate embryo attachment. Although no functional information is available, the presence of apical adhesion molecules could suggest a role in the interaction with the embryo. If so, the variety of different receptors present could indicate functional redundancy.

### *'Bridging' vs Direct Binding*

Several integrins whose constituent subunits have been detected in the epithelium bind extracellular ligands including fibronectin, vitronectin and others (TABLE 1),[52] and are not known to interact directly with other cell surfaces. This

TABLE 1. Ligand Specificities of Integrin Heterodimers Containing Subunits Detected in Endometrial Epithelium

| Integrin | Extracellular Ligands |
| --- | --- |
| $\alpha 1\beta 1$ | collagens, laminin |
| $\alpha 2\beta 1$ | collagens, laminin |
| $\alpha 3\beta 1$ | fibronectin, laminin, collagens |
| $\alpha 4\beta 1$ | fibronectin |
| $\alpha 6\beta 4$ | laminin? |
| $\alpha v\beta 1$ | fibronectin, vitronectin |
| $\alpha v\beta 3$ | fibronectin, vitronectin, fibrinogen, collagen, osteopontin, thrombospondin, von Willebrand factor |
| $\alpha v\beta 5$ | vitronectin, fibronectin |

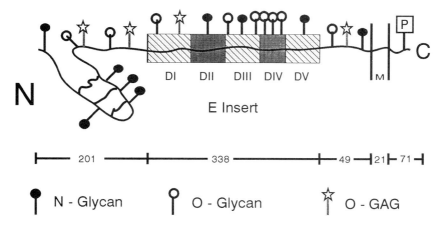

**FIGURE 10.** Structure of CD44. The isoform lacking the E insert is known as CD44H. Various isoforms of CD44E are found and contain different combinations of the domains illustrated. *Numbers* in the bars represent amino acids. M is the transmembrane domain.

might suggest the need for a bifunctional 'bridging' ligand between the two cell surfaces. Other endometrial receptors including integrins $\alpha 2\beta 1$ and $\alpha 3\beta 1$ are known to act in homotypic cell-cell attachment as well as attachment to extracellular matrix.[60] There has also been a suggestion that trophectodermal cell surface heparan sulphate may participate in binding to appropriate receptors on the endometrium.[61]

*Steric Hindrance by MUC-1*

If the reasonable assumption is made that endometrial MUC-1 takes on a highly extended conformation at the cell surface, its polypeptide core is expected to extend much further from the cell surface than conventional glycoprotein receptors of the integrin or CD44 families. Experiments by Hilkens and co-workers[62,63] have shown that when lymphoblastoid cells are transfected with cDNA for MUC-1 and high levels of expression at the cell surface are achieved, the cells lose the ability to aggregate spontaneously in shaker culture. Similarly, cell attachment to substrates containing extracellular matrix components, an integrin-mediated phenomenon, is inhibited if MUC-1 is expressed at the cell surface. In principle therefore, MUC-1 could act to hinder sterically the approach of molecules or cells to the endometrial epithelium. If the pattern of MUC-1 expression in luminal cells is the same as in the glands, there is likely to be maximal steric hindrance to implantation 7 days after the LH peak, that is, at precisely the time that implantation is thought to occur. Furthermore, the polyanionic character of MUC-1, which contains both sulphate and sialic acid, is likely to lead to Coulombic repulsion of the negatively charged trophectodermal surface.

*Glycan Ligand/Neutrophil Extravasation Model*

It is possible (by analogy with the attachment of neutrophils to endothelial surfaces at sites of inflammation)[64] that the endometrial surface presents a specific

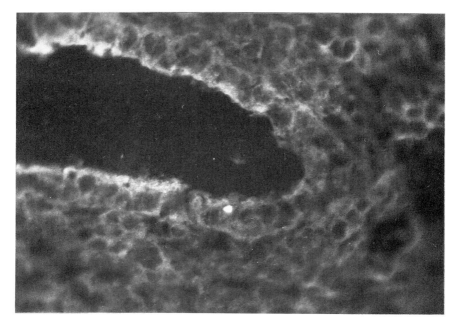

**FIGURE 11.** Immunofluorescence of CD44 in endometrial tissue demonstrating localisation in both epithelial and stromal cells. Monoclonal antibody PIG12.

glycan ligand to the embryo which acts as a 'first stage' point of attachment, later leading to a higher affinity integrin-mediated interaction. Kimber and Lindenberg have direct evidence for carbohydrate-mediated recognition in mouse.[43] The glycan ligand could be presented by MUC-1 or another component of the glycocalyx.

*Embryonic Microenvironment*

Given a generally nonadhesive maternal surface, the embryo might need to create a suitable microenvironment for close approach. This might require proteolytic[65] or other enzymic modification to the glycocalyx in advance of interaction with an integrin.

*Embryo-Epithelial Stimulation*

It is possible that the embryo produces local signals either to stimulate expression of new surface adhesion molecules or to cause loss of cell surface polarity in the epithelium at the site of attachment. The latter idea was first suggested by Denker.[66] It might lead to laterally disposed adhesion molecules gaining rapid access to the apical surface. It might also lead to a redistribution of inhibitory MUC-1 from the apical to lateral surfaces with dilution of its putative inhibitory effect on embryo attachment.

*Apoptosis of the Endometrial Epithelium Prior to Implantation*

It is by no means certain that embryo attachment is mediated by direct binding of trophectoderm to maternal epithelial cells. Although observations *in vitro* suggest such an interaction is possible,[59] there is no recorded instance of such an interaction being observed *in vivo*. In the rat, interstitial implantation occurs following spontaneous cell death of the uterine epithelium; the loss of the luminal cells occurs in the absence of direct contact with trophectoderm and allows the embryo to interact with the underlying stroma and vasculature.[67–69]

Since MUC-1, integrins and CD44 are products of glandular as well as surface epithelial cells, it should not be forgotten that interactions between invading trophoblast and endometrial glands occur during early implantation and placental morphogenesis and throughout the first trimester of pregnancy. In this period, gland cells continue their secretory activity and their products are capable of transfer into fetal tissue compartments.[70,71] There is evidence that during the first trimester, the maternal vascular circuit supplying the intervillous space is not fully open, so that placentation in this period is deciduochorial rather than hemochorial.[72,73] The abundance of MUC-1 and adhesion molecules in gland cell surfaces may also have some functional significance in pregnancy.

## SUMMARY

The cell surface mucin MUC-1 is present in endometrial epithelial cells and their associated apical glycocalyx and is also released into gland lumens as a secretory product. MUC-1 mRNA and core protein are found at low levels in the proliferative phase of the cycle, but their abundance increases after ovulation. Endometrial MUC-1 has been found to carry sialokeratan sulphate chains and these show a dramatically increased abundance in cells and secretions in the post-ovulatory phase of the cycle, reaching a maximum in secretions 6–7 days after the LH peak. The apical epithelium also contains adhesion receptor molecules of the integrin and CD44 families. MUC-1 is large and highly glycosylated and probably extends farther from the cell surface than these 'conventional' glycoprotein receptors. It has the potential to inhibit sterically receptor-mediated cell-cell adhesion. However, it is also possible that MUC-1 displays specific (*e.g.*, glycan) recognition structures for the initial attachment of the blastocyst or that the embryo may create a specialised microenvironment in which to implant.

## REFERENCES

1. DEVINE, P. & I. F. C. MCKENZIE. 1992. Mucins: structure, function and association with malignancy. BioEssays **14:** 619–625.
2. STROUS, G. J. & J. DEKKER. 1992. Mucin-type glycoproteins. Crit. Rev. Biochem. Mol. Biol. **27:** 57–92.
3. GUM, J. R., J. C. BYRD, J. W. HICKS, N. W. TORIBARA, D. T. A. LAMPORT & Y. S. KIM. 1989. Molecular cloning of human intestinal mucin cDNAs. Sequence analysis and evidence for genetic polymorphism. J. Biol. Chem. **264:** 6480–6487.
4. GENDLER, S. J., C. A. LANCASTER, J. TAYLOR-PAPADIMITRIOU, T. DUHIG, N. PEAT, J. BURCHELL, L. PEMBERTON, E. LALANI & D. WILSON. 1990. Molecular cloning

and expression of human tumour-associated polymorphic epithelial mucin. J. Biol. Chem. **265:** 15286-15293.
5. LAN, M. S., S. K. BATRA, W.-N. QI, R. S. METZGAR & M. A. HOLLINGSWORTH. 1990. Cloning and sequencing of a human pancreatic tumor mucin cDNA. J. Biol. Chem. **265:** 15294-15299.
6. LIGTENBERG, M. J. L., H. L. VOS, A. M. C. GENNISSEN & J. HILKENS. 1990. Episialin, a carcinoma-associated mucin, is generated by a polymorphic gene encoding splice variants with alternative amino termini. J. Biol. Chem. **265:** 5573-5578.
7. CARRAWAY, K. L., N. FREGIEN, K. L. CARRAWAY III & C. A. C. CARRAWAY. 1992. Tumor sialomucin complexes as tumor antigens and modulators of cellular interactions and proliferation. J. Cell Sci. **103:** 299-307.
8. DEVINE, P., G. T. LAYTON, B. A. CLARK, G. W. BIRRELL, B. G. WARD, P.-X. XING, & I. F. C. MCKENZIE. 1991. Production of MUC1 and MUC2 mucins by human tumour cell lines. Biochem. Biophys. Res. Commun. **178:** 593-599.
9. DAHIYA, R., K.-S. KWAK, J. C. BYRD, S. HO, W.-H. YOON & Y. S. KIM. 1993. Mucin synthesis and secretion in various human epithelial cancer cell lines that express the MUC1 mucin gene. Cancer Res. **53:** 1437-1443.
10. SHEEHAN, J. K., R. P. BOOT-HANDFORD, E. CHANTLER, I. CARLSTEDT & D. J. THORNTON. 1991. Evidence for shared epitopes within the naked protein domains of human mucus glycoproteins. Biochem. J. **274:** 293-296.
11. SHEEHAN, J. K. & I. CARLSTEDT. 1990. Electron microscopy of cervical mucus glycoproteins and fragments therefrom. Biochem. J. **265:** 169-178.
12. VAN KOOIJ, R. J., H. J. M. ROELOFS, G. A. M. KATHMAN & M. F. KRAMER. 1982. Synthesis of a mucous glycoprotein in the human uterus. Eur. J. Obstet. Gynecol. Reprod. Biol. **14:** 191-197.
13. CODINGTON, J. F. & S. HAAVIK. 1992. Epiglycanin—a carcinoma-specific mucin-type glycoprotein of the mouse TA3 tumour. Glycobiology **2:** 173-180.
14. ARKLIE, J., J. TAYLOR-PAPADIMITRIOU, W. BODMER, M. EGAN & R. MILLS. 1981. Differentiation antigens expressed by epithelial cells in the lactating breast are also detectable in breast cancers. Int. J. Cancer **28:** 23-29.
15. XING, P.-X., J. J. TJANDRA, S. A. STACKER, J. G. TEH, C. H. THOMPSON, P. J. MCLAUGHLIN & I. F. C. MCKENZIE. 1989. Monoclonal antibodies reactive with mucin expressed in breast cancer. Immunol. Cell Biol. **67:** 183-195.
16. BRAGA, V. M. M. & S. J. GENDLER. 1993. Modulation of Muc-1 mucin expression in the mouse uterus during the estrus cycle, early pregnancy and placentation. J. Cell Sci. **105:** 397-405.
17. SHENG, Z., K. WU, K. L. CARRAWAY & N. FREGIEN. 1992. Molecular cloning of the transmembrane component of the 13762 mammary adenocarcinoma sialomucin complex. J. Biol. Chem. **267:** 16341-16346.
18. GENDLER, S. J., J. M. BURCHELL, T. DUHIG, D. LAMPORT, R. WHITE, M. PARKER & J. TAYLOR-PAPADIMITRIOU. 1987. Cloning of partial cDNA encoding differentiation and tumor-associated mucin glycoproteins expressed by human mammary epithelium. Proc. Natl. Acad. Sci. USA **84:** 6060-6064.
19. GENDLER, S. J., J. TAYLOR-PAPADIMITRIOU, T. DUHIG, J. ROTHBARD & J. BURCHELL. 1988. A highly immunogenic region of a human polymorphic epithelial mucin expressed by carcinomas is made up of tandem repeats. J. Biol. Chem. **263:** 12820-12823.
20. WILLIAMS, C. J., D. H. WRESCHNER, A. TANAKA, L. TSARFATY, L. KEYDAR & A. S. DION. 1990. Multiple protein forms of the human breast tumor-associated epithelial membrane antigen are generated by alternative splicing and induced by hormonal stimulation. Biochem. Biophys. Res. Commun. **170:** 1331-1338.
21. LIGTENBERG, M. J. L., L. KRUISHAAR, F. BUIJS, M. V. MEIJER, S. V. LITVINOV & J. HILKENS. 1992. Cell-associated episialin is a complex containing two proteins derived from a common precursor. J. Biol. Chem. **267:** 6171-6177.
22. BOSHELL, M., E.-N. LALANI, L. PEMBERTON, J. BURCHELL, S. GENDLER & J. TAYLOR-PAPADIMITRIOU. 1992. The product of the human MUC1 gene when secreted by mouse cells transfected with the full length cDNA lacks the cytoplasmic tail. Biochem. Biophys. Res. Commun. **185:** 1-8.

23. BURCHELL, J., S. GENDLER, J. TAYLOR-PAPADIMITRIOU, A. GIRLING, A. LEWIS & R. MILLS. 1987. Development and characterisation of breast cancer reactive monoclonal antibodies directed to the core protein of the human milk mucin. Cancer Res. **47:** 5476-5482.
24. BURCHELL, J., J. TAYLOR-PAPADIMITRIOU, M. BOSHELL, S. GENDLER & T. DUHIG. 1989. A short sequence within the amino acid tandem repeat of a cancer-associated mucin contains immunodominant epitopes. Int. J. Cancer **44:** 691-696.
25. HOADLEY, M. E., M. W. SEIF & J. D. APLIN. 1990. Menstrual cycle-dependent expression of keratan sulphate in human endometrium. Biochem. J. **266:** 757-763.
26. HEY, N. A., R. A. GRAHAM, M. W. SEIF & J. D. APLIN. 1994. The polymorphic epithelial mucin MUC1 in human endometrium is hormonally regulated with maximal expression in the implantation phase. J. Clin. Endocrinol. Metab. **78:** 337-342.
27. GIRLING, A., J. BARTKOVA, J. BURCHELL, S. GENDLER, C. GILLETT & J. TAYLOR-PAPADIMITRIOU. 1989. A core protein epitope of the polymorphic epithelial mucin detected by the monoclonal antibody SM3 is selectively exposed in a range of primary carcinomas. Int. J. Cancer **43:** 1072-1076.
28. DEVINE, P. L., J. A. WARREN, B. G. WARD, I. F. C. MACKENZIE & G. T. LAYTON. 1990. Glycosylation and the exposure of tumor-associated epitopes on mucins. J. Tumor Marker Oncol. **5:** 11-26.
29. GRAHAM, R. A. 1992. Ph.D. Thesis. University of Manchester.
30. CAMPBELL, S., M. W. SEIF, J. D. APLIN, S. J. RICHMOND, P. HAYNES & T. D. ALLEN. 1988. Expression of a secretory product by microvillous and ciliated cells of the human endometrial epithelium *in vivo* and *in vitro*. Hum. Reprod. **3:** 927-934.
31. ABE, M. & D. KUFE. 1993. Characterisation of cis-acting elements regulating transcription of the human DF3 breast carcinoma-associated antigen. Proc. Natl. Acad. Sci. U.S.A. **90:** 282-286.
32. PARRY, G., J. LI, J. STUBBS, M. J. BISSELL, C. SCHMIDHAUSER, A. P. SPICER & S. J. GENDLER. 1992. Studies of Muc-1 mucin expression and polarity in the mouse mammary gland demonstrate developmental regulation of Muc-1 glycosylation and establish the hormonal basis for mRNA expression. J. Cell Sci. **101:** 191-199.
33. HILKENS, J. & F. BUIJS. 1988. Biosynthesis of MAM-6, an epithelial sialomucin. J. Biol. Chem. **263,** 4215-4222.
34. HANISCH, F.-G., G. UHLENBRUCK, J. PETER-KATALINIC, H. EGGE, J. DABROWSKI & U. DABROWSKI. 1989. Structures of neutral O-linked polylactosaminoglycans on human skim milk mucins. A novel type of linearly extended poly-N-acetyllactosamine backbones with Gal$\beta$(1-4)GlcNAc$\beta$(1-6) repeating units. J. Biol. Chem. **264:** 872-883.
35. APLIN, J. D. 1991. Glycans as biochemical markers of human endometrial secretory differentiation. J. Reprod. Fertil. **91:** 525-541.
36. CARSON, D. D., J. Y. TANG, J. JULIAN & S. R. GLASSER. 1988. Vectorial secretion of proteoglycans by polarised rat uterine epithelial cells. J. Cell Biol. **107:** 2425-2434.
37. JULIAN, J., D. D. CARSON & S. R. GLASSER. 1992. Polarised rat uterine epithelium *in vitro*: constitutive expression of estrogen-induced proteins. Endocrinology **130:** 79-87.
38. DUTT, A., J.-P. TANG & D. D. CARSON. 1988. Estrogen preferentially stimulates lactosaminoglycan-containing oligosaccharide synthesis in mouse uteri. J. Biol. Chem. **263:** 2270-2279.
39. DUTT, A. & D. D. CARSON. 1990. Lactosaminoglycan assembly, cell surface expression, and release by mouse uterine epithelial cells. J. Biol. Chem. **265:** 430-438.
40. BABIARZ, B. S. & H. J. HATHAWAY. 1988. Hormonal control of the expression of antibody-defined lactosaminoglycans in the mouse uterus. Biol. Reprod. **39:** 699-706.
41. KIMBER, S. J., S. LINDENBERG & A. LUNDBLAD. 1988. Distribution of some Gal$\beta$1-3(4)GlcNAc related carbohydrate antigens on the mouse uterine epithelium in relation to the peri-implantational period. J. Reprod. Immunol. **12:** 297-313.
42. KIMBER, S. J. & S. LINDENBERG. 1990. Hormonal control of a carbohydrate epitope involved in implantation in mice. J. Reprod. Fertil. **89:** 13-21.
43. LINDENBERG, S., K. SUNDBERG, S. J. KIMBER & A. LUNDBLAD. 1988. The milk

oligosaccharide, lacto-N-fucopentaose I, inhibits attachment of mouse blastocysts on endometrial monolayers. J. Reprod. Fertil. **83:** 149–158.
44. SEIF, M. W., J. D. APLIN, L. J. FODEN & V. R. TINDALL. 1989. A novel approach for monitoring the endometrial cycle and detecting ovulation. Am. J. Obstet. Gynecol. **160:** 357–362.
45. SMITH, R. A., M. W. SEIF, A. W. ROGERS, T.-C. LI, P. DOCKERY, I. D. COOKE & J. D. APLIN. 1989. The endometrial cycle: the expression of a secretory component correlated with the luteinising hormone peak. Hum. Reprod. **4:** 236–242.
46. GRAHAM, R. A., T.-C. LI, M. W. SEIF, J. D. APLIN & I. D. COOKE. 1991. The effects of the antiprogesterone RU486 (Mifepristone) on an endometrial secretory glycan: an immunocytochemical study. Fertil. Steril. **55:** 1132–1136.
47. APLIN, J. D., M. E. HOADLEY & M. W. SEIF. 1988. Hormonally regulated secretion of keratan sulphate by human endometrial epithelium. Biochem. Soc. Trans. **17:** 136–137.
48. LESSEY, B. A., L. DAMJANOVICH, C. COUTIFARIS, A. CASTELBAUM, S. M. ALBELDA & C. A. BUCK. 1992. Integrin adhesion molecules in the human endometrium. Correlation with the normal and abnormal menstrual cycle. J. Clin. Invest. **90:** 188–195.
49. TABIBZADEH, S. 1992. Patterns of expression of integrin molecules in human endometrium during the menstrual cycle. Hum. Reprod. **7:** 876–882.
50. KLENTZERIS, L. D., J. N. BULMER, L. K. TREDOSIEWICZ, L. MORRISON & I. D. COOKE. 1993. Beta-1 integrin cell adhesion molecules in the endometrium of fertile and infertile women. Hum. Reprod. **8:** 1223–1230.
51. SONNENBERG, A., J. CALAFAT, H. JANSSEN, H. DAAMS, L. M. H. VAN DER RAAIJ-HELMER, R. FALCIONI, S. J. KENNEL, J. D. APLIN, J. BAKER, M. LOIZIDOU & D. R. GARROD. 1991. Integrin alpha 6/beta 4 complex is located in hemidesmosomes, suggesting a major role in epidermal cell-basement membrane adhesion. J. Cell Biol. **113:** 907–917.
52. HYNES, R. O. 1992. Integrins: versatility, modulation and signalling in cell adhesion. Cell **69:** 11–25.
53. BROWN, T. A., T. BOUCHARD, T. ST. JOHN, E. WAYNER & W. G. CARTER. 1991. Human keratinocytes express a new CD44 core protein as a heparan sulphate intrinsic membrane proteoglycan with additional exons. J. Cell Biol. **113:** 207–221.
54. ARUFFO, A., I. STAMENKOVIC, M. MELNICK, C. B. UNDERHILL & B. SEED. 1990. CD44 is the principal cell surface receptor for hyaluronate. Cell **61:** 1303–1313.
55. GOLDSTEIN, L. A., D. F. H. ZHOU, L. J. PICKER, C. N. MINTY, R. F. BARGATZE, J. F. DING & E. C. BUTCHER. 1989. A human lymphocyte homing receptor, the hermes antigen, is related to cartilage proteoglycan core and link proteins. Cell **56:** 1063–1072.
56. SCREATON, G. R., M. V. BELL, D. G. JACKSON, F. B. CORNELIS, U. GERTH & J. I. BELL. 1992. Genomic structure of DNA encoding the lymphocyte homing receptor CD44 reveals at least 12 alternatively spliced exons. Proc. Natl. Acad. Sci. USA **89:** 12160–12164.
57. STAMENKOVIC, I., A. ARUFFO, M. AMIOT & B. SEED. 1991. The hematopoietic and epithelial forms of CD44 are distinct polypeptides with different adhesion potentials for hyaluronate-bearing cells. EMBO J. **10:** 434–438.
58. GUNTHERT, U., M. HOFMANN, W. RUDY, S. REBER, M. ZOLLER, I. HAUSSMAN, S. MATZKU, A. WENZEL, H. PONTA & P. HERRLICH. 1991. A new variant of glycoprotein CD44 confers metastatic potential to rat carcinoma cells. Cell **65:** 13–24.
59. LINDENBERG, S., S. J. KIMBER & L. HAMBURGER. 1990. Embryo-endometrium interaction. *In* From Ovulation to Implantation. J. H. L. Evers & M. J. Heineman, Eds. Elsevier Biomedical. Amsterdam.
60. SYMINGTON, B. E., Y. TAKADA & W. G. CARTER. 1993. Interaction of integrins $\alpha 2\beta 1$ and $\alpha 3\beta 1$: potential role in keratinocyte intercellular adhesion. J. Cell Biol. **120:** 523–536.
61. RABOUDI, N., J. JULIAN, L. H. ROHDE & D. D. CARSON. 1992. Identification of cell surface heparin/heparan sulphate-binding proteins of a human uterine epithelial cell line (RL95). J. Biol. Chem. **267:** 11930–11939.

62. HILKENS, J., M. J. L. LIGTENBERG, H. L. VOS & S. V. LITVINOV. 1992. Cell membrane-associated mucins and their adhesion-modulating property. TIBS **17:** 359–363.
63. LIGTENBERG, M. J. L., F. BUIJS, H. L. VOS & J. HILKENS. 1992. Suppression of cellular aggregation by high levels of episialin. Cancer Res. **52:** 2318–2324.
64. BUTCHER, E. C. 1991. Leukocyte-endothelial cell recognition: three or more steps to specificity and diversity. Cell **67:** 1033–1036.
65. DENKER, H.-W. 1982. Proteases of the blastocyst and of the uterus. *In* Proteins and Steroids in Early Pregnancy. H. M. Beier & P. Karlson, Eds. 183–208. Springer-Verlag. Berlin.
66. DENKER, H.-W. 1990. Trophoblast-endometrial interactions at embryo implantation: a cell biological paradox. *In* Trophoblast Invasion and Endometrial Receptivity: Novel Aspects of the Cell Biology of Embryo Implantation. H.-W. Denker & J. D. Aplin, Eds. Trophoblast Res. **4:** 3–29.
67. WELSH, A. O. & A. C. ENDERS. 1985. Light and electron microscopic examination of mature decidual cells of the rat with emphasis on the antimesometrial decidua and its degeneration. Am. J. Anat. **172:** 1–29.
68. WELSH, A. O. & A. C. ENDERS. 1987. Trophoblast-decidual cell interactions and establishment of maternal blood circulation in the parietal yolk sac placenta of the rat. Anat. Rec. **217:** 203–219.
69. WELSH, A. O. & A. C. ENDERS. 1991. Chorioallantoic placenta formation in the rat: II. Angiogenesis and maternal blood circulation in the mesometrial region of the implantation chamber prior to placenta formation. Am. J. Anat. **192:** 347–365.
70. APLIN, J. D. 1989. Cellular biochemistry of the endometrium. *In* Biology of the Uterus. R. M. Wynn & W. P. Jollie, Eds. 89–129. Plenum Press. New York.
71. APLIN, J. D. 1991. Implantation, trophoblast differentiation and haemochorial placentation: mechanistic evidence *in vivo* and *in vitro*. J. Cell Sci. **99:** 681–692.
72. HUSTIN, J. & J.-P. SCHAAPS. 1987. Echocardiographic and anatomic studies of the maternotrophoblastic border during the first trimester of pregnancy. Am. J. Obstet. Gynecol. **157:** 162–168.
73. HUSTIN, J. 1992. The maternotrophoblastic interface: uteroplacental blood flow. *In* The First Twelve Weeks of Gestation. E. R. Barnea, J. Hustin & E. Jaunieux, Eds. 97–110. Springer-Verlag. New York.

# Human Trophoblast Invasion

## Autocrine Control and Paracrine Modulation[a]

MICHAEL T. McMASTER,[b] KATHRYN E. BASS,[b]
AND SUSAN J. FISHER[b-e]

*Departments of [b]Stomatology; [c]Obstetrics, Gynecology, and
Reproductive Sciences; [d]Anatomy; and
[e]Pharmaceutical Chemistry
University of California, San Francisco
3rd and Parnassus Avenue
San Francisco, California 94143-0512*

## INTRODUCTION

Human embryonic development depends on the ability of fetal cells to gain access to the maternal circulation. This is accomplished by the transient expression of invasive behavior by trophoblast cells that invade deeply into the uterine wall and breach the uterine spiral arterioles. Invasion occurs throughout the first and early second trimesters of pregnancy, declining rapidly thereafter.[1,2] This unique interaction between genetically distinct populations of cells (*i.e.*, maternal and fetal) must involve elaborate control mechanisms that first allow, and then limit, the invasion of trophoblasts. However, the nature of these control mechanisms is largely unknown.

The invasive subpopulation of cytotrophoblasts arises as a consequence of trophoblast differentiation. In the first trimester of pregnancy, chorionic villi contain cytotrophoblast stem cells that can differentiate to form either syncytiotrophoblasts or mononuclear cytotrophoblasts that invade the uterus. In floating chorionic villi, stem cells fuse to form the syncytium that covers the villus. Lying at the maternal-fetal interface, these cells are bathed by maternal blood and perform gas and nutrient exchange. In anchoring chorionic villi, cytotrophoblasts break through the syncytium and form multilayered columns of nonpolarized cells that attach to, and subsequently invade, the uterine wall (FIG. 1A). These cells, also referred to as intermediate trophoblasts, are found in the pregnant endometrium (deciduum) and the first third of the myometrium (collectively called the placental bed). A subpopulation also invades uterine blood vessels.

To study trophoblast differentiation, we have used two complementary approaches. Immunolocalization studies of placental bed biopsy specimens containing cytotrophoblasts that have invaded the uterus have yielded information about the expression of relevant molecules that are differentially regulated during trophoblast invasion *in vivo* (*e.g.*, adhesion molecules, MHC class I proteins). This approach, however, only gives a static view of a complex and dynamic process.

---

[a] This work was supported by grants from the National Institutes of Health (HD26732 and HD30367) and a Postdoctoral Graduate Research Training Fellowship from the March of Dimes Birth Defects Foundation (#18-92-1148).

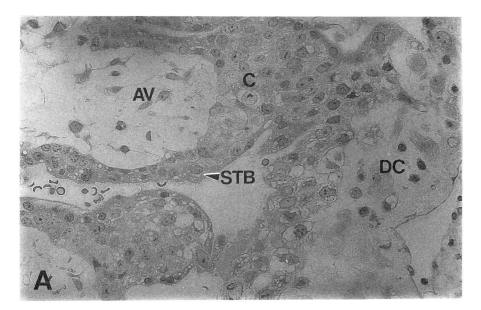

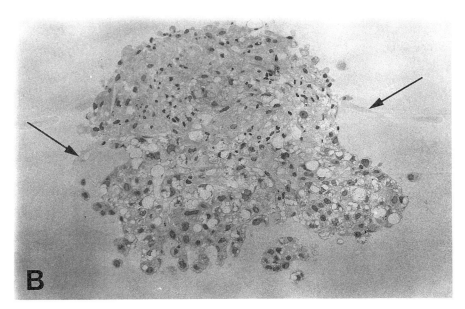

**FIGURE 1.** Appearance of invasive cytotrophoblasts *in vivo* and *in vitro*. (**A**) Frozen section of the maternal-fetal interface at 20 weeks of gestation, stained with hematoxylin and eosin. Maternal blood cells can be seen in the intervillus space at the *lower left* of the micrograph. AV, anchoring villus; C, cytotrophoblast cell column; STB, syncytiotrophoblast; DC, deciduum. (**B**) Cross section of cytotrophoblasts isolated from first trimester placentas, plated on Matrigel and incubated for 72 h. Cells from the aggregate have penetrated the surface of the Matrigel (*arrows*) and are morphologically similar to cell columns observed *in vivo*. (Stained with hematoxylin and eosin.)

We therefore developed procedures for isolating cytotrophoblasts from placentas of different gestational ages.[3,4] These highly purified cell preparations have allowed us to dissect the molecular components of trophoblast invasion *in vitro*. As discussed in the following sections, we have uncovered evidence for both autocrine and paracrine control mechanisms that play an important role in regulating the invasiveness of these unusual cells.

## *Comparison of Trophoblast Invasion in Vivo and in Vitro: Evidence for Autocrine Regulation*

Histological examination of sections of the placental bed stained with anti-cytokeratin antibodies (which label only trophoblasts in this tissue) showed that near the end of the first trimester, many anchoring villi connect the placenta to the uterine wall via extensive cell columns. Cytokeratin-positive cytotrophoblasts in these cell columns have an elongated shape consistent with their migratory character. At this time, trophoblasts have invaded only the superficial portions of uterine blood vessels. During the early portion of the second trimester, cell columns still contain trophoblasts with elongated shapes, indicating that they continue migrating away from the column toward the deeper portions of the uterus (FIG. 1A). By this time they have replaced the muscular coat and endothelial lining of uterine blood vessels as far as the superficial layers of the myometrium (not shown), the limit of trophoblast invasion in normal pregnancy. By the third trimester, cell columns are completely gone, although numerous trophoblasts are present in the decidua and the adjacent myometrium. These late-gestation cells have a rounded shape consistent with their loss of migratory character.

To determine whether trophoblast cells isolated from 1st, 2nd and 3rd trimester placentas also exhibit gestation-related loss of invasiveness, we developed an *in vitro* model of invasion.[4] Briefly, purified cytotrophoblasts are plated on the laminin (Ln)-rich extracellular matrix substrate, Matrigel (Collaborative Research Inc., Bedford, MA). An important advantage of this approach is that soluble factors (*e.g.*, growth factors, cytokines, proteinase inhibitors, function-perturbing antibodies) can be co-polymerized with the Matrigel to investigate their effects on the cells. To observe invasion by light microscopy, cells are plated on Matrigel plugs formed in capsules. After various times the Matrigel plugs are fixed, washed, embedded, and sectioned. To quantify invasion, cytotrophoblasts are plated on Transwell inserts (6.5 mm) containing polycarbonate filters with pores of defined sizes. The upper surface of the filters is coated with 10 $\mu$l of Matrigel and overlaid with cytotrophoblasts ($2 \times 10^5$). After incubation (2–96 h), the Transwell inserts are processed for scanning electron microscopy and invasion is quantified by estimating the surface area of the filter covered by invasive cells.[5] The ability of many types of cells to penetrate the Matrigel and/or migrate through pores of defined sizes has been positively correlated with invasive potential.[6-10]

When plated on Matrigel or other basement membrane preparations, first trimester cytotrophoblasts rapidly formed large, multicellular aggregates and invaded these substrates (FIG. 1B).[3,4] Between 24 h and 48 h in culture the cells progressively invaded the underlying matrix, forming finger-like columns. These invasive cells were highly vacuolated, as *in vivo,* and expressed appropriate markers for intermediate trophoblasts. For example, intermediate cytotrophoblasts in tissue sections of the uterus stain brightly with anti-human placental lactogen (hPL) antibodies.[11] Using sections of Matrigel plugs, we demonstrated that cytotrophoblasts invading basement membrane *in vitro* also stain with anti-hPL antibodies.

Purified cytotrophoblasts *in vitro* also secreted human chorionic gonadotropin (hCG) and progesterone.[4]

Cells isolated from placentas >20 weeks of gestation formed much smaller aggregates that were interspersed among single cells and did not penetrate the surface of the Matrigel on which they were plated. Quantitative invasion assays confirmed that second and third trimester cytotrophoblast cells had greatly reduced invasive potential compared with early-gestation cells.[4] Thus, cultured cytotrophoblasts retain the developmental regulation of invasion they demonstrate *in vivo*.

Subsequently we expanded these initial descriptive studies to examine the role of specific molecules implicated in other invasive processes (*e.g.*, proteinases, adhesion molecules, growth factors, cytokines). For example, the ability of a cell to invade an extracellular matrix (ECM) barrier depends on the production of degradative enzymes. These include plasminogen activators, which are members of the serine proteinase family, and matrix-degrading metalloproteinases (MMPs).[12-14] We have shown, using gelatin substrate gel zymography, that cytotrophoblasts synthesize a variety of metalloproteinases, including both the 72- and the 92-kDa type IV collagenases.[3] However, only production of the 92-kDa type IV collagenase paralleled the invasive properties of the cells; the levels detected were highest in first trimester cells and greatly reduced at term. MMP inhibitors and a function-perturbing antibody specific for the 92-kDa metalloproteinase completely inhibited cytotrophoblast invasion *in vitro*.[4] These experiments demonstrated that the 92-kDa type IV collagenase is rate-limiting for human cytotrophoblast inasion *in vitro* and, therefore, probably plays an important role in invasion *in vivo*. Immunolocalization studies are in progress to determine whether this proteinase is also expressed as cytotrophoblasts invade the uterus.

The adhesive characteristics of cells also correlate with invasiveness. For this reason we used immunocytochemical techniques to examine the expression of integrin adhesion receptors and their ECM ligands by differentiating cytotrophoblasts in tissue sections of the placental bed.[15] Polarized cytotrophoblasts that adhere to the villus basement membrane expressed α6 and β4 integrin subunits (the combination of which is thought to act as a Ln receptor). These cells also stained for multiple forms of Ln, suggesting that they produce this basement membrane constituent as well as a cognate receptor. As these cells leave the villus basement membrane and enter cytotrophoblast cell columns, they modulate their integrin repertoire, expressing primarily the fibronectin (Fn) receptor, α5/β1. Cytotrophoblast clusters in the uterine wall stained for α1 (Ln/collagen receptor), β5 and β1 integrins, but not for most of the ECM ligands with which these receptors interact. These data suggest that invasive cytotrophoblasts interact primarily with surrounding maternal cells and matrices. Furthermore, the dramatic modulation of integrin expression by trophoblasts in the placental bed is evidence that the development of the appropriate adhesion phenotype is critical to the invasion process.

To study the functional role of specific adhesion components, we used our *in vitro* model of trophoblast invasion. Antibodies against type IV collagen (Col IV) and Ln inhibited invasion, but antibodies against Fn had the opposite effect. Consistent with these results, anti-α5/β1 enhanced invasion 2.5-fold. In contrast, antibodies against the α1/β1 Col/Ln receptor reduced invasion by 60%. Taken together, these data suggest that interactions between α5/β1 and Fn may inhibit invasion, whereas interactions of α1/β1 and α6/β1 with Ln and Col IV may promote invasion.[16]

The importance of adhesion molecule expression is further suggested by our studies showing that abnormal regulation of trophoblast integrin expression is associated with preeclampsia.[17] This condition is characterized by abnormally shallow penetration of the decidua by trophoblasts, suggesting that a defect in invasion is involved (for a review see Friedman et al., 1991).[18] Discovery of the dramatic alterations in integrin expression as trophoblast cells differentiate along the invasive pathway led us to postulate that a defect in this process may occur in preeclampsia. By immunohistological staining, we showed that the characteristically shallow invasion consistently seen in preeclampsia is accompanied by abnormalities in integrin expression.[17] The downregulation of $\alpha 6/\beta 4$ and upregulation of $\alpha 5/\beta 1$ and $\alpha 1/\beta 1$ as trophoblasts leave the villus basement membrane, enter cell columns and subsequently invade the uterine wall was not observed in preeclamptic placental beds.[17] The failure of trophoblasts to undergo the integrin transition in preeclampsia suggests a defect in the differentiation of these cells. While factors controlling integrin expression by cytotrophoblasts are unknown, it is possible that aberrant expression of regulatory molecules by maternal cells is responsible for the abnormalities in integrin expression seen in preeclampsia.

Finally, the specialized case of trophoblast invasion requires that the genetically dissimilar fetus and extraembryonic tissues avoid maternal immune rejection during pregnancy. The recent discovery that cytotrophoblasts in culture express a unique class I major histocompatibility complex protein (HLA-G)[19,20] represents significant progress toward an understanding of maternal tolerance at the molecular level. Unlike the highly polymorphic classical class I molecules, expressed on the surface of virtually all other nucleated cells, HLA-G is apparently nonpolymorphic. Thus, it is tempting to speculate that placental HLA-G expression plays an important role in maternal immune tolerance of the fetus by restricting fetal class I expression to a nonpolymorphic molecule, which does not stimulate MHC-restricted rejection by maternal effector cells.

To determine whether HLA-G expression is a consequence of differentiation along the invasive pathway *in vivo*, we again performed immunolocalization studies using an HLA-G–specific monoclonal antibody produced in this laboratory. The results showed that HLA-G was not expressed by any cells in the floating chorionic villus and was first detected in an intermediate zone of the cytotrophoblast cell column (FIG. 2B). In addition, all placental bed cytotrophoblasts, including those which invaded blood vessels, stained brightly with this antibody. Thus, HLA-G expression in the *in vitro* model of invasion parallels the expression observed *in vivo*.

In summary, we have shown that the invasive potential of isolated cytotrophoblasts correlates with their behavior *in vivo*. In addition, we have identified several molecules that mediate important functions relative to the invasion process. These include the 92-kDa type IV collagenase, several adhesion molecules and their ECM ligands, as well as HLA-G. Furthermore, cytotrophoblast expression of these molecules is modulated during invasion, both *in vivo* and *in vitro*. These results suggest that, within the limitations of our assays, removal of the cells from their normal milieu and the influences of uterine cells has surprisingly little effect on cytotrophoblast differentiation along the invasive pathway. Therefore, we postulate that many features of this differentiation pathway are part of a developmental program that, once initiated, may be largely under autocrine control. As discussed in the following section, we hypothesize that the paracrine effects of uterine factors that modulate this process are superimposed upon the intrinsic invasiveness of cytotrophoblasts.

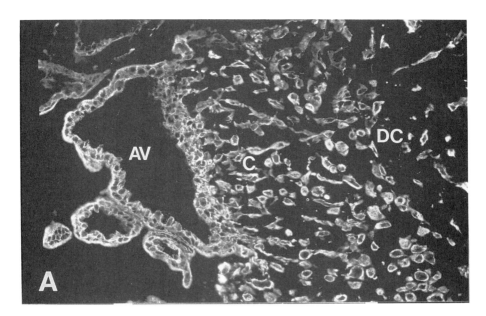

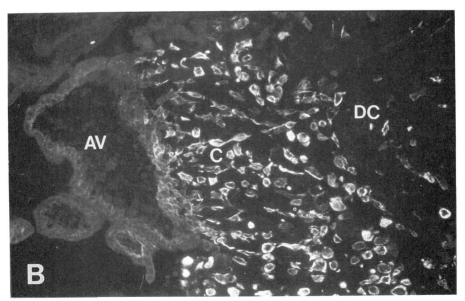

**FIGURE 2.** HLA-G expression by invasive cytotrophoblasts *in vivo*. Frozen sections of the maternal-fetal interface of a normal 20-week placenta were double-stained with anti-cytokeratin **(A)** and anti-HLA-G **(B)**, which were localized with fluorescein- and rhodamine-conjugated secondary antibodies, respectively. AV, anchoring villus; C, cytotrophoblast cell column; DC, deciduum.

## Uterine-Derived Factors Modify the Invasiveness of Trophoblast Cells: Evidence for Paracrine Regulation

Ample evidence suggests that paracrine interactions between trophoblast and uterine cells are an important part of development. For example, it has long been recognized that, beginning at implantation, trophoblasts (trophectoderm) induce significant changes in the endometrium that result in decidual cell proliferation and differentiation. Conversely, trophoblast invasion is controlled and limited by the uterus; thinning of the endometrium is associated with abnormally deep trophoblast invasion (*e.g.*, placenta accreta).

It is likely that a significant proportion of these paracrine effects are mediated by cytokines and growth factors. For example, the CSF-1 receptor is present on human intermediate cytotrophoblasts and syncytiotrophoblasts,[21] whereas the ligand for this receptor is produced by uterine glandular epithelium and endothelial cells.[22] There is an increase in levels of placental mRNA for both CSF-1 and its receptor as gestation proceeds, as well as increased levels of the protein in amniotic fluid.[23] Thus, it is likely that paracrine networks at the maternal-fetal interface involving CSF-1 play an important role in the growth and differentiation of the placenta.

The situation with regard to placental and uterine production of many other growth factors, cytokines and their receptors is far less clear (for reviews see references 24 and 25). Often it is not certain which cells, among the various cell types that constitute these tissues, produce and/or respond to these factors. To begin to understand some of these interactions, our laboratory has used a variety of techniques to identify the repertoire of growth factors, cytokines and their receptors expressed by cytotrophoblasts at different stages of differentiation. Principally, we used the reverse transcriptase-polymerase chain reaction (RT-PCR) to analyze mRNA from highly purified cytotrophoblasts and, when possible, ELISAs to assay protein levels.

Particularly striking among the results we obtain were our findings concerning epidermal growth factor (EGF) and EGF receptor expression by cytotrophoblasts. Other investigators have shown that EGF increases trophoblast production of hCG and hPL[26,27] and induces the differentiation of term cells, as evidenced by syncytium formation.[28] Whether or not these effects are mediated by autocrine and/or paracrine mechanisms is unknown. In an attempt to resolve this question, we used a radioreceptor assay and RT-PCR to examine EGF production by first trimester and term cytotrophoblasts. These experiments showed that neither EGF, transforming growth factor-$\alpha$ (TGF-$\alpha$) nor any other ligands for the EGF receptor are produced by cytotrophoblasts in culture (Bass *et al.*, in preparation). Therefore, the source of EGF receptor ligand is likely maternal, suggesting that EGF may be involved in paracrine (maternal) regulation of cytotrophoblast differentiation.

Interestingly, the human situation seems to parallel that which occurs in the mouse. EGF production by mouse uterine epithelial cells has been demonstrated at the protein and mRNA levels,[29] and significant effects of this growth factor have been demonstrated on the development of mouse embryos *in vitro*.[30] Furthermore, EGF receptors have been identified on the surface of mouse blastocysts[31] but not in the uterine luminal epithelium.[32] Although the mouse blastocyst produces TGF-$\alpha$,[33] it is unlikely to interact with the uterine epithelium which lacks the appropriate receptors. Thus, despite the significant morphological differences between placentation in rodent species and humans, the paracrine action of uterine EGF on trophoblast cells appears to be conserved.

It seems likely that other cytokines and growth factors will have both autocrine and paracrine effects. For example, we and others have shown that cytotrophoblasts produce IL-1$\beta$.[34] Recently, we found that this cytokine is produced by cytotrophoblasts in a developmentally regulated manner, with the highest levels detected during the first trimester of pregnancy. We also showed that cytotrophoblasts express the type I IL-1 receptor, suggesting that they have the potential to both produce and respond to this cytokine. Furthermore, IL-1$\beta$ dramatically affects trophoblast differentiation *in vitro*, as evidenced by a severalfold stimulation of invasion.[35] Since the cells of the pregnant uterus, including the large number of bone-marrow-derived cells that populate the decidua, also have the potential to respond to IL-1$\beta$, it is likely that this cytokine affects differentiation of both maternal and fetal components within the placenta.

## CONCLUSIONS AND FUTURE DIRECTIONS

In conclusion, we showed that the signals necessary for early gestation cytotrophoblasts to invade basement membranes *in vitro* are present in our cultures that lack maternal cells. These results suggest that cytotrophoblasts have an intrinsic pace of invasiveness that does not depend on uterine factors. However, experiments that were aimed at determining which growth factors, cytokines and receptors are produced by cytotrophoblasts suggest that in some cases (*e.g.*, EGF) cytotrophoblasts respond to ligands of maternal origin. Thus, we hypothesize that the primary function of the uterine environment is to modulate trophoblast invasion.

Future studies will concentrate on identifying the molecular basis of autocrine mechanisms that regulate trophoblast differentiation and invasion. These studies will be significantly aided by our ability to precisely define stages of differentiation by using the complex patterns of antigen switching that cytotrophoblasts undergo during invasion *in vivo* and *in vitro*. Thus, one important approach will be to determine which sets of molecules (*e.g.*, MMPs, adhesion molecules, HLA-G) are regulated by cytotrophoblast growth factors and cytokines acting either individually or in concert. Studies of paracrine regulation of invasion are hampered by the difficulty of duplicating the specialized uterine environment *in vitro*. Nevertheless, significant progress is possible as more reagents become available.

## SUMMARY

Development of the human placenta involves rapid invasion of the uterine wall by fetal trophoblasts, a process with certain similarities to tumor cell invasion. Unlike tumor invasion, however, this unique interaction between genetically dissimilar trophoblast and uterine cells is closely regulated and limited both temporally and spatially by mechanisms that are largely unknown. We have used a combination of two experimental approaches to study this process: immunolocalization using tissue sections to investigate trophoblast invasion *in vivo,* and a cell culture model that allows manipulation of the invasion process *in vitro*. The results show that invading trophoblasts express activated forms of metalloproteinases, adhesion molecules and the novel class I histocompatibility antigen, HLA-G, in a highly regulated manner during invasion. The behavior of cytotrophoblasts *in vitro,* removed from the influences of uterine cells, closely parallels their behavior *in vivo,* suggesting the existence of autocrine control mechanisms. However, studies examining the effect of growth factors and cytokines on trophoblast invasion suggest that molecules of uterine origin can modify this process. Thus, we hypothesize that the intrinsic invasiveness of these cells is controlled, at least in part, by the specialized environment of the uterus. Future studies will concentrate on identifying these factors and the specific trophoblast functions they modify.

## REFERENCES

1. BROSENS, I. & H. G. DIXON. 1966. Anatomy of the maternal side of the placenta. J. Obstet. Gynaecol. Br. Commonw. **73:** 357–363.
2. BOYD, J. D. & W. J. HAMILTON. 1970. The Human Placenta. Heffer and Sons. Cambridge, UK.
3. FISHER, S. J., T. CUI, L. ZHANG, L. HARTMAN, K. GRAHL, G. ZHANG, J. TARPEY & C. H. DAMSKY. 1989. Adhesive and degradative properties of human placental cytotrophoblast cells *in vitro.* J. Cell Biol. **109:** 891–902.
4. LIBRACH, C., Z. WERB, M. L. FITZGERALD, K. CHIU, N. CORWIN, R. ESTEVES, D. GROBELNY, R. GALARDY, C. H. DAMSKY & S. J. FISHER. 1991. 92-kD type IV collagenase mediates invasion of human cytotrophoblasts. J. Cell Biol. **112:** 437–449.
5. WEIBEL, E. & R. BOLENDER. 1973. Stereological techniques for electron microscope morphology. *In* Principles and Techniques for Electron Microscopy. M. A. Hayat, Ed. Vol. 3: 237–261. Van Nostrand Co. Inc. New York, NY.
6. TULLBERG, K. & M. BURGER. 1985. Selection of B16 melanoma cells with increased metastatic potential and low intercellular cohesion using Nucleopore filters. Invasion Metastasis **5:** 1–15.
7. KRAMER, R., K. BENSCH & J. WONG. 1986. Invasion of reconstituted basement membrane matrix by metastatic human tumor cells. Cancer Res. **46:** 1980–1989.
8. ALBINI, A., Y. IWAMOTO, H. KLEINMAN, G. MARTIN, S. AARONSON, J. KOZLOWSKI & T. MCEWEN. 1987. A rapid *in vitro* assay for quantitating the invasive potential of tumor cells. Cancer Res. **47:** 3239–3245.
9. HENDRIX, M., E. SEFTOR, R. SEFTOR & I. FIDLER. 1987. A simple quantitative assay for studying the invasive potential of high and low metastatic variants. Cancer Lett. **38:** 137–147.
10. REPESH, L. 1989. A new *in vitro* assay for quantitating tumor cell invasion. Invasion Metastasis **9:** 192–208.
11. KURMAN, R., C. MAIN & H. CHEN. 1984. Intermediate trophoblast: a distinctive form of trophoblast with specific morphological, biochemical and functional features. Placenta **5:** 349–369.
12. ALEXANDER, C. & Z. WERB. 1989. Proteinases and extracellular matrix remodeling. Curr. Opin. Cell Biol. **1:** 1974–1982.
13. MATRISIAN, L. 1990. Metalloproteinases and their inhibitors in matrix remodeling. Trends Genet. **6:** 121–125.
14. HENDRIX, M., E. SEFTOR, T. GROGAN, R. SEFTOR, E. HERSH & E. BOYSE. 1992. Expression of type IV collagenase correlates with the invasion of human lymphoblastoid cell lines and pathogenesis in SCID mice. Mol. Cell Probes **6:** 59–65.
15. DAMSKY, C., M. FITZGERALD & S. FISHER. 1992. Distribution patterns of extracellular matrix components and adhesion receptors are intricately modulated during first trimester cytotrophoblast differentiation along the invasive pathway *in vivo.* J. Clin. Invest. **89:** 210–222.
16. LIBRACH, C., S. J. FISHER, M. L. FITZGERALD & C. H. DAMSKY. 1991. Cytotrophoblast-Fn and cytotrophoblast-laminin interactions have distinct roles in cytotrophoblast invasion. J. Cell Biol. **115:** 6a. (Abstr.)
17. ZHOU, Y., C. H. DAMSKY, K. CHIU, J. M. ROBERTS & S. J. FISHER. 1993. Preeclampsia is associated with abnormal expression of adhesion molecules by invasive cytotrophoblasts. J. Clin. Invest. **91:** 950–960.

18. FRIEDMAN, S. A., R. N. TAYLOR & J. M. ROBERTS. 1991. Pathophysiology of preeclampsia. Clin. Perinatol. **18:** 661–682.
19. KOVATS, S., E. MAIN, C. LIBRACH, M. STUBBLELINE, S. FISHER & R. DEMARS. 1990. A class I antigen, HLA-G, expressed in human trophoblasts. Science **248:** 220–223.
20. ELLIS, S. A., M. S. PALMER & A. J. MCMICHAEL. 1990. Human trophoblast and the choriocarcinoma cell line BeWo express a truncated HLA class I molecule. J. Immunol. **144:** 731–735.
21. PAMPFER, S., E. DAITER, D. BARAD & J. W. POLLARD. 1992. Expression of the colony-stimulating factor-1 receptor (c-fms proto-oncogene product) in the human uterus and placenta. Biol. Reprod. **46:** 48–57.
22. DAITER, E., S. PAMPFER, Y. G. YEUNG, D. BARAD, E. R. STANLEY & J. W. POLLARD. 1992. Expression of colony-stimulating factor-1 in the human uterus and placenta. J. Clin. Endocrinol. Metab. **74:** 850–858.
23. RINGLER, G. E., C. COUTIFARIS, J. F. STRAUSS, J. I. ALLEN & M. GEIER. 1989. Accumulation of colony-stimulating factor-1 in amniotic fluid during human pregnancy. Am. J. Obstet. Gynecol. **160:** 655–656.
24. CASEY, M. L. & P. C. MACDONALD. 1993. Cytokines in the human placenta, fetal membranes, uterine decidua and amniotic fluid. In Molecular Aspects of Placental and Fetal Membrane Autocoids. E. G. Rice & S. P. Brenneke, Eds. 361–394. CRC Press Inc. Boca Raton, FL.
25. HAN, V. K. M. 1993. Growth factors in placental growth and development. In Molecular Aspects of Placental and Fetal Membrane Autocoids. E. G. Rice & S. P. Brenneke, Eds. 395–445. CRC Press Inc. Boca Raton, FL.
26. BARNEA, E. R., D. FELDMAN, M. KAPLAN & D. W. MORRISH. 1990. The dual effect of epidermal growth factor upon human chorionic gonadotropin secretion by the first trimester placenta in vitro. J. Clin. Endocrinol. Metab. **71:** 923–928.
27. MORRISH, D. W., L. H. HONORE & D. BHARDWAJ. 1992. Partial hydatidiform moles have impaired differentiated function (human chorionic gonadotropin and human placental lactogen secretion) in response to epidermal growth factor and 8-bromocyclic adenosine monophosphate. Am. J. Obstet. Gynecol. **166:** 160–166.
28. MORRISH, D. W., D. BHARDWAJ, L. DABBAGH, H. MARUSYK & O. SIY. 1987. Epidermal growth factor induces differentiation and secretion of human chorionic gonadotropin and placental lactogen in normal human placenta. J. Clin. Endocrinol. Metab. **65:** 1282–1290.
29. HUET-HUDSON, Y. M., C. CHAKRABORTY, S. K. DE, Y. SUZUKI, G. K. ANDREWS & S. K. DEY. 1990. Estrogen regulates the synthesis of epidermal growth factor in mouse uterine epithelial cells. Mol. Endocrinol. **4:** 510–523.
30. PARIA, B. C. & S. K. DEY. 1990. Preimplantation embryo development in vitro: cooperative interactions among embryos and role of growth factors. Proc. Natl. Acad. Sci. USA **87:** 4756–4760.
31. PARIA, B. C., H. TSUKAMURA & S. K. DEY. 1991. Epidermal growth factor-specific protein tyrosine phosphorylation in preimplantation embryo development. Biol. Reprod. **45:** 711–718.
32. DAS, S. K., X. WANG, M. KLAGSBRUN, J. ABRAHAM & S. K. DEY. 1993. Heparin-binding epidermal growth factor-like growth factor gene is expressed in the periimplantation mouse uterus and regulated by progesterone and estrogen. Biol. Reprod. **48**(Suppl. 1): 76.
33. RAPPOLEE, D. A., C. A. BRENNER, R. SCHULTZ, D. MARK & Z. WERB. 1988. Developmental expression of PDGF, TGF-$\alpha$ and TGF-$\beta$ genes in preimplantation mouse embryos. Science **241:** 1823–1825.
34. PAULESU, L., A. KING, Y. W. LOKE, M. CLINTORINO, E. BELLIZZI & D. BORASCHI. 1991. Immunohistochemical localization of IL-1 alpha and IL-1 beta in normal human placenta. Lymphokine Cytokine Res. **10:** 443–448.
35. LIBRACH, C. L., S. L. FEIGENBAUM, T. CUI, N. VERASTAS & S. J. FISHER. 1993. Interleukin-1$\beta$ regulates human cytotrophoblast metalloproteinase activity and invasion in vitro. Submitted.

# Negative Regulation of Placental Fibronectin Expression by Glucocorticoids and Cyclic Adenosine 3′,5′-Monophosphate[a,b]

SETH GULLER,[c,d,e] ROBERT WOZNIAK,[d]
MATTHEW I. LEIBMAN,[d] AND CHARLES J. LOCKWOOD[d]

[d]Department of Obstetrics, Gynecology
and Reproductive Science
and
[e]Department of Biochemistry
Mount Sinai Medical Center
One Gustave L. Levy Place
New York, New York 10029-6574

## INTRODUCTION

The fibronectins (FNs) are a group of large extracellular matrix (ECM) glycoproteins which play a vital role in cell adhesion.[1,2] Previous studies have demonstrated that the placenta expresses a FN known as oncofetal FN that is generated by the transfer of α-N-acetylgalactosamine (NAG) from uridine diphosphate (UDP) to a single threonine residue in the third connecting segment (IIICS) of FN by α-N-acetylgalactosaminyl transferase.[3-5] The monoclonal antibody (MAb) FDC-6 differentiates between onfFN and adult forms of FN in extracts of placental tissue, amniotic fluid and cancer cell lines.[4] The presence of onfFN in cervical and vaginal secretions of women at 21 to 37 weeks of gestation was used to identify women who were at risk for preterm delivery.[6] The immunohistochemical localization of onfFN to regions of contact between the placenta and uterus suggested that it is an important mediator of uterine-placental adherence.[6,8] We[7] and others[8] have demonstrated that all FNs released to the culture medium by cytotrophoblasts isolated from human term placentas contained the oncofetal epitope.

---

[a] This work was supported in part by a Mount Sinai Medical Center Seed Grant (to S.G.).
[b] The abbreviations used are: ECM, extracellular matrix; FN, fibronectin; onfFN, oncofetal fibronectin; DEX, dexamethasone; cAMP, cyclic adenosine 3′,5′-monophosphate; 8-bromo-cAMP, 8-bromo-cyclic adenosine 3′,5′-monophosphate; CRH, corticotropin-releasing hormone; E2, estradiol; MPA, medroxyprogesterone acetate; DHT, dihydrotestosterone; DOC, deoxycorticosterone; hCG, human chorionic gonadotropin; hPL, human placental lactogen; NAG, α-N-acetylgalactosamine; NAGT, α-N-acetylgalactosaminyl transferase; SCS medium, culture medium supplemented with 2% charcoal-stripped calf serum; GR, glucocorticoid receptor; GRE, glucocorticoid response element; CRE, cAMP response element; CREB, cAMP response element binding protein.
[c] To whom correspondence should be sent.

Cortisol and corticotropin releasing-hormone (CRH) have been associated with the initiation of parturition based on their profound increase in concentration in maternal plasma and amniotic fluid near parturition whether occurring prior to or at term.[9–12] We have previously reported that glucocorticoids profoundly and specifically inhibit FN and laminin expression in cytotrophoblasts isolated from human term placentas.[13] Based on these data we proposed a model in which we suggested that a pathological rise in glucocorticoids preterm may suppress ECM protein expression and reduce uterine-placental adherence. This could promote aberrant separation of the placenta from the uterus resulting in *abruptio placentae*,[14] membrane rupture and preterm delivery. During normal parturition we suggested that increased levels of cortisol near parturition could similarly reduce ECM protein expression and be associated with separation of the uterus and placenta following expulsion of the fetus.[13]

In the present study we have further evaluated glucocorticoid-mediated suppression of placental FN expression by examining individual and combined effects of glucocorticoids, CRH, estrogens and progestins on FN expression in cytotrophoblasts isolated from human term placentas. Since cyclic adenosine 3′,5′-monophosphate (cAMP) was observed to profoundly regulate FN expression,[2] we examined the effects of cAMP and relaxin, *i.e.*, a peptide produced by placenta that is known to increase intracellular concentrations of cAMP,[15,16] on onfFN expression in cytotrophoblasts. Thus, we tested the effects of glucocorticoids on placental ECM protein expression in the presence of other physiologic compounds associated with human pregnancy. The ECM has been demonstrated to markedly influence the effects of hormones on protein and gene expression.[17,18] Therefore, we also determined whether composition of the ECM alters the pattern of glucocorticoid-mediated effects on FN expression in cytotrophoblasts.

## MATERIALS AND METHODS

### Materials

Tissue culture media, media supplements, and plasticware were obtained from previously described sources.[7,13] Twenty-four-well culture dishes coated with human fibronectin, murine laminin, or rat tail collagen I, and the media supplement ITS$^+$ (containing insulin, transferrin and selenium) were obtained from Collaborative Research (Bedford, MA). The synthetic progestin OD-14 was a gift from Organon (Oss, The Netherlands). RU486 was a gift from Roussel-Uclaf (Romainville, France). Other steroids used in this study were obtained from Sigma (St. Louis, MO) or from Steraloids, Inc. (Wilton, NH). Corticotropin-releasing hormone (CRH) and 8-bromo-cAMP were also obtained from Sigma. Recombinant human relaxin (hRLX-2) was a gift from Genentech, Inc. (South San Francisco, CA). Reagents employed in the isolation of cytotrophoblasts from human term placentas were purchased from previously published sources.[7,13] The ELISA kit utilizing FDC-6 MAb to detect onfFN was a gift from Adeza Biomedical (Sunnyvale, CA). cDNA to human FN was obtained from the American Type Culture Collection (Bethesda, MD). The murine cyclophilin cDNA was generously supplied by Dr. J. Gregor Sutcliffe (Scripps Clinic, La Jolla, CA).

## Methods

### Cell Culture

We isolated cytotrophoblasts from human term placentas with purities of ≥95%[7,13] by a modification of the method of Douglas and King[19] which is based on earlier procedures described by Kliman et al.[20] For experiments, term placentas were obtained from women undergoing uncomplicated cesarean section. Digestion of villous tissue, isolation of cytotrophoblasts on percoll gradients, and procedures employing immunomagnetic microspheres were carried out as we have previously described.[7,13]

Following isolation, cytotrophoblasts were resuspended in SCS medium, a formulation containing a 1 : 1 mixture of phenol red-free Ham's F12 and Dulbecco's Modified Eagle's medium supplemented with 2% charcoal-stripped calf serum and ITS$^+$ (a supplement used to obtain a final concentration of insulin of 6.25 $\mu$g/ml, bovine serum albumin 1.25 mg/ml, transferrin 6.25 $\mu$g/ml, linoleic acid 5.35 $\mu$g/ml, and selenous acid 6.25 ng/ml). Cells were inoculated in SCS medium with or without the indicated compounds at a density of $0.5 \times 10^6$ cells per well of a 24-well dish for ELISA studies and at $7 \times 10^6$ cells per 6-cm dish for Northern blotting analysis.

### Immunoassay for onfFN

We previously measured levels of onfFN in culture media by a sensitive immunoassay (Adeza Biomedical, Sunnyvale CA) using FDC-6 MAb.[7,13] Briefly, for assay, culture media were added to 96-well dishes coated with FDC-6 MAb. After washing and incubation with goat anti-human plasma FN Ab and phenolphthalein monophosphate substrate, optical densities at 550 nm were determined. Sample levels of onfFN were derived from a standard curve employing known concentrations of onfFN.[7] In the current study, intraassay and interassay errors were less than 10% as we have previously reported.[7,13]

Media levels of onfFN were normalized based on the level of cell protein. Cells were scraped and lysed in a solution of 0.2% SDS, 1% (w/v) sodium cholate, 10 mM Tris-HCl, pH 7.4, and nuclei and cell debris were removed by centrifugation ($10,000 \times g$, 5 min). The concentration of supernatant cell protein was measured using the Micro BCA Protein kit from Pierce (Rockford, IL). Alternatively, for experiments in which we examined onfFN expression in cells maintained on tissue culture plastic coated with ECM proteins, results were normalized to levels of total DNA, determined in a fluorometric assay that we previously described.[21]

### Northern Blotting and Detection of FN mRNA

Total RNA was extracted from cytotrophoblasts as we previously described[7,13] using the RNAzol B method, which is a modification of the protocols described by Chomczynski and Sacchi.[7,13] Twenty $\mu$g of total RNA (determined by optical absorbance at 260 nm) per sample was separated on a 1% (w/v) agarose gel containing 2.2 M formaldehyde.[13,23] Following transfer of RNA to Zeta Probe Nylon membranes (BIO-RAD, Richmond, CA), levels of FN and cyclophilin mRNA were determined using $^{32}$P-labeled cDNA probes generated by random primer synthesis.[24] The FN cDNA was 5.6 kb in size consisting of insert and plasmid.[25] cDNA insert for cyclophilin (0.8 kb) was obtained following digestion of plasmid with EcoRI.[26] Separation and purification of plasmids and inserts on agarose gels were carried out as we previously described.[23,27] Autoradiography and densitometry of Northern blots were carried out according to published procedures.[23,27]

## RESULTS

Cytotrophoblasts isolated from human term placentas were maintained in SCS medium with or without DEX (100 nM), CRH (200 nM), E2 (10 nM) and MPA (1000 nM), and after 2 and 5 days of culture, levels of onfFN in the culture medium were measured by immunoassay. As shown in FIGURE 1, DEX treatment reduced levels of onfFN approximately 85% relative to controls. The presence of CRH, MPA or E2 did not affect the DEX-mediated suppression of onfFN expression. CRH had less than a 30% effect on levels of onfFN when employed alone or in combination with DEX, E2 or MPA treatments (FIG. 1). This suggested that CRH did not mediate the glucocorticoid induced suppression of onfFN expression, and that glucocorticoids can reduce onfFN expression in the presence of high concentrations of steroids and peptide paracrine effectors.

Steroid specificity studies demonstrated that, relative to controls, the glucocorticoids DEX, cortisol, and corticosterone promoted a dose-dependent, 65–92% reduction in media levels of onfFN in cytotrophoblast cultures (TABLE 1). Androgens (testosterone and DHT), progestins (progesterone and the synthetic progestins OD-14 and norethynodrel) and the estrogen estradiol (E2) had less than a 30% effect on levels of onfFN without a consistent pattern of dose-dependence (TABLE 1). The mineralocorticoid aldosterone did elicit a dose-dependent reduction in levels of onfFN (TABLE 1). Similarly, glucocorticoid-like effects of aldosterone have been noted in other systems.[28] Interestingly, the progestin MPA promoted a marked (50–75%) reduction in onfFN expression (TABLE 1). MPA has been demonstrated to have glucocorticoid-like activity *in vivo* based on antiinflammatory properties and inhibition of ACTH synthesis.[29] The synthetic steroid RU486 has been found to elicit antiglucocorticoid/antiprogestin effects on gene expression in many systems.[30] We found that RU486 treatment reduced onfFN expression 50% relative to controls (TABLE 1), indicating that it had weak glucocorticoid-like activity in our system. Similarly, steroid agonistic properties of RU-486 have also been demonstrated in other systems.[30]

To determine the effect of ECM composition on glucocorticoid-mediated reduction of onfFN expression, cytotrophoblasts were maintained for 3 days in SCS medium with or without 100 nM DEX on untreated tissue culture wells, or on wells coated with the ECM proteins FN, laminin or collagen I (FIG. 2). We observed that DEX treatment promoted approximately an 80% reduction in media levels of onfFN under all culture conditions. For this experiment, onfFN levels were normalized to cellular levels of DNA and not protein, since use of detergents during extraction of cells could solubilize the exogenous ECM protein coat from the culture well and lead to artifactually high protein values. These results indicated that the presence of an exogenous matrix is not required for glucocorticoids to reduce onfFN expression in cytotrophoblasts.

To examine the effect of cAMP on levels of FN expression in cytotrophoblasts, cells were maintained for 3 days in SCS medium alone, or in medium supplemented with 8-bromo-cAMP (10–1500 nM). As shown in FIGURE 3, the presence of

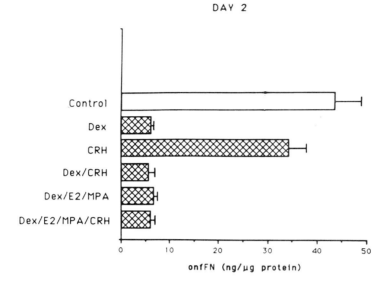
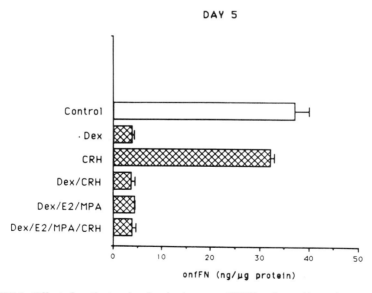

**FIGURE 1.** Effect of corticotropin releasing hormone (CRH) and steroids on glucocorticoid-mediated suppression of onfFN expression in cytotrophoblasts. Cytotrophoblasts isolated from human term placentas were maintained in SCS medium without (Control) or with 100 nM dexamethasone (DEX), 200 nM corticotropin-releasing hormone (CRH), 10 nM estradiol (E2), and 1000 nM medroxyprogesterone acetate (MPA). After 2 and 5 days, levels of onfFN in culture media were measured by immunoassay as described in *Materials and Methods*. Data are presented as a mean ± SD of determinations performed in triplicate.

TABLE 1. Glucocorticoid-Specific Suppression of onfFN Expression in Cytotrophoblasts Isolated from Human Term Placentas[a]

| Steroid Tested | $EC_{50}$ (nM) | Maximal Response (% Inhibition of Control) |
|---|---|---|
| Dexamethasone | 2 | 85–92% |
| Cortisol | 16 | 75–90% |
| Corticosterone | 20 | 65–90% |
| Cortisone | N.D. | <30% |
| MPA | 30 | 50–75% |
| Progesterone | N.D. | <30% |
| Norethynodrel | N.D. | <30% |
| OD-14 | N.D. | <30% |
| E2 | N.D. | <30% |
| Testosterone | N.D. | <30% |
| DHT | N.D. | <30% |
| Aldosterone | 70 | 65–80% |
| DOC | N.D. | <30% |
| RU486 | 110 | 40–60% |

[a] Cytotrophoblasts isolated from human term placentas were incubated for 3 days in SCS medium without (Control) or with the indicated steroids, and levels of onfFN in culture media were determined by immunoassay and standardized based on the level of cell protein. $EC_{50}$s were determined by examining steroid effects in triplicate culture wells at concentrations ranging from 0.1 to 1000 nM. Steroid-induced suppression of onfFN was normalized based on control levels within the same experiment. DEX, dexamethasone; MPA, medroxyprogesterone acetate; E2, estradiol; DHT, dihydrotestosterone; DOC, deoxycorticosterone; N.D., $EC_{50}$s that were not determined because these compounds did not show a clear dose-dependent inhibition of onfFN expression.

8-bromo-cAMP promoted a dose-dependent reduction in media levels of onfFN to approximately 3% of control levels with an $EC_{50}$ of approximately 150 nM.

Cytotrophoblasts were maintained for 3 days in SCS medium with or without 100 nM DEX, 1 mM 8-bromo-cAMP, or 2 nM relaxin, a peptide hormone produced by the placenta that increases intracellular concentrations of cAMP.[15,16] Levels of FN mRNA were estimated following Northern blotting and hybridization of a $^{32}$P-labeled FN cDNA (FIG. 4). Compared with control, treatment of cells with DEX, 8-bromo cAMP, or relaxin promoted a ≥90% reduction in levels of FN mRNA (FIG. 4) based on normalization to levels of cyclophilin mRNA (not shown).

Our results suggest that glucocorticoids and agents that elevate intracellular concentrations of cAMP may profoundly suppress placental FN expression, reduce uterine-placental adherence and influence the poise that exists between maintenance of pregnancy and parturition.

## DISCUSSION

Increased maternal serum levels of glucocorticoids are associated with human parturition whether occurring prior to or at term.[9,12] Levels of CRH are also known to rise dramatically near parturition.[10,11] Although serum levels of estrogens and progestins do not show a dramatic change at parturition, their levels increase throughout pregnancy largely due to synthesis by the placenta.[31] To provide a physiologic context for our studies of glucocorticoid-mediated suppression of ECM protein expression in the human placenta, in the current study we examined glucocorticoid effects on cytotrophoblast onfFN expression in the presence of estrogens, progestins, and CRH. Since glucocorticoids were previously found to dramatically increase placental synthesis of CRH,[32,33] we also determined whether or not CRH treatment alone affected cellular levels of onfFN.

In the present study, our ELISA data indicated that estrogens and progestins do not affect glucocorticoid-mediated suppression of onfFN expression in cytotrophoblasts isolated from term placentas (FIG. 1). We presently (TABLE 1) and previously[7] demonstrated that estrogens and progestins alone do not markedly affect onfFN expression, supporting our hypothesis that steroid suppression of placental ECM protein synthesis is a glucocorticoid-specific process.[7,13] CRH treatment was not found to affect onfFN levels whether employed alone or in combination with DEX (FIG. 1), suggesting that glucocorticoid effects on FN expression were not mediated by CRH. In addition, our results indicated that glucocorticoid-mediated downregulation of FN expression does not require, and is not markedly influenced by the presence of an exogenous ECM (FIG. 2), suggesting that this is a constitutive response in cytotrophoblasts.

We observed that, like glucorticoids, the presence of 8-bromo cAMP profoundly suppressed FN expression in cytotrophoblasts (FIGS. 3 and 4). In many human cell systems cAMP has been observed to markedly increase FN synthesis.[2] Our results are consistent with cAMP-mediated negative regulation of FN expression in human cytotrophoblasts[8] and bovine granulosa cells.[34] Our finding that relaxin, a peptide hormone that increases intracellular concentrations of cAMP,[16]

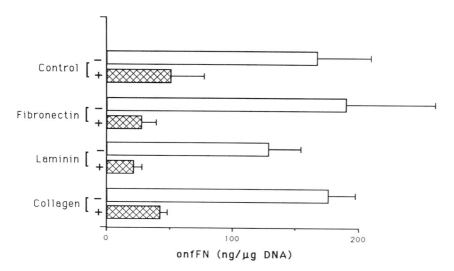

**FIGURE 2.** Influence of extracellular matrix (ECM) protein composition on glucocorticoid-induced reduction of onfFN expression in cytotrophoblast cultures. Cytotrophoblasts were maintained for 3 days in SCS medium with (+) or without (−) 100 nM DEX on untreated tissue culture plastic (Control), or on plastic coated with fibronectin, laminin or collagen I. Media levels of onfFN were quantitated by immunoassay and are presented as a mean ± SD of determinations carried out in triplicate.

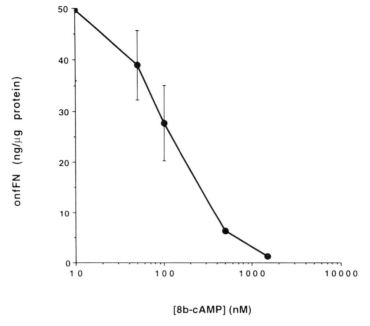

**FIGURE 3.** Dose-dependent inhibition of onfFN expression by 8-bromo-cAMP. Cytotrophoblasts were incubated for 3 days in SCS medium supplemented with the indicated concentration of 8-bromo-cAMP. Media levels of onfFN, obtained by immunoassay, are expressed as a mean ± SD of determinations carried out in triplicate. Control values were 54.9 ± 5.4 ng onfFN/$\mu$g cell protein.

also downregulated FN expression (FIG. 4) may be significant, since this compound is made by the human placenta.[15] Thus, relaxin could regulate placental FN synthesis through an autocrine pathway.

Since the human placenta expresses glucocorticoid receptor (GR),[33,35] it is likely that glucocorticoid-mediated regulation of FN expression observed in the present study was mediated through interaction of the GR with the FN gene. It has been shown that after binding hormone, the GR stimulates gene transcription through interaction with a classic glucocorticoid response element (GRE).[36] Negative regulation of gene expression by glucocorticoids has been suggested to be elicited through binding of GR to negative or composite hormone response elements distinct from classical GREs.[36] cAMP-mediated stimulation of gene expression occurred through a cAMP response element (CRE) in cAMP-activated genes, which increased transcription after binding of the CRE binding protein (CREB).[37] In bovine granulosa cells cAMP inhibited FN gene expression by antagonizing binding to a CRE and by promoting binding of negative regulators of transcription at sites flanking a CRE.[34] Whether glucocorticoids and cAMP reduce FN expression in cytotrophoblasts through analogous mechanisms remains to be elucidated.

The results of the present study indicate that glucocorticoids and peptides that elevate intracellular concentrations of cAMP may be important negative physiologic regulators of placental ECM expression. Thus, increased levels of glucocorticoids and/or increased intracellular levels of cAMP near parturition may suppress FN synthesis, reduce uterine-placental adherence and be associated with the separation of the placenta from the uterus.

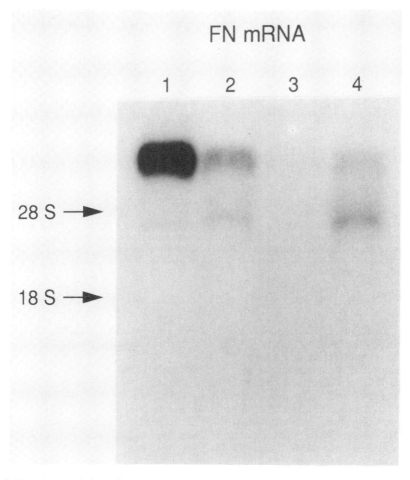

**FIGURE 4.** Regulation of levels of FN mRNA by DEX, 8-bromo cAMP and relaxin. Cytotrophoblasts were maintained for 3 days in SCS medium alone (*lane* 1) or in SCS medium supplemented with 100 nM DEX (*lane* 2), 1 mM 8-bromo-cAMP (*lane* 3) or 2 nM relaxin (*lane* 4). RNA was extracted from cells and 15 μg of total RNA was separated on a 1% agarose gel containing 2.2 M formaldehyde. After transfer of RNA to nylon membranes, levels of FN mRNA were detected using a $^{32}$P-labeled cDNA to human FN. Level of FN mRNA was normalized based on the level of cyclophiln mRNA (not shown) following autoradiography and densitometry.

## SUMMARY

Fibronectin is a ubiquitous extracellular matrix (ECM) protein known to play a critical role in cell adhesion. In the present study we dissected the effects of glucocorticoids and cyclic adenosine 3′,5′-monophosphate (cAMP) on FN expression in cultures of cytotrophoblasts isolated from human term placentas to identify compounds which may influence uterine-placental adherence. Based on immunoassay data, relative to controls, glucocorticoid treatment (1–1000 nM) of cytotrophoblasts specifically inhibited media levels of oncofetal FN (*i.e.*, FNs bearing an oncofetal epitope) 65–92%. Treatment of cytotrophoblasts with androgens, estrogens, and progestins (1–1000 nM) did not markedly affect onfFN expression. Corticotropin-releasing hormone (CRH) treatment (200 nM) alone had no effect on levels of onfFN. In combination experiments using 100 nM dexamethasone (DEX), 1000 nM medroxyprogesterone acetate (MPA), 10 nM estradiol (E2) and 200 nM corticotropin-releasing hormone CRH, we observed that DEX treatment also promoted approximately an 85% reduction in media levels of onfFN. This indicated that glucocorticoids profoundly suppress FN expression in the presence of high concentrations of other steroids and pregnancy-associated paracrine effectors. To examine the influence of ECM protein composition on glucocorticoid-mediated suppression of onfFN expression, cells were inoculated on untreated culture wells or on wells coated with FN, laminin, or collagen I. We observed that DEX treatment downregulated onfFN levels 70–85% under each of these conditions, suggesting that glucocorticoid effects on FN expression were not dependent on the presence of an exogenous ECM. Treatment of cytotrophoblasts with 8-bromo-cAMP resulted in a dose-dependent reduction in onfFN expression to 3% of control levels with an $EC_{50}$ of 150 nM. Based on Northern blotting, treatment of cytotrophoblasts with 100 nM DEX, 1 mM 8-bromo-cAMP, or 2 nM relaxin inhibited steady state levels of FN mRNA approximately 90% relative to controls. Our results suggest that during pregnancy glucocorticoids and compounds that alter intracellular concentrations of cAMP may profoundly suppress FN expression and therefore may have dramatic effects on uterine-placental adherence.

## ACKNOWLEDGMENTS

We would like to thank Rebeca Caze for her technical assistance and Dr. L. Tax of Organon International B.V. for supplying Org OD-14.

## REFERENCES

1. HYNES, R. 1985. Ann. Rev. Cell. Biol. **1:** 67–90.
2. SCHWARZBAUER, J. E. 1991. Curr. Opin. Cell. Biol. **3:** 786–791.
3. MATSUURA, H. & S. HAKOMORI. 1985. Proc. Natl. Acad. Sci. USA **82:** 6517–6521.
4. MATSUURA, H., K. TAKIO, K. TITANI, T. GREENE, S. B. LEVERY, M. K. E. SALYAN & S. HAKOMORI. 1988. J. Biol. Chem. **263:** 3314–3322.
5. MATSUURA, H., T. GREENE & S. HAKOMORI. 1989. J. Biol. Chem. **264:** 10472–10476.
6. LOCKWOOD, C. J., A. E. SENYEI, M. R. DISCHE, D. CASAL, K. D. SHAH, S. N. THUNG, L. JONES, L. DELEGDISH & T. GARITE. 1991. N. Engl. J. Med. **325:** 669–674.
7. GULLER, S., N. C. LACROIX, G. KRIKUN, R. WOZNIAK, L. MARKIEWICZ, E.-Y. WANG, P. KAPLAN & C. J. LOCKWOOD. 1993. J. Steroid Biochem. Mol. Biol. **46:** 1–10.

8. FEINBERG, R. F., H. J. KLIMAN & C. J. LOCKWOOD. 1991. Am. J. Pathol. **138:** 537–543.
9. DORMER, R. A. & J. T. FRANCE. 1973. Steroids **21:** 497–510.
10. BROOKS, A. N. & J. R. G. CHALLIS. 1988. Can. J. Physiol. Pharmacol. **66:** 1106–1112.
11. RILEY, S. C. & J. R. G. CHALLIS. 1991. Placenta **12:** 105–119.
12. DORR, H. G., A. HELLER, H. T. VERSMOLD, W. G. SIPPELL, M. HERRMANN, F. BIDLINGMAIER & D. KNORR. 1989. J. Clin. Endocrinol. Metab. **68:** 863–868.
13. GULLER, S., R. WOZNIAK, G. KRIKUN, J. M. BURNHAM, P. KAPLAN & C. J. LOCKWOOD. 1993. Endocrinology. **133:** 1139–1146.
14. SAFTLAS, A. F., D. R. OLSON, H. K. ATRASH, R. ROCHAT & D. ROWLEY. 1991. Obstet. Gynecol. **78:** 1081–1086.
15. BRYANT-GREENWOOD, G. D. 1991. Mol. Cell. Endocrinol. **79:** C125–C132.
16. FEI, D. T. W., M. C. GROSS, J. L. LOFGREN, M. MORA-WORMS & A. B. CHEN. 1990. Biochem. Biophys. Res. Commun. **170:** 214–222.
17. GATMAITAN, Z., D. M. JEFFERSON, N. RUIZ-OPAZO, L. BIEMPICA, I. M. ARIAS, G. DUDAS, L. A. LEINWAND & L. M. REID. 1983. J. Cell Biol. **97:** 1179–1190.
18. LIN, C. Q. & M. J. BISSELL. 1993. FASEB J. **7:** 737–743.
19. DOUGLAS, G. C. & B. F. KING. 1989. J. Immunol. Meth. **119:** 259–268.
20. KLIMAN, H. J., J. E. NESTLER, E. SERMASI, J. M. SANGER & J. F. STRAUSS III. 1986. Endocrinology **118:** 1567–1582.
21. LOCKWOOD, C. J., Y. NEMERSON, S. GULLER, G. KRIKUN, M. ALVAREZ, V. HAUSKNECHT, E. GURPIDE & F. SCHATZ. 1993. J. Clin. Endocrinol. Metab. **76:** 231–236.
22. CHOMCZYNSKI, P. & N. SACCHI. 1992. Anal. Biochem. **162:** 156–159.
23. GULLER, S., D. L. ALLEN, R. E. CORIN, C. J. LOCKWOOD & M. SONENBERG. 1992. Endocrinology **130:** 2609–2616.
24. SAMBROK, J., E. F. FRITSCH & T. MANIATIS. 1989. Molecular Cloning. A Laboratory Manual. 2nd edit. 7.37–7.45. Cold Spring Harbor Laboratory Press. New York.
25. KORNBLIHTT, A. R., K. VIBE-PEDERSON & F. E. BARALLE. 1984. Nucleic Acids Res. **12:** 5853–5868.
26. SUTCLIFFE, J. G. & K. W. HASEL. 1990. Nucleic Acids Res. **18:** 4019.
27. GULLER, S., R. E. CORIN, K.-Y. WU & M. SONENBERG. 1991. Endocrinology **129:** 527–533.
28. ROUSSEAU, G. G. & J. D. BAXTER. 1979. Glucocorticoid receptors. *In* Glucocorticoid Hormone Action. J. D. Baxter & G. G. Rousseau, Eds. 55. Springer-Verlag. New York.
29. TAUSK, M. & J. DE VISSER. 1972. Pharmacology of orally active progestational compounds: animal studies. *In* Pharmacology of the Endocrine System & Related Drugs: Progesterone, Progestational Drugs & Antifertility Agents. M. Tausk, Ed. Vol. 2: 160. Pergamon Press. New York.
30. MEYER, M.-E., A. PORNON, J. JI, M.-T. BOCQUEL, P. CHAMBON, & H. GRONEMEYER. 1990. EMBO J. **9:** 3923–3932.
31. RYAN, K. J. 1980. Placental synthesis of steroid hormones. *In* Maternal-Fetal Endocrinology. D. Tulchinsky & K. J. Ryan, Eds. 10. W. B. Saunders Company. Philadelphia.
32. JONES, S. A., A. N. BROOKS & J. R. G. CHALLIS. 1989. J. Clin. Endocrinol. Metab. **68:** 825–830.
33. ROBINSON, B. G., R. L. EMANUEL, D. M. FRIM & J. A. MAJZOUB. 1988. Proc. Natl. Acad. Sci. USA **85:** 5244–5248.
34. BERNATH, V. A., A. F. MURO, A. D. VITULLO, M. A. BLEY, J. LINO & A. R. KORNBLIHTT. 1990. J. Biol. Chem. **205:** 18219–18226.
35. SPEEG, JR., K. V. & R. W. HARRISON. 1979. Endocrinology **104:** 1364–1368.
36. FUNDER, J. W. 1993. Science **259:** 1132–1133.
37. YAMAMOTO, K. R., G. A. GONZALEZ, W. H. BIGGS & M. R. MONTMINY. 1988. Nature **334:** 494–498.

# Hormone Regulation and Hormone Antagonist Effects on Protein Patterns of Human Endometrial Secretion during Receptivity[a]

KARIN BEIER-HELLWIG, KARL STERZIK,[b]
BARBARA BONN, ULRIKE HILMES,
MARC BYGDEMAN,[c] KRISTINA GEMZELL-DANIELSSON,[c]
AND HENNING M. BEIER

*Department of Anatomy and Reproductive Biology*
*RWTH University of Aachem*
*D-52057 Aachen, Germany*

[b]*Department of Obstetrics and Gynecology*
*University of Ulm*
*D-89075 Ulm, Germany*

[c]*Department of Obstetrics and Gynecology*
*Karolinska Hospital*
*S-10401 Stockholm, Sweden*

## INTRODUCTION

In the diagnosis and treatment of infertility, knowledge accumulated by intense endocrine monitoring has improved the outcome of viable embryos, yet no appropriate attention has been paid to endometrial reactions. Implantation rates remain low. In view of the fact that 65–90% of apparently normal embryos fail to implant after embryo transfer,[1,2] monitoring of endometrial function in diagnostic as well as in treatment cycles is clearly essential.

So far, the histological evaluation of the endometrium according to Noyes, Hertig and Rock[3] is still the main approach to assessing endometrial quality. However, it has the disadvantage of retrospective insight, since tissue is taken at the end of a given cycle. New research approaches applying the technique of morphometric analysis, related to the LH peak allow evaluation at any time within the luteal phase and promise more precision.[4-7] More and more, detailed information is accumulating to indicate that there is no clinical benefit in luteal phase evaluation from histological dating of the endometrium alone. Balasch *et al.*[8] have clearly shown that histological endometrial adequacy or inadequacy in the

---

[a] The work performed in Aachen, Germany was supported by Schering Aktiengesellschaft, Dept. Fertility Control and Hormone Therapy Research, Berlin, Germany; the investigations performed in Stockholm, Sweden were supported by grants from The Knut & Alice Wallenberg Foundation, Stockholm.

cycle of conception or in previous cycles is unrelated to the outcome of pregnancy in infertile patients.

Higher resolution of morphological structures by transmission or scanning electron microscopy of the epithelial surface so far does not contribute substantially to the interpretation of adequacy of the endometrium and cannot give a prospective judgement either.[9] Consequently, reproductive biologists are searching for a method to assess a receptive endometrium, which goes beyond the information that ultrasound measurement, by now routinely applied in the clinical procedure, can offer.[10-12] Such a new diagnostic method should prove to be reliable, easy and, if necessary, repeatable, and should consequently allow for prospective interpretation in a therapeutic cycle.

Based on our reproductive biological research in several animal models, we have developed techniques that permit protein analyses of the uterine milieu, which is the site where attachment and implantation actually start. From animal models we know that implantation only succeeds in a favorable uterine milieu as a result of an adequate endometrial transformation, which yields a characteristic composition of the proteins in uterine secretion. After electrophoresis, the protein patterns allow for a significant prediction of implantation success. By means of biochemical analysis of the uterine proteins only, we have been able to diagnose and define numerous changes of the endocrine system. For instance, the phenomenon of delayed secretion, initiated by postcoital injection of estrogens revealed that assessment of protein patterns in uterine secretion is a reliable tool.[13,14] This tool has made it possible to predict the proper time at which embryo transfer of viable embryos, *e.g.*, in the rabbit, will succeed in implantation. In addition, a further intriguing experimental approach has shown the reliability of prediction by protein pattern evaluation of uterine secretion in our rabbit model. Postovulatory application of progesterone antagonists (Lilopristone, onapristone, mifepristone) initiates a protein-biochemical alteration of uterine secretion, giving rise to delayed secretion of 4 to 5 days, which in turn does not permit a timely implantation. However, reduction of the progesterone antagonists influences the secretion pattern in such a way that it normalizes gradually, and finally, after a delay of 4 to 5 days, is again ready for implantation. The favorable point of time for embryo transfer in this experimental model could also be predicted precisely.[15-17]

### *Human Endometrial Secretion*

In the human uterus also, the fluid layer on the inner surfaces of the lumen contains a considerable amount of protein. These proteins are transudates of serum origin and products of local glandular secretion.[14] Both components, transudate and secretion material vary in composition and amount during the menstrual cycle dependent on hormonal control. Due to steroid hormone influence, viscosity and biochemical composition in terms of electrolyte concentration, glucoseaminoglycanes, glycogen, peptide and protein contents change. Estrogen decreases the viscosity of uterine secretion, while progesterone stimulates an increase of viscosity.

From cell kinetic studies it is known that cellular proliferation of the endometrial epithelium and glands initiates synthesis and immediate apocrine secretion into the lumen. A significant increase in macromolecules, predominantly proteins, characterizes the preimplantation milieu, in which facilitation for implantation takes place. Production and transformation of the protein composition in uterine secretion regularly are generated strictly dependent on ovarian hormonal control.[18]

However, in up to 30% of patients, endometrial histology appears not to correspond with steroid hormonal regulation in the physiological way, resulting in a defective luteal phase.[19]

Almost two decades ago, we presented the first protein biochemical analyses of human uterine secretion.[20,21] At that time, uterine fluid with an amount of protein large enough for electrophoretical resolution was gained by gently flushing the uterine lumen after hysterectomy. The methodological improvements in the analysis of minute volumes today allows PAGE resolution, reliable and repeatable, as of amounts of protein in the range between 60 and 80 $\mu$g. SDS-treatment of proteins further permits high resolution of protein patterns. As described earlier, the protein biochemical analysis reveals numerous characteristic variations and alterations of protein patterns of uterine secretion in patients of the infertility clinic, the definition of which should lead to more accuracy in diagnosing normality or deficiency of endometrial performance.

## Patients and Methods

So far, we have investigated more than 300 patients from the infertility clinic of the Department of Gynecology of the University of Ulm, Germany. Another small group of 4 patients has been investigated in a clinical study at the Department of Gynecology and Obstetrics of the Karolinska Hospital, Stockholm, Sweden, using mifepristone (RU 486) for treatment at Day +2 after LH. We obtained the samples for investigation after informed consent. A one-way-device was introduced into the uterus to pick up small amounts of uterine secretion out of the cavity. This technique and the "Prevical$^R$" instrument used have been described in detail elsewhere.[22,23] Further, we subjected the protein samples to SDS-PAGE electrophoresis on ultra-thin gradient gels, also described elsewhere in detail.[23] These gels were scanned by a laser densitometer and assessed as "uterine secretion electrophoretic" patterns (USE patterns).

## Biochemical Analysis of the Uterine Secretion Proteins

After SDS-treatment of the protein samples, there appears a considerable number of protein bands in acrylamide gel electrophoresis, particularly among the lower molecular weight fractions. This area is represented by the bands between 68,000 MW (68 kD, Marker Albumin) and 6,500 MW (6.5 kD, Marker Trypsin-Inhibitor from the lung). The totally expressed electrophoretical pattern is comprised of some 60–70 protein bands, the most pronounced and heavy staining of which are the albumin fraction at 68 kD and that of the a-globin fraction at 12.5 kD. The bands below 68 kD are in focus of our investigation. They are characterized by forming 3 groups of very similarly sized, partly faintly staining bands. Group A is represented by bands between 45 and 34 kD, group B between 29 and 25 kD, group C between 18 and 12 kD (FIG. 1).

The protein patterns of various stages of the menstrual cycle represent a dynamic spectrum of appearing and disappearing bands reaching a maximum of individual bands together with the most intensely staining fractions during the time period between the 15th and 24th day of the ideal cycle. All protein patterns analyzed for the "normal" cycle were obtained from patients without hormonal stimulation.[23]

It is obvious that during the beginning of the menstrual cycle, Day 1 to 5, and

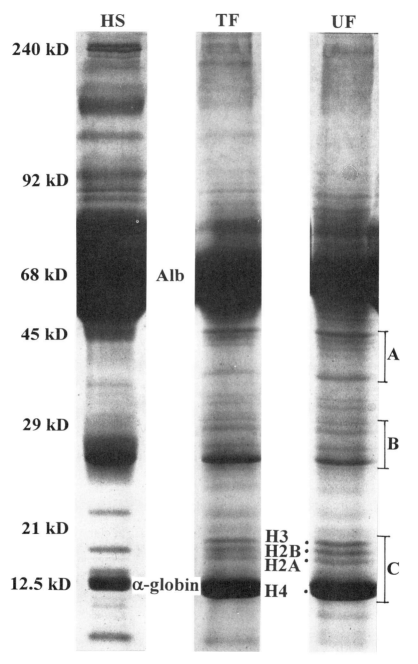

**FIGURE 1.** Protein patterns of human blood serum (HS), human tubal fluid (TF), and human uterine fluid (UF). These patterns demonstrate the similarity of the protein patterns

also at the end of the cycle, Days 25 to 28, there are a number of bands missing while others are only very weakly expressed, except albumin and the 12.5-kD fraction. Particularly, group A and group C lack various bands. These patterns are both considered as "quiescence patterns," and together they form a sort of intermediate phase between the end of secretory and the beginning of proliferative phase patterns, reinforcing that the physiologic cycle is divided into three functional states instead of two.[24-26]

During the period of endometrial proliferation, the protein patterns develop several more intensely staining bands. Finally at Day 14 the pattern of "complete proliferation" is reached. Groups A and B are strongly expressed now, whereas group C has not reached its completion.

Postovulation, there already appears a fully expressed protein pattern with a maximum of bands at all regions of the molecular weight spectrum. Particular attention must be paid to the 3 intensely staining protein bands within group C at the MW range of 14 to 18 kD. The 12.5-kD protein fraction decreases in width and staining intensity during the periovulatory period and stays less prominent for the whole luteal phase. Within all other regions, however, increasingly staining bands appear right from the day after ovulation and comprise a stable pattern over a period of up to 9–10 days. This typical pattern, stable up to Day 24 of the ideal cycle of 28 days, is defined as luteal phase pattern. It seems as if during these 9–10 days of an ideal menstrual cycle there is no decrease or vanishing of components of the protein patterns which may be considered as the patterns of endometrial receptivity.[23]

### Identification of Significant Protein Bands

The most obvious changes during the luteal phase comprise individual protein bands in group C, the molecular weight range between 14.0 and 18.0 kD. After SDS-PAGE using 15% PAA gels, the resolved proteins were transferred to a Millipore Immobilon-P membrane using the discontinuous semidry blotting method for 45 min at 5 mA/cm$^2$ at 15°C. After staining with Commassie Blue G250, the three bands between 14.0 and 18.0 kD were excised and frozen at $-20$°C. These samples were processed for amino acid sequencing using the Applied Biosystems 477A pulsed liquid protein sequencer (Dr. Dietmar Linder, Biochemical Institute, University of Giessen, Germany). The sequence [Pro-Glu-Pro-Ala-Lys-X-Ala-Pro-Ala-Pro] resulted, after the comparison of these 10 amino acid positions, clearly in the identification of histone H2B.

Further investigations using comigration of histones H2A, H2B, H3 and H4 (commercially available from Boehringer Comp., Mannheim, Germany) in SDS-PAGE-electrophoresis revealed convincing evidence (FIG. 2) that all these his-

---

of the genital tract material compared to the significantly different protein pattern of the blood serum. Particularly, the lower molecular weight protein fractions exhibit a clear organ-specific differentiation compared to the compartment of the blood. Both genital tract samples were obtained during the first half of the luteal phase of the menstrual cycle. Particular "families" of protein bands are indicated by the areas of group A, group B, and group C. The molecular weight ranges are shown at the *left margin* of the figure; histones H2A, H2B, H3, and H4, as well as albumin (Alb) and $\alpha$-globin are indicated. SDS-PAGE electrophoresis was performed in a polyacrylamide gradient of 8.3–16.6%.

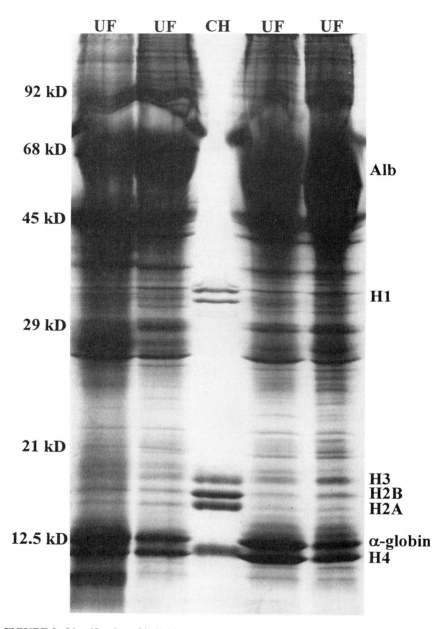

**FIGURE 2.** Identification of individual protein bands of protein patterns of four individual uterine secretion samples (UF) obtained during luteal phases. The USE patterns are demonstrated in comparison with comigrating histones (CH) H1, H2A, H2B, H3, and H4, commercially available from Boehringer Comp., Mannheim, Germany. SDS-PAGE electrophoresis was performed in a high density gel (15% PAA). Alb = albumin, α-globin = monomeric chain of hemoglobin.

tones had corresponding protein bands in the uterine secretion samples.[27] Finally, we were able to present definite proof of molecular identity by immunological identification using polyclonal antibodies directed specifically to histones H2A, H2B, H3 and H4. These antibodies had been produced in rabbits, and were provided by courtesy of Dr. Sylviane Muller, Institute of Molecular and Cellular Biology, CNRS, Strasbourg, France. We used diluted antisera for H2A (1:1000), H2B (1:1500), H3 (1:1500), and H4 (1:1800) in blocking solution. The AP-conjugated secondary goat-anti rabbit antibody was diluted 1:5000. There were no cross-reactions with human blood serum samples and with uterine secretion samples from the beginning of the follicular phase. Since we had no antibodies against histone H1 available, we can only speculate after comigration, using the commercial histone H1 preparations, that these histone bands may also be components of the uterine secretion protein pattern during the luteal phase (FIG. 2).

## *Assessment of USE Patterns*

Monitoring of menstrual cycle quality in the clinical procedure so far lacks any reliable and significant assessment of the "endometrial factor," which might serve as a useful predictive parameter for a receptive endometrium, which is capable of supporting implantation successfully. Regularly, the endometrium reacts as target tissue to the ovarian hormones. Consequently histological dating proved to be a sensitive indicator of ovarian function, reflecting perturbations of the physiological balances of ovarian steroids.[28,29] However, conversely, the assumption that normal or rather sufficient steroid hormone levels measured in blood plasma would guarantee a normal endometrial development is false.

There are numerous reports in the literature[30-35] indicating that despite a normal progesterone output during the luteal phase, there might be an insufficient histological transformation of the endometrium. Even an atrophic endometrium can rarely be present together with normal ovarian function.[36-38] G. S. Jones was the first to discuss a defective endometrial response to hormonal stimulation as cause of luteal inadequacy.[39] As mentioned above, as a rule, endometrial transformation is absolutely dependent on steroid hormone control of the ovary. The dynamic process of transformation is paralleled by a remarkable and characteristic secretory activity. Circumstantially, the endometrial reaction can be segregated from hormonal control. Under such conditions the physiological dependency is broken down, the endometrium turns out to be completely refractory or provides partial response only in that proliferation and/or transformation are not completed. Thus, the endometrium loses the capacity of building up the necessary full composition of protein patterns in uterine secretion which seems to be a prerequisite for the support of implantation. The physiological cycle appears as a dynamic sequence of a continuously changing protein release, which in turn can be analysed by the sequentially changing protein patterns seen in PAGE.

Furthermore, pathological alterations of USE patterns in patients of the infertility clinic can be sensitively assessed. We investigated, for example, protein patterns from stimulated cycles of patients who presented with the tubal factor and underwent stimulation for IVF treatment, but could not receive embryo transfer. In such examples of follicular growth stimulation, we could observe different individual endometrial responses: (a) Physiological luteal phase patterns with *adequate endometrial preparation*. The endometrium of such patient is considered to be in a *receptive stage*. (b) USE pattern, reflecting the *quiescence phase* of the

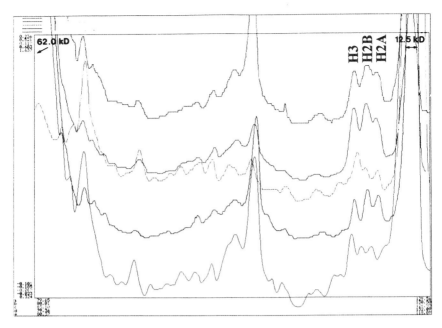

**FIGURE 3.** Laser densitometric assessment of human uterine secretion electrophoretic samples from the second day of the luteal phase (2nd day after LH peak). This figure demonstrates five USE resolutions within segments of the molecular weight ranges from 12.5 to 62.0 kD. The samples express the typical "adequate" luteal phase patterns within the cycle of conception. Each patient experienced a normal clinical pregnancy which began in this cycle. SDS-PAGE was performed in a polyacrylamide gel gradient of 8.3 to 16.6%; laser densitometry was performed by Helium-Neon-Laser at 633 nm. Histones H2A, H2B, and H3 are indicated.

physiological cycle. In this case there *is no endometrial response* to stimulation. (c) USE pattern diagnosis reveals a protein pattern which is *pseudo-proliferative*. The endometrium is capable of *partial response only*, appropriate transformation was not achieved. (d) USE pattern diagnosis reveals an assessment, where *abortive secretion* is found only. The endometrium is *not capable of answering* the steroid hormone stimulation.

Intensive work on determination and interpretation of protein patterns of uterine secretion under various stimulation conditions (HMG, GnRHa) is in progress in our laboratory. We have evidence that densitometric tracing of the SDS-PAGE samples of USE-protein patterns will serve as promising means for clinical evaluation.[16,23] It may eventually lead to new approaches for luteal phase management. Even within a cycle of conception assessment of USE protein patterns is possible. Diagnostic analyses of samples, obtained at the 2nd day after the LH peak, expressed patterns of "adequate" luteal phases. These samples were taken from patients in conception cycles, who went on to normal clinical pregnancies (FIG. 3).

## Progesterone Regulates the Luteal Phase and the Expression of Single Proteins

According to our experience in research on rabbit endometrial proteins, particularly uteroglobin,[15,16] we used the competitive receptor antagonists to progesterone for more detailed studies of progesterone effects on human endometrial proteins. Since mifepristone (RU 486) is the only registered progesterone antagonist that is permitted for clinical application in France, England and Sweden, this compound was studied in its effect on the human luteal phase. Earlier investigations at the Karolinska Hospital[40,41] on dose finding and classical clinical parameters had demonstrated, that a single dose of 200 mg of RU 486 given orally at the second day after the LH peak, inhibited the establishment of pregnancy and allowed an undisturbed menstrual bleeding.[41] Also, along this protocol it has been found that RU 486 was effective in lowering the progesterone receptor concentration in the endometrium, and in turn retarding endometrial maturation, but it did not alter the serum concentration of FSH, estradiol, and progesterone.[40]

Following the same protocol, we started a collaboration to study the effect of a single administration of 200 mg RU 486 on the uterine secretion protein pattern assessed by USE. From the 4 patients, each uterine secretion sample was obtained at day 6 after LH peak in a non-treated control cycle. The following cycle served as treatment cycle, when 200 mg of RU 486 were given at day LH +2, and again the uterine secretion sample was obtained at day LH +6 according to the method described elsewhere.[23] The most striking changes following mifepristone treatment occurred among the histone bands in group C of the USE pattern (FIG. 4). Two of the patients showed significant reduction of the H2A and H3 peaks, whereas the H2B peak revealed only partial reduction compared to the control. Some additional protein bands of group A and group B appeared markedly changed after progesterone antagonist application. However, more detailed information will be available only after more patients will have been investigated. Two of the four patients showed only a relatively weak response to RU 486. Those two patients displayed a significantly abnormal cycle history, beginning already with an unusually extended control cycle. Consequently, we need to include more individuals into this study. However, preliminary evidence already shows that progesterone-dependent events in the luteal phase of the human cycle can be altered by progesterone antagonists, particularly the expression of several single endometrial proteins can be inhibited partly or totally.

## Prediction of the Stage of Receptivity

From animal models we have learned that a histologically normally transformed endometrium must offer an adequate luminal secretion milieu to the preimplantational blastocyst to ensure a stage of "receptivity" which in turn facilitates implantation.[13,16,18,42,44] A complete understanding of the mechanism by which "receptivity" acts to promote implantation requires the identification, and also the isolation and purification of molecules which are the essential components of this uterine luminal milieu, defined as "receptive."

When electrophoretical, chromatographic, and biological means became extremely sensitive, several research groups started independently the isolation and identification of single uterine proteins which reacted immunologically identical to the placental proteins PP12 and PP14. These two proteins soon were characterized as endometrial proteins.[45-65]

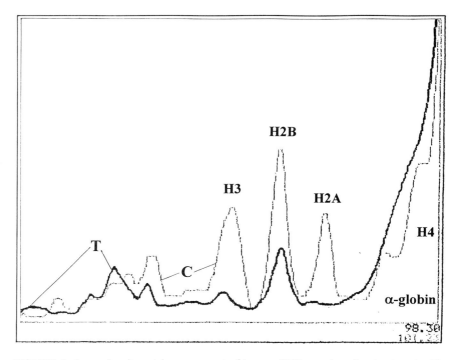

**FIGURE 4.** Laser densitometric assessment of human USE samples after treatment with the progesterone antagonist mifepristone (RU 486), 200 mg at day 2 after the LH surge. The uterine secretion sample was obtained at day 6 after the LH peak. The control sample was assessed equally after collection at day 6 after the LH peak of the preceding nontreated control cycle. Significant changes appear in the histone bands H2A, H2B, and H3. SDS-PAGE was performed in a high density gel (15% PAA). Segment of laser densitometry is shown between molecular weight range of 12.5 kD ($\alpha$-globin) and about 24 kD. Laser densitometric tracing of sample from the treated cycle (T) is printed out in bold compared to the tracing of the control sample (C).

Since the success of the radioimmunological determination of these endometrial proteins within peripheral blood plasma, there have been concepts proposed to develop "blood tests" for diagnostic procedures which should predict the functional stage of the endometrium. So far, however, there is no such reliable blood test available, partly because other sources of synthesis and release of these proteins have been identified in the human body, and partly because circumstantial evidence is against the hypothesis that peripheral blood plasma levels would accurately reflect a substantial synthesis and lumenal release of endometrial proteins. The cellular and histological compartmentation of the endometrium most likely suggests that specific secretory proteins are not released at the same time and at the same quantities into the peripheral circulation. On the contrary, all cell biological evidence on the compartmentation of epithelium, stroma, glands and microcirculation points to the conclusion that those specific protein concentrations of the blood plasma are different from their origin in the endometrium.[43,66-68]

Here again a comparative aspect by the rabbit preimplantation model must be recalled. We are faced with the experimental facts that one single uterine protein alone could never be used as a marker for receptivity. It had turned out that the protein *patterns* always provide the reliable information for the diagnosis of receptivity for implantation.[15,17,43,69,70]

## SUMMARY

Endometrial receptivity is a particular stage of maturation during the luteal phase to permit implantation. We have studied endometrial protein secretion and its patterns evaluated by SDS-PAGE, laser densitometry and Western blots. Uterine secretion electrophoresis (USE) permits highly sophisticated analyses of the intrauterine milieu and allows clinical determination of the receptive stage of the endometrium. This technique reveals direct parameters by patterns of numerous individual protein bands, mainly resolved between 68.0 and 6.5 kD. Characteristic bands appear during the typical functional states of the menstrual cycle presenting evidence on the diagnostic capacity of this method to identify stages of adequate (= normal) or inadequate (= defective) luteal phase maturation. Several individual protein bands appear as characteristic markers for the receptive stage of the luteal phase. We have isolated and molecularly identified several of these proteins: histones H2A, H2B, H3 and H4. In order to identify the endocrine dependency of the protein bands, which significantly contribute to the "receptive stage pattern," patients were treated with the progesterone antagonist RU 486 at day LH +2. The assessment 4 days later revealed deficient USE patterns, particularly diminished and missing bands of the H2A-, H2B-, and H3-histones. These results demonstrate progesterone-dependent components of the endometrium at the receptive stage, which can be used as useful markers for an improved precision in luteal phase diagnostics. On the other hand, essential parts of the protein pattern may serve as new targets for successful contraceptive interventions ("endometrial contraception").

## REFERENCES

1. MACNAMEE, M. C., R. G. EDWARDS & C. M. HOWLES. 1988. The influence of stimulation regimes and luteal phase support on the outcome of IVF. Reprod. **3**(Suppl. 2): 43–52.
2. ROGERS, P. A., B. J. MILNE & A. O. TROUNSON. 1986. A model to show human uterine receptivity and embryo viability following ovarian stimulation for *in vitro* fertilization. J. In Vitro Fertil. Embryo Transfer **3**: 93–98.
3. NOYES, R. W., A. T. HERTIG & J. ROCK. 1950. Dating the endometrial biopsy. Fertil. Steril. **1**: 3–25.
4. JOHANNISSON, E., B.-M. LANDGREN & E. DICZFALUSY. 1987. Endometrial morphology and peripheral hormone levels in women with regular menstrual cycles. Fertil. Steril. **48**: 401–408.
5. JOHANNISSON, E., R. A. PARKER, B.-M. LANDGREN & E. DICZFALUSY. 1982. Morphometric analysis of the human endometrium in relation to peripheral hormone levels. Fertil. Steril. **38**: 564–571.
6. KONINCKX, P. R., P. G. GODDEERIS, J. M. LAUWERYNS, R. C. DE HERTOGH & I. A. BROSENS. 1977. Accuracy of endometrial biopsy dating in the relation of the midcycle luteinizing hormone peak. Fertil. Steril. 28: 443–445.
7. LI, T.-C., A. W. ROGERS, P. DOCKERY, E. A. LENTON & I. D. COOKE. 1988. A new method of histologic dating of human endometrium in the luteal phase. Fertil. Steril. **50**: 52–60.

8. BALASCH, J., F. FABREGUES, M. CREUS & J. A. VANRELL. 1992. The usefulness of endometrial biopsy for luteal phase evaluation in infertility. Hum. Reprod. **7:** 973–977.
9. SUNDSTRÖM, P., O. NILSSON & P. LIEDHOLM. 1983. Scanning electron microscopy of human preimplantation endometrium in normal and clomiphene/human chorionic gonadotropin-stimulated cycles. Fertil. Steril. **40:** 642–647.
10. FLEISCHER, A. C., D. E. PITTAWAY & L. BEARD. 1983. Sonographic depiction of endometrial changes in spontaneous and stimulated cycles. New York: 28th Annual Meeting of the American Society for Sonography, Abstracts Vol.
11. HACKELÖER, B.-J. 1984. The role of ultrasound in female infertility management. Ultrasound Med. Biol. **10:** 35–50.
12. HANSMANN, M., B.-J. HACKELÖER & A. STAUDACH. 1985. Ultraschalldiagnostik in Geburtshilfe und Gynäkologie. Springer-Verlag. Berlin, Heidelberg, New York.
13. BEIER, H. M. 1973. Die hormonelle Steuerung der Uterussekretion und frühen Embryonalentwicklung. 1–216. Habilitationsschrift, Medizinische Fakultät der Christian-Albrechts-Universität Kiel, Kiel, Germany.
14. BEIER, H. M. 1974. Oviductal and uterine fluids. J. Reprod. Fertil. **37:** 221–237.
15. BEIER, H. M., W. ELGER & C. HEGELE-HARTUNG. 1987. Effects of antiprogestins on the endometrium during the luteal phase after postovulatory treatment. *In* The Control of Follicle Development, Ovulation and Luteal Function: Lessions from *in Vitro* Fertilization. F. Naftolin & A. De Cherney, Eds. 331–343. Raven Press. New York.
16. BEIER, H. M., W. ELGER, C. HEGELE-HARTUNG, U. MOOTZ & K. BEIER-HELLWIG. 1991. Dissociation of corpus luteum, endometrium and blastocyst in human implantation research. J. Reprod. Fert. **92:** 511–523.
17. HEGELE-HARTUNG, C., U. MOOTZ & H. M. BEIER. 1992. Luteal control of endometrial receptivity and its modification by progesterone antagonists. Endocrinology **131:** 2446–2460.
18. BEIER, H. M. & U. MOOTZ. 1979. Significance of maternal uterine proteins in the establishment of pregnancy. *In* Maternal Recognition of Pregnancy. 111–140. Ciba Foundation Series, 64. Excerpta Medica. Amsterdam.
19. CROSIGNANI, P. G. 1988. The defective luteal phase. Hum. Reprod. **3:** 157–160.
20. BEIER, H. M. & K. BEIER-HELLWIG. 1973. Specific secretory protein of the female genital tract. Acta Endocrinol. (Copenhagen) (Suppl.) **180:** 404–425.
21. BEIER, H. M., G. PETRY & W. KÜHNEL. 1970. Endometrial secretion and early mammalian development. *In* Mammalian Reproduction. H. Gibian & E. J. Plotz, Eds. 264–285. Kolloquium der Gesellschaft für Biologische Chemie, Mosbach. Springer-Verlag. Berlin, Heidelberg, New York.
22. BEIER-HELLWIG, K., H. M. BEIER, B. BONN & C. GOECKE. 1987. Diagnostik der Proteinsekretion des Uterus durch Abradul-Mikroproben-Entnahme. Arch. Gynecol., **242:** 192–194.
23. BEIER-HELLWIG, K., K. STERZIK & H. M. BEIER. 1988. Zur Rezeptivität des Endometriums: Die Diagnostik der Proteinmuster des menschlichen Uterussekretes. Fertilität **4:** 128–134.
24. BARTELEMEZ, A. W. 1957. The phases of the menstrual cycle and their interpretation in terms of the pregnancy cycle. Am. J. Obstet. Gynec., **74:** 931.
25. FORBES, J. A. & J. C. HEINZ. 1953. Glycogen synthesis in human endometrium. A histochemical study using frozen dried material. Aust. N. Z. J. Surg. **22:** 297.
26. STRAUSS, G. 1962. Zur Histochemie der Kohlenhydrate in den Endometriumdrüsen des Menschen. Arch. Gynäk **197:** 524.
27. HILMES, U., K. BEIER-HELLWIG, K. STERZIK, J. KLUG & H. M. BEIER. 1993. Identification of histones in human uterine secretion samples. J. Reprod. Fertil. Abstr. Ser. **12:** 43.
28. DALLENBACH-HELLWEG, G. 1981. Endometrium. Pathologische Histologie in Diagnostik und Forschung, 2. Aufl. Springer-Verlag. Berlin, Heidelberg, New York.
29. STERZIK, K., C. DALLENBACH, V. SCHNEIDER, V. SASSE & G. DALLENBACH-HELLWEG. 1988. *In vitro* fertilization: the degree of endometrial insufficiency varies with the type of ovarian stimulation. Fertil. Steril. **50:** 457–462.
30. JONES, G. S. & V. MADRIGAL-CASTRO. 1970. Hormonal findings in association with

abnormal corpus luteum function in the human: the luteal phase defect. Fertil. Steril. **21:** 1–12.
31. KELLER, D. W., W. G. WIEST, F. B. ASKIN, L. W. JOHNSON & R. C. STRICKLER. 1979. Pseudocorpus luteum insufficiency: a local defect of progesterone action on endometrial tissue. J. Clin. Endocrinol. Metab. **48:** 127.
32. ROSENBERG, S. M. 1980. Inappropriateness of single midluteal progesterone for diagnosis of corpus luteum defect. Obstet. Gynecol. **56:** 267.
33. ROSENFELD, D. L. & C.-R. GARCIA. 1976. A comparison of endometrial histology with simultaneous plasma progesterone determinations in infertile women. Fertil. Steril. **27:** 1256.
34. WENTZ, A. C., C. M. HERBERT, W. S. MAXSON & C. H. GARNER. 1984. Outcome of progesterone treatment of luteal phase inadequacy. Fertil. Steril. **41:** 856–862.
35. WENTZ, A. C., C. M. HERBERT, W. S. MAXSON, G. A. HILL & D. E. PITTAWAY. 1986. Cycle of conception endometrial biopsy. Fertil. Steril. **46:** 196–199.
36. ENFINGER, H. 1952. Zur Frage des Menstruationsmechanismus. Geburtsh. Frauenheilkd. **12:** 1014.
37. PLOTZ, J. 1950. Der Wert der Basalttemperatur für die Diagnose der Menstruationsstörungen. Arch. Gynäk., **177:** 521.
38. STIEVE, H. 1952. Angeblich sterile Zeiten im Leben geschlechstüchtiger Frauen. Z. Geburtsh. Gynäk **136:** 117.
39. JONES, G. S. 1949. Some newer aspects of the management of infertility. J. Am. Med. Assoc., **141:** 1123.
40. SWAHN, M. L., M. BYGDEMAN, S. CEKAN, S. XING, B. MASIRONI & E. JOHANNISSON. 1990. The effect of RU 486 administered during the early luteal phase on bleeding pattern, hormonal parameters and endometrium. Hum. Reprod. **5:** 402–408.
41. SWAHN, M. L., K. GEMZELL & M. BYGDEMAN. 1991. Contraception with mifepristone. Lancet **338:** 942–943.
42. BEIER, H. M. 1978. Physiology of uteroglobin. *In* Novel Aspects of Reproductive Physiology. C. H. Spilman & J. W. Wilks, Eds. Vol. 8: 219–248. SP Medical & Scientific Books. New York.
43. BEIER, H. M. 1982. Uteroglobin and other endometrial proteins: biochemistry and biological significance in beginning pregnancy. *In* Proteins and Steroids in Early Pregnancy. H. M. Beier & P. Karlson, Eds. 38–71. Springer-Verlag. Berlin, Heidelberg, New York.
44. BEIER, H. M. & P. KARLSON. 1982. Proteins and steroids in early pregnancy. Springer-Verlag. Berlin, Heidelberg, New York.
45. BELL, S. C. 1986. Secretory endometrial and decidual proteins: studies and clinical significance of a maternally derived group of pregnancy-associated serum proteins. Hum. Reprod. **1:** 129–143.
46. BELL, S. C. 1986. Purification of human secretory "pregnancy-associated endometrial $\alpha_2$-globulin" from cytosol of first trimester pregnancy endometrium. Hum. Reprod. **1:** 313–318.
47. BELL, S. C. & H. BOHN. 1985. Immunochemical and biochemical relationship between human pregnancy-associated secreted endometrial $\alpha_1$ and $\alpha_2$-globulins ($\alpha_1$- and $\alpha_2$-PEG) and the soluble placental proteins 12 and 14 (PP12 and PP14). Placenta **7:** 283–294.
48. BELL, S. C., S. R. PATEL, P. H. KIRWAN & J. O. DRIVE. 1986. Protein synthesis and secretion by the human endometrium during the menstrual cycle and the effect of progesterone *in vitro*. J. Reprod. Fertil **72:** 221–231.
49. BELL, S. C., M. W. HALES, S. PATEL, P. H. KIRWAN & J. W. DRIVE. 1985. Protein synthesis and secretion by the human endometrium and decidua during early pregnancy. Br. J. Obstet. Gynaecol. **92:** 793–803.
50. BELL, S. C., S. PATEL, M. W. HALES, P. H. KIRWAN & J. O. DRIFE. 1985. Immunochemical detection and characterization of pregnancy-associated endometrial $\alpha_1$- and $\alpha_2$-globulins secreted by the human endometrium. J. Reprod. Fertil. **74:** 261–270.
51. BOHN, H. & W. KRAUS. 1980. Isolierung und Charakterisierung eines neuen plazentaspezifischen Proteins (PP12). Arch. Gynecol. **229:** 279–281.
52. BOHN, H., W. KRAUS & W. WINCKLER. 1982. New soluble placental tissue proteins:

their isolation, characterization, localization and quantification. Placenta (Suppl.) **4:** 67–81.
53. JOSHI, S. G. 1983. A progestagen-associated protein of the human endometrium: basic studies and potential clinical applications. J. Steroid Biochem. **19:** 751–757.
54. JOSHI, S. G., K. M. EBERT & D. P. SWARTZ. 1980. Detection and synthesis of a progestagen-dependent protein in the human endometrium. J. Reprod. Fertil. **59:** 273–285.
55. JOSHI, S. G., J. E. BANK, E. S. HENRIQUES, A. MARARACHI & G. MATTIES. 1982. Serum levels of progestagen-associated endometrial protein during the menstrual cycle and pregnancy. J. Clin. Endocrinol. Metab. **56:** 642–648.
56. JOSHI, S. G., R. RAO, E. E. HENRIQUES, R. S. RAIKAR & M. GORDON. 1986. Luteal phase concentration of a progestagen-associated endometrial protein (PEP) in the serum of cyclic women with adequate or inadequate endometrium. J. Clin. Endocrinol. Metab. **63:** 1247–1249.
57. JULKUNEN, M. 1986. Human decidua synthesizes placental protein 14 (PP14) *in vitro*. Acta Endocrinol. (Copenhagen) **112:** 271–277.
58. JULKUNEN, M., R. KOSTINEN, J. SJÖBERG, E.-M. RUTANEN, T. WAHLSTRÖM & M. SEPPÄLÄ. 1986. Secretory endometrium synthesizes placental protein 14. Endocrinology **118:** 1782–1786.
59. JULKUNEN, M., E.-M. RUTANEN, A. KOSKIMIES, T. RANTA, H. BOHN & M. SEPPÄLÄ. 1985. Distribution of placental protein 14 in tissue and body fluids during pregnancy. Br. J. Obstet. Gynaecol. **93:** 1145–1151.
60. KOISTINEN, R., N. KALINEN, M.-L. HUHTALA, M. SEPPÄLÄ, H. BOHN & E.-M. RUTANEN. 1986. Placental protein 12 is a decidual protein that binds somatomedin and has an identical N-terminal amino acid sequence with somatomedin-binding protein from human amniotic fluid. Endocrinology **118:** 1375–1378.
61. RUTANEN, E.-M., H. BOHN & M. SEPPÄLÄ. 1982. Radioimmunoassay of placental protein 12: levels in amniotic fluid, cord blood and serum of the healthy adults, pregnant women and patients, with trophoblastic disease. Am. J. Obstet. Gynecol. **144:** 460–463.
62. SEPPÄLÄ, M., T. WAHLSTRÖM, A. L. KOSKIMIES, A. TENHUNEN, E.-M. RUTANEN, R. KOISTINEN, I. HUBTANIEMI, H. BOHN & U.-H. STENMAN. 1984. Human preovulatory follicles, and corpus luteum contain placental protein 12. J. Clin. Endocrinol. Metab. **58:** 505–510.
63. SUTCLIFFE, R. G., S. G. JOSHI, W. F. PATERSON & J. F. BANK. 1982. Serological identity between human alpha uterine protein and human progestagen-dependent endometrial protein. J. Reprod. Fertil. **65:** 207–209.
64. SUTCLIFFE, R. G., A. E. BOLTON, F. SHARPO, L. V. B. NICHOLSON & R. MACKINNON. 1980. Purification of human alpha uterine protein. J. Reprod. Fertil. **58:** 435–442.
65. THAN, G. N., H. BOHN & D. G. SZABO. 1993. Advances in pregnancy-related protein research. Functional and clinical applications. CRC Press. Boca Raton, Ann Arbor, London, Tokyo.
66. MCRAE, A. C. 1988. The blood-uterine lumen barrier and exchange between extracellular fluids. J. Reprod. Fertil. **82:** 857–873.
67. WAITES, G. T., P. L. WOODD, R. A. WALTER & S. C. BELL. 1988. Immunohistological localization of human endometrial secretory protein "pregnancy-associated endometrial $\alpha_2$-globulin" ($\alpha_2$-PEG) during the menstrual cycle. J. Reprod. Fertil. **82:** 665–672.
68. TODOROW, S., E. SIEBZEHNRÜBL, K. BEIER-HELLWIG, U. MEYER, M. BÜHNER, A. TULUSAN, L. WILDT & N. LANG. 1993. PP14 and PP12 determination in human uterine fluid: a less invasive method to monitor endometrial maturity. J. Reprod. Fertil. Abstr. Ser. **12:** 127.
69. BEIER, H. M. 1986. Hormone and Hormonantagonisten in der Implantationsforschung. Fortschr. Fertilitätsforsch. **13:** 2–15.
70. HEGELE-HARTUNG, C. & H. M. BEIER. 1986. Distribution of uteroglobin in the rabbit endometrium after treatment with an anti-progesterone (ZK 98.734): an immunocytochemical study. Hum. Reprod. **1:** 497–505.

# The Role of Leukemia Inhibitory Factor (LIF) and Other Cytokines in Regulating Implantation in Mammals

COLIN L. STEWART

*The Roche Institute of Molecular Biology*
*Roche Research Center*
*340 Kingsland Street*
*Nutley, New Jersey 07110*

## INTRODUCTION

Implantation is the time at which the blastocyst becomes physically more intimately associated with the maternal uterine tissues and is a critical stage in embryonic development. At this time the embryo which has been developing autonomously becomes directly dependent on the maternal environment for its continued development.

Many studies have shown that the uterus plays a central role in regulating the timing of implantation. This has best been illustrated by the phenomenon of delayed implantation, the process by which both the development and implantation of the blastocyst can be arrested for days or even weeks with the duration of delay depending on the species. This form of arrested development occurs quiet widely in many mammalian species.[1,2] Elegant studies involving the transfer of embryos to the uteri of females undergoing implantational delay have showed that it is the uterus rather than the blastocyst that determines the onset of implantation.[3,4]

How implantation is regulated and brought about is still not understood. It has long been recognized that the cells that comprise the endometrium of the uterus, the glandular and luminal epithelium, the stroma and hemopoietic cells, undergo a well described series of proliferative and differentiative changes in anticipation of implantation.[5] Furthermore, it is equally clear that these cellular changes arise in response to the synthesis and secretion of steroid hormones, the estrogens and progesterones. In rodents such as rats and mice an increase in estrogen levels before ovulation results in proliferation of the glandular and luminal epithelial cells of the endometrium. Upon ovulation the levels fall accompanied by a cessation in proliferation. Progesterone, produced by the corpus luteum, inhibits proliferation and also induces differentiation of the epithelial cells to a secretory phenotype. A subsequent brief burst of estrogen, (the nidatory pulse), which in the mouse occurs on the third day of pregnancy results in a further round of proliferation, this time predominantly in the stromal cells of the endometrium. This second round of proliferation is accompanied by further differentiative changes, which are essential for the uterus to become receptive to the embryo, allowing it to implant.[6-8]

In the human, similar changes in cellular proliferation of the uterus occur in response to the steroid hormones, although the details are slightly different. As in the rodent, estrogen induces extensive proliferation in the endometrium and following ovulation progesterone transforms the endometrium into a secretory tissue. However, in contrast to a brief nidatory pulse of estrogen, estrogen levels rise, plateau and then fall over a period of 10–14 days, before either the next cycle begins or pregnancy is initated by implantation.[9]

Clearly the steroid hormones play a central role in regulating the preparation of the uterus for implantation, yet it is becoming increasingly apparent that another group of bioregulatory molecules, namely cytokines or growth factors, play an essential role and may also be the effectors of the steroid hormones.

### *Cytokines in the Regulation of Uterine Cell Proliferation and Implantation*

Many reviews have already extensively documented the changes in the levels and patterns of expression of a multitude of cytokines and growth factors that are found in the uterus throughout the reproductive cycle.[10,11] However, only recently has it become possible to demonstrate their requirement in pregnancy due to the derivation or identification of mice lacking specific factors and because of the availability of experimentally useful amounts of recombinant protein.

At present four cytokines have been shown by experimental means to have a variety of roles during the reproductive cycle, from regulating cell proliferation in the uterus prior to implantation, to controlling the onset of implantation. These are Epidermal Growth Factor (EGF), Colony-Stimulating Factor-1 (CSF-1), Interleukin-1 (IL-1) and Leukemia Inhibitory Factor (LIF). The functions of the first three will be briefly reviewed and a more detailed description of the role LIF will be presented, because it is necessary for regulating implantation.

### *EGF*

Prior to ovulation, EGF is expressed in the uterine epithelium with levels rising following an increase in estrogen. Because estrogen can induce an increase in EGF levels, EGF has been implicated in the regulation of cellular proliferation in the uterus.[12] The evidence for this comes from mice that had been surgically implanted with slow-release pellets containing an antibody against EGF. These mice exhibited a 60–70% reduction in the levels of uterine epithelial proliferation following injection of estradiol. In contrast, ovariectomized mice (thus unable to produce estrogen) that received pellets containing EGF showed significantly increased levels of proliferation in the uterine luminal epithelial cells, in the absence of estradiol.[12,13]

### *CSF-1*

CSF-1 is expressed in the luminal epithelium of the uterus with the levels rising throughout pregnancy so that at term the concentration of CSF-1 is 1000-fold greater than in the nonpregnant uterus. In the early stages of gestation CSF-1 expression is induced by the synergistic action of estrogen and progesterone.[14] The receptor for CSF-1 (CSF-1R) or the proto-oncogene *v-fms* is initially detected in the primary decidua especially in areas adjacent to the ectoplacental cone of the embryo.[15–17] Throughout the remainder of pregnancy uterine expression occurs predominately in the macrophages and to some extent in the placenta. In the embryo, CSF-1R expression is first detectable in the mural trophoblast of the ectoplacental cone of the 10-day embryo where it persists with the levels increasing throughout the remainder of gestation.[18,19] That CSF-1 has a critical role in pregnancy was shown by the existence of a naturally occurring null mutation in the CSF-1 gene, the *op/op* or osteopetrotic mouse.[20,21] Females homozygous for this mutation when crossed to fertile homozygous males fail to produce any viable offspring. Although CSF-1 is clearly required during pregnancy it is not clear at what point during the reproductive cycle this is critical. An additional rather puzzling observation is that female homozygotes mated to heterozygous males show reduced fertility rather than a complete absence of embryos, which would be characteristic of a maternal effect mutation. It has been suggested that some factor present in the seminal fluid or in the heterozygous embryos can compensate for the deficiency in CSF-I.[22]

## *IL-1*

Interleukin-1 is a cytokine that is involved in mediating many inflammatory, physiological, metabolic, hemopoietic and immunological processes.[23,24] Interleukin-1 in fact consists of at least 2 ligands, IL-1$\alpha$ and $\beta$,. There are also 2 receptors, only 1 of which (type 1) has been shown to act as a signal transducer. There is also a naturally occurring antagonist (IL-1rA) that shares sequence homology with IL-1$\beta$ and prevents ligand binding to the receptors. In mice both IL-1$\alpha$ and IL-1$\beta$ are expressed in uterine tissues, with the most abundant expression occurring on the first day of pregnancy. Thereafter, expression falls and reaches basal levels by the fourth day of pregnancy.[25] In the human, IL-1$\beta$ is expressed in the endothelial cells of the spiral capillaries and by the macrophages present in the stroma.[26,27] The type 1 receptor is present on the luminal epithelium with the levels increasing during the post-ovulatory or secretory phase of the cycle.

The evidence that IL-1 may be an essential regulatory factor for early pregnancy or implantation is suggested by the observation that intraperitoneal injection into pregnant mice of high levels of the IL-1 antagonist, starting on the third day of pregnancy results in a significant drop in the number of implantation sites, implying that IL-1 may be a necessary requirement for implantation and that elevated antagonist levels are detrimental to a successful pregnancy.[28]

## *LIF*

Leukemia inhibitory factor was originally cloned and characterized because it induced the differentiation of one myeloid leukemia cell line, M1.[29] Since its discovery LIF has been found to be a member of a family of ligands that show loose structural homology to one another, but can under varying circumstances bind to each other's receptors resulting in similar effects in a variety of biological systems.[30,31] These other members of the LIF family are Interleukin-6 (IL-6), Oncostatin M (OSM) and Ciliary Neurotrophic Factor.[32]

LIF has multiple effects on a variety of different cell types and tissues,[33] and these include the induction of the acute phase response proteins in hepatocytes and liver,[34] regulating bone resorbtion[35] and adipocyte formation,[36] as well as influencing neuronal phenotype and viability in tissue culture.[37,38] However, one of LIF's most striking characteristics is its requirement for inhibiting the differentiation of embryonic stem cells derived from mouse embryos.[39-41]

Embryonic stem (ES) cells are pluripotent cells isolated from the inner cell mass (ICM) of cultured mouse blastocysts.[42] They have attracted much interest, both as a means of studying the molecular basis of early mouse development[43] and as a route to genetically manipulating the genome of mice.[44,45] Their maintenance as stem cells *in vitro* is dependent on their growth on a fibroblast feeder cell layer. Subsequently it was shown that this requirement existed because the feeders produced LIF, which prevented the ES cells from differentiating.[39–41] These observations were, at the time, of particular interest and significance, since LIF was the first protein identified that influenced the differentiation of cells of the early mouse embryo. Subsequent studies have revealed that its influence on the embryo is, surprisingly, mediated through the maternal-uterine environment.

LIF transcripts are found at low levels in a wide variety of different tissues, both in adult and embryonic stages, including the preimplantation embryo.[46–48] Higher levels are detected in the uterus, with 2 distinct peaks of expression: the first at estrous, prior to ovulation[49] and the second on the fourth day of pregnancy (day 1 = day copulation plug),[46] where expression is confined to the endometrial glands. On the fifth day following implantation and decidua formation, the glands degenerate and stop transcribing LIF.[46] The location of LIF expression in the uterus during estrous has not yet been determined.

This pattern of expression was particularly intriguing, because the second peak of expression on the fourth day coincided with the presence of the blastocyst in the uterine lumen. This suggested that LIF expression might be induced by some signal originating from the embryo. However, an alternative possibility is that LIF expression may be independent of the embryo and be under maternal control. By analyzing LIF expression in pseudopregnant females and in females undergoing delayed implantation it was possible to distinguish between these two alternatives.

In mice, copulation is essential for physiologically stimulating the female into preparing for pregnancy by maintaining the corpus luteum so that progesterone levels remain high, thus prolonging the luteal phase of the estrous cycle. Therefore, when a female mates with a vasectomized male, the same changes are initiated in her that are associated with the onset of pregnancy, but because there are no fertilized eggs present, she is referred to as being pseudopregnant.[5] LIF expression in the uteri of these pseudopregnants was the same as that observed in normal pregnant females, showing that LIF expression on the fourth day of pregnancy was not dependent on the presence of viable embryos.[46]

Further evidence that LIF expression is under maternal control came from analyzing its expression in mice undergoing embryonic diapause or delayed implantation. Delayed implantation can be induced experimentally in mice by ovariectomizing a female on the third day of pregnancy, so preventing ovarian production of the nidatory surge of estrogen that is necessary for implantation. Providing that the females are maintained on a relatively high dose of progesterone the blastocysts will enter into a state of delay and will not implant until the females receive a small dose of estrogen. Under natural circumstances, delayed implantation can occur following birth of a litter, since after parturition a female mouse almost immediately ovulates. If she mates with a male then, she then has two sets of offspring to sustain. However, the suckling stimulus of the newborn litter inhibits the ovarian nidatory pulse of estrogen, so preventing implantation of the second set of embryos and the blastocysts enter into a state of delay. Once the suckling stimulus starts to fall, either due to weaning or the loss of the first litter, estrogen expression occurs and the blastocysts implant. In both the ovariectomized and lactating females, in which viable but delayed blastocysts were present in the uteri on the fourth–seventh days following fertilization, no LIF expression was observed. However, as soon as delay was interrupted, by either removing the suckling pups, or by giving a single injection of estrogen, LIF expression was detected within 18–24 hours. These results showed that LIF expression is under maternal control and that it always precedes implantation.[46] Furthermore, because the 2 peaks of LIF expression in the reproductive cycle coincide with elevated levels of estrogen, or can be induced following a single injection of estrogen, these results suggest that LIF expression might be under the direct control of this hormone.

Direct evidence for LIF regulating implantation was obtained with the derivation of mice lacking a functional LIF gene. This was achieved by targeted mutagenesis using homologous recombination to disrupt the LIF gene in ES cells, which were than used to introduce the mutated allele into the germ line of mice. Homozygotes were initially identified at the expected frequency of 25% following heterozygous matings. The homozygotes were overtly normal, except that they were 25–30% smaller in body size.

When the homozygotes were test-mated, the males were found to be fertile, while the females, despite repeated matings with homozygous or wild type males, never produced offspring. However, a closer examination of the female homozygotes following mating, revealed that they were fertile in that overtly normal blastocysts could be recovered from their uteri on the fourth day of pregnancy. Furthermore, blastocysts were also recovered from the uteri on the seventh day of gestation. However, there was no indication in these mice that implantation had been initiated. Morphologically the blastocysts resembled those undergoing delayed implantation with loss of the *zona pellucida* and an elongated shape. By transplanting the embryos to wild type pseudopregnant recipients, it was shown that blastocysts that had developed in a completely LIF-deficient environment were able to develop normally to term if placed in an environment in which LIF was present. Thus the failure of implantation was maternal in origin and not due to abnormalities associated with the blastocysts.[40]

How LIF regulates implantation is at present unclear. It could be acting on the uterus by, for instance, mediating cell proliferation in the epithelial or stromal cells. Or it could be acting on the blastocyst, or both. Currently, we favor the last possibility for the following reasons. We have evidence that LIF receptors are expressed in the uterus, although their exact cellular distribution has not yet been determined. The cellular and proliferative changes that occur in the stromal and epithelial cells of the uterus as a response to the steroid hormones appear to be indistinguishable in the LIF-deficient females from that of wild type controls, indicating that LIF is not involved in mediating these changes in preparation of the uterus for implantation. However, it is well established that the proliferative and differentiative response of the endometrium that occurs with implantation (the decidual response) can be experimentally induced in normal mice by subjecting the uterus at the appropriate time (*i.e.*, fourth–fifth day of pregnancy) to a stimulus of a nonspecific nature (*e.g.*, the injection of a small amount of paraffin oil into the uterine lumen). Attempts to induce this in the LIF-deficient females (mated to vasectomized males) failed to produce a decidual response, whereas all heterozygous controls responded by undergoing decidua formation (E. Cullinan and C. L. Stewart, in preparation). Thus LIF may, therefore, be involved in "priming" of the uterus so making it responsive to implantation signals. However, we believe that LIF may also affect the embryo. The evidence for this is that there are LIF receptors on the trophectoderm, suggesting that LIF produced and secreted from the endometrial glands might have a direct effect on the blastocyst. Furthermore, there is evidence that treating blastocysts with LIF induces gene expression (S. Heyner and C. L. Stewart, in preparation).

The results from these studies have shown that LIF is not essential for overt differentiation of the preimplantation mouse embryo. Rather, its function may have more to do with regulating proliferation in the pre-implantation/peri-implantation embryo. Since LIF may interact with and affect both the uterus and blastocyst, it is an effective means for synchronizing the interaction between these two tissues, so ensuring that the changes in maternal physiology that are associated with pregnancy are co-ordinated with development of the embryo.

## *Implications for Reproduction in Other Mammals*

The LIF gene has been cloned from a variety of other mammalian species, including the human, sheep, cow and pig.[50,51] Therefore, it is of interest to determine whether LIF has a similar role in regulating implantation in these other species as in the mouse. In the sheep, LIF transcripts are detected in the uterus,[52] and the addition of LIF to the medium used to culture pre-implantation stages resulted in a significant increase in the numbers of viable offspring born following uterine transfer, indicating that LIF may have a positive growth stimulus on sheep embryos.[53,54]

In the human LIF transcripts are absent from the uterus during the pre-ovulatory or proliferative phase of the cycle. However, they are expressed in the endometrium during the secretory or post-ovulatory phase, with expression starting around days 18–21 of the cycle. An antibody raised against human LIF was used to localize the expression in the endometrium during the secretory stage and this revealed that it was largely restricted, as in the mouse, to the endometrial glands (C. L. Stewart and B. Lessey, in preparation).

Thus in the human the pattern of LIF expression is similar in timing and distribution to that in the mouse suggesting that it may have a similar role in regulating implantation as in the mouse.

## CONCLUSIONS

There is now good evidence that cytokines are important for the regulation of many of the physiological proliferative and differentiative changes that are associated with maternal-fetal interactions that occur during the reproductive cycle in mammals. Advances in the techniques of molecular biology, especially in the ability to manipulate the expression of genes in the whole animal should make it feasible to gain an accurate description of how these cytokines function. This should provide a better comprehension of how maternal-fetal relationships are regulated during pregnancy and result in a deeper understanding of the causes of infertility and how fertility can be regulated.

## ACKNOWLEDGMENTS

I would like to thank Jeff Pollard for advice on some of the points covered and Alisoun Carey for critical reading of the manuscript.

## REFERENCES

1. RENFREE, M. B. 1978. Embryonic diapause in mammals—a developmental strategy. In Dormancy and Developmental Arrest. M. E. Clutter, Ed. 1–46. Academic Press. New York.
2. RENFREE, M. B. & J. H. CALABY. 1981. Background to delayed implantation and embryonic diapause. J. Reprod. Fertil. (Suppl.) **29:** 67–78.
3. DICKMANN, Z. & V. J. DEFEO. 1967. The rat blastocyst during normal pregnancy and during delayed implantation, including an observation on the shedding of the *zona pellucida*. J. Reprod. Fertil. **13:** 3–9.
4. PSYCHOYOS, A. 1977. Hormonal control of uterine receptivity for nidation. J. Reprod. Fertil. **49:** 355–357.
5. FINN, C. A. & L. MARTIN. 1974. The control of implantation. J. Reprod. Fertil. **39:** 195–206.
6. FINN, C. A. & L. MARTIN. 1969. Hormone secretion during early pregnancy in the mouse. J. Endocrinol. **45:** 57–65.
7. MARTIN, L., C. A. FINN & G. TRINDER. 1973. DNA synthesis in the endometrium of progesterone-treated mice. J. Endocrinol. **56:** 303–307.
8. MARTIN, L., R. M. DAS & C. A. FINN. 1973. The inhibition by progesterone of uterine epithelial proliferation in the mouse. J. Endocrinol. **57:** 549–554.
9. KNOBIL, E. & J. HOTCHKISS. 1988. The menstrual cycle and its neuroendocrine control. The Physiology of Reproduction. E. Knobil & J. D. Neill, Eds. Vol. 2: 1971–1994. Raven Press.
10. TABIBZADEH, S. 1991. Human endometrium: an active site of cytokine production and action. Endocr. Rev. **12:** 272–290.
11. PAMPFER, S., R. J. ARCECI & J. W. POLLARD. 1991. Role of colony stimulating factor-1 (CSF-1) and other lympho-hematopoietic growth factors in mouse pre-implantation development. Bioassays **13:** 535–540.
12. IGNAR, T. D. M., K. G. NELSON, M. C. BIDWELL, S. W. CURTIS, T. F. WASHBURN, J. A. MCLACHLAN & K. S. KORACH. 1992. Coupling of dual signaling pathways: epidermal growth factor action involves the estrogen receptor. Proc. Natl. Acad. Sci. USA **89:** 4658–4662.
13. NELSON, K. G., T. TAKAHASHI, N. L. BOSSERT, D. K. WALMER & J. A. MCLACHLAN. 1991. Epidermal growth factor replaces estrogen in the stimulation of female genital-tract growth and differentiation. Proc. Natl. Acad. Sci. USA **88:** 21–25.
14. POLLARD, J. W., A. BARTOCCI, R. ARCECI, A. ORLOFSKY, M. B. LADNER & E. R. STANLEY. 1987. Apparent role of the macrophage growth factor, CSF-1, in placental development. Nature **330:** 484–486.
15. ARCECI, R. J., F. SHANAHAN, E. R. STANLEY & J. W. POLLARD. 1989. Temporal expression and location of colony-stimulating factor 1 (CSF-1) and its receptor in the female reproductive tract are consistent with CSF-1-regulated placental development. Proc. Natl. Acad. Sci. USA **86:** 8818–8822.
16. DAITER, E., S. PAMPFER, Y. G. YEUNG, D. BARAD, E. R. STANLEY & J. W. POLLARD. 1992. Expression of colony-stimulating factor-1 in the human uterus and placenta. J. Clin. Endocrinol. Metab. **74:** 850–858.
17. PAMPFER, S., S. TABIBZADEH, F. C. CHUAN & J. W. POLLARD. 1991. Expression of colony-stimulating factor-1 (CSF-1) messenger RNA in human endometrial glands during the menstrual cycle: molecular cloning of a novel transcript that predicts a cell surface form of CSF-1. Mol. Endocrinol. **5:** 1931–1938.
18. REGENSTREIF, L. J. & J. ROSSANT. 1989. Expression of the c-fms protooncogene and of the cytokine, CSF-1, during mouse embryogenesis. Dev. Biol. **133:** 284–294.
19. PAMPFER, S., E. DAITER, D. BARAD & J. W. POLLARD. 1992. Expression of the colony-stimulating factor-1 receptor (c-fms protooncogene product) in the human uterus and placenta. Biol. Reprod. **46:** 48–57.
20. YOSHIDA, H., S. HAYASHI, T. KUNISADA, M. OGAWA, S. NISHIKAWA, H. OKAMURA, T. SUDO, L. D. SHULTZ & S. NISHIKAWA. 1990. The murine mutation osteopetrosis is in the coding region of the macrophage colony stimulating factor gene. Nature **345:** 442–444.

21. WIKTOR, J. W., A. BARTOCCI, A. W. J. FERRANTE, A. A. AHMED, K. W. SELL, J. W. POLLARD & E. R. STANLEY. 1990. Total absence of colony-stimulating factor 1 in the macrophage-deficient osteopetrotic (op/op) mouse. Proc. Natl. Acad. Sci. USA **87:** 4828–4832.
22. POLLARD, J. W., J. S. HUNT, J. W. WIKTOR & E. R. STANLEY. 1991. A pregnancy defect in the osteopetrotic (op/op) mouse demonstrates the requirement for CSF-1 in female fertility. Dev. Biol. **148:** 273–283.
23. DINARELLO, C. A. 1991. Interleukin-1 and interleukin-1 antagonism. Blood **77:** 1627–1652.
24. DINARELLO, C. A. 1992. Role of interleukin-1 in infectious diseases. Immunol. Rev. **127:** 119–146.
25. MCMASTER, M. T., R. C. NEWTON, S. K. DEY & G. K. ANDREWS. 1992. Activation and distribution of inflammatory cells in the mouse uterus during the preimplantation period. J. Immunol. **148:** 1699–1705.
26. SIMON, C., G. N. PIQUETTE, A. FRANCES, L. M. WESTPHAL, W. L. HEINRICHS & M. L. POLAN. 1993. Interleukin-1 type I receptor messenger ribonucleic acid expression in human endometrium throughout the menstrual cycle. Fertil. Steril. **59:** 791–796.
27. SIMON, C., G. N. PIQUETTE, A. FRANCES & M. L. POLAN. 1993. Localization of interleukin-1 type I receptor and interleukin-1 beta in human endometrium throughout the menstrual cycle. J. Clin. Endocrinol. Metab. **77:** 549–555.
28. SIMON, C., G. N. PIQUETTE, A. FRANCES, I. EL-DANASSOURI & M. L. POLAN. 1993. Interleukin-1 receptor antagonist (IL-1ra): a novel immune mediator prevents embryonic implantation. Abstract from the American Fertility.
29. HILTON, D. J., N. A. NICOLA & D. METCALF. 1988. Purification of a murine leukemia inhibitory factor from Krebs ascites cells. Anal. Biochem. **173:** 359–367.
30. IP, N. Y., S. H. NYE, T. G. BOULTON, S. DAVIS, T. TAGA, Y. LI, S. J. BIRREN, K. YASUKAWA, T. KISHIMOTO, D. J. ANDERSON & G. D. YANCOPOULOS. 1992. CNTF and LIF act on neuronal cells via shared signaling pathways that involve the IL-6 signal transducing receptor component gp130. Cell **69:** 1121–1132.
31. GEARING, D. P., M. R. COMEAU, D. J. FRIEND, S. D. GIMPEL, C. J. THUT, J. MCGOURTY, K. K. BRASHER, J. A. KING, S. GILLIS, B. MOSLEY & D. COSMAN. 1991. The IL-6 signal transducer, gp130: an oncostatin M receptor and affinity converter for the LIF receptor. Science **255:** 1434–1437.
32. BAZAN, J. F. 1991. Neuropoietic cytokines in the hematopoietic fold. Cell **67:** 197–211.
33. HILTON, D. J. 1992. LIF: lots of interesting functions. Trends Biochem. Sci. **17:** 72–76.
34. BAUMANN, H. & G. G. WONG. 1989. Hepatocyte-stimulating factor III shares structural and functional identity with leukemia-inhibitory factor. J. Immunol. **143:** 1163–1167.
35. ABE, E., H. TANAKA, Y. ISHIMI, C. MIYAURA, T. HAYASHI, H. NAGASAWA, M. TOMIDA, Y. YAMAGUCHI, M. HOZUMI & T. SUDA. 1986. Differentiation-inducing factor purified from conditioned medium of mitogen-treated spleen cell cultures stimulates bone resorption. Proc. Natl. Acad. Sci. USA **83:** 5958–5962.
36. MORI, M., K. YAMAGUCHI & K. ABE. 1989. Purification of a lipoprotein lipase-inhibiting protein produced by a melanoma cell line associated with cancer cachexia. Biochem. Biophys. Res. Commun. **160:** 1085–1092.
37. MURPHY, M., K. REID, M. A. BROWN & P. F. BARTLETT. 1993. Involvement of leukemia inhibitory factor and nerve growth factor in the development of dorsal root ganglion neurons. Development **117:** 1173–1182.
38. YAMAMORI, T., K. FUKADA, R. AEBERSOLD, S. KORSCHING, M. J. FANN & P. H. PATTERSON. 1989. The cholinergic neuronal differentiation factor from heart cells is identical to leukemia inhibitory factor. Science **246:** 1412–1416.
39. WILLIAMS, R. L., D. J. HILTON, S. PEASE, T. A. WILLSON, C. L. STEWART, D. P. GEARING, E. F. WAGNER, D. METCALF, N. A. NICOLA & N. M. GOUGH. 1988. Myeloid leukaemia inhibitory factor maintains the developmental potential of embryonic stem cells. Nature **336:** 684–687.
40. STEWART, C. L., P. KASPAR, L. J. BRUNET, H. BHATT, I. GADI, F. KONTGEN & S. J. ABBONDANZO. 1992. Blastocyst implantation depends on maternal expression of leukaemia inhibitory factor. Nature **359:** 76–79.

41. SMITH, A. G., J. K. HEATH, D. D. DONALDSON, G. G. WONG, J. MOREAU, M. STAHL & D. ROGERS. 1988. Inhibition of pluripotential embryonic stem cell differentiation by purified polypeptides. Nature **336:** 688–690.
42. EVANS, M. J. & M. H. KAUFMAN. 1981. Establishment in culture of pluripotential cells from mouse embryos. Nature **292:** 156–158.
43. MUMMERY, C. L., D. E. V. R. A. J. VAN, A. FEIJEN, E. FREUND, E. HULSKOTTE, J. SCHOORLEMMER & W. KRUIJER. 1990. Expression of growth factors during the differentiation of embryonic stem cells in monolayer [published erratum appears in Dev. Biol. 1991 May; 145(1): 203]. Dev. Biol. **142:** 406–413.
44. CAPECCHI, M. R. 1989. Altering the genome by homologous recombination. Science **244:** 1288–1292.
45. KOLLER, B. H. & O. SMITHIES. 1992. Altering genes in animals by gene targeting. Proc. Natl. Acad. Sci. USA **89:** 6070–6074.
46. BHATT, H., L. J. BRUNET & C. L. STEWART. 1991. Uterine expression of leukemia inhibitory factor coincides with the onset of blastocyst implantation. Proc. Natl. Acad. Sci. USA **88:** 11408–11412.
47. CONQUET, F. & P. BRULET. 1990. Development expression of myeloid leukemia inhibitory factor gene in preimplantation blastocysts and in extraembryonic tissue of mouse embryos. Mol. Cell. Biol. **10:** 3801–3805.
48. MURRAY, R., F. LEE & C. P. CHIU. 1990. The genes for leukemia inhibitory factor and interleukin-6 are expressed in mouse blastocysts prior to the onset of hemopoiesis. Mol. Cell. Biol. **10:** 4953–4956.
49. SHEN, M. M. & P. LEDER. 1992. Leukemia inhibitory factor is expressed by the preimplantation uterus and selectively blocks primitive ectoderm formation *in vitro*. Proc. Natl. Acad. Sci. USA **89:** 8240–8244.
50. WILLSON, T. A., D. METCALF & N. M. GOUGH. 1992. Cross-species comparison of the sequence of the leukaemia inhibitory factor gene and its protein. Eur. J. Biochem. **204:** 21–30.
51. GOUGH, N. M., D. P. GEARING, J. A. KING. T. A. WILLSON, D. J. HILTON, N. A. NICOLA & D. METCALF. 1988. Molecular cloning and expression of the human homologue of the murine gene encoding myeloid leukemia-inhibitory factor. Proc. Natl. Acad. Sci. USA **85:** 2623–2627.
52. POWELL, A. M., C. E. J. REXROAD, N. C. TALBOT & S. OGG. 1993. Leukemia inhibitor factor (LIF) expression in the uterus of the ewe during early pregnancy. 85th Annual Meeting of the American Society of Animal Science. Spokane, WA.
53. FRY, R. C., P. A. BATT, R. J. FAIRCLOUGH & R. A. PARR. 1992. Human leukemia inhibitory factor improves the viability of cultured ovine embryos. Biol. Reprod. **46:** 470–474.
54. FRY, R. C. 1992. The effect of leukaemia inhibitory factor (LIF) on embryogenesis. Reprod. Fertil. Dev. **4:** 449–458.

# Formation of the Chorio-Decidual Interface of Human Fetal Membranes

## Is It Analogous to Anchoring Villi Development in the Placenta?[a]

S. C. BELL AND T. M. MALAK

*Department of Obstetrics and Gynaecology*
*Clinical Sciences Building*
*Leicester Royal Infirmary*
*P.O. Box 65*
*Leicester, LE2 7LX, United Kingdom*

The fetal membranes contain a large chorio-decidual interface. Recent evidence suggests that instability and degradation of this interface is associated with the process of birth at term[1,2] and preterm.[2] It is therefore possible that failure of formation of this interface may result in its premature degradation which may contribute to preterm birth. This interface is formed by attachment and fusion of the cytotrophoblast of the fetal membranes to the decidua parietalis during the second trimester of pregnancy. The mechanisms and control of this process are unknown. However during early pregnancy cytotrophoblasts (CTB) emerge from villous tips and invade the decidua to form the 'anchoring villi' which form part of the placental decidual interface. Recently a pattern of integrins has been reported to reflect the pathway of cytotrophoblastic differentiation during this process.[3] We have therefore examined the distribution of these components in the fetal membranes to determine whether the interface at these sites involves similar mechanisms.

## MATERIAL AND METHODS

Multiple specimens of fetal membranes were obtained after term vaginal deliveries. Cryostat sections were stained with monoclonal antibodies against $\alpha_1$ (TS2/7), $\alpha_3$ (P1B5), $\alpha_5$ (P1D6), $\alpha_6$ (GoH3), $\beta_1$ (102DF5) and $\beta_4$ (3E11) integrin subunits and polyclonal antibody against placental alkaline phosphatase (PLAP). Antibodies were obtained as generous gifts (M. Hemler, A. Sonnenberg and J. Ylanne) or from Bioquote Limited. Tissue sections were examined using a confocal laser scanning microscopy.

## RESULTS

The interface between the CTB and decidua is not clearly demarcated; CTB infiltrate, but not deeply, the underlying decidua. PLAP expression has identified

---

[a] This work was supported by WellBeing, UK.

two CTB subpopulations (FIG. 1): [a] Basal CTB (PLAP$^+$) predominately located towards the chorionic basement membrane (CBM). It is formed of a single layer attached to the CBM and of a variable number of layers of detaching cells. [b] Superficial CTB (PLAP$^-$) predominately located towards the decidua. The basal CTB were $\alpha_6\beta_4{}^+$, $\alpha_5\beta_1{}^-$, $\alpha_3\beta_1{}^{-/+}$, $\alpha_1\beta_1{}^-$ while the superficial CTB were $\alpha_6\beta_4{}^-$, $\alpha_5\beta_1{}^+$, $\alpha_3\beta_1{}^+$, $\alpha_1\beta_1{}^+$ (TABLE 1).

## DISCUSSION

In the chorion of fetal membranes integrin and PLAP[4] expression characterized two CTB subpopulations. In comparison to integrin expression of the CTB of the anchoring villi[3] (TABLE 1); the CTB attached to basement membranes were identical whether in anchoring villi (Zone I, villous) or chorion, *i.e.*, $\alpha_6\beta_4{}^+$, $\alpha_5\beta_1{}^-$. In the chorion the layers of detaching CTB were also referred to as 'basal' since they were PLAP$^+$ and their integrin expression was similar to that of the CTB attached to basement membrane. This relation is similar to that between Zone I and Zone II CTB of the anchoring villi. In the anchoring villi Zone III CTB at the cytotrophoblast-decidual interface appeared to be phenotypically intermediate between Zone I/II cells ($\alpha_6\beta_4{}^+$, $\alpha_5\beta_1{}^-$) and the 'invasive' Zone IV CTB ($\alpha_6\beta_4{}^-$, $\alpha_5\beta_1{}^+$) except the latter uniquely express $\alpha_1\beta_1{}^+$. In contrast the superficial CTB

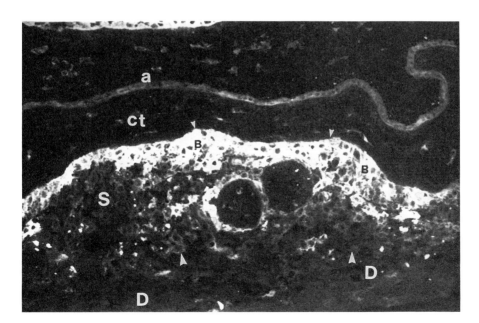

**FIGURE 1.** PLAP (placental alkaline phosphatase)-stained cryostat sections of the fetal membranes. PLAP expression has identified two CTB subpopulations: basal (B) (PLAP$^+$) and superficial (S) (PLAP$^-$). a: amniotic epithelium; ct: connective tissue layer; *small arrow head:* chorionic basement membrane; *large arrow head:* chorio-decidual interface and D: decidua.

TABLE 1. Integrin Expression in the Cell Layers of the Fetal Membranes and the Corresponding Cell Population in the First Trimester Anchoring Villi (+: Positive Staining; −: Negative Staining; −/+: Faint Staining

| Cell Layers of the Fetal Membranes | PLAP | $\alpha_1\beta_1$ | $\alpha_3\beta_1$ | $\alpha_5\beta_1$ | $\alpha_6\beta_4$ | Corresponding Cell Populations in 1st Trimester Anchoring Villi[3] |
|---|---|---|---|---|---|---|
| Cytotrophoblast | | | | | | |
| Basal layer | + | − | −/+ | − | + | cytotrophoblast zones: |
| I: Attached to BM | | | | | | I: villous |
| II: Detaching cells | | | | | | II: proximal column |
| Superficial layer | − | + | + | + | − | cytotrophoblast zone: IV: invasive CTB |
| Decidua | | | | | | |
| Fetal aspect | − | + | + | + | − | |
| Maternal aspect | − | + | + | − | − | |

expressed the 'invasive' Zone IV phenotype. It would appear therefore that paradoxically CTB of the superficial layer have completed their 'invasive' pathway of differentiation yet have not invaded the decidua. Indeed interstitial CTB are less frequently detected in the decidua of the fetal membranes compared to the placental bed. We suggest that fusion of the amniochorion to the decidual parietalis may be analogous to the process involved in the development of anchoring villi although in the former the extent of decidual infiltration is restricted. Defects in this process may result in suboptimal attachment at this site and may underlie premature instability of this interface in preterm birth.

## REFERENCES

1. MALAK, T. & S. BELL. 1993. Contemp. Rev. Obstet. Gynaecol. **5:** 117–123.
2. LOCKWOOD, C., A. SENYEI, M. DISCHE et al. 1991. N. Engl. J. Med. **325:** 669–674.
3. DAMSKY, C., M. FITZGERAID & S. FISHER. 1992. J. Clin. Invest. **89:** 210–222.
4. BULMER, J. & P. JOHNSON. 1985. Placenta **6:** 127–140.

# Morphology of the Human Endometrium in the Peri-Implantation Period

T. C. LI,[a] M. A. WARREN,[c] C. J. HILL,[c]
AND H. SARAVELOS[b]

[a]*Consultant Gynaecologist*
[b]*Biomedical Research Unit*
*Jessop Hospital for Women*
*Leavygreave Road*
*Sheffield S3 7RE, United Kingdom*

and

[c]*Department of Biomedical Science*
*University of Sheffield*
*Western Bank*
*Sheffield S10 2TN, United Kingdom*

## INTRODUCTION

The endometrium is a complex mixture of tissues separating the uterine lumen from the strong muscular supporting layers of the myometrium and delicate perimetrium. It is composed of three distinct compartments; luminal epithelium, glandular epithelium and stroma. Parts of all three contribute to the two functional layers, the functionalis (thought to be shed and renewed every month of reproductive life), and the basalis (the germinal layer from which renewal occurs.[1] This cyclical process is directed by changes in circulating levels of the ovarian hormones, oestradiol and progesterone, themselves under central control.

### *Glandular Epithelium*

As soon as menstruation has ended, the growing ovarian follicle produces oestrogen which stimulates proliferation of cells in the endometrium. Mitoses are seen in both stroma and epithelial compartments and, unlike in intestinal glands where cell division is strictly localised to the basal regions, occur throughout uterine glands. Once the ovarian follicle has matured and released its egg, about 18 hours after the peak in luteinizing hormone (LH),[2] the resulting corpus luteum produces progesterone which causes the most dramatic changes in the cells of the endometrial glands. Mitoses are less common in this luteal or secretory phase than earlier in the cycle and the glands undergo a series of precisely controlled morphological changes, apparently in preparation for blastocyst implantation. Johannisson[3] has reported that the volume of secretion and transudation across the endometrium is greater during the proliferative phase than the secretory phase and peaks about ovulation. This may be due to an oestrogen-induced increase in capillary permeability and blood flow.[4] An overall reduction of fluid from the uterine cavity, which may be related to the early stages of blastocyte-epithelial

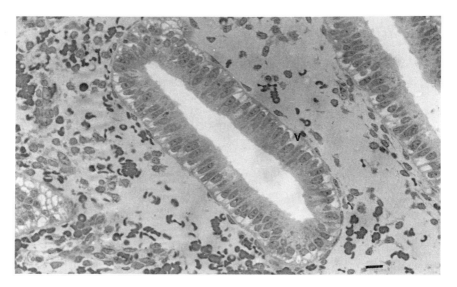

**FIGURE 1.** Light micrograph of endometrium from the early luteal phase showing subnuclear vacuoles of glycogen (V). *Bar* = 10 um.

apposition, begins shortly after ovulation, possibly related to a sodium-led water resorption.[3] Perhaps more important than overall changes in secretory volume are specific modifications to the quality of the secretion. The content, concentration and viscosity of uterine secretions change during the cycle, particularly around the peri-implantation phase, and show strong correlations to changes in cell morphology.[5-8]

During the late proliferative phase cell mitoses are over three times as common as at LH+3 (3 days after the periovulatory peak in LH), decreasing from 23 per 1000 to 7 per 1000.[9] During this time the endometrium thickens, the glands become longer and more tortuous and the average gland lumen increases from about 50 um at LH+0 to 100 um by LH+8.[10,3] Gland cell nuclei in the proliferative phase are unremarkable, being small and round in profile. Changes occur in the early luteal phase when the nucleus becomes oval, rounded and euchromatic. At this time there is an accumulation of storage material in the basal region of the cells so that at day LH+3 distinct subnuclear vacuoles are visible which displace the cell nuclei apically. Since this occurs at slightly different times in adjacent cells, the glandular epithelium acquires a 'pseudo-stratified' appearance (FIGS. 1, 2).[10] By day LH+4 over 10% of the gland cell is occupied by glycogen-containing vacuoles, much more than the 2.5% seen at day LH+2.[11]

These secretions have been shown to contain glycogen-like material by electron microscopic immunohistochemistry[12] and a peptide-associated sialyted oligosaccharide which binds to the monoclonal antibody D9B1[6] and lipid-containing vacuoles, amongst other things.

During the next few days this secretory material passes through vacuoles and the endoplasmic reticulum, eventually to be liberated, at the apical cell surface, into the gland lumen.[6,13] A similar pattern of secretion has also been reported by

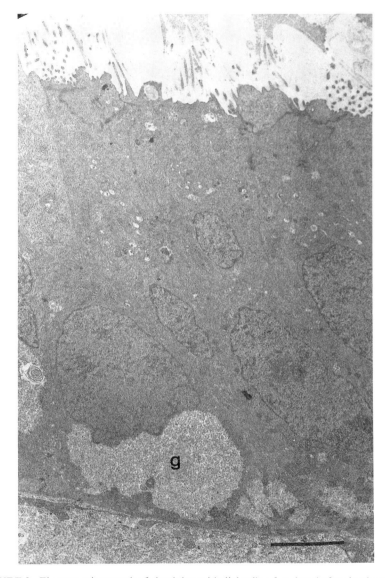

**FIGURE 2.** Electron micrograph of glandular epithelial cells a few days before implantation might occur. Deposits of glycogen (g) are seen basally. *Bar* = 2.5 um.

Klentzeris et al.[5] for the lectins Wheat Germ Agglutinin (WGA) and Concanavalin A (ConA) visualized by an avidin-biotin complex reaction. Interestingly, the staining patterns for both lectins and the D9B1 epitope seen in normal women of proven fertility are disrupted in women classified as unexplained infertile.[14,5] Morphologically the secretory vacuoles may be detected by a decrease in the relative proportion of the cell made up nucleus, although the nucleus itself does not change substantially in volume between days $LH+4$ ($288.1 \pm 20.0$ um$^3$, mean $\pm$ standard error) and $LH+6$ ($260.8 \pm 24.6$ um$^3$).[11] By day $LH+7$, the time at which implantation of the blastocyst would occur, the secretions have largely passed into the glandular lumen and the vacuoles have almost disappeared (making up under 2% of the cell volume) and the nuclei are positioned in the basal part of the cells.

Cyclical changes of the glandular epithelium described above, which clearly illustrate the dynamic nature of the endometrium throughout the menstrual cycle, have a number of implications. Firstly, the morphology of the endometrium throughout the menstrual cycle must be carefully documented in control subjects to establish the normal ranges of measurements in order that any deviation from normality could be measured with confidence. Secondly, in view of the rapid changes of the endometrial morphology throughout the menstrual cycle, any biopsy specimens obtained for study must be timed precisely with reference to a defined reference point, for example ovulation or the luteinizing hormone surge.[2] Otherwise, it may be impossible to conclude that any observed deviation of the morphology from what is expected is a consequence of an underlying endometrial defect, or merely a reflection of the endometria sample being obtained in a different stage of the cycle. It is therefore important that all endometrial samples be precisely timed according to the LH surge, or follicular rupture as observed on serial ultrasonography, either of which is significantly better than that based on the onset of the next menstrual period.[2]

### *Ultrastructure*

During the early luteal phase many other morphological changes occur in the endometrial cells in addition to those described in connection with secretion. These are best seen by electron microscopy.[11,13,15,16] Microvilli increase in length due to elevated oestrogen levels and, in the peri-implantation period of the rat, become irregular with their plasma membranes exhibiting changed molecular dynamics which are essential for implantation.[17] Two other features characterize human glandular epithelial cells around the time of implantation: nuclear channel systems (ncs; FIG. 3) and 'giant' mitochondria (FIG. 4). The ncs is commonly seen in gland cell nuclei at day $LH+4$, while their frequency declines from about day $LH+7$.[13,18] They appear to be complex tubular systems (lumenal diameter about 500–600 nm) with a lumen continuous with the peri-nuclear space.[19] Although several profiles of ncs may be seen in one nucleus it is unknown whether this represents several ncs or one ncs sectioned several times. Kohorn and others[20] reported that the 17-B-position on the D-ring of progesterone is essential for ncs formation. Although ncs do not appear to be essential for secretion they may affect the quality of the secretion. It has been suggested that they influence the transport of recently synthesized mRNA from nucleus to cytoplasm,[19] although they could also affect the process of implantation.[21] In both *in vivo* and *in vitro* studies, exogenous oestrogen has been reported to cause ncs to disappear from gland cell nuclei.[22,23]

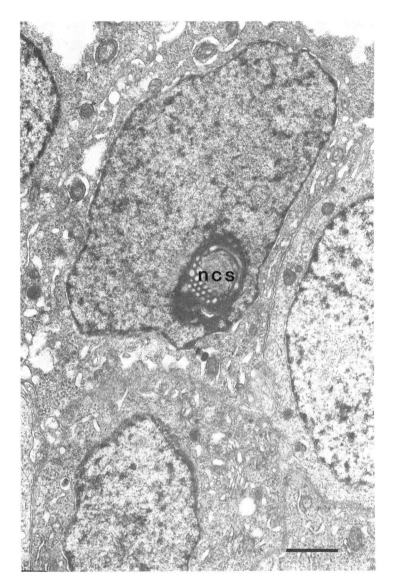

**FIGURE 3.** A large euchromatic nucleus from a gland cell shows a prominent nuclear channel system (ncs) typical of peri-implantation endometrium. *Bar* = 1 um.

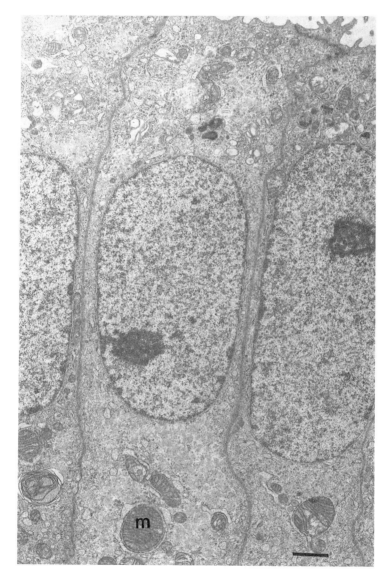

**FIGURE 4.** An electron micrograph showing gland cells at day LH+5. Profiles of giant mitochondria (m) are visible. *Bar* = 1 um.

Giant mitochondria are large, branched organelles with tubular cristae[18] (FIG. 4). They are frequently enveloped in semi-rough endoplasmic reticulum and are thought to develop due to the action of progesterone on the mitochondrial DNA.[12,24] Their function is unknown, but it is likely to be related to the energy requirements of the active endometrium and its need to respond to rapid fluxes in progesterone.

Changes are seen also in the ultrastructure of the Golgi apparatus in the peri-implantation period. Just after ovulation stacks of Golgi are seen to lie parallel to the apical cell surface. By day LH+6 these cisternae have enlarged and are oriented along the long axis of the cell;[13] they then degenerate if pregnancy does not occur.[25]

There is little doubt that ultrastructural study helps to further understand the cellular biology of the endometrium. In addition, it is possible that ultrastructural study may detect subtle changes in the endometrium not otherwise detectable at the light microscopic level. For example, in our recent study on the impact of growth hormone on endometrial morphology in the peri-implantation period in the artificial cycle, although we were unable to detect any significant changes in the endometrium at the light microscopic level, defined changes at the ultrastructural level were observed (Li and Warren, unpublished data).

## *Luminal Epithelium*

Most previous studies on endometrial morphology concentrate on the glandular epithelium. In contrast, luminal epithelium has received relatively little attention although it is the first contact with the embryo during the process of implantation.

The changes reported in glandular epithelial cells around the time of implantation are generally mirrored by luminal epithelial cells,[26] although luminal cells are much less responsive than gland cells.[16] This is probably due to them having fewer steroid receptors than gland cells.[26] Johannisson[3] reports that luminal cells undergo delayed morphological changes compared to gland cells, although they produce glycogen vacuoles a little earlier than in glands. Luminal cells show ncs, although with less frequency than gland cells, but do not seem to form giant mitochondria.[13]

Normal fertile women at day LH+6 have $22.8 \pm 1.8\%$ of their gland cells occupied by nucleus,[11] compared to $42.2 \pm 1.9\%$ of their luminal epithelium.[27] However, comparison between these two values should be made with some caution since the gland cells were measured on 0.5 um semithin sections while luminal cells were examined on 2-um-thick JB4 sections. Using similar material, the mean nuclear profile diameter of glandular cells at day LH+6 was $8.5 \pm 0.5$ um compared to $6.0 \pm 0.1$ um for luminal cells. For comparison, stromal cell nuclear profile diameter at day LH+6 in a group of previous fertile women was about 8 um.[28]

## *Stromal Component*

Similarly, the stromal component of the endometrium is generally less well studied than the epithelium. Even so it undergoes cyclical changes which are largely independent of those in the epithelium but may be just as important for successful pregnancy.[29] Mitoses of stromal cells reach a maximum (of about 10 per 1000) around the time of ovulation.[3] They are reduced to almost zero over the peri-implantation period, increasing again near menses.[10] The stroma prepares for implantation by increasing its mean nuclear profile diameter by 24% between

LH+2 and LH+8.[28] From day LH+2 to LH+6 stromal cell density increased by about 30% before falling to day LH+2 values at LH+8. At day LH+8 the cells were less densely packed than at any other time measured and oedema was maximal. This may well represent preparation of the endometrium for its erosion by the implanting embryo. Also at this time other potentially preparative events occur, such as the formation of pseudo-decidual or pre-decidual[3] cells close to blood vessels. Although their function is unclear, they may be nutritive (since they contain glycogen, although this may be unrelated to hormonal stimulation),[29] or they may form a physical barrier for immunological protection or to help in mechanical support of the growing embryo.[30] These cells are also secretory to some extent, producing, for example, decidual prolactin; however the function of this secretion is uncertain.[3] Other ultrastructural and immunological changes relevant to continued and successful pregnancy have also been reported.[13,16,31]

Although the endocrinological control of endometrial development is fairly well studied, the paracrine control of the different components of the human endometrium, *i.e.*, luminal epithelium, glandular epithelium and stromal component, is poorly understood. It is likely that the co-ordinated development of the three components is crucial for normal physiological function leading to successful implantation. To explore the paracrine relationship between these several components, it may be necessary to employ *in vitro* endometrial cell culture studies.

## In Vitro *Studies*

Experimental study and investigation of the function of the endometrium *in vivo* are necessarily limited by ethical and practical constraints. A successful *in vitro* model of the endometrium would overcome many of these limitations and permit further research into fertilization, implantation and early development of the embryo. Traditional monolayer cell and tissue culture produces cells which have a flattened, squamous morphology (FIG. 5) irrespective of the original cell type. By using cells grown on artificial cell matrices in bi-cameral culture systems it is possible to produce cells which have a morphology very similar to their original phenotype[32,33] (FIG. 6). It is a basic biological assumption that cells which have the appropriate cell morphology are likely to behave and function in a more realistic way than cells which have an altered structure. With this in mind we have been developing a tissue culture model of the female reproductive tract which allows for cell growth in an anatomically correct and polarized manner (preliminary report in Hill *et al.*[34]). This model makes use of an artificial extracellular matrix (Matrigel, Uniscience, London, UK) coated on to millicell inserts (Millipore HA culture inserts, Millipore, Watford, UK) and placed in multiwell tissue culture plates (Falcon, UK). Fresh endometrial tissue is collected in HBSS and immediately transferred to the tissue culture laboratory. Following mechanical and enzymatic dissociation the suspension is washed and the fraction containing gland fragments collected. This fraction is pipetted on to Matrigel-coated millicell inserts, which sit in the multiwell plate, where they are grown in DMEM/F-12 medium in an humidified atmosphere of 95% air/5% $CO_2$ at 37°C. Cells can be grown under these conditions for several weeks if the medium is changed every 2–3 days.

Tissue treated in this way produced epithelial cells which are columnar in profile, have apical membrane specialisations such as microvilli and contain secretory vesicles (FIG. 6). Qualitative descriptions of carefully selected cells may be misleading, and therefore in an attempt to make objective comparison of the cultured cells with those from *in vivo* preparations we have conducted some

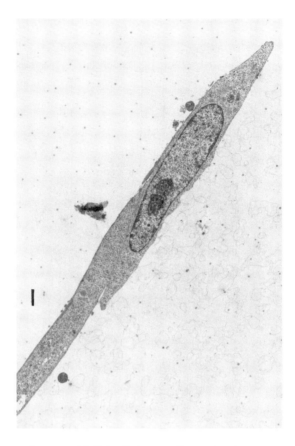

**FIGURE 5.** Even columnar epithelial cells become flattened and squamous when grown in traditional monolayer culture. *Bar* = 1 um.

preliminary quantitative experiments using fields of view which were systematic random samples of the sections obtained. The volume faction (proportion of the cell occupied by nucleus) of glandular epithelial cells grown for 15 days under polarising conditions was (mean ± standard error, n = 3) 0.251 ± 0.110, compared with a value of 0.261 ± 0.020 for the original *in vivo* tissue. Similarly, the surface to volume ($S_v$) ratio of nuclear membrane to nucleus was 89.2 ± 11.0 for cultured cells and 95.8 ± 11.2 for the original biopsy. Although the variances appear relatively large, there is a very close agreement between the mean values for all features measured for cells taken from the original *in vivo* biopsy and cells of the same biopsy grown *in vitro* for over two weeks. Further work on this model is needed, but the potential for utilizing what, at least morphologically, appears to be a very realistic model of the *in vivo* situation is great. It is already clear that these cells are able to secrete and are responsive to the addition of exogenous steroid hormones. We intend to use this model in our studies of the female reproductive system.[32,35,36]

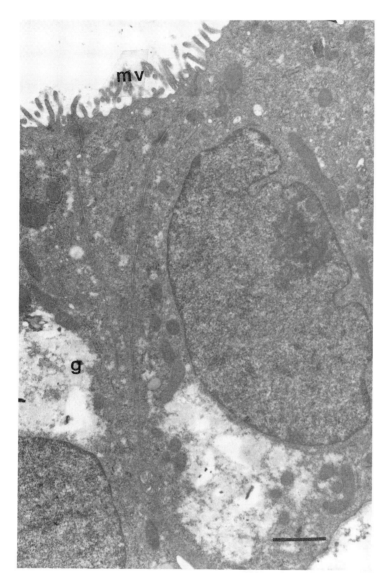

**FIGURE 6.** Cells from the same tissue biopsy as that shown in FIGURE 5 grown on Matrigel-coated millicell inserts have a morphology similar to *in vivo* specimens (FIGS. 2–4). Glycogen deposits (g) and microvilli (mv) are prominent. *Bar* = 1 um.

## Heterogeneity

It is well known that given a particular biopsy specimen, the endometrial morphology may vary significantly in different parts of the specimen. It is important to remember that the endometrium is composed of two layers, the functional layer and the basal layer. The functional layer is more responsive to steroid hormones whereas the basal layer is less responsive because it has a reduced number of oestrogen and progesterone receptors. For the same reason, the endometrium from the upper or fundal part of the uterus is also more responsive than the lower or isthmic part of the uterus to steroid hormones. In general, the study of endometrial morphology should be confined to the functional layer from the upper part of the uterus, as inclusion of the basal layer or the isthmic part of the uterus will introduce unnecessary variance to the result of any study and should therefore be avoided. The basal layer or isthmic sample contains a more compact stroma and the glands are at an earlier stage of development in comparison with the functional layer, which should be easily distinguished. Microheterogeneity, which refers to the variation of morphology within the functional layer, has also been recognized, but the biological significance of such phenomenon is not well understood.

For the above reasons, endometrial biopsy specimens should always be obtained from the upper or fundal part of the uterus and great care should be taken to exclude the basal layer or the isthmic specimens. We have observed that measurements confined to the functional layer of the endometrium have much reduced variance[12] when compared to measurements of the concentration of endometrial protein PP14 in homogenized specimens in which it was not possible to differentiate the basal/functional layer, and the fundal/isthmic specimens.[37]

## Correlation between Morphological and Functional Studies

In recent years, the application of immunohistochemical techniques has permitted the study of the expression of specific proteins in the endometrium, including placental protein 12,[38] placental protein 14,[39] 24 K protein,[40] CA125,[41] prolactin,[42] a keratin sulphate 5DU,[43] laminin,[44] a sialo-glycoprotein D9B1 epitope,[45] 17-beta hydroxysteroid dehydrogenase,[46] a stromal protein desmin,[47] and the use of lectin binding to study glycoproteins.[5] Many of these epitopes are hormone dependent and have variable expressions throughout the menstrual cycle. It is likely that the study of specific proteins or epitopes in the endometrium using immunohistochemical techniques will complement the information obtained from morphological study using either the traditional dating criteria or morphometric techniques. We examined the endometrium of women with unexplained infertility and found that they have not only morphological evidence of abnormal development,[48] but also defective production of specific endometrial proteins, including D9B1 epitope,[14] and glycoprotein production as studied by the use of lectin binding techniques.[5]

In order to study these functional changes, we developed a technique of washing the uterine cavity with 10 mls of normal saline solution using a size 8 (paediatric) Foley catheter. After inserting it into the uterine cavity, the balloon of the catheter was inflated with 1 ml of normal saline solution. Following this 2 ml of physiological saline solution was gradually flushed into the uterine cavity via the opening connected to the inner lumen; afterwards gentle suction via the same opening was applied to recover the fluid. The flushing was carried out slowly over approximately

TABLE 1. The Results of Progesterone (P) Measurements in Subjects with Retarded Endometrial Development

| Authors | Number of Subjects with Retarded Endometrium | Proportion with | |
|---|---|---|---|
| | | Normal P | Subnormal P |
| Shangold et al.[52] | 20 | 45% | 55% |
| Zorn et al.[53] | 37 | 78% | 22% |
| Balasch and Vanrell[54] | 42 | 86% | 14% |
| Li et al.[55] | 15 | 87% | 13% |

15 seconds and the procedure was repeated 5 times, each time using a fresh sample of 2 ml of physiological saline solution. Thus a total of 10 ml of saline solution was used to carry out the procedure. We observed that uterine washing resulted in a significantly reduced amount of discomfort experienced by women when compared to that of endometrial biopsy and may be repeated serially in the same cycle. The procedure is simple and noninvasive and carries a number of other advantages, including the measurement of a number of proteins in the washings. We were able to recover more than 90% of the fluid used to wash the uterine cavity in 90% of cases.[49] We measured the PP14 levels in the uterine flushings throughout the menstrual cycle of normal fertile women and found that the concentration rises rapidly after day LH+6, with a doubling time of only 6.6 to 14.6 hours in the mid-luteal phase. In addition, we observed that the concentration of PP14 in uterine flushing were over 100 times higher than the corresponding plasma samples in the late luteal phase.[50]

We correlated the result of PP14 concentration in uterine washings with those of histological dating and morphometric measurements of the endometrial glands. We found that PP14 concentration in uterine flushings was consistently below the sensitivity of the assay when histological dating was less than day LH+5, or when the gland lumen was less than 20% of the gland volume.[51]

Thus, there appeared to be significant correlation between the results of the morphological study and the expression of specific endometrial proteins both in biopsy specimens and in uterine flushings. Of course, these two types of studies are not mutually exclusive but complementary to each other. Uterine flushings may be performed just prior to endometrial biopsy, and the endometrial biopsy specimens obtained could be examined morphologically as well as with the use of immunohistochemical techniques for expression of specific endometrial proteins.

### *Primary and Secondary Abnormality*

Abnormal endometrial development in the peri-implantation period may be secondary to suboptimal levels of circulating steroid hormones, including oestrogen and progesterone, or it might be due to inadequate response of the endometrium to the hormones (primary abnormality). A number of studies suggest that the majority of women with abnormal endometrium in the luteal phase was associated with normal progesterone levels, indicating that the abnormality lies in the responsiveness of the endometrium to steroid hormones[52-55] (TABLE 1). We also observed that women with Turner's syndrome had significantly reduced endometrial responsiveness to defined doses of steroid hormones when compared to women with idiopathic premature ovarian failure.[56] Additionally, we found that endometrial responsiveness in the luteal phase may be influenced by oestrogen priming in the follicular phase of the same cycle.[57] In a group of women (n = 11) with persistent endometrial abnormality in the luteal phase, by downregulating the hypothalamic-pituitary ovarian axis, followed by the administration of exogenous steroid hormones to produce an artificial cycle, we found that endometrial development was normalized in all the eleven subjects studied.[58] It seems that inadequate endometrial response to steroid hormones producing abnormal endometrial development in the luteal phase is likely to have an endocrine basis as it could be consistently corrected by endocrine manipulation.

## SUMMARY

Although the histology and ultrastructure of the human endometrium are well documented, it is clear that morphometry can reveal subtle changes in cellular biology, especially when combined with suitable sampling and dating of the specimen. These changes reflect functional events, such as protein secretion, which may be studied using the endometrial flushing technique. Although it is likely that further insights into the basic cell physiology of the reproductive tract will result from the use of appropriate *in vitro* models, the role of endometrial biopsy for clinical monitoring remains essential.

## REFERENCES

1. FERENCZY, A. 1976. Studies on the cytodynamics of human endometrial regeneration. I. Scanning electron microscopy. Am. J. Obstet. Gynecol. **124:** 64–74.
2. LI, T. C., A. W. ROGERS, E. A. LENTON, P. DOCKERY & I. D. COOKE. 1987. A comparison between two methods of chronological dating of human endometrial biopsies during the luteal phase and the correlation and histologic dating. Fertil. Steril. **48:** 928–932.
3. JOHANNISSON, E. 1985. Endocrine responses in the female genital tract. *In* Clinical Reproductive Endocrinology. R. P. Shearman, Ed. 128–140. Churchill-Livingstone. Edinburgh.
4. CLARK, J. H. & B. M. MARKEVERICH. 1981. Relationships between type I and type II estradiol binding sites and estrogen induced responses. J. Steroid Biochem. **15:** 49–54.
5. KLENTZERIS, L. D., J. N. BULMER, T. C. LI, L. MORRISON, M. A. WARREN & I. D. COOKE. 1991. Lectin binding of endometrium in women with unexplained infertility. Fertil. Steril. **56:** 660–667.
6. SMITH, R. A., M. W. SEIF, A. W. ROGERS, T. C. LI, P. DOCKERY, I. D. COOKE & J. APLIN. 1989. The endometrial cycle: the expression of a secretory component correlated with the luteinizing hormone peak. Hum. Reprod. **4:** 236–242.
7. APLIN, J. A., M. E. HOADLEY & M. W. SEIF. 1989. Hormonally regulated secretion of keratin sulphate by human endometrial epithelium. Biochem. Soc. Trans. **17:** 136–137.
8. LI, T. C., C. DALTON, A. E. BOLTON, E. LING, M. A. WARREN & I. D. COOKE. 1992. An analysis of the variation of plasma concentrations of placental protein 14 in artificial cycles. Fertil. Steril. **57:** 776–782.
9. JOHANNISSON, E., R. A. PARKER, B-M. LANDGREN & E. DICZFALUSY. 1982. Morphometric analysis of the human endometrium in relation to peripheral hormone levels. Fertil. Steril. **38:** 564–571.

10. Noyes, R. W., A. T. Hertig & J. Roack. 1950. Dating the endometrial biopsy. Fertil. Steril. **1:** 3–25.
11. Dockery, P., K. Pritchard, A. Taylor, T. C. Li, M. A. Warren & I. D. Cooke. 1993. The fine structure of the human endometrial glandular epithelium in cases of unexplained infertility: a morphometric study. Hum. Reprod. **8:** 667–673.
12. Dockery, P., T. C. Li, A. W. Rogers, I. D. Cooke & E. A. Lenton. 1988. The ultrastructure of the glandular epithelium in the timed endometrial biopsy. Hum. Reprod. **3:** 826–834.
13. Dockery, P. & A. W. Rogers. 1989. The effects of steroids on the fine structure of the endometrium. Balliere's Clin. Obstet. Gynaecol. **3:** 227–248.
14. Graham, R. A., M. W. Seif, J. D. Aplin, T. C. Li, I. D. Cooke, A. W. Rogers & P. Dockery. 1990. An endometrial factor in unexplained infertility. Br. Med. J. **300:** 1428–1431.
15. Kohorn, E. I., S. I. Rice, S. Hemperly & M. Gordon. 1972. The relation of the structure of progestational steroids to nucleolar differentiation in human endometrium. J. Clin. Endocrinol. Metab. **34:** 257–264.
16. Cornillie, F. J., J. M. Lauweryns & I. A. Brosens. 1985. Normal human endometrium. Gynecol. Obstet. Invest. **20:** 113–129.
17. Murphy, C. R. & V. F. Turner. 1991. Glycocalyx carbohydrates of uterine epithelial cells increase during early pregnancy in the rat. J. Anat. **177:** 109–115.
18. More, I. A. R., E. M. Armstrong, D. McSeveney & W. R. Chatfield. 1974. The morphogenesis and fate of the nucleolar channel system in the human endometrial glandular cell. J. Ultrastruct. Res. **47:** 74–85.
19. Terzakis, J. A. 1965. The nucleolar channel system of human endometrium. J. Cell Biol. **27:** 293–304.
20. Kohorn, E. I., S. I. Rice & M. Gordon. 1970. In vitro production of nucleolar channel system by progesterone in human endometrium. Nature (London) **228:** 671–672.
21. Luginbuhl, W. H. 1968. Electron microscopic studies of the effects of tissue culture on human endometrium. Am. J. Obstet. Gynecol. **102:** 192–201.
22. Gordon, M., E. I. Kohorn, B. Z. Gore & S. I. Rice. 1973. Effect of postovulatory oestrogens on the fine structure of the epithelial cells in the human endometrium. J. Reprod. Fertil. **34:** 375–378.
23. Dehou, M. F., B. Lejeune, C. Airjis & F. Leroy. 1987. Endometrial morphology in stimulated in vitro fertilisation cycles and after steroid replacement therapy in cases of primary ovarian failure. Fertil. Steril. **48:** 995–1000.
24. Coaker, T., T. Downie & I. A. R. More. 1982. Complex giant mitochondria in the endometrial glandular cell: serial sectioning, high voltage electron microscopy and three dimensional reconstruction studies. J. Ultrastruct. Res. 78: 283–291.
25. Verma, V. 1983. Ultrastructural changes in human endometrium at different phases of the menstrual cycle and their functional significance. Gynecol. Obstet. Invest. **15:** 193–212.
26. Williams, T. & A. W. Rogers. 1983. Morphometric studies of the response of the luminal epithelium in the rat uterus to exogenous hormones. J. Anat. **130:** 867–881.
27. Saleh, M. I. A. Personal communication.
28. Dockery, P., M. A. Warren, T. C. Li, A. W. Rogers, I. D. Cooke & J. Mundy. 1990. A morphometric study of the human endometrial stroma during the peri-implantation period. Hum. Reprod. **5:** 112–116.
29. More, I. A. R., E. M. Armstrong, M. Carty & D. McSeveney. 1974. Cyclical changes in the ultrastructure of the normal human endometrial stromal cell. J. Obstet. Gynaecol. Br. Commonw. **81:** 337–347.
30. Johnson, M. & B. Everitt, Eds. 1984. Implantation and the establishment of the placenta. In Essential Reproduction. 2nd edit. 215–242. Blackwell Scientific Publications. Oxford.
31. Bulmer, J. N., L. Morrison, M. Longfellow, A. Ritson & D. Pace. 1991. Granulated lymphocytes in human endometrium histochemical and immunohistochemical studies. Hum. Reprod. **6:** 791–798.
32. Glasser, S. R., J. Julian, G. L. Decker, J. P. Tang & D. D. Carson. 1988.

Development of morphological and functional polarity in primary cultures of immature rat uterine epithelial cells. J. Cell Biol. **107:** 2409–2423.
33. RINEHART, C. A., B. D. LYN-COOK & D. G. KAUFMANN. 1988. Gland formation from human endometrial cells *in vitro*. Dev. Biol. **24:** 1037–1041.
34. HILL, C. J., M. A. WARREN, T. C. LI & I. D. COOKE. 1993. Polarised growth of human endometrial cell *in vitro*. J. Anat. **182:** 149–150.
35. LINDENBERG, S., J. G. LAURISTEN, M. H. NIELSEN & J. F. LARSEN. 1984. Isolation and culture of human endometrial cells. Fertil. Steril. **41:** 625–650.
36. BONGSO, A., S-C. NG, C-Y. FONG & R. RATNAM. 1991. Cocultures: a new lead in embryo quality improvement for assisted reproduction. Fertil. Steril. **56:** 179–191.
37. LI, T. C., G. POCKLEY, A. E. BOLTON & I. D. COOKE. 1991. The variation of endometrial protein PP14 in different parts of the human endometrium. Int. J. Gynecol. Obstet. **34:** 257–260.
38. BELL, S. C., S. PATEL, M. W. HALES, P. H. KIRWAN & J. O. DRIFE. 1985. Immunocytochemical detection and characterization of pregnancy-associated endometrial alpha$_1$ and alpha$_2$-globins secreted by the human endometrium. J. Reprod. Fertil. **74:** 261–270.
39. JULKUNEN, M., R. KOLISTEINEN, A. M. SUIKKARI, M. SEPPALA & O. A. JANNE. 1990. Identification by hybridization histochemistry of human endometrial cells expressing mRNA encoding a uterine beta-lactoglobulin homologue and insulin-like growth factor-binding homologue and insulin-like growth factor-binding protein-1. Mol. Endocrinol. **4:** 700–707.
40. CIOCCA, D. R., R. H. ASCH, D. J. ADAMS & W. L. MCGUIRE. 1983. Evidence for modulation of a 24K protein in human endometrium during the menstrual cycle. J. Clin. Endocrinol. Metab. **57:** 496–499.
41. KABAWAT, S. E., R. C. BAST, A. K. BHAN, W. WELCH, R. C. KNAPP & R. B. COLVIN. 1983. Tissue distributoin of a coelomic-epithelium-related antigen recognised by the monoclonal antibody CA125. Int. J. Gynecol. Pathol. **2:** 275–285.
42. KAUMA, S. & A. Sharpio. 1986. Immunoperoxidase localisation of prolactin in endometrium during normal menstrual luteal phase defect and corrected luteal phase defect cycles. Fertil. Steril. **46:** 37–41.
43. APLIN, J. D., M. E. HOADLEY & M. W. SEIF. 1988. Hormonally regulated secretion of keratin sulphate by human endometrial epithelium. Biochem. Soc. Trans. **17:** 136–137.
44. APLIN, J. D., A. K. CHARLTON & S. AYAD. 1988. An immunohistochemical study of the human endometrial extracellular matrix during the menstrual cycle and first trimester of pregnancy. Cell Tissue Res. **253:** 231–240.
45. SEIF, M. W., J. D. APLIN, I. I. FODEN & V. R. TINDALL. 1989. A novel approach for monitoring the endometrial cycle and detecting ovulation. Am. J. Obstet. Gynecol. **160:** 357–362.
46. MAENTAUSTA, O., H. PEKTOKETO, V. OSOMAE, P. JOUPPILA & R. VIHKO. 1990. Immunological measurement of human 17 beta-hydroxysteroid dehydrogenase. J. Steroid Biochem. **36:** 673–680.
47. HALPERIN, R., G. FLEMINGER, P. F. KRAICER & E. HADAS. 1991. Desmin as an immunochemical marker of human decidual cells and its expression in menstrual fluid. Hum. Reprod. **6:** 186–189.
48. LI, C., P. DOCKERY & I. D. COOKE. 1990. A quantitative study of endometrial development in the luteal phase: comparison between women with unexplained infertility and normal fertility. Br. J. Obstet. Gynaecol. **97:** 576–582.
49. LI, T. C., A. MACKENNA & R. ROBERTS. 1993. The techniques and complications of outpatient uterine washing in the assessment of endometrial function. Hum. Reprod. **8:** 343–346.
50. LI, T. C., E. LING, C. DALTON, A. E. BOLTON & I. D. COOKE. 1993. Concentration of endometrial protein PP14 in uterine flushings throughout the menstrual cycle in normal, fertile women. Br. J. Obstet. Gynaecol. **100:** 460–464.
51. LI, T. C., C. DALTON, K. S. HUNJAN, A. E. BOLTON & M. A. WARREN. The correlation of endometrial protein PP14 concentrations in uterine flushings and endometrial morphology in the peri-implantation period. Hum. Reprod. In press.

52. SHANGOLD, M., A. BERKELEY & J. GRAY. 1983. Both midluteal serum progesterone levels and late luteal endometrial histology should be assessed in all infertile women. Fertil. Steril. **40:** 627–630.
53. ZORN, J. R., L. CEDARD, C. NESSMAN & M. SEVALE. 1984. Delayed endometrial maturation in women with normal progesterone levels. The dysharmonic luteal phase syndrome. Gynecol. Obstet. Invest. **17:** 157–162.
54. BALASCH, J. & J. A. VANRELL. 1987. Corpus luteum insufficiency and fertility: a matter of controversy. Hum. Reprod. **2:** 557–567.
55. LI, T. C., P. DOCKERY & I. D. COOKE. Endometrial development in the luteal phase of women with various types of infertility: comparison with women of normal fertility. Hum. Reprod. **6:** 325–330.
56. LI, T. C., P. DOCKERY, S. S. RAMSEWAK, L. D. KLENTZERIS, E. A. LENTON & I. D. COOKE. 1991. The variation of endometrial response to a standard hormone replacement therapy in women with premature ovarian failure. An ultrasonographic and histological study. Br. J. Obstet. Gynaecol. **98:** 656–661.
57. LI, T. C., I. D. COOKE, M. A. WARREN, M. GOOLAMALLEE, R. A. GRAHAM & J. D. APLIN. 1992. Endometrial responses in artificial cycles: a prospective study comparing four different oestrogen dosages. Br. J. Obstet. Gynaecol. **99:** 751–756.
58. LI, T. C., M. A. WARREN & I. D. COOKE. The artificial cycle as an effective treatment of persistently retarded endometrium in the luteal phase. Hum. Reprod. In press.

# Human Endometrial Lymphocytes in Normal Pregnancy and Pregnancy Loss

JUDITH N. BULMER[a]

*Division of Pathology*
*School of Pathological Sciences*
*University of Newcastle upon Tyne*
*Newcastle upon Tyne NE1 4LP, United Kingdom*

## ENDOMETRIAL LYMPHOCYTES IN NORMAL PREGNANCY

### Introduction

Leucocytes form a substantial proportion of the constituent cells of human endometrial stroma accounting for around 7% of stromal cells in proliferative endometrium and increasing to over 30% in early pregnancy. Macrophages are present in nonpregnant endometrium, increasing in number premenstrually, and in both decidua basalis and decidua parietalis throughout gestation.[1–3] Although endometrial macrophages may play a role in successful implantation and fetoplacental development with reports of immunosuppressive activity, accessory cell function and cytokine production,[4–7] recent attention has focused primarily on investigation of the lymphoid populations in the human uterus. The endometrium differs from other mucosal sites such as the gastrointestinal tract, respiratory tract and cervix by its scarcity of B cells and plasma cells, the predominant lymphocytes being T cells and phenotypically unusual granulated lymphocytes.

### T Lymphocytes

T cells are present within both the stroma and the epithelium of human endometrium. Stromal T cells show little variation in number and distribution during the menstrual cycle and in early pregnancy decidua, although they account for a lower proportion of the total endometrial leucocyte population in the late luteal phase and early pregnancy, when granulated lymphocytes increase in number.[1,8] T lymphocytes are scattered throughout the stroma, sometimes forming small aggregates. In contrast with peripheral blood T cells, most endometrial stromal T cells express the CD8 suppressor-cytotoxic subset marker, only 25–35% expressing CD4.[1,8]

Considerable interest has been focused on expression of the $\gamma\delta$ heterodimeric form of T cell receptor (TcR) by T lymphocytes at mucosal sites. However, despite evidence of preferential localisation of $\gamma\delta$ T cells in mouse intestine,

---

[a] Correspondence: Dr. Judith N. Bulmer, Division of Pathology, University of Newcastle upon Tyne, Royal Victoria Infirmary, Newcastle upon Tyne NE1 4LP, UK.

immunohistochemical studies have not revealed selective accumulation of $\gamma\delta$ T cells in the normal human small intestine.[9] There are conflicting reports of expression of $\alpha\beta$ and $\gamma\delta$ T cell receptors in human endometrium. Dietl et al.[10] were unable to detect either $\alpha\beta$ or $\gamma\delta$ TcR on T lymphocytes in normal first trimester human decidua, causing speculation about alternative pathways of T cell activation.[11] In contrast, Mincheva-Nilsson et al.[12] reported expression of $\gamma\delta$ TcR on around 30% of cells in early pregnancy decidua, although results with two of the four antibodies used differed between flow cytometric and immunohistochemical analysis. An increased proportion of $\gamma\delta$ T cells compared with $\alpha\beta$ T cells has also been reported in third trimester decidua, although the proportions were lower with a less than threefold increase compared with peripheral blood.[13] Between these extremes are other reports that the proportion of T cells bearing the $\gamma\delta$ heterodimer parallels that in peripheral blood.[14–16] The explanation for these diverse results is not clear but most probably relates to the specificity of the monoclonal antibodies used and their suitability for use both in flow cytometric analysis of living cells and in immunohistochemical techniques applied to frozen sections.

Intraepithelial T cells in human endometrium are almost exclusively of the CD8 subset, with a substantial proportion having cytoplasmic granules.[17] CD3-negative granulated lymphocytes are also present in an intraepithelial position. Intraepithelial lymphocytes are infrequent in normal endometrium and to date their detailed distribution in endometrial pathology has not been reported. However, immunohistochemical studies of both pregnant and nonpregnant endometrium show no selective localisation of $\gamma\delta$ T cells within normal endometrial epithelium.[14,18]

The function of T cells in human endometrium is not known. Most in vitro studies have focused on early pregnancy decidua in which T cells account for less than 20% of the leucocytes.[1] The lack of variation in their numbers between different cycle stages may also explain the relative neglect of the T lymphocyte population. Nevertheless, alterations in the numbers of CD4 and CD8-positive T cells in endometrium from women suffering unexplained infertility[19] may stimulate further interest in their function.

CD8-positive T cells may function as suppressor cells and immunosuppressive activity of both endometrium and decidua has been reported.[20,21] Furthermore, a hormone-dependent suppressor cell expressing suppressor T cell surface antigens has been described in the mouse uterus.[22] However, several cell types have been implicated in local intrauterine immunosuppression in both murine and human pregnancy and the relative importance of the various cell types implicated remains obscure.

CD8-positive T cells can also function as cytotoxic cells recognising targets in association with class I MHC antigens. Evidence of in vivo cytotoxicity in human decidua is lacking and the expression of the nonpolymorphic HLA-G molecule by the invasive extravillous trophoblast and lack of a polymorphic class I MHC molecule should prevent recognition of the invasive trophoblast by maternal T cells.

T lymphocytes can also secrete a wide range of cytokines, including several which have been implicated in regulation of placental growth.[23] A wide variety of cytokine receptors have been localised in human utero-placental tissues with cytokine production by cells in both decidua and placenta.[24] Despite evidence for autocrine and paracrine control of placental growth, with cytokine networks operating within uteroplacental tissues, the precise role of cytokines in vivo remains obscure and their cellular site of origin is often disputed. Improved methods for positive selection of cells to yield highly purified viable populations, together with studies of pathological tissues may enhance understanding of the *in vivo* role of endometrial T cells.

## Granulated Lymphocytes

The most abundant lymphoid cell population in human endometrium in the late luteal phase of the cycle and early pregnancy are phenotypically unusual granulated lymphocytes.[1,8] The presence of granulated cells in human endometrium has been recognised for many years but their identification as a leucocyte has been recent.[25] The phenotype (CD56+ CD16− CD3− CD2±) resembles that of a minor population of peripheral blood lymphocytes which have been considered as a differentiation stage of natural killer (NK) cells.[26]

Endometrial granulated lymphocytes (eGL), identified by expression of the NK cell antigen CD56, are present in endometrium throughout the menstrual cycle but increase in number dramatically during the late luteal phase[1,8] and again in early pregnancy decidua.[1] In proliferative and early luteal phase endometrium, CD56-positive cells are scattered throughout the stratum basalis and stratum functionalis. In late luteal phase endometrium they form aggregates scattered within the endometrial stroma and also adjacent to glands and vessels. Although there may be some influx of CD56-positive cells from peripheral blood, numbers of circulating CD56-positive, CD16-negative cells being higher in women of reproductive age,[27] the bulk of the sudden increase in eGL numbers appears to be due to proliferation *in situ*,[8,28] although the stimulus is not known. Single and double immunohistochemical studies indicate that endometrial lymphocytes do not express progesterone receptor[19,29] and the large increase in eGL numbers premenstrually occurs at a time when progesterone levels are falling. The apparent progesterone dependence of these cells may be indirect, reflecting their close association with decidualised stromal cells which themselves express progesterone receptor.

The *in vivo* role of eGL is unknown: their increase in the late luteal phase of the menstrual cycle in the days which would immediately follow implantation in a fertile cycle, and their persistence in the first trimester of pregnancy followed by a rapid decline subsequently has suggested that these cells may play a role in implantation and placental development. Furthermore, granulated leucocytes have been identified in endometrium and decidua in a number of animal species, including rat and mouse, where the granulated metrial gland (GMG) cells show phenotypic and functional similarities to granulated lymphocytes in human endometrium.[30,31]

*In vitro* functional studies of eGL enriched from human first trimester decidua using a range of techniques including density gradient centrifugation, flow cytometry and panning onto immunoglobulin-coated plates, have consistently detected NK cell activity using the classical target K562.[32–35] It has been suggested that eGL may control trophoblast invasion by cytotoxicity of individual aberrant or unduly invasive cells;[36] direct evidence for such a role is, however, not present in placental bed tissues and invasion of uterine tissues by extravillous trophoblast terminates in the myometrium, a site at which eGL are absent.

Time lapse video studies of cocultures of mouse or rat GMG cells with labyrinthine trophoblast of the appropriate species reveal direct lysis of occasional labyrinthine trophoblast by GMG cells.[30,31] Light microscope and ultrastructural studies suggest a functional relationship between mouse GMG cells and layer 1 labyrinthine trophoblast cells. There is no morphological evidence for a functional interaction between GMG cells and interstitial invasive trophoblast in decidua in experimental animal species, such as rat and field vole, which show prominent trophoblast invasion.[37] Nevertheless, *in vitro* studies have demonstrated that eGL are able to lyse human trophoblast cells after activation with IL-2, reflecting their capacity to act as lymphokine-activated killer (LAK) cells.[38,39] Evidence in both murine and human decidua suggests local suppression of IL-2 activity in normal pregnancy: killing of trophoblast after IL-2 activation may, however, reflect a mechanism of pregnancy loss.

Despite consistent reports of NK cell activity, eGL are poor effectors compared with peripheral blood NK cells and an *in vivo* role for a function defined by an *in vitro* assay should not be overestimated. Christmas *et al.*[40] failed to detect NK activity in CD3-negative CD56-positive CD16-negative clones prepared from first trimester human decidua and proposed that the cytotoxicity noted in other studies[32-35] may be due to the presence in the enriched populations of 'classical' CD16-positive CD56-positive NK cells from peripheral blood within the decidual tissue. Although there have been reports of killing of the NK cell target Yac-1 by mouse GMG cells after stimulation with high doses of IL-2,[41,42] GMG cells from both mouse and rat decidua and metrial gland are unable to lyse Yac-1 targets without IL-2 activation even after *in vivo* stimulation of NK activity with polyinosilic cytidilic acid (polyIC).[43,44]

The presence of small granulated non-T non-B suppressor lymphocytes in murine decidua acting by secretion of a TGF $\beta$2-like molecule has been reported.[45] Evidence that eGL act as immunosuppressive cells in human decidua is scanty. Although supernatants from decidual cell suspensions enriched for eGL were able to suppress lymphocyte proliferation in response to mitogens, suppression was lower than in the comparable unfractionated decidual cell suspension, and responses in the mixed lymphocyte reaction were often stimulatory.[46] *In vitro* studies of human endometrium and decidua have so far revealed several cell types apparently capable of mediating immune suppression, their relative *in vivo* importance remaining undetermined.

Suppressive and stimulatory activity in lymphoproliferative assays may be explained by cytokine production and there is evidence that complex intrauterine cytokine networks are active in normal pregnancy. Clones of CD3-negative CD56-positive CD16-negative decidual lymphocytes produce TNF$\alpha$, TGF$\beta$ and IFN$\gamma$.[40] mRNA and production of G-CSF, M-CSF, GM-CSF, TNF$\alpha$, IFN$\gamma$ and LIF by eGL freshly isolated from decidua has also been reported.[47]

Natural killer cells mediate non-MHC restricted cytotoxicity and are considered to play an important role in innate anti-viral and anti-tumour immunity. The human feto-placental unit is susceptible to a wide variety of micro-organisms, both ascending via the vagina and travelling via the bloodstream. Local immune responses within the uterus may be suppressed during pregnancy and there is evidence that some infections, notably malaria, are commoner in pregnancy, particularly in primigravidae.[48] The large population of granulated lymphocytes which appears conserved in a wide range of species may be responsible for a first line of defence against infectious agents which would otherwise harm the fetoplacental unit.

## ENDOMETRIAL LYMPHOCYTES IN PREGNANCY PATHOLOGY

Despite phenotypic characterisation and *in vitro* functional studies, the role of endometrial lymphocytes in normal human pregnancy remains unknown. Study of pathological tissues provides an alternative approach which may provide clues to cell function.

## Primary Unexplained Infertility

Subtle morphological abnormalities have been demonstrated in luteal phase endometrium from infertile women using morphometric techniques applied to endometrial biopsies precisely timed from the luteinising hormone (LH) surge.[49] Abnormalities in the distribution of glycoconjugates have also been demonstrated using lectin histochemistry.[50] Similar timed biopsies of luteal phase endometrium have been used to examine stromal leucocyte populations. Frozen sections of endometrial biopsies taken 4, 7, 10 and 13 days following the LH surge (LH+4, +7, +10, +13) were stained with a panel of monoclonal antibodies against leucocyte subsets. Compared with normal women, the endometrium from women with unexplained infertility contained increased numbers of CD4-positive T cells, decreased numbers of CD8-positive T cells and decreased numbers of CD56-positive granulated lymphocytes throughout the luteal phase. Furthermore, a lower proportion of CD56-positive eGL co-expressed CD2 compared with normal endometrium. The numbers of macrophages, B cells and 'classical' CD16-positive NK cells did not differ between fertile and infertile endometrium.[19]

Although the role of both T cells and granulated lymphocytes is not clear these results provide some support for the concept that the endometrial lymphoid populations play an important role in early pregnancy. Abnormalities in leucocyte populations could cause disruption of cytokine networks essential for successful implantation and early development of the placenta. Alternatively, decreased secretion of TGF$\beta$ or of other soluble factors could lead to deficient immunoregulatory activity within the endometrium.

The mechanisms underlying the leucocyte abnormalities are not known, although recent studies have suggested possible explanations. Granulated lymphocytes normally proliferate very actively in premenstrual endometrium. The stimulus for this proliferation is unknown and is only indirectly related to progesterone since CD56-positive eGL do not express progesterone receptor.[18] Placental protein 14 (PP14) is produced by secretory phase endometrium and both serum and uterine PP14 levels are reduced in endometrium from infertile women which shows retarded development.[51] PP14 is a candidate for stimulation of eGL proliferation and differentiation, relative deficiency or delayed production leading to reduced eGL numbers. PP14 also suppresses the NK cell function of decidual granulated lymphocytes;[52] deficiency of PP14 could thus lead to loss of a normal regulatory mechanism and inappropriately high levels of lytic activity by eGL.

The factors which govern the recruitment of eGL into endometrium and their distribution within the tissue with aggregation around vessels and glands are unknown. Cell adhesion molecules play a fundamental role in the immune response affecting lymphocyte homing and both intercellular and cell-matrix interactions. Luteal phase endometrium from women suffering primary unexplained infertility shows a deficiency of $\alpha_4\beta_1$ (VLA-4) integrin expression by epithelial cells:[53] such a deficiency could lead to failure of attachment of the blastocyst via fibronectin to its counter-receptor on endometrium at implantation. A proportion of eGL express the adhesion molecules CD2, CD11a and $\alpha_4\beta_1$, respectively, whose counter-receptors are LFA-3(CD58), ICAM-1(CD54) and VCAM.[14,54,55] Expression of ICAM-1 and VCAM by endometrial vascular endothelium may stimulate recruitment of eGL into tissues, although local proliferation appears to account for most of the premenstrual increase[27,28] and may also influence their distribution around vessels. Reactivity of scattered stromal cells for ICAM-1 has been observed associated with CD11a-positive lymphoid aggregates.[14,54] Similarly, expression of LFA-3 by glandular and surface epithelium and in a perivascular position may stimulate accumulation of CD2-positive eGL around glands.[14]

## *Spontaneous Abortion*

Despite the reported successful treatment of women suffering recurrent miscarriage with paternal lymphocytes, there is essentially no concrete evidence that immune mechanisms play a role in early pregnancy loss in humans. However, evidence from murine models has led to the proposal that NK cells are involved in pregnancy loss. In CBA/J × DBA/2 matings, the normally high rate of spontaneous resorption can be reduced by treatment with anti-asialoGM1 and increased by *in vivo* stimulation of NK cell activity by injection of polyIC[56] and the implantation site in resorbing pregnancies is infiltrated by asialoGM1-positive cells.[57]

Mouse trophoblast cannot be lysed by cytotoxic T cells or NK cells grown under standard conditions, but is susceptible to IL-2-activated LAK cells.[58] Human trophoblast is also susceptible to decidual NK cells activated by IL-2.[38,39] Evidence has suggested that IL-2 responses are suppressed within the uterus during normal pregnancy, although the precise mechanism remains disputed. Loss of this normal regulation of IL-2 responses could lead to generation of IL-2-activated LAK cells capable of direct attack on placental trophoblast.

Evidence that NK cells play a role in human pregnancy loss is scanty. A mononuclear cell infiltrate noted in decidua in pregnancies aborting on an IVF programme was not characterised phenotypically or morphologically.[59] A study of decidua from spontaneously aborting pregnancies revealed lymphocytes with large ($>1$ $\mu$m) granules in normal pregnancies and lymphocytes with small ($<1$ $\mu$m) granules in miscarriages with an associated deficiency of decidual immunosuppression.[60] Studies of spontaneous abortion in humans are hampered by the frequency of superimposed secondary inflammation with consequent difficulty in distinguishing cause and effect.

In both mouse and human it is unclear whether cytolytic attack on trophoblast would be due to resident decidual NK cells—the eGL in human and the GMG cells in mouse—or to infiltrating 'classical' NK cells from peripheral blood. Indeed, any deficiency in the resident decidual granulated lymphocyte population would be obscured by an infiltrate of NK cells causing the pregnancy loss.

T lymphocytes within decidua could also play a role in spontaneous pregnancy loss. T cell-derived cytokines may be fundamental for fetoplacental development, depletion of T cells leading to pregnancy loss.[23] Deficiency of decidual T cells could lead to an unfavourable cytokine environment for placental development. Further studies are required to clarify the role of granulated lymphocytes and T cells in pregnancy loss in humans. Such investigations are hampered by the presence of secondary inflammation and by the likely heterogeneity of causes of spontaneous abortion in humans.

## SUMMARY

Leucocytes are a major component of decidualised endometrium in normal human pregnancy but despite numerous *in vitro* studies the *in vivo* role of the two major lymphocyte populations in implantation and early placental development remains uncertain. Although there is evidence from animal studies that NK cells play a role in pregnancy loss, further studies are required to clarify mechanisms of pregnancy loss in humans.

## REFERENCES

1. BULMER, J. N., L. MORRISON, M. LONGFELLOW, A. RITSON & D. PACE. 1991. Hum. Reprod. **6:** 791–798.
2. KAMAT, B. R. & P. G. ISAACSON. 1987. Am. J. Pathol. **127:** 66–73.
3. BULMER, J. N., J. C. SMITH, L. MORRISON & M. WELLS. 1988. Placenta **9:** 237–246.
4. PARHAR, R. S., T. G. KENNEDY & P. K. LALA. 1988. Cell. Immunol. **116:** 392–410.
5. OKSENBERG, J. R., S. MOR YOSEF, Y. EZRA & C. BRAUTBAR. 1988. Am. J. Reprod. Immunol. Microbiol. **16:** 151–158.
6. VINCE, G., S. SHORTER, P. STARKEY, J. HUMPHREYS, L. CLOVER, T. WILKINS, I. SARGENT & C. REDMAN. 1992. Clin. Exp. Immunol. **88:** 174–180.
7. SHORTER, S., G. S. VINCE & P. M. STARKEY. 1992. Immunology **75:** 468–474.
8. KLENTZERIS, L. D., J. N. BULMER, M. A. WARREN, L. MORRISON, T. C. LI & I. D. COOKE. 1992. Am. J. Obstet. Gynecol. **167:** 667–674.
9. TREJDOSIEWICZ, L. K., C. J. SMART, D. J. OAKES, P. D. HOWDLE, G. MALIZIA, D. CAMPANA & A. W. BOYLSTON. 1989. Immunology **68:** 7–12.
10. DIETL, J., H. P. HORNY, P. RUCK, K. MARZUSCH, E. KAISERLING, H. GRIESSER & D. KOBELITZ. Am. J. Reprod. Immunol. **24:** 33–36.
11. CLARK, D. A. 1990. Am. J. Reprod. Immunol. **24:** 37–39.
12. MINCHEVA-NILSSON, L., S. HAMMASTROM & M. L. HAMMASTROM. 1992. J. Immunol. **149:** 2203–2211.
13. DITZIIAN-KADANOFF, R., J. GARON, M. S. VERP & M. ZILBERSTEIN. 1993. Am. J. Obstet. Gynecol. **168:** 831–836.
14. BULMER, J. N., L. MORRISON, M. LONGFELLOW & A. RITSON. 1991. Colloque INSERM **212:** 189–196.
15. YEH, C-J. G., J. N. BULMER, B-L. HSI, W-T. TIAN, C. RITTERHAUS & S. H. IP. 1990. Placenta **11:** 253–261.
16. DIVERS, M., J. N. BULMER, D. MILLER & R. J. LILFORD. Submitted for publication.
17. PACE, D., M. LONGFELLOW & J. N. BULMER. 1991. J. Reprod. Fertil. **91:** 165–174.
18. MORRISON, L. 1992. Studies of the granules, phenotypic heterogeneity and distribution of endometrial granulated lymphocytes. M. Phil. Thesis. University of Leeds.
19. KLENTZERIS, L. D., J. N. BULMER, M. A. WARREN, L. MORRISON, T. C. LI & I. D. COOKE. 1994. Hum. Reprod. **9:** 646–652.
20. WANG, H. S., H. KANZAKI, M. YOSHIDA, S. SATA, M. TOKUSHIGE & T. MORI. 1987. Am. J. Obstet. Gynecol. **157:** 956–963.
21. NAKAYAMA, E., S. ASANO, H. KODO & S. MIWA. 1985. J. Reprod. Immunol. **8:** 25–31.
22. BRIERLEY, J. & D. A. CLARK. 1987. J. Reprod. Immunol. **10:** 201–208.
23. WEGMANN, T. G. 1988. Immunol. Lett. **17:** 297–302.
24. HAMPSON, J., P. J. MCLAUGHLIN & P. M. JOHNSON. 1993. Immunology **79:** 485–490.
25. BULMER, J. N., D. HOLLINGS & A. RITSON. 1987. J. Pathol. **153:** 281–287.
26. NAGLER, A., L. L. LANIER, S. CWIRLA & J. H. PHILLIPS. 1989. J. Immunol. **143:** 3183–3991.
27. KING, A., N. BALENDRAN, P. WOODING, N. P. CARTER & Y. W. LOKE. 1991. Dev. Immunol. **1:** 169–190.
28. PACE, D., L. MORRISON & J. N. BULMER. 1989. J. Clin. Pathol. **42:** 35–39.
29. TABIBZADEH, S. & P. G. SATYASWAROOP. 1989. Am. J. Clin. Pathol. **91:** 656–663.
30. STEWART, I. J. 1991. J. Leuk. Biol. **50:** 198–207.
31. PEEL, S. 1989. Adv. Anat. Embryol. Cell Biol. **115:** 1–112.
32. RITSON, A. & J. N. BULMER. 1989. Clin. Exp. Immunol. **77:** 263–268.
33. KING, A., C. BIRKBY & Y. W. LOKE. 1989. Cell. Immunol. **118:** 337–344.
34. MANASEKI, S. & R. F. SEARLE. 1989. Cell. Immunol. **121:** 166–173.
35. FERRY, B. L., P. M. STARKEY, I. L. SARGENT, G. M. O. WATT, M. JACKSON & C. W. G. REDMAN. 1990. Immunology **70:** 446–452.

36. KING, A. & Y. W. LOKE. 1991. Immunol. Today **12:** 432–435.
37. STEWART, I. J. & J. R. CLARKE. 1993. Placenta **14:** A75.
38. FERRY, B. L., I. L. SARGENT, P. M. STARKEY & C. W. G. REDMAN. 1991. Cell. Immunol. **132:** 140–149.
39. KING, A. & Y. W. LOKE. 1990. Cell. Immunol. **129:** 435–448.
40. CHRISTMAS, S. E., J. N. BULMER, A. MEAGER & P. M. JOHNSON. 1990. Immunology **71:** 182–189.
41. CROY, B. A., N. REED, B.-A. MALASHENKO, K. KIM & B. S. KWON. 1991. Cell. Immunol. **133:** 116–126.
42. LINNEMEYER, P. A. & S. B. POLLACK. 1991. J. Immunol. **147:** 2530–2535.
43. STEWART, I. J. & S. PEEL. 1993. J. Reprod. Immunol. **24:** 165–171.
44. STEWART, I. J. & S. PEEL. 1993. J. Reprod. Fertil. **98:** 489–494.
45. LEA, R. G., K. C. FLANDERS, C. B. HARLEY, J. MANUEL, D. BANWATT & D. A. CLARK. 1992. J. Immunol. **148:** 778–787.
46. BULMER, J. N., M. LONGFELLOW & A. RITSON. 1991. Ann. N.Y. Acad. Sci. **622:** 57–68.
47. SAITO, S., K. NISHIKAWA, T. MORII, M. ENOMOTO, N. NARITA, K. MOTOYOSHI & M. ICHIJO. 1993. Int. Immunol. **5:** 559–563.
48. MCGREGOR, I. A., M. E. WILSON & W. Z. BILLEWICZ. 1983. Trans. R. Soc. Trop. Med. Hyg. **77:** 232–244.
49. LI, T. C., P. DOCKERY, A. E. ROGERS & I. D. COOKE. 1990. Br. J. Obstet. Gynaecol. **97:** 576–582.
50. KLENTZERIS, L. D., J. N. BULMER, T. C. LI, L. MORRISON, A. WARREN & I. D. COOKE. 1991. Fertil. Steril. **56:** 660–667.
51. KLENTZERIS, L. D., J. N. BULMER, M. SEPPALA, T. C. LI, M. A. WARREN & I. D. COOKE. 1993. Hum. Reprod. **8:** 1223–1230.
52. OKAMOTO, N., A. UCHIDA, K. TAKAKURA, Y. KARIYA, H. KANZAKI, L. RITTINEN, R. KOISTINEN, M. SEPPALA & T. MORI. 1991. Am. J. Reprod. Immunol. **26:** 137–142.
53. KLENTZERIS, L. D., J. N. BULMER, L. K. TREJDOSIEWICZ, L. MORRISON & I. D. COOKE. 1993. Hum. Reprod. **8:** 1223–1230.
54. MARZUSCH, K., P. RUCK, A GEISELHART, R. HANDGRETINGER, J. A. DIETL, E. KAISERLING, H-P. HORNY, G. VINCE & C. W. G. REDMAN. 1993. Hum. Reprod. **8:** 1203–1208.
55. BURROWS, T. D., A. KING & Y. W. LOKE. 1993. Cell. Immunol. **147:** 81–94.
56. DE FOUGEROLLES, A. R. & M. G. BAINES. 1987. J. Reprod. Immunol. **11:** 147–153.
57. GENDRON, R. L. & M. G. BAINES. 1988. Cell. Immunol. **113:** 261–267.
58. DRAKE, B. L. & J. R. HEAD. 1989. J. Immunol. **143:** 9–14.
59. NEBEL, L. 1986. Colloque INSERM **154:** 303–312.
60. MICHEL, M., J. UNDERWOOD, D. A. CLARK, J. F. MOWBRAY & R. W. BEARD. 1989. Am. J. Obstet. Gynecol. **161:** 409–414.

# Is Controlled Ovarian Stimulation Associated with Adverse Endometrial Effects?

ARIE BIRKENFELD[a]

*The Diamond Institute for Infertility and Menopause*
*Irvington and Millburn, New Jersey 07111*
*and*
*Department of Obstetrics, Gynecology and*
*Reproductive Science*
*Mount Sinai School of Medicine*
*New York, New York 10029*

Fundamental questions still remain unanswered and are the focus of research and speculations. First, is the decline in fecundability observed with age related to a decline in egg and embryo quality, endometrial receptivity, or both? Secondly, are we inducing adverse endometrial effects while using "infertility drugs" for the purpose of controlled ovarian stimulation (COS) thus compromising conception rates? Finally, what are the best criteria to assess endometrial function and receptivity and how can we prevent or reverse undesirable effects? Subclinical or early embryonical losses in normal cycles are hard to detect and are estimated to range between 20–30%.[1,2] Unknown numbers of embryos are wasted prior to implantation and biochemical recognition. *In vitro* fertilization (IVF) together with embryo transfer (ET) provides a unique model to evaluate preimplantation and early postimplantation loss. Following IVF/ET, most embryos are lost prior to the chemical recognition and, therefore, probably fail to implant. Slightly more than 10% are defined as chemical pregnancies,[3] and therefore implanted but failed to reach clinical detection. Thus, with normal physiologic conception, even embryos of lesser quality may implant but later fail to progress, and following IVF even better quality embryos probably fail to implant. In addition, pregnancy rates following ET of embryos after IVF of donated eggs are significantly higher then IVF results with own eggs even for the younger age groups.[4] Therefore, based upon these observations, endometrial receptivity following COS may be a crucial factor affecting conception rates.

The effect of clomiphene citrate on early embryonic development, the endometrium and implantation was reviewed by us previously.[5] In general, clomiphene citrate, a synthetic drug with both estrogenic and antiestrogenic properties, has been used in fertility clinics for more then two decades. Clomiphene is mainly used for the induction of follicular maturation and ovulation as treatment of hypothalamic-pituitary dysfunction, but in recent years its use has been applied alone or in combination with gonadotropin preparations for COS for all ramifications of assisted reproductive technologies. Almost all authors and clinics reporting

---

[a] Correspondence address: Arie Birkenfeld, M.D., The Diamond Institute for Infertility and Menopause, 1387 Clinton Avenue, Irvington, NJ 07111.

results with clomiphene citrate have reached the same conclusions: although ovulation rates are relatively high and reach 80% and higher, pregnancy rates only range between 15 and 60% with probably a higher rate of miscarriage.[6,7] Also, subclinical pregnancy loss following stimulation with clomiphene has been showed to be significantly higher than in spontaneous conception.[8] At least part of this discrepancy may be explained by an effect of clomiphene on the endometrium and as a result, on the process of implantation. Following the administration of 0.01 to 10 mg/kg per day of clomiphene to female nulliparous rabbits, secretory changes were detected in both the oviductal and uterine mucosa.[9] We concluded that these histologic changes observed by light and electron microscopy may reflect with oviductal and endometrial dysfunction. In a consecutive study evaluating the effect of clomiphene on blastocyst development and implantation in the rabbit, we transferred 4-day-old blastocysts from untreated donors to clomiphene treated pseudopregnant recipients. When recipients were treated with clomiphene before ovulation induction, implantation rates were reduced to 18.8% and were significantly ($p < 0.0002$) lower than implantation rates (62%) in the controls.[10]

Although these results may indicate a direct antiestrogenic effect of clomiphene on the endometrium, endocrine studies demonstrated that when compared with a control group, clomiphene-primed pseudopregnant rabbits had significantly lower progesterone levels after ovulation, and therefore an effect of clomiphene on ovarian corpus luteum function and progesterone production should not be excluded.[11] Trying to characterize the effect of clomiphene on the human endometrium, we have performed follicular phase endometrial biopsies 24–48 hours following routine clomiphene administration.[12] In 10 of the 19 biopsy specimens, local or diffuse signs of early secretory events were demonstrated by the presence of subnuclear vacuolization and glycogen in the glandular epithelial cells. Scanning electron microscopical evaluation corroborated these findings of advanced secretory changes. Progesterone levels at the time of biopsy were either undetectable or lower than 1.1 ng/ml. The low progesterone levels indicating the lack of luteinization suggested a possible direct antiestrogenic effect of clomiphene on the endometrium.

Other investigators have pointed out possible relations between clomiphene treatment and the incidence of luteal phase abnormalities.[13] Yet, others recommend the use of clomiphene to treat luteal phase defects.[14] In addition to a possible antiestrogenic effect evident during the proliferative phase, and closer to the time of administration, the function of the endometrium at later stages of the cycle may be altered as well and therefore in our opinion clomiphene is more likely to cause rather than treat luteal phase defects. Abortive biochemical secretory profile following clomiphene treatment was also demonstrated.[15]

Late follicular phase levels of 17-bestradiol (E2) and progesterone in serum were studied during the induction of follicular maturation with human menopausal gonadotropin (hMG) (n = 23) and hMG-clomiphene (n = 18), between 6 days to 2 hours before administration of human chorionic gonadrotropin (hCG).[16] Ultrasonographic follicular measurement at the time of evaluation demonstrated preovulatory ovarian follicles of various numbers and sizes in all patients studied. Sixteen endometrial biopsies were performed at the time of ovulation (eight for each subgroup) before hCG administration. Mean late follicular phase levels of E2 did not differ significantly between the two groups (436 ± 348 and 475 ± 267 pg/ml for the hMG and hMGcc groups, respectively). The mean progesterone levels in the hMGcc group (1.233 ± 0.67 ng/ml) was significantly higher than that for the hMG group of (0.86 ± 0.55 ng/ml, $p \leq 0.04$). The mean interval between evaluation and hCG administration for the two groups was 2.5 and 2.4 days for the hMG and hMG-clomiphene groups, respectively. In all eight biopsies taken from the hMG group, various stages of proliferative endometrium were demonstrated. Premature glandular secretory transformation and edematous stroma were observed in three out of eight biopsy specimens obtained from the hMG-clomiphene group. We concluded that subtle or full premature luteinization in the late follicular phase occurs more frequently with the use of hMG-clomiphene.

Subtle premature luteinization may have a profound and unique effect on stromal maturation causing stromal advancement resulting in asynchronous grandular-stromal transformation. Seventy patients underwent COS with GnRH agonist-hMG regime and had endometrial biopsies performed on the day of egg retrieval (hCG day +2). Sixty patients (86%) had biopsies that showed asynchrony between glands and stroma with stromal advancement greater than 2 days (mean $5.6 \pm 1.1$, range 3–8 days). Again, as demonstrated above, in this group, too, mean progesterone (P) levels over a 3-day period extending up to the day of hCG administration were $1.2 \pm 0.8$ ng/ml compared to $0.8 \pm 0.4$ ng/ml in patients with synchronized glandular and stromal development ($p < 0.05$). Serum E2 values over the same period were remarkably similar between the two groups; $2221 \pm 1062$ pg/ml, and $2242 \pm 1124$ pg/ml for the synchronous and asynchronous groups, respectively. No significant difference could be detected in E2/P ratios between the two groups.[17] To further elucidate hormonal contribution to endometrial pathology, areas under the curve (AUC) were calculated throughout the follicular and periovulatory phases. The abnormal-asynchronous endometria had a significantly higher P exposure ($5.5 \pm 2.9$ ng/ml/day) than those with normal morphological evaluation ($3.6 \pm 1.8$ ng/ml/day, $p < 0.05$).

In addition to dating criteria established in 1950 by Noyes *et al.*,[18] transmission electron microscopy may be used to refine endometrial dating and detect nucleolar channel systems (NCS). The nucleolar channel system, or nucleolar basket, is a highly organized structure found most frequently on days 17–20 of the normal cycle. NCS consists of a labyrinth of membrane bound channels confluent with the cell cytoplasm through nuclear pores. More than one NCS may often be present in the same nucleolus.[19] The function of this structure is still obscure, although there is some evidence that it may function as a nucleoluscytoplasm transport system of ribosome-like particles.

Of particular interest is the correspondence between the time and duration of NCS appearance and the presumptive endometrial window of implantation. In 3 out of 5 days 17 biopsies obtained during GnRH-a/hMG COS we were unable to detect NCS further supporting a possible functional derangement. As the morphological changes observed may reflect biochemical and functional changes, we have studied possible markers of endometrial transformation and stromal decidualization in an attempt to demonstrate biochemical changes in conjunction with the morphological observation. Using immunohistochemical staining, we evaluated the expression of prolactin, placental protein 12 (PP12) insulin-like growth factor-1 binding protein, 24 protein, stress responsive protein 27, and desmin as well as transferrin in the same samples evaluated in the morphological study. The immunohistochemical procedure was carried out in formalin fixed, paraffin-embedded tissue samples. Antibody binding was visualized using the avidin-biotin immunoperoxidase technique, graded semiquantitatively, and analyzed by percentile scattergrams. Stromal positive staining for PP12 was detected in 10% of the samples of synchronous endometrium, as compared to 60% positive PP12 staining in asynchronous endometrium with advanced stroma. Glands staining for PP12 demonstrated the same pattern (15% vs 55% in synchronized and asynchronized glands, respectively ($p < 0.01$)). The same trend was observed with stromal 24K protein.

Neither prolactin nor desmin demonstrated different expression patterns in synchronous versus asynchronous stroma, though a higher percentage of asynchronous glands than synchronous glands exhibited positive staining for prolactin. Again, in this subgroup mean serum P on the day of hCG administration was significantly higher in the asynchronous (n = 28) group as compared to the synchronous group (n = 21) (1.414 ± 0.535 ng/ml and 0.812 ± 0.316 ng/ml, respectively, $p < 0.01$). In particular, advanced stromal events may affect the endometrial environment receptivity and synchronized development. In synchronized early secretory phase biopsies, a positive stromal transferrin reaction was evident in 16/16 samples as compared to 5/16 positive reactions in glands.[20] In asynchronized biopsies' positive reaction was observed in 23/23 stromal samples as compared to 16/23 positive reaction in glands. Advanced stroma demonstrated more intensive staining as compared to early secretory stroma. In both synchronized and asynchronized samples the stroma stained earlier and more intensely than glands.

## CONCLUSIONS

Pregnancy rates and early pregnancy loss following COS are compromised. Assisted reproductive technologies apply the use of various combinations of cc, hMG and GnRH-a for COS and result in impressive follicular response and egg yield. However, even when supraphysiological numbers of embryos are transferred into the uterine cavity and pregnancy rates are calculated per embryo transfers, most embryos are lost prior to or during the peri-implantation phase.

Although so far the interest has been focused in the luteal phase and most endometrial studies were done during this period, earlier events may lead to "proliferative phase" and peri-ovulatory phase," endometrial defects which in turn may affect consequent endometrial function. In particular, advanced asynchronous stromal development may affect endometrial function and receptivity.

Morphological criteria are currently used to examine endometrial adequacy, but a biochemical profile that will reflect endometrial function throughout the cycle is missing. As morphological dating does not always correlate with clinical results, the future use of a biochemical profile may provide a better way for clinical assessment.

The endocrine pathophysiology leading to adverse endometrial effects may include supraphysiological estrogen levels and subtle to full premature luteinization. The clinician should test for these events and take them into consideration while planning clinical interventions in assisted reproductive technologies.

## REFERENCES

1. BOKLAGE, C. E. 1990. Survival probability of human conception from fertilization to term. Int. J. Fertil. **35:** 75–94.
2. WILCOX, A. J., C. R. WEINBERG, J. F. O'CONNOR et al. 1988. Incidence of early loss of pregnancy. **319:** 189–194.
3. EDWARDS, R. G. & P. C. STEPTOE. 1983. Current status of in vitro fertilization and implantation of human embryos. Lancet **2:** 1265.
4. NAVOT, D., P. A. BERGH, M. A. WILLIAMS, G. J. GARRISI, I. GUZMAN, B. SANDLER & L. GRUNFELD. 1991. Poor oocyte quality rather than implantation failure as a cause of age-related decline in female fertility. Lancet **337:** 1375–1377.
5. BIRKENFELD, A., H. M. BEIER & J. G. SCHENKER. 1986. The effect of clomiphene

citrate on early embryonic development, endometrium and implantation. Hum. Reprod. **1:** 387–395.
6. GARCIA, J., G. S. JONES & A. C. WENTZ. 1979. The use of clomiphene citrate. Fertil. Steril. **28:** 707.
7. TALBERT, L. M. 1983. Clomiphene citrate induction of ovulation. Fertil. Steril. **39:** 742.
8. BATEMAN, B. G., L. A. KOLP, W. C. NUNLEY, JR., R. FELDER & B. BURKETT. 1992. Subclinical pregnancy loss in clomiphene citrate-treated women. Fertil. Steril. **57:** 25–27.
9. BIRKENFELD, A., M. WEBER-BENNDORF, U. MOOTZ & H. M. BEIER. 1985. Effect of clomiphene on the functional morphology of oviductal and uterine mucosa. Ann. N.Y. Acad. Sci. **442:** 153–167.
10. BIRKENFELD, A., U. MOOTZ & H. M. BEIER. 1985. The effect of clomiphene citrate on blastocysts development and implantation in the rabbit. Cell Tissue Res. **241:** 495–503.
11. MEYER-WITTKOPF, M., A. BIRKENFELD & H. M. BEIER. 1989. Die pseudograviditat des kaninchens als lutealphasenmodell: Steroid und proteohormonspiegel nach clomiphencitrat-behandlung. Arch. Gynecol. Obstet. **245:** 1030–1032.
12. BIRKENFELD, A., D. NAVOT, I. S. LEVIJ, N. LAUFER, K. BEIR-HELLWIG, C. GOECKE, J. G. SCHENKER & H. M. BEIER. 1986. Advanced secretory changes in the proliferative human endometrial epithelium following clomiphene citrate treatment. Fertil. Steril. **45:** 462–468.
13. JONES, G. S., R. D. MAFFEZZOLI, C. A. STROTT, G. T. ROSS & G. KAPLAN. 1970. Pathophysiology of reproductive failure after clomiphene induced ovulation. Am. J. Obstet. Gynecol. **108:** 847–867.
14. DOWNS, K. A. & M. GIBSON. 1983. Clomiphene citrate therapy for luteal phase defect. Fertil. Steril. **39:** 34–38.
15. BEIER-HELLWIG, K., K. STERZIK, B. BONN & H. M. BEIER. 1989. Contribution to the physiology and pathology of endometrial receptivity: the determination of protein in human uterine secretions. Hum. Reprod. **4:** 115–120.
16. BIRKENFELD, A., S. J. MOR, J. EZRA, A. SIMON & D. NAVOT. 1990. Preovulatory luteinization during induction of follicular maturation with menotropin and mentropin-clomiphene combination. Hum. Reprod. **5:** 561–564.
17. BERGH, P. A., M. DREWS, S. MASUKU, G. E. HOFMANN, A. BIRKENFELD & D. NAVOT. 1991. Controlled ovarian hyperstimulation may result in profound stromal advancement and is linked to subtle premature luteinization. (Abstract) 47th Annual Meeting of the American Fertility Society. Orlando, FL. October 21–24, 1991.
18. NOYES, R. W., A. T. HERTIG & J. ROCK. 1950. Dating the endometrial biopsy. Fertil. Steril. **1:** 3–25.
19. GORDON, M. 1975. Cyclic changes in the fine structure of the epithelial cells of human endometrium. Int. Rev. Cytol. **42:** 127.
20. BIRKENFELD, A., S. TABANELLI, L. ROBERTS, E. GURPIDE, D. DELIGDISCH, D. HELLER & D. NAVOT. 1991. Immunohistochemical demonstration and localization of transferrin in the human endometrium. (Abstract) 7th Annual Meeting of the European Society of Human Reproduction and Embryology. Paris, France. June 28–30, 1991.

# The Use of the Donor Oocyte Program to Evaluate Embryo Implantation

JEROME H. CHECK[a]

*The University of Medicine and Dentistry of New Jersey*
*Robert Wood Johnson Medical School at Camden*
*Cooper Hospital/University Medical Center*
*Department of Obstetrics and Gynecology*
*Division of Reproductive Endocrinology & Infertility*
*Camden, New Jersey, 08103*

## INTRODUCTION

The first pregnancy resulting from donor oocyte fertilization was described by Lutjen *et al.*[1] Initially the oocytes for other donor oocyte programs were obtained from women undergoing tubal ligation who were willing to be hyperstimulated, or women willing to give up extra oocytes at the time of their own retrieval (before most programs had cryopreservation).[2-5] Other sources of oocytes included sisters or other non-anonymous donors provided by the recipient,[6-9] or anonymous donors provided by the *in vitro* fertilization (IVF) program itself.[10]

Another source of oocytes is the shared oocyte program where a woman needing IVF-embryo transfer (ET) herself gives 50% of the oocytes retrieved back in exchange for sharing the costs of the procedure.[11] The transfer of embryos derived from the same pool of oocytes, but transferred to two different uteri, offers a great opportunity to evaluate the importance of the endometrial factors contributing to the success or failure of certain procedures for solving problems with infertility.

Most centers have found a higher pregnancy rate (PR) in their donor oocyte program than conventional IVF. One obvious question is, can the difference in PRs be explained solely by high quality oocytes from known fertile donors in the non-shared programs? Other possible explanations are: the endometria of donors may not be as receptive, possibly related to chronic endometritis; or the estrogen used in the luteal phase by the recipients may improve uterine receptivity; or, somehow elevated gonadotropins improve receptivity; or, the hyperstimulation regimen has an adverse effect on the endometrium, *e.g.*, by advancing the endometrium too much because of subtle rise of progesterone (P) or, possibly, by adversely effecting endometrial thickness and/or echo pattern.

Preliminary data were presented where 28 donors shared oocytes with 22 recipients in 38 cycles. Though a mean of 2.7 embryos was transferred for donors vs 2.8 for recipients, there was a higher PR in recipients (28.9%) vs donors (10.5%).[12] We suggested that the hyperstimulation regimen might have had an adverse effect on the PR to explain these data.[12] But, we also suggested an alternative hypothesis of improved receptivity of the recipients or diminished receptivity of the donors.[13]

---

[a] Reprint requests to: Jerome H. Check, M.D., 7447 Old York Road, Melrose Park, PA 19027.

However, a significant negative role for the hyperstimulation regimen as the etiologic factor was provided by the data from deZiegler and Frydman, in which they demonstrated a higher PR from the transfer of cryopreserved-thawed embryos originating from donor oocytes than from those cryopreserved embryos from women undergoing hyperstimulation in previous cycles for standard IVF.[14] Their data would suggest that the better results with recipients were related either to superior quality oocytes or to differences in uterine receptivity. When the shared donor oocyte data and the frozen data are combined, the common denominator to explain the superior PR for recipients appears to be uterine receptivity.

Presented herein are four separate studies in which important information was acquired about the endometrium and implantation using the donor oocyte IVF-ET program; for these studies a shared-oocyte program was used.[1] For the first two studies only the shared program could have provided the proper experimental design to obtain these data.

*Study 1.* The aim was to corroborate or refute the preliminary data demonstrating that PRs in recipients are superior to those in donors but evaluating a larger series in a different time period.

*Study 2.* This study tried to determine if the adverse effect of a subtle rise in P at the time of human chorionic gonadotropin (hCG) injection is related to an adverse effect on the oocyte or endometrium.

There have been studies demonstrating, that, even when using a controlled ovarian hyperstimulation (COH) employing luteal phase gonadotropin releasing hormone agonist (GnRHa) plus gonadotropins followed by hCG, a subtle rise in P prior to hCG injection may lead to a decreased PR.[15-17] The premature rise of P prior to full follicular maturation in unstimulated cycles has been reported to adversely affect PR(s).[18] There are data to support the concept that premature luteinization adversely affects the oocyte.[19-21] One study reported that high P levels increased the incidence of polyspermy, suggesting that post-maturity occurs in response to premature luteinization.[22]

However, Fanchin *et al.* hypothesized that

> pre-hCG increases in plasma P that sporadically occurs in IVF-ET cycles might alter IVF-ET outcome primarily by affecting endometrium receptivity to embryo implantation. It is, indeed, conceivable that a pre-hCG elevation in plasma P could advance the secretory transformation of the endometrium, thereby leading to a premature closure of the window of receptivity before embryos are available for transfer.[23]

These authors based their hypothesis on data from their own studies and studies by Silverberg,[16] in which there was an equal number of embryos available for transfer in both high and low P groups.[23] They concluded that, ultimately, studying the outcome of transfers of cryopreserved embryos originating from IVF-ET, where P at the time of hCG was either high or low, could test the hypothesis that the adverse effect of elevated P is on the endometrium rather than embryo quality.

However, another method of testing this hypothesis is to study the outcome of embryo transfers to recipients according to the level of serum P in the oocyte donors, as in the present study. Furthermore, if one uses a shared oocyte program, noting a decreased PR in donors with high P, but no reduction in recipients from the same donor, would strongly suggest that the adverse affect of P is on the endometrium.

*Study 3.* The use of the donor oocyte program to help understand the importance of endometrial sonographic studies before hCG or the luteinizing hormone (LH) surge.[24]

The importance of achieving a minimum endometrial thickness following COH prior to the hCG injection has been found in females whose COH regimen was clomiphene citrate (CC)-human menopausal gonadotropin (hMG),[25] or, the use of the GnRHa leuprolide acetate (LA) in the luteal phase followed by hMG.[26] Similarly, an adverse effect of a pre-hCG homogeneous hyperechogenic endometrial sonographic pattern was seen with these two COH regimens in PRs during IVF-ET.[27,28]

However, no adverse effect of a thin or homogeneous echo-dense endometrium measured prior to LH surge was found in non-IVF cycles.[29] This leads to the question as to whether these abnormal endometrial signs are only important when COH is used in preparation for IVF-ET or may it be related to direct transfer of embryos to the uterus rather than the normal pathway through the fallopian tubes. Might the endometrium have more time to adjust if the embryo arrives at the proper time or may the fallopian tubes provide substances that better enable the embryo to implant, even if the uterus is not quite ready?

Evaluation of PRs following donor oocyte fertilization and subsequent embryo transfer may provide answers to the above question. A poor PR with thin endometria or homogeneous echo-dense endometrial patterns in recipients would favor the theory that timing or mode of reaching the uterine cavity requires a more perfect endometrium than the normal transtubal arrival.

*Study 4.* The use of the donor oocyte program to test whether advancing age leads to a senescent uterus, or, is the reduction in fertility potential strictly related to the oocyte factor?[30,31]

Recently, pregnancies have even been achieved in women over the age of 50.[32] This fact, coupled with the reports of success of donor oocyte programs with aged recipients,[33-35] has lead to the conclusion that the general decline of fertility with advancing age is not related to uterine senescence.[36,37]

However, the possibility exists that aging does decrease endometrial receptivity but that the defects may be reversible. For example, there is some indirect evidence that the uterus becomes less sensitive to P with advancing age. Meldrum initially found only an 8% PR in his oocyte recipient population >40 years compared to 43% in those ≤40;[38] however, when he increased the luteal phase support dosage of P from the conventional 50 mg/day to 100 mg/day intramuscular (IM) there was no longer a difference in PRs between older and younger recipients.[39]

The study herein evaluated whether part of uterine senescence might be manifested by thinner endometria pre-hCG. If in fact this was found and a reduced PR was seen, the next part of the study would be to see if adjustments for endometrial thickness could raise the PR. These studies would all be performed at the lower 50 mg/day IM P dosage.

## MATERIALS AND METHODS

### Study 1

A different time period (1/1/92 to 12/31/92) was evaluated than was previously reported; there was no overlap. During this time interval there were some patients who provided their own donors, but they were excluded from these data. The clinical and viable PR per transfer was calculated. Statistical evaluation was performed using Chi-square analysis.

The large majority of donors used the luteal phase LA-hMG COH protocol.[39] Treatment protocols for donor and recipients have been previously described.[24]

## Study 2

All women undergoing IVF-ET who shared oocytes between 11/1/91 and 8/19/92 were evaluated. These data were chosen because at that time the serum P assay was the same one used when a higher PR was found to be associated with low levels of P measured by the Amerlex-M radioimmunoassay (RIA) (Amersham Inc., Arlington Heights, IL). Donors were given the luteal phase LA-hMG regimen as in Study 1.

The clinical and viable PRs were calculated in both donors and recipients according to sera $P \leq 1$ ng/mL or $> 1$ ng/mL. Statistical evaluation used Chi-square analysis.

## Study 3

This study evaluated endometrial thickness and echo pattern pre-hCG in 44 donor oocyte recipients undergoing a total of 58 transfer cycles at the Cooper Institute for IVF-ET. The details of the methodology were previously presented.[24]

## Study 4

There were two parts to the study: the first one included 78 consecutive donor oocyte transfer cycles and PRs were compared related to age <40 or 40 or more. Though endometrial thickness prior to the hCG injection of the donor was measured no therapeutic decisions were made based on these measurements. More specific details of this first part were previously described.[30]

The second part of the study included 121 consecutive donor-oocyte transfers from 9/88 to 9/92. During these cycles adjustments were made for endometrial thickness. If the donor reached criteria suitable for giving hCG and stopping hMG, but the recipient had not reached a minimal 10 mm endometrial thickness, the estradiol ($E_2$) was increased by 2 mg in the recipient while the donor's hMG was continued for one to two days. If, despite this adjustment, the minimal thickness was not achieved, the recipients' embryos were cryopreserved and transferred on a subsequent cycle when adequate thickness was achieved (the $E_2$ dosage would be started at 4 mg instead of 2 mg and the increments would be the same).[24]

## RESULTS

### Study 1

The clinical PR observed in the shared oocyte program during 1992 was 23.6% (17 of 72 cycles) for the donors and 34.6% (26 or 75) for the recipients (Chi-square, $p > 0.05$). Since the mean age of the donors was only 32 years as compared to 40 years for the recipients ($p < 0.05$, $t$ test), the age-specific PRs were computed for those recipients ≤40 years and those >40 years (note, only donors <40 years old are eligible to participate in this program). The clinical PR for recipients ≤40 years of age was 44.1% as compared to 26.8% for the older recipients. Chi-square

TABLE 1. Pregnancy Rates from the Shared Oocyte Program in 1992

|  | Donors | All Recipients[a] | Recipients ≤40[b] | Recipients >40[c] |
|---|---|---|---|---|
| # Transfers | 72 | 75 | 34 | 41 |
| # Pregnancies | 26 (36.1%) | 28 (37.3%) | 16 (47.1%) | 12 (29.2%) |
| # Viable pregnancies | 17 (23.6%) | 26 (34.6%) | 15 (44.1%) | 11 (26.8%) |
| Average age | 32 | 39.8 | 36.3 | 42.8 |

[a] All donors vs all recipients, not significant.
[b] All donors to recipients ≤40, $p < 0.05$.
[c] All donors to recipients ≥40, not significant.

analysis demonstrated that the PRs are similar for donors and older recipients, but are significantly higher for the younger recipients compared to donors (TABLE 1).

## Study 2

For those recipients who received oocytes from donors whose sera P level on the day of hCG administration was ≤1 ng/mL, the clinical PR per transfer was 17.3% as compared to 17.5% (Chi-square, $p > 0.05$) for those recipients who received their oocytes from donors whose sera P level was >1 ng/mL on day of hCG. The rates for the donors in these two groups were 15.9% and 11.6% (Chi-square, $p > 0.05$). The viable PR was the same (14.4%) for the two recipient groups, but was lower ($p < 0.05$) in the donor group with high serum P (7.2%) than the donor group with lower pre-hCG P levels (12.7%).[40]

## Study 3

For the 58 recipient cycles evaluated in terms of sonographic endometrial conditions, the clinical PR/transfer of 9% (2 of 22) observed for patients whose endometrium measured less than 10 mm was significantly lower than the 38.7% rate (14 of 36) observed for patients whose endometrium was greater than 10 mm (Chi-square, $p < 0.01$). However, no relationship was found between the echo pattern observed on day of donor's hCG and subsequent PR: the PRs were 16.7% (1 of 6) for the hypoechogenic pattern; 31% (9 of 39) for the isoechogenic pattern; and 26.1% (6 of 23) for the hyperechogenic pattern (Chi-square, $p > 0.05$).[24]

## Study 4

For the first 78 cycles evaluated no clinical intervention was made for endometrial thickness. The clinical PR per transfer for older recipients (over 40 years old) was 8.6% (2 of 23 cycles). This rate was much lower than the 25.4% rate (14 of 55) observed in the younger recipients (Chi-square, $p < 0.05$). The endometrial thickness was thin (<10 mm) for 61% of the older recipients, as compared to only 29% of the younger recipients (Chi-square, $p < 0.05$).[30]

Based on these findings, the protocol for all subsequent recipient cycles was modified to take into account the endometrial thickness. The clinical PRs per transfer for all IVF-ET cycles in which fresh embryos were transferred was 29.6% (16 of 54) for the younger recipients and 25.4% (17 of 67) for the older recipients (Chi-square, $p > 0.05$). The PRs for the donors was 15.1% for those who donated to the younger recipients (8 of 53) and 14.3% for those who donated to the older recipients.[31]

## DISCUSSION

Combining all four studies from the donor oocyte program the following hypothesis may be drawn. The uterus of recipients seems to provide a better tissue for implantation than the normal population undergoing IVF-ET. Since this could be related to chronic endometritis in the group undergoing conventional IVF-ET with a high rate of previous pelvic infection, *e.g.*, salpingitis, more interest may be generated into special culturing techniques or even empirical use of prophylactic antibiotics prior to transfer in this group.

However, the possibility exists that one factor reducing the PR might be the serum P level at the time of hCG. The fact that the PR was similar in recipients obtaining oocytes from donors with higher vs lower pre-hCG sera P levels suggests that the adverse effect of subtle rise of P is not on oocyte quality. Though the PR was not as high during this study as in the previous one, when $P \leq 1$ ng/mL, nevertheless, the lower viable PR in the donor group with higher pre-hCG P levels supports the concept of subtle rise in P adversely effecting embryo implantation, possibly by advancing the secretory endometrium. One advantage to the recipient, obviously, is that the P is low prior to the donor's hCG. Further randomized studies are now in progress in our laboratory to see if there is any adverse effect of the serum P from 1.1 to 1.5 ng/mL pre-hCG by delaying transfer in half the patients and cryopreserving the other embryos with transfer in a subsequent cycle (our cryopreservation PR of 2 pronuclear embryos is equal to our fresh transfer rates).

The data from other studies finding the older donor oocyte recipient with improved PRs with increased P dosage in the luteal phase has to make one wonder whether some patients undergoing IVF-ET may need a higher dosage of P for luteal phase supplementation. Perhaps late luteal phase endometrial biopsies should be obtained if the beta hCG levels are negative and dosage adjusted for the next cycle. Indeed Ben-Nun *et al.* found an improved PR by increasing the P dosage in the luteal phase of patients undergoing IVF-ET.[41] Check *et al.* were unable to confirm Ben-Nun's data and, in fact, the higher P dosage resulted in a lower PR;[42] however, the possibility exists that if we would have merely increased the luteal phase P dosage rather than also starting IM P on the day of hCG (and thus maybe advancing the secretory endometrium) we may have obtained an even greater PR.

Study 3 also showed poor PRs with thin endometria in donor-oocyte recipients not receiving COH (but no adverse effect of a homogeneous echo-dense endometrium), suggesting that the importance of an adequate thickness is essential when embryos are transferred to the uterus, but, possibly not when the embryos arrive through the fallopian tubes. Furthermore, Study 4 suggests that one of the uterine senescent factors might be reduced endometrial thickness; when adjustments are made, a markedly improved PR results. The possibility exists that increasing the dosage of P support may overcome this defect.

Of course, the higher percentage of older patients who do not develop adequate thickness following COH or the hormone replacement regimen used for donor oocyte replacement and their subsequent reduced PRs might only apply to assisted reproductive technology (ART) since we did not demonstrate any adverse effect for non-IVF cycles.[29] However, in that study there was not a high percentage of women with very thin endometria and the possibility exists that a study of older patients in non-IVF cycles might demonstrate thinner endometria than younger patients; perhaps the critical thickness for a natural cycle is significantly less than for a cycle with uterine transfers of embryos.

All of the conclusions and suggestions accrued from these four studies are based on the assumption that the basic premises are correct. All studies are not unanimous that the endometrial thickness influences the PR in ART;[43] also, some centers believe that the endometrial thickness does influence PRs even from non-IV cycles.[44,45]

Similarly, there is not universal agreement that a subtle rise in P pre-hCG predicts a reduced PR.[46] In fact, we were unable to confirm our original data;[47] however, for the second study a non-isotopic method rather than an RIA to measure P was used and although the coefficient of variation (CV) was low at mid-luteal and pregnancy levels, the CV was poor in the very low ranges of 1 ng/mL or less. Similarly, the Pantex assay used by Edelstein *et al.* was criticized for the very high CV.[48,49]

All these data need to be confirmed by other centers with larger numbers of cases. The shared donor oocyte program especially has the potential to help elucidate even more information about oocyte vs endometrial receptivity factor and even help learn about male factor (comparing fertilization by donor's vs recipient's husband), yet at the same time two people get the opportunity to conceive at one time who may not have had the opportunity otherwise. There has not been a reduction in PRs in those who donate vs those not choosing to do so, except for donors over age 35.[50]

## SUMMARY

Pregnancy rates (PRs) are generally higher in most IVF programs when embryos derived from donor oocytes are transferred compared to the PRs of women undergoing IVF-ET. DeZiegler *et al.*, using the transfer of frozen embryos (either patient or donor derived) in natural cycles, found a higher PR following donor oocyte derived ET and thus concluded that the lower PR in the non-donor cycles was not related to the controlled ovarian hyperstimulation (COH) regimen. Their data thus suggested the improved PR with donor embryos may be related to better quality oocytes used for recipients; however, a more receptive endometrium in the oocyte recipients could also explain the data. The studies presented herein further evaluated the latter hypothesis of improved endometrial environment for recipients by comparing PRs in donors vs recipients in a shared oocyte program. Also the study would determine if endometrial echo patterns (EP) and/or thickness (ET) help predict better PRs as they do in stimulated cycles. Finally studies would be performed to compare PRs in older vs younger oocyte recipients to see if there may be a uterine senescence in humans as in other animals and to see if age has an adverse effect on the endometrium as evidenced by sonographic studies. Study 1 compared the clinical PRs in donors vs recipients in a shared program from 1/1/92 to 12/31/92. PR for donors was 23.6% (17 pregnant in 72 transfers) compared to 34.6% for recipients (26/75). Mean age of the donors was 32 compared to 39.8 for recipients. If recipients >40 were eliminated the PR for recipients was 44.1%

(15/34). Study 2 evaluated PRs according to ET and EP in 58 transfers using donor oocytes (44 patients). There were only 2 clinical pregnancies of 22 transfers (9%/cycle) when ET was <10 mm at the time of the donor's hCG injection compared to 14 pregnant of 36 transfers (38.7%) when ET was ≥10 mm ($p < 0.01$). However, there were no differences in PR when the endometrium compared to myometrium was hypoechogenic, isoechogenic, or hyperechogenic. The respective PRs were 16.7% (1/6), 31% (9/39) and 26.1% (6/23). Study 3 evaluated PRs in donor oocyte recipients according to age (<40 vs ≥40 years). After evaluating PRs after the first 58 ETs to recipients of shared oocytes we found a much lower PR in women ≥40 (2/23, 8.6%/cycle) vs 14/55 (25.4%) in those <40. The ET was <10 mm in 61% of those patients ≥40 vs only 29% in those <40 at time of donor's hCG. We then evaluated PRs in donor oocyte recipients in 121 consecutive shared oocyte ETs from 9/88 to 9/92; when adjustments were made to try to get ET improved to 10 mm by increasing and prolonging estrogen exposure to recipients and by cancellation of fresh ET and performing frozen ET (FET) in a subsequent cycle, the combined fresh and FET clinical PRs in women <40 was 29.6% (16/54) vs 25.4% (17/67) in those ≥40. Meldrum had previously found only an 8% PR in recipients over 40 which increased to 43% when the IM progesterone (P) dosage was doubled from 50 to 100 mg (we used only 50 mg IM daily). Asch found a higher PR in donor oocyte recipients using GIFT rather than IVF. We did not find a different PR in women with ET < 10 mm in non-IVF cycles. These data may support the hypothesis that improved PRs may be present in donor oocyte recipients related to better endometria (perhaps greater chance of chronic endometritis in women with nonpatent tubes related to salpingitis). There is reduced endometrial receptivity with advancing age but this may be compensated for by adjusting for ET, increasing the luteal phase dosage or delaying the time the embryo reaches the endometrial cavity (GIFT, 3-day transfer, co-culture, etc.).

## REFERENCES

1. LUTJEN, P., A. TROUNSON, J. LEETON, J. FINDLAY, C. WOOD & P. RENOV. 1984. The establishment and maintenance of pregnancy using *in vitro* fertilization and embryo donation in a patient with primary ovarian failure. Nature **307:** 174–175.
2. ROSENWAKS, Z., L. L. VEECK & H. C. LIU. 1986. Pregnancy following transfer of *in vitro* fertilized donated oocytes. Fertil. Steril. **45:** 417–420.
3. NAVOT, D., W. LAUFER, J. KOPOLOVIC, R. RABINOWITZ, A. BIRKENFELD, A. LEWIN, M. GRANAT, E. MARGALIOT & J. G. SHENKER. 1986. Artificially induced endometrial cycles and establishment of pregnancies in the absence of ovaries. N. Engl. J. Med. **314:** 806–811.
4. LUTJEN, P. J., J. F. LEETON & J. K. FINDLAY. 1985. Oocyte and embryo donation in IVF programs. Clin. Obstet. Gynaecol. **12:** 799–813.
5. DEVROEY, P., A. WISANTO, M. CAMUS, L. V. WAESBERGHE, C. BOURGAIN, I. LIEBAERS & A. C. VAN STEIRTEGHEM. 1988. Oocyte donation in patients without ovarian function. Hum. Reprod. **3:** 699–704.
6. LEETON, J., L. CHAN, A. TROUNSON & J. HARMAN. 1986. Pregnancy established in an infertile patient after transfer of an embryo fertilized *in vitro* where the oocyte was donated by the sister of the recipient. J. *In Vitro* Fert. Embryo Transfer **3:** 379–382.
7. ROSENBERG, S. M., J. M. EAST, S. C. WOOD & J. J. CRAIN. 1989. Ovum donation by sisters in ovarian failure simplified primary and early withdrawal of exogenous support. J. *In Vitro* Fert. Embryo Transfer **6:** 228–237.
8. SAUER, M., I. A. RODI, M. SCROOC, M. BUSTILLO & J. E. BUSTER. 1988. Survey of attitudes regarding the use of siblings for gamete donation. Fertil. Steril. **49:** 721–722.
9. SAUER, M. V., R. J. PAULSON, T. M. MACASO, M. FRANCES-HERNANDEZ & R. A.

LOBO. 1989. Establishment of a nonanonymous donor oocyte program: preliminary experience at the University of Southern California. Fertil. Steril. **52:** 433–436.
10. SAUER, M. V., R. J. PAULSON & R. A. LOBO. 1992. Reversing the natural decline in human fertility. JAMA **268:** 1275–1279.
11. CHECK, J. H., K. NOWROOZI, J. CHASE, A. NAZARI & C. BRAITHWAITE. 1992. Comparison of pregnancy rates following *in vitro* fertilization-embryo transfer between the donors and the recipients in a donor oocyte program. J. Assist. Reprod. Genet. **9:** 248–250.
12. CHECK, J. H., K. NOWROOZI, J. S. CHASE, A. NAZARI, C. BRAITHWAITE & G. GOLDSMITH. 1990. Evidence supporting the hyperstimulation regimen as a negative factor for *in vitro* fertilization pregnancies. (Abstr. P-143) Presented at the 46th Annual Meeting of the American Fertility Society, Washington, D.C., October 13–18, 1990. Published by The American Fertility Society, Birmingham, Alabama, in the Program Supplement, 1990, p. S125.
13. CHECK, J. H., D. DE ZIEGLER & R. FRYDMAN. 1991. Uterine receptivity in subjects with ovarian failure. Fertil. Steril. **55:** 1208–1209.
14. DE ZIEGLER, D. & R. FRYDMAN. 1990. Different implantation rates after transfers of cryopreserved embryos originating from donated oocytes or from regular *in vitro* fertilization. Fertil. Steril. **54:** 682–688.
15. SCHOOLCRAFT, W., E. SINTON, T. SCHLENKER, D. HUYNH, F. HAMILTON & D. R. MELDRUM. 1991. Lower pregnancy rate with premature luteinization during pituitary suppression with leuprolide acetate. Fertil. Steril. **55:** 563–566.
16. SILVERBERG, K. M., W. N. BURNS, D. L. OLIVE, R. M. RIEHL & R. S. SCHENKEN. 1991. Serum progesterone levels predict success of *in vitro* fertilization/embryo transfer in patients stimulated with leuprolide acetate and human menopausal gonadotropins. J. Clin. Endocrinol. Metab. **73:** 797–803.
17. CHECK, J. H., D. LURIE, H. A. ASKARI, L. HOOVER & C. LAUER. 1993. The range of subtle rise in serum progesterone levels following controlled ovarian hyperstimulation associated with lower *in vitro* fertilization pregnancy rates is determined by the source of manufacturer. Eur. J. Obstet. Gynecol. Reprod. Biol. In press.
18. CHECK, J. H., J. S. CHASE, K. NOWROOZI & C. J. DIETTERICH. 1991. Premature luteinization: treatment and incidence in natural cycles. Hum. Reprod. **6:** 190–193.
19. LEUNG, P. C. S., A. LOPATA, G. N. KELLOW, W. I. H. JOHNSTON & M. J. GRONOW. 1983. A histochemical study of cumulus cells for assessing the quality of preovulatory oocytes. Fertil. Steril. **39:** 853–855.
20. DLUGI, A. M., N. LAUFER, M. L. POLAN, A. H. DE CHERNEY, B. C. TARLATZIS, N. J. MACLUSKY & H. R. BEHRMAN. 1984. 17B-estradiol and progesterone production by human granulosa-luteal cells isolated from human menopausal gonadotropin-stimulated cycles for *in vitro* fertilization. J. Clin. Endocrinol. Metab. **59:** 986–992.
21. HARTSHORNE, G. M. 1989. Steroid production by the cumulus: relationship to fertilization *in vitro*. Hum. Reprod. **4:** 742–745.
22. EDWARDS, R. G. 1985. *In vitro* fertilization and embryo replacement. Ann. N.Y. Acad. Sci. **442:** 1–24.
23. FANCHIN, R., D. DE ZIEGLER, J. TAIEB, A. HAZOUT & R. FRYDMAN. 1993. Premature elevation of plasma progesterone alters pregnancy rates of *in vitro* fertilization and embryo transfer. Fertil. Steril. **59:** 1090–1094.
24. CHECK, J. H., K. NOWROOZI, J. CHOE, D. LURIE & C. DIETTERICH. 1993. The effect of endometrial thickness and echo pattern on *in vitro* fertilization outcome in donor oocyte-embryo transfer cycle. Fertil. Steril. **59:** 72–75.
25. GONEN, Y., R. F. CASPER, W. JACOBSON & J. BLANKIER. 1989. Endometrial thickness and growth during ovarian stimulation: a possible predictor of implantation in *in vitro* fertilization and embryo transfer. Fertil. Steril. **52:** 446–450.
26. CHECK, J. H., K. NOWROOZI, J. CHOE & C. DIETTERICH. 1991. Influence of endometrial thickness and echo patterns on pregnancy rates during *in vitro* fertilization. Fertil. Steril. **56:** 1173–1175.
27. GONEN, Y. & R. F. CASPER. 1990. Prediction of implantation by the sonographic appearance of the endometrium during controlled ovarian stimulation for *in vitro* fertilization (IVF). J. *In Vitro* Fert. Embryo Transfer **7:** 146–152.

28. CHECK, J. H., D. LURIE, C. DIETTERICH, C. CALLAN & A. BAKER. 1993. Adverse effect of a homogeneous hyperechogenic endometrial sonographic pattern, despite adequate endometrial thickness on pregnancy rates following *in vitro* fertilization. Hum. Reprod. **8:** 1293-1296.
29. CHECK, J. H., C. DIETTERICH, D. LURIE, J. S. CHASE & K. NOWROOZI. 1993. The relationship of endometrial thickness and echo patterns and pregnancy rates in non-IVF cycles. (Abstr. P-013) Presented at the 41st Annual Meeting of the Pacific Coast Fertility Society, April 14-18, 1993. Indian Wells, CA.
30. CHECK, J. H., H. A. ASKARI, J. K. CHOE, A. BAKER & H. G. ADELSON. 1993. The effect of the age of the recipients on pregnancy rates following donor-oocyte replacement. J. Assist. Reprod. Genet. **10:** 137-140.
31. CHECK, J. H., H. A. ASKARI, C. FISHER & L. VANAMAN. 1993. The use of a shared donor oocyte program to evaluate the effect of uterine senescence. Fertil. Steril. In press.
32. CHECK, J. H., K. NOWROOZI, E. R. BARNEA, K. J. SHAW & M. V. SAUER. 1992. Successful delivery after age 50: a report of two cases as a result of oocyte donation. Obstet. Gynecol. **81:** 835-836.
33. ROMEU, A., S. S. MUASHER, A. A. ACOSTA, L. L. VEECK, J. DIAZ, G. S. JONES, H. W. JONES, JR. & Z. ROSENWAKS. 1987. Results of IVF attempts in women 40 years of age and older, the Norfolk experience. Fertil. Steril. **47:** 130-136.
34. SAUER, M. V., R. J. PAULSON & R. A. LOBO. 1990. A preliminary report on oocyte donation extending reproductive potential to women over 40. N. Engl. J. Med. **323:** 1157-1160.
35. SAUER, M. V., R. J. PAULSON & R. A. LOBO. 1992. Reversing the natural decline in human fertility. JAMA **268:** 1275-1279.
36. TALBERT, G. B. 1968. Effect of maternal age on the reproductive capacity. Am. J. Obstet. Gynecol. **102:** 451-477.
37. TULANDI, T., G. H. ARROVET & R. A. MCINNES. 1981. Infertility in women over the age of 36. Fertil. Steril. **35:** 611-614.
38. MELDRUM, D. R. 1993. Female reproduction aging-ovarian and uterine factors. Fertil. Steril. **59:** 1-5.
39. MELDRUM, D. R., A. WISOT, F. HAMILTON, A. L. GUTLAY, W. KEMPTON & D. HUYNH. 1989. Routine pituitary suppression with leuprolide before ovarian stimulation for oocyte retrieval. Fertil. Steril. **51:** 455-459.
40. CHECK, J. H., C. HOURANI, J. K. CHOE, C. CALLAN & H. G. ADELSON. 1993. Pregnancy rates in donors versus recipients according to the serum progesterone level at time of human chorionic gonadotropin (hCG) in a shared oocyte program. Fertil. Steril. In press.
41. BEN-NUN, I., Y. GHETLER, R. JAFFE, A. SIEGAL, H. KANETI & M. FEJGIN. 1990. Effect of preovulatory progesterone administration on the maturation and implantation rate after *in vitro* fertilization and transfer. Fertil. Steril. **53:** 276-281.
42. CHECK, J. H., K. NOWROOZI, J. S. CHASE, A. NAZARI & C. CALLAN. 1991. Comparison of luteal phase support with high and low-dose progesterone therpay on pregnancy rates in an *in vitro* fertilization program. J. *In Vitro* Fert. Embryo Transfer **8:** 173-175.
43. FLEISCHER, A. C., C. M. HERBERT, G. A. SACKS, A. C. WENTZ, S. S. ENTMAN & A. E. JAMES, JR. 1986. Sonography during conception and non-conception cycles of *in vitro* fertilization and embryo transfer. Fertil. Steril. **46:** 442-447.
44. SHOHMAN, Z., C. DiCAROLO, A. PATEL, G. S. CONWAY & H. S. JACOBS. 1991. Is it possible to run a successful ovulation induction program based solely on ultrasound monitoring? The importance of endometrial measurements. Fertil. Steril. **56:** 836-841.
45. COHEN, B. M., L. BERRY, V. ROETHEMEYER & D. SMITH. 1992. Sonographic assessment of late proliferative phase endometrium during ovulation induction. J. Reprod. Med. **37:** 685-690.
46. EDELSTEIN, M. C., H. G. SELTMAN, B. J. COS, S. M. ROBINSON, R. A. SHAW & S. J. MUASHER. 1990. Progesterone levels on the day of human chorionic gonadotropin administration in cycles with gonadotropin-releasing hormone agonist suppression are not predictive of pregnancy outcome. Fertil. Steril. **54:** 853-857.

47. CHECK, J. H., D. LURIE, J. S. CHASE, L. HOOVER, L. STUMPO & D. SUMMERS. 1993. Progesterone levels prior to hCG determined by RIA method superior to enzyme immunoassay method in predicting which IVF patients are more likely to conceive. Presented at the 41st Annual Pacific Coast Fertility Meeting (Abstr. P-030).
48. SILVERBERG, K. M., D. L. OLIVE & R. S. SCHENKEN. 1991. Statistical scuds. Fertil. Steril. **56:** 153–154.
49. MELDRUM, D. R. 1991. Letter to the Editor. Fertil. Steril. **56:** 154–155.
50. CHECK, J. H., J. CHOE, H. ADELSON & C. FISHER. 1992. Effect of age of oocyte donors on pregnancy rates in a shared-oocyte *in vitro* fertilization (IVF) program. Presented at the 48th Annual Meeting of the American Fertility Society (Abstr. O-092).

# Hormonal Control of Endometrial Receptivity

## The Egg Donation Model and Controlled Ovarian Hyperstimulation

DOMINIQUE DE ZIEGLER,[a] RENATO FANCHIN,[a]
MARC MASSONNEAU,[b] CHRISTINE BERGERON,[c]
RENÉ FRYDMAN,[a] AND PHILIPPE BOUCHARD[d]

[a]*Department of Obstetrics and Gynecology*
*Hôpital A. Béclère*
*Clamart, France*

[b]*IôDP*
*Image Analysis*
*Paris, France*

[c]*Institut de Pathologie et de Cytologie Appliquée-CERBA*
*St. Ouen, France*

[d]*Department of Endocrinology*
*Hôpital St. Antoine*
*Paris, France*

## INTRODUCTION

Embryo implantation has remained a stumbling block hampering success rates in *in vitro* fertilization (IVF) and other assisted reproductive techniques (ART). Recent years have witnessed spectacular progress in mastering induction of multiple ovulation with exogenous gonadotropins (hMG and/or hFSH), most often in various forms of association with agonist or antagonist analogs of GnRH. This satisfactory control of follicular maturation has been associated with parallel improvements in *in vitro* techniques leading to reliable yields of multiple-morphologically acceptable embryos available for transfer. Low embryo implantation rates, however, have remained the bottleneck of all ART systems that cripples pregnancy rates severely. Originally meant to be merely a minor by-product of IVF, egg donation has since blossomed into an unexpectedly successful clinical tool and has become a primary source of information to clarify how hormones control endometrial receptivity.

A belief that has been widely shared states that of all ovarian products, only estradiol ($E_2$) and progesterone (P) carry significant effects on the endometrium. This concept has been the basis for including only $E_2$ and P in replacement cycles conceived for egg donation recipients, a practice rapidly encouraged by spectacular success rates which reward egg donation programs worldwide. The conclusion drawn from egg donation results, however, should not be erroneously confused with the reciprocal assertion that ovarian factors other than $E_2$ and P are incapable of affecting the endometrium. Yet this error has been de facto implied when only the high $E_2$ levels of COH have been considered as potentially harmful to receptivity in IVF and most forms of ARTs. On the contrary, the possible endometrial impact of a variety of other ovarian factors such as androgens and peptides, whose production is also enhanced by ovarian hyperstimulation with exogenous gonadotropins, have been remarkably ignored.

In the present review, we shall analyze the lessons taught by egg donation about hormonal control of endometrial receptivity. In doing so, the emphasis will be put on the role of the $E_2/P$ ratio as well as on the dose-effect relationships that govern the endometrial effects of P. Also, we shall attempt to establish a parallel between the situation observed in egg donation and that prevailing in regular IVF. For this we shall discuss recent studies which look extensively at the hormonal profiles brought by the two actors of COH, hMG and hCG. In the discussion, we shall ponder the possible merits and limitations of the new *third factor* theory proposed to account for some of the counterperformances in embryo implantation seen in IVF. In keeping with this concept we shall try to substantiate the allegation that a purported ovarian factor, other than $E_2$ or P, (or *third factor*) produced excessively in COH may adversely affect endometrial receptivity.

## *The Egg Donation Model: When Less Appears Better*

The possibility of offering egg donation to young women prematurely deprived of ovarian function has come as a direct spin off directly evolving from mastering extra corporeal fertilization of human eggs. At first glance, egg donation was perceived as a nearly heroic endeavor because of the seemingly complex tasks it involved.[1,2] Indeed, to succeed egg donation required that oocyte maturation in the donor be synchronized with endometrial transformations induced in the recipient with exogenous hormones. Yet, it has rapidly become apparent that egg donation was universally rewarded by excellent pregnancy rates[3-8] that by and large exceeded results of corresponding regular IVF programs.[9-12] On top of being gratifying to its participants, the high pregnancy rates have validated egg donation hormonal replacement regimens as a study model for elucidating the physiology and physiopathology of the hormonal control of endometrial receptivity.

One domain in which egg donation replacement cycles have been particularly informative is in understanding the advantages and limitations of the various hormone delivery systems. Estradiol can be administered orally,[1,2] vaginally[13] or transdermally[14,15] for the purpose of inducing physiological estrogen priming of the endometrium. When administered orally, the $E_2$ doses that need to be administered to duplicate physiological levels of $E_2$ seen in the menstrual cycle, range from 4 to 8 mg/day.[1,2,5,7] These amounts are approximately 10 times higher than the corresponding $E_2$ production rates seen in the menstrual cycle. Hence, the differences between ovarian production rates and $E_2$ treatment delivery rates required in egg donation mock cycles reflect the massive $E_2$ inactivation that occurs by metabolism in the digestive mucosa and liver.[16] When administered orally, $E_2$ is readily metabolized into the lesser active estrone ($E_1$) in the mucosal cells of the digestive tract.[17] Part of the newly formed $E_1$ is reconverted in the liver and elsewhere in the body into $E_2$. Yet, kinetic characteristics of 17$\beta$-hydroxylase, the enzyme governing the $E_2 \rightarrow E_1$ conversion, are such that egg donation replacement cycles achieving menstrual cycle levels of $E_2$ also result in $E_1$ levels 10 times higher than encountered normally.[17] Aside from the conversion of $E_2$ into $E_1$ in the digestive epithelium, orally ingested estrogen must transit through the liver before reaching any other target organ. During its obligatory transit through the liver, a fraction of the estrogen load undergoes sulfation or conjugation (namely, glucuronidation) yielding more polar derivatives that are excreted in the urine and bile. The practical consequence of the functional overload of the liver is an elevation in the circulating levels of a variety of estrogen sensitive proteins, a phenomenon commonly referred to as the liver first-pass effect. Despite this intense liver and digestive metabolism requiring doses of oral $E_2$ to be tenfold higher than ovarian production rates and resulting in high plasma $E_1$ levels, the endometrial effects of egg donation mock cycles using oral, vaginal and transdermal $E_2$ are remarkably similar.[9,12,18,19] In a prospective randomized cross-over trial we compared the endometrial effects of oral and transdermal $E_2$ administered in amounts duplicating the menstrual cycle pattern of plasma $E_2$ levels in association with vaginal P administration. We previously observed that the two forms of $E_2$ treatment resulted in indistinguishable day 26 endometrial biopsies.[20]

Attempting to simplify the hormonal replacement regimens prescribed for egg donation recipients, numerous investigators have questioned whether it is necessary to reproduce the cyclical increase in $E_2$ levels that normally takes place just prior to ovulation in the menstrual cycle.[21] In the menstrual cycle, it has been amply documented that the cyclical increase in $E_2$ exerts a facilitatory role on the neuro-endocrinological mechanisms governing the pre-ovulatory LH surge.[21] The classical reproductive endocrinology reference texts, however, usually remain silent about the possibility that the pre-ovulatory increase in $E_2$ has any associated endometrial effects. The report by Craft et al.[19] which shows excellent pregnancy rates after egg donation recipients received constant doses of $E_2$, has seriously challenged the possibility that the endometrium benefits from specific endometrial priming brought by the preovulatory pattern of $E_2$ increase. Hence, looking at egg donation data it appears that sufficient estrogen priming (time and dose wise) is all that is needed as prerequisite for P to trigger proper endometrial receptivity.

Egg donation protocols have also enriched our understanding of the therapeutic dilemmas pertaining to P administration. Here, the situation differs slightly from that experienced with $E_2$ treatment because oral P administration has rightfully not been attempted for priming endometrial receptivity. Indeed, the extremely poor bioavailability of orally administered P[22,23] and the lack of secretory changes it induces in the endometrium[24-26] would have in all likelihood made the oral P option ill fated for egg donation. Analyzing the remaining options for P administration in egg donation, namely, the intramuscular (IM) and transvaginal routes, revolves around establishing the correlations existing between plasma P levels and endometrial effects. This will be the object of a specific section later in this review, which surveys the dose-effect relationship of P action.

A corollary to the excellent pregnancy rates observed after transferring embryos in women whose endometrium has been prepared solely with exogenous hormone is that ovarian factors other than $E_2$ and P are not strictly necessary for triggering prime endometrial receptivity. Aside from being particularly helpful for treating egg donation recipients simply yet successfully, the observation that only $E_2$ and P are necessary for triggering endometrial receptivity raises puzzling queries about the physiological significance of the multitude of newly discovered nonsteroidal ovarian factors. Expressed in simple terms as far as endometrial priming is concerned, "less," i.e., $E_2$ and P only, not only suffice for triggering optimal endometrial receptivity but may also benefit from avoiding potentially deleterious effects on the endometrium of other ovarian factors such as androgens. This possibility will be further explored later in the paper when comparing endometrial receptivity in egg donation and regular IVF.

## The Plasma $E_2/P$ Ratio

Historically, great importance has been attributed to the plasma $E_2/P$ ratio because of the strongly held belief that deviations from ideal values of this ratio might affect the chances for successful embryo implantation.[27,28] This extraordinarily persistent, if dubious, paradigm has led many to conceptualize that plasma P levels need to be raised in proportion to actual levels of $E_2$ to induce proper endometrial effects when $E_2$ levels are markedly higher than normal, as in COH cycles induced for IVF. This concept is rooted in the anti-estrogenic properties that P exerts by lowering $E_2$ receptors (ER) and stimulating $17\beta$-dehydrogenase,[29] as stated earlier.

We realized that little was known about the physiological role of one of its constituents, $E_2$ produced by the corpus luteum, or luteal $E_2$. Hence, to clarify the physiological significance of luteal $E_2$, we undertook to modify mock egg donation replacement cycles as follows: from day 1 to 14, young women 20 to 40 years of age, deprived of ovarian function received progressively increasing amounts of $E_2$ administered transdermally (from 0.1 to 0.4 mg/day), to duplicate the $E_2$ levels encountered during the follicular phase of the menstrual cycle as previously reported.[30] From day 15 to 28 these women received 300 mg/day of micronized P vaginally, a regimen shown to induce full secretory transformation of the endometrium in these patients.[31] The physiological replacement regimen was modified, however, in that the $E_2$ supply was abruptly interrupted on the morning of day 15 by requesting patients to remove their transdermal therapeutic systems. Despite plasma $E_2$ returning to menopausal levels as early as 24 h later endometrial biopsies performed on days 20 and 24 were not different[32] from findings made in controls who continued to receive $E_2$ through day 28. In another experiment, opposite changes in the plasma $E_2/P$ ratio were induced by administrating 5 mg of $E_2$ benzoate ($E_2$-B), BID, from day 15 onwards.[33] This hefty estrogen treatment led to mean plasma $E_2$ levels that nearly reached the 3000 pg/mL mark thereby duplicating the highest of $E_2$ levels encountered in COH. This regimen, too, failed to have any repercussion on endometrial morphology, a finding that came much to our surprise.[33] Both these sets of data suggest that the levels of luteal $E_2$ exert little, if any, endometrial effects, throwing serious doubt on the long held belief that alterations in $E_2/P$ ratio affect endometrial morphology. Great caution is warranted for not leaping too hastily to conclude that changes in $E_2/P$ ratio do not affect endometrial receptivity. Indeed, it is conceivable that such changes in hormonal levels may affect the potential for embryo implantation by altering endometrial biochemistry without carrying obvious morphological stigmata of these effects. The current state of the art is that P supplementation during the luteal phase remains warranted in view of the existing clinical data supporting such practices.

## Endometrial Action of P: Dose/Effect Relationship and First Uterine Pass Effect of P Administered Transvaginally

Classically, the physiological effects of P have been difficult to establish with precision because they were believed to depend at least in part on the amount of prior $E_2$ exposure ($E_2$ priming) as well as on the concurrent $E_2$ levels ($E_2/P$ ratio). The egg donation model offered study paradigms that can account for both these variables. Globally, egg donation results have indicated that when $E_2$ priming and the $E_2/P$ ratio are kept within reasonable limits, neither affects endometrial morphology achieved by P.[19,34,35] These results leave P as sole agent affecting endometrial morphology at the time of endometrial implantation. Hence, we became interested in studying the role played by levels of plasma P. It has been established that endometrial data obtained in egg donation mock cycles using IM or transvaginal P administration show similar histological findings despite markedly different plasma P levels.[36] After vaginal administration of 300 mg of micronized P, plasma P levels range from 8 to 12 ng/mL, while IM administration of 25 to 30 mg of P leads to plasma P levels in excess of 20 ng/mL.

Two distinct hypotheses may be put forth to unravel this apparent paradox. First, plasma P levels equal or inferior to those achieved by transvaginal administration (8–12 ng/mL) may suffice to induce full secretory transformation of the endometrium. This putative concept implies that plasma P levels achieved in the menstrual cycle (from 10 to 30 ng/mL) far exceed the minimum marks required for inducing full endometrial effects. In keeping with the idea that an overshooting of plasma P levels exists in the menstrual cycle is the notorious lack of correlation described in several clinical studies between plasma P levels and endometrial anomalies, such as luteal phase defects (LPD). The second hypothesis capable of explaining that vaginal P administration induces full secretory transformation of the endometrium despite relatively low P levels proposes a specific uterine selectivity of P effects inherently linked to the transvaginal route of administration. This concept infers that the apparent uterine selectivity of transvaginally administered P results from the hormone transiting first through the uterus before reaching the general circulation. To shed new light on this provocative concept, we undertook to analyze the consequences resulting from modulating the dose of P administered either IM, or transvaginally.

In a series of experiments we studied the effects resulting from lowering plasma P levels by administrating mini IM doses of P. For this, we applied an experimental design first described by Chang and Jaffe[37] in which IM administration of 1.25 mg BID had been shown to raise plasma P to between 1 to 2 ng/mL. To modify mock luteal phases, egg donation candidates receiving physiological $E_2$ supply as previously described[38] also received mini IM doses of P (1.25 mg every 12 h) from day 15 to 28. Endometrial biopsies performed on day 20 were not different from women receiving full scale P treatment, thereby indicating an exquisite sensitivity of endometrial glands to P. On day 24, however, we observed a marked delay in the development of stromal changes.[38] These data were interpreted as indicative of different glandular and stromal sensitivities to P.

To address the issue of a possible *first uterine pass* effect of transvaginally administered P we were also interested in conducting a dose-effect study with this route of P administration. We used a newly designed sustained release system (SRS) for transvaginal P administration developed by Columbia Laboratories, New York, COL-1620. We analyzed the effects of COL-1620 containing 3 P doses (45, 90 and 180 mg) administered transvaginally every other day from day 15 to 28. The sustained release properties of this new vaginal delivery system are based on bioadhesion of the COL-1620 gel (and the P it contains) to the cell surface of the vaginal mucosa. In our egg donation model, the 3 P doses of COL-1620 prevented uterine bleeding until at least day 27 in all but one patient who started to bleed on day 25.[39] Plasma P levels peaked 7 h after insertion of COL-1620 and decreased progressively thereafter. Mean P levels were higher in women receiving 180 and 90 mg of P every other day than in those receiving 45 mg.[39] In the latter group the median peak P levels were 3.0 ng/mL (95% confidence interval: 2.2 to 6.5 ng/mL) while median trough levels were 0.9 ng/mL (95% confidence interval: 0.85 to 1.4 ng/mL). Despite these low P levels full secretory transformation of endometrial stroma was observed in all but one (n = 24) of the day 24 biopsies, irrespective of the P dose administered. One patient belonging to the 45 mg dose group showed hemorrhagic changes in her endometrial biopsy and bled by day 25. Plasma P levels observed in this later patient suggested that she may not have received the 2 first COL-1620 doses.

Another potential parameter for studying P effects on the endometrium is to analyze the changes in appearance it induces on high resolution transvaginal ultrasounds, referred to as endometrial echogenicity. It has now been clearly established, including by analyses conducted in the egg donation model,[39] that the relatively hypoechogenic endometrium (by comparison to the surrounding myometrium) observed in the late follicular phase becomes hyperechogenic under the influence of P. Yet the mechanisms at play are still elusive. Because of the tightly controlled hormonal environment that pertains to egg donation mock cycles, this model offers advantages for studying the echographic expression of the changes in endometrial morphology induced by P. In an attempt to delineate the morpho-echographic correlations underlying the hyperechogenic transformations of endometrium exposed to P, we added an echographic arm to the study described above. In our analysis of the effects of 3 P doses, 45, 90 and 180 mg, we recorded daily 15-min echographic scans of the endometrium on s-VHS tapes during the first 6 days of P administration. The dose-effect relationships pertaining to the echographic manifestations of P exposure were then evaluated with an off-line gray scale analysis using an appropriate computerized system (IôDP Imaging, Paris, France). Preliminary data from this study[40] indicated a progressive and linear increase in relative endometrial vs myometrial echogenicity during the first 6 days of P exposure. No difference could be noted between the 3 doses. In this study the echographic manifestations of P treatment paralleled the morphological findings in the lack of differences seen between the 3 P dose groups. Further, based on the chronology of the endometrial changes in echogenicity we observed (during the first 6 days of P exposure) we were led to hypothesize that the changes in echogenicity induced by P are a reflection of the secretory transformations occurring in endometrial glands. According to this hypothesis it would be the coiling of the endometrial glands filled with sonoluscent mucus that would increase the number of interfaces encountered by the sound beam, itself responsible for the increase in endometrial echogenicity. Potentially, the increase in endometrial echogenicity induced by P may serve to monitor the action of P on endometrial glands, the endometrial component prone to undergo hyperplastic and potentially carcinomatous changes in response to $E_2$-only treatment.

That profound endometrial effects were observed despite low plasma P levels has been the starting point for conceiving that this apparent paradox might be grounded in a *first uterine pass effect* of transvaginally administered P. Speaking strongly in support of the propounded *first uterine pass* of substances administered transvaginally is a report made by Kullander and Svanberg in 1985.[41] In their ingenious experimental design, these authors observed salbutamol levels that were markedly higher in the uterine veins than in general circulation when performing hysterectomies shortly after vaginal administration of salbutamol.[41]

The transport mechanisms potentially involved in a *first uterine pass* of transvaginally administered P are far from limpid. Three presumptive mechanisms may account for the direct transport of P from the vagina to the uterus, namely: 1. direct circulatory loops resulting in portal like flow from the vagina to the uterus before reaching the general circulation; 2. transit through lymphatic pathways; and 3. direct substance diffusion between cells of vaginal and cervical epithelium and/ or through the uterine canal. Different experimental designs must be developed to test the validity of each of these respective working hypotheses before one can come to the fore with a reasonable experimental explanation. Based on its high efficacy, transvaginal P administration offers prospects for sound clinical applications in infertility as well as for menopause treatment. The use of a SRS such as COL-1620 offers the advantage of limiting the number of transvaginal applications needed (every other day or possibly less often), a characteristic that should render the vaginal route of administration more readily acceptable to women contemplating hormonal replacement therapy (HRT).

Further, the possibility of counteracting the proliferative effects that $E_2$ exerts on the endometrium while elevating plasma P only minimally, as seen with COL-1620, can satisfy the newly defined *minimal P exposure* concept.[42] This new approach has been proposed to define a therapeutic objective that some authors recommend striving for because of the fear of an association between P exposure and breast cancer incidence,[43-45] a finding, however, that is debated.[46] The concern about a possible link between breast cancer and P is rooted in epidemiological[47] and biological data showing that in the breast mitoses culminate on day 25 of the menstrual cycle, *i.e.*, when the endometrium is exposed to the highest P levels. In keeping with the possibility that P might promote mitosis or even cancer in breast tissue, epidemiological data on the incidence of breast cancer in OC pill users at the two extremes of reproductive life suggest that breast cancer risk may increase with the number of cyclical exposures to P or progestins.[44,47] So far, the clinical options offered to satisfy the *minimal P exposure* objective have revolved around regimens offering less than monthly exposure to progestins.[42] While cogent in theory, every 3 or 4 month progestin administration, however, results in longer and possibly cumbersome withdrawal bleeding episodes.

Alternative options to satisfy the *minimal P exposure* objective were already conceived by Pike *et al.*[47] In the comments concluding their article, these authors expressed that a possibly better option to minimize breast exposure to P without jeopardizing endometrial protection against the risk of $E_2$ induced hyperplasia and cancer would be "to deliver a progestogen solely to the endometrium." Ideally, continued the authors, this purported regimen would result in "a significant reduction in the incidence of breast, ovarian and endometrial cancer."[47] From our results it can be postulated that transvaginal administration of P doses as little as 45 mg every other day made possible by COL-1620, offers such a viable therapeutic option for keeping breast exposure at a minimum while respecting the monthly secretory transformation of the endometrium. Further epidemiological data should clarify the still inconspicuous and obscure ties that may link female hormones and breast cancer. In the meantime, the circumspect *minimal P exposure* option may satisfy the sheer admonition recommended when treating patients at higher risk for breast cancer. Another conclusion elicited by our studies with COL-1620 is that no correlation can be drawn between plasma P levels and endometrial effects when P is administered transvaginally.

### *Endometrial Receptivity in IVF:* the **Third Factor** *Hypothesis*

As previously mentioned, a deleterious effect of high plasma $E_2$ levels and the related changes in $E_2/P$ ratio had originally been put forth as accounting for the suboptimal endometrial receptivity that seems to overwhelm IVF results. This vision, however, was seriously impugned lately by reports indicating that high $E_2$ levels were not as ominous as originally thought.[48] Moreover, recent uterine

Doppler data have suggested different lines of thought for explaining why endometrial receptivity might be suboptimal in IVF.

In women deprived of ovarian function, Doppler studies of uterine artery resistance have shown results that are interpretable by a simple $E_2$-dependent vasodilation paradigm. Untreated women whose ovaries are inactive as a result of premature[30] or normally occurring menopause[49] display high resistance status. In both cases, initiating estrogen replacement resulted in profound and persistent changes of uterine artery Doppler flow waves (appearance of a persistent diastole flow signal) that evoked a marked decrease in vascular impedance.

In COH cycles, the findings reported cannot be explained solely by the vasodilative properties of $E_2$. Steer et al.[50] have shown that a sizable fraction of women undergoing IVF had uterine artery Doppler flow waves that evoked high resistance as expressed by high (>3) pulsatility index (PI) values on the day of oocyte retrieval. As these women were exposed to the markedly elevated $E_2$ levels characteristic of COH cycles, a mechanism other than $E_2$ must partake in the final resistance status of uterine arteries during COH. Steer's data indicated that women with elevated uterine artery PI values failed to become pregnant, an observation that unpublished data from our own group tend to confirm. Hence, it can be inferred that the factor responsible for elevating uterine artery resistance also affects endometrial receptivity (unless the vascular status itself directly affects receptivity). An incidental observation made in PCOD patients led us to suspect that ovarian factors other than $E_2$ and P, namely, androgens, may affect uterine flow and endometrial receptivity in COH.[51] In 14 women combining clinical, biological and echographic stigmata characteristic of PCOD, uterine artery PI values were markedly higher than would be expected on the sole basis of $E_2$ levels.[51] In a fraction of these women (n = 5) undergoing ovarian suppression with a GnRH agonist (GnRH-a) followed by $E_2$ add back therapy, we observed a perfect normalization of uterine Doppler values. This observation led us to postulate that in PCOD a gonadotropin-dependent ovarian factor (suppressible by GnRH-a) interferes with the vasodilative properties of $E_2$ or carries vasoactive effects of its own. Because of the common understanding of PCOD's physiopathology, it is reasonable to consider that the elevated ovarian androgens are the most likely candidates for the putative ovarian factor interfering with the vasodilative properties of $E_2$. Some similarity may exist between PCOD and COH cycles as Cedars et al.[52] have shown that plasma $\Delta^4$ androstenedione ($\Delta^4$) and testosterone (T) increased markedly more in IVF than previously reported in the menstrual cycle.[54] This led us to formulate the working hypothesis that, as in PCOD, an elevation in ovarian androgens might also affect uterine vascular status and endometrial receptivity in some women undergoing COH, a concept we called the *third factor hypothesis*.

To test the premise that ovarian androgens might actually exert potentially deleterious effects on the endometrium pertaining to the *third factor hypothesis*, we undertook an in-depth analysis of post hMG and hCG hormonal profiles.[55,56] The effects of hMG on ovarian androgens were analyzed by collecting repeated blood samples (every hour for 4 h and after 3 h for the remaining fraction of 24 h) starting immediately after the last hMG injection (225 IU), *i.e.*, 24 h before hCG administration.[55] A preliminary analysis of the results indicated that plasma $\Delta^4$ and T increased significantly after hMG, peaking 12 h after the injection. Hence, it can be inferred that the ≥2.5 fold increase in $\Delta^4$ and T observed between baseline and the day of hCG reflect stepwise accumulation of the effects of each hMG injection necessary for completing multiple follicular maturation.

In contradiction with the androgen pattern seen after hMG, much to our surprise, hCG failed to further elevate plasma $\Delta^4$ and T above the levels achieved at the end of the hMG stimulation.[56] The lack of effect of hCG on androgens is puzzling because of the widely admitted androgen-stimulating properties attributed to LH and the LH-like activity of hCG. Hence, our data speak either for specific differences in the effects of LH and hCG on ovarian androgens or for the ovaries becoming refractory to the LH-like properties of hCG at the end of COH.

Overall, our data on the post hMG and hCG hormonal profiles support the *third factor hypothesis*. Simply stated this tentative assumption proposes that an ovarian substance produced in excessive amounts as a result of COH may interfere with endometrial receptivity, at least in some individuals. Hence, it is possible that nonsteroidal anti-androgen compounds may prove to be clinically helpful for optimizing endometrial receptivity, particularly in women who have experienced repeated embryo transfer failures.

## CONCLUSION

Because of its successes, the egg donation model has elegantly proved that optimal endometrial receptivity to embryo implantation can be induced in women whose ovaries are inactive with the sole replacement of $E_2$ and P. While $E_2$ can indifferently be administered orally, vaginally or transdermally, P can only be administered transvaginally or by IM injections. Transvaginal P administration has revealed a paradox between fairly low (subphysiological) levels of P and marked endometrial efficacy (complete predecidual transformation and embryo implantation rates). This discrepancy between low plasma levels and high endometrial efficacy has been the basis for postulating a *first uterine pass effect* of transvaginally administered P. In COH, endometrial receptivity appears inferior to that seen in egg donation. Yet even extreme alterations in the plasma $E_2/P$ ratio remained without affecting endometrial morphology at the time of presumed implantation (day 20) or at the end of the luteal phase (day 24). This led us to formulate that in COH an ovarian factor other than $E_2$ and P but also produced excessively as a result of hMG treatment, may alter endometrial receptivity, a speculation referred to as *the third factor hypothesis*. Our preliminary data on post hMG hormonal profiles speak for ovarian androgens playing the stipulated *third factor* role. Surprisingly, however, we observed that hCG did not elevate plasma androgen further above the levels achieved at the end of hMG treatment. Further work is needed to determine the clinical value of using nonsteroidal androgens and/or 5 alpha reductase inhibitors to prevent possibly deleterious effects of COH-dependent androgens on the endometrium.

## REFERENCES

1. LUTJEN, P., A. TRAUNSON, J. LEETON, J. FINDLAY, C. WOOD & P. RENOW. 1984. The establishment and maintenance of pregnancy using *in vitro* fertilization and embryo donation in a patient with primary ovarian failure. Nature **307:** 174–175.
2. NAVOT, D., N. LAUFER, J. KOPOLOVIC *et al.* 1984. Artificially induced endometrial cycles and establishment of pregnancies in the absence of ovaries. N. Engl. J. Med. **314:** 806–811.
3. ROSENWAKS, Z. 1987. Donor eggs: their application in modern reproductive technologies. Fertil. Steril. **47:** 895–909.

4. FRYDMAN, R., H. LETUR-KÖNIRSCH, D. DE ZIEGLER, D. BYDLOWSKI, A. RAOUL-DUVAL & J. SELVA. 1990. A protocol of satisfying the ethical issues raised by oocyte donation: the free, anonymous, and fertile donors. Fertil. Steril. **53:** 666–672.
5. SAUER, M. V., R. J. PAULSON & R. A. LOBO. 1990. A preliminary report on oocyte donation extending reproductive potential to women over 40. N. Engl. J. Med. **323:** 1157–1160.
6. ASCH, R., J. P. BALMACEDA, T. ORD et al. 1988. Oocyte donation and gamete intrafallopian transfer in premature ovarian failure. Fertil. Steril. **49:** 263–267.
7. NAVOT, D., R. T. SCOTT, K. DROESCH, L. L. VEECK, H. C. LIU & Z. ROSENWAKS. 1991. The window of embryo transfer and the efficiency of human conception *in vitro*. Fertil. Steril. **55:** 114–118.
8. DEVROEY, P., A. WISANTO, M. CAMUS, L. VAN WAEBERGHE, C. BOURGAIN, I. LIEBARS & A. C. VAN STEIRTEGHEM. 1988. Oocyte donation in patients without ovarian function. Hum. Reprod. **3:** 399–704.
9. EDWARDS, R. G., S. MORCOS, M. MACNAMEE, J. P. BALMACEDA, D. E. WALTERS & R. ASCH. 1991. High fecundity of amenorrheic women in embryo-transfer programmes. Lancet **338:** 292–294.
10. EDWARDS, R. G. 1992. Why are agonadal and post-amenorrheic women so fertile after oocyte donation? Hum. Reprod. **7:** 773–774.
11. SAUER, M. V., R. J. PAULSON & R. A. LOBO. 1992. Reversing the natural decline in human fertility: an extended clinical trial of oocyte donation to women of advanced reproductive age. JAMA **268:** 1275–1279.
12. BEN NUN, I., R. JAFFE, M. D. FEJGIN & Y. BEYTH. 1992. Therapeutic maturation of endometrium in *in vitro* fertilization and embryo transfer. Fertil. Steril. **57:** 953–962.
13. STEINGOLD, K., P. STUMPF, D. KREINER, H. C. LIU, D. NAVOT & Z. ROSENWAKS. 1989. Estradiol and progesterone replacement regimens for the induction of endometrial receptivity. Fertil. Steril. **52:** 756–760.
14. DROESCH, K., D. NAVOT, R. T. SCOTT, D. KREINER & Z. ROSENWAKS. 1988. Transdermal estrogen replacement in ovarian failure for ovum donation. Fertil. Steril. **50:** 931–934.
15. SCHMIDT, C. L., D. DE ZIEGLER, C. L. GAGLIARDI, R. W. MELLON, F. H. TANEY, M. J. KUHAR, J. M. COLON & G. WEISS. 1988. Transfer of cryopreserved-thawed embryos: the natural cycle versus controlled preparation of the endometrium with gonadotropin-releasing hormone agonist and exogenous estradiol and progesterone (GEEP). Fertil. Steril. **49:** 609–616.
16. DE ZIEGLER, D. 1991. Is the liver a target organ for estrogen? *In* The Menopause and Replacement Therapy: Facts, Controversies. R. Sitruk-Ware & W. Utian, Eds. 201. Marcel Dekker. New York.
17. YEN, S. S. C., P. L. MARTIN, A. M. BURNIER et al. 1975. Circulating estradiol, estrone, and gonadotropin levels following the administration of orally active 17$\beta$-estradiol on postmenopausal women. J. Clin. Endocrinol. Metab. **40:** 518.
18. LEETON, J., P. ROGERS, C. KING & D. HEALY. 1991. A comparison of pregnancy rates for 131 donor oocyte transfers using either a sequential or fixed regimen of steroid replacement therapy. Hum. Reprod. **6:** 299–301.
19. SERHAL, P. F. & I. L. CRAFT. 1987. Ovum donation—a simplified approach. Fertil. Steril. **48:** 265–269.
20. STEINGOLD, K. A., D. W. MATT, D. DE ZIEGLER, J. E. SEALEY, M. FRATKIN & S. REZNIKOV. 1991. Comparison of transdermal to oral estradiol administration on hormonal and hepatic parameters in women with premature ovarian failure. J. Clin. Endocrinol. Metab. **73:** 275–280.
21. HOFF, J. D., M. E. QUIEGLEY & S. S. C. YEN. 1983. Hormonal dynamics at midcycle: a reevaluation. J. Clin. Endocrinol. Metab. **57:** 792–796.
22. NAHOUL, K., L. DHEMIN & R. SCHOLLER. 1987. Radioimmunoassay of plasma progesterone after oral administration of micronized progesterone. J. Steroid Biochem. **26:** 241–249.
23. NAHOUL, K., L. DHEMIN, M. JONDET & M. ROGER. 1993. Profiles of plasma estrogens, progesterone and their metabolites after oral or vaginal administration of estradiol and progesterone. Maturitas **16:** 185–202.

24. WHITEHEAD, M. I., P. T. TOWNSEND, D. K. GILL, W. P. COLLINS & S. CAMPBELL. 1985. Absorption and metabolism of oral progesterone. Br. Med. J. **280:** 825–827.
25. LANE, G., N. C. SIDDLE, T. A. RYDER, J. PRYSE-DAVIES, R. J. B. KING & M. I. WHITEHEAD. 1983. Dose dependent effects of oral progesterone on the oestrogenized postmenopausal endometrium. Br. Med. J. **287:** 1241.
26. PADWICK, M. L., J. ENDACOTT, C. MATSON & M. I. WHITEHEAD. 1986. Absorption and metabolism of oral progesterone when administered twice daily. Fertil. Steril. **46:** 402–407.
27. MUASHER, S., A. A. ACOSTA, J. E. GARCIA, G. S. JONES & H. W. JONES, JR. 1984. Luteal phase serum estradiol and progesterone in *in vitro* fertilization. Fertil. Steril. **41:** 838.
28. CORSAN, G. H. & E. KEMMANN. 1991. The role of superovulation in ovulatory infertility: a review. Fertil. Steril. **55:** 468–477.
29. TSENG, L. & E. GURPIDE. 1975. J. Clin. Endocrinol. Metab. **41:** 402.
30. DE ZIEGLER, D., R. BESSIS & R. FRYDMAN. 1991. Vascular resistance of uterine arteries: physiological effects of estradiol and progesterone. Fertil. Steril. **55:** 775–779.
31. DE ZIEGLER, D., C. CORNEL, C. BERGERON, A. HAZOUT, P. BOUCHARD & R. FRYDMAN. 1991. Controlled preparation of the endometrium with exogenous estradiol and progesterone in women having functioning ovaries. Fertil. Steril. **56:** 851–855.
32. DE ZIEGLER, D., C. BERGERON, C. CORNEL, D. A. MÉDALIE, M. R. MASSAI, E. MILGROM, R. FRYDMAN & P. BOUCHARD. 1992. Effects of luteal estradiol on the secretory transformation of human endometrium and plasma gonadotropins. J. Clin. Endocrinol. Metab. **74:** 322–331.
33. DE ZIEGLER, D., C. CORNEL, C. BERGERON, R. FANCHIN, R. FRYDMAN & P. BOUCHARD. 1992. The role of plasma $E_2/P$ ratio on endometrial morphology: effects of very high levels of luteal $E_2$. Presented at the Society for Gynecologic Investigations (SGI), San Antonio, Texas, March 1992.
34. YOUNIS, J. S., N. MORDEL, G. LIGOVETZKY, A. LEWIN, J. G. SCHENKER & N. LAUFER. 1991. The effect of a prolonged artificial follicular phase on endometrial development in an oocyte donation program. J. *In Vitro* Fert. Embryo Transf. **8:** 84–88.
35. NAVOT, D., T. L. ANDERSON, K. DROESCH, R. T. SCOTT, D. KREINER & Z. ROSENWAKS. 1989. Hormonal manipulation of endometrial maturation. J. Clin. Endocrinol. Metab. **68:** 801–807.
36. LI, T. C., P. DOCKERY & I. D. COOKE. 1991. Effect of exogenous progesterone administration on the morphology of normally developing endometrium in the pre-implantation period. Hum. Reprod. **6:** 641–644.
37. CHANG, R. J. & R. B. JAFFE. 1978. Progesterone effects on gonadotropin release in women pretreated with estradiol. J. Clin. Endocrinol. Metab. **47:** 119–125.
38. DE ZIEGLER, D., C. CORNEL, M. R. MASSAI, C. BERGERON, R. FRYDMAN & P. BOUCHARD. 1992. The role of plasma $E_2/P$ ratio on endometrial morphology: Effects of lowering plasma P levels. Presented at the Society for Gynecologic Investigation (SGI), San Antonio, Texas, March 1992.
39. GRUNFELD, L., B. WALKER, P. A. BERGH, B. SANDLER, G. HOFMANN & D. NAVOT. 1991. High-resolution endovaginal ultrasonography of the endometirum: a noninvasive test for endometrial adequacy. Obstet. Gynecol. **78:** 200–204.
40. BERGERON, C., R. FANCHIN, P. BOUCHARD, R. FRYDMAN & D. DE ZIEGLER. 1993. Transvaginal administration of progesterone (P) using a new sustained release system, COL 1620: dose-effect analysis of P action on endometrial morphology. Oral communication. This conference.
41. KULLANDER, S. & L. SVANBERG 1985. On resorption and the effects of vaginally administered terbutaline in women with premature labor. Acta Obstet. Gynecol. Scand. **64:** 613–616.
42. SPICER, D. V. & M. C. PIKE. 1992. The prevention of breast cancer through reduced ovarian steroid exposure. Acta Oncol. **31:** 167–174.
43. BERGKVIST, L., H. O. ADAMI, I. PERSSON, R. HOOVER & C. SCHAIRER. 1989. The risk of breast cancer after estrogen and estrogen-progestin replacement. N. Engl. J. Med. **321:** 293–297.

44. HENDERSON, B. E. 1989. Endogenous and exogenous endocrine factors. Hematol. Oncol. Clin. North Am. **3:** 577–598.
45. BERGKVIST, L., H. O. ADAMI, I. PERSSON, R. BERGSTROM & U. B. KRUSEMO. 1989. Prognosis after breast cancer diagnosis in women exposed to estrogen and estrogen-progestogen replacement therapy. Am. J. Epidemiol. **130:** 221–228.
46. BARRETT CONNOR, E. 1989. Postmenopausal estrogen replacement and breast cancer. N. Engl. J. Med. **321:** 319–320.
47. PIKE, M. C., R. K. ROSS, R. A. LOBO, T. J. KEY, M. POTTS & B. E. HENDERSON. 1989. LHRH agonists and the prevention of breast and ovarian cancer. Br. J. Cancer **60:** 142–148.
48. CHENETTE, P. E., M. V. SAUER & R. J. PAULSON. 1990. Very high serum estradiol levels are not detrimental to clinical outcome of *in vitro* fertilization. Fertil. Steril. **00:** 858.
49. BOURNE, T., T. C. HILLARD, M. I. WHITEHEAD, D. CROOK & S. CAMPBELL. 1990. Oestrogens, arterial status, and postmenopausal women. Lancet **335:** 1471–1472.
50. STEER, C. V., S. CAMPBELL, S. L. TAN, T. CRAYFORD, C. MILS, B. A. MASON & W. P. COLLINS. 1992. The use of transvaginal color flow imaging after *in vitro* fertilization to identify optimum uterine conditions before embryo transfer. Fertil. Steril. **57:** 372–376.
51. DE ZIEGLER, D. & C. LINH. 1992. A gonadotropin dependent ovarian factor elevates uterine artery resistance in polycystic ovary disease (PCOD) despite a normal response of uterine arteries to E2. Presented at the Society for Gynecologic Investigation (SGI), San Antonio, Texas, March 1992.
52. CEDARS, M. I., E. SUREY, F. HAMILTON, P. LAPOLT & D. R. MELDRUM. 1990. Leuprolide acetate lowers circulating bioactive luteinizing hormone and testosterone concentrations during ovarian stimulation for oocyte retrieval. Fertil. Steril. **53:** 627.
54. JUDD, H. L. & S. S. C. YEN. 1973. Serum androstenedione and testosterone levels during the menstrual cycle. J. Clin. Endocrinol. Metab. **36:** 475.
55. FANCHIN, R., D. CASTRACANE, J. TAIEB, F. OLIVENNES, R. FRYDMAN, P. BOUCHARD & D. DE ZIEGLER. 1993. The hormonal profile of control ovarian hyperstimulation (COH): the effect of human menopausal gonadotropin (hMG). The American Fertility Society, Montreal Canada, Oct. 12, 1993.

# Endometrial and Embryonic Factors Involved in Successful Implantation[a]

C. BULLETTI, V. POLLI, F. LICASTRO,[b]
AND R. PARMEGGIANI

*Reproductive Medicine Unit*
*Department of Obstetrics and Gynecology*
[b]*Department of Pathology*
*University of Bologna*
*Via Massarenti, 13*
*40138 Bologna, Italy*

## INTRODUCTION

Implantation of the embryo in the predecidualized endometrium is modulated by many factors.[1] Adequate embryo-endometrial interaction depends on synchronization of the embryo's developmental stage with endometrial maturation.

After passing through the fallopian tubes, embryos enter the uterine cavity at the 6-to-12 cell stage. Before attaching to the endometrium the embryo grows and differentiates to become a blastocyst; only at this stage is it able to invade and penetrate the endometrium itself.

During the menstrual cycle, the endometrium undergoes proliferative and differentiation events, evident from morphological and biochemical changes. There is a strict temporal relation between embryo implantation and endometrial receptivity, which in humans is confined to days 16–19 of a 28-day cycle.[2-3]

Low/high levels of circulating steroid hormones and/or inadequate endometrial response to hormonal stimulation might be the cause of an abnormal endometrial development in the perimplantation period.[4-7] The endometrial changes may reflect functional events, such as protein secretion, which in turn may influence the first step of embryo-endometrial interaction. The endometrial output into the uterine lumen includes vascular exudate, glandular secretion, etc. The embryo survives in this fluid from fertilization until the blastocyst stage, without maternal blood supply. The present study assessed factors that influence both maturation of the embryonic and endometrial tissue and control the embryo's capability to invade the endometrium including transforming growth factor $\beta 1$ (TGF $\beta 1$), leukemia inhibitory factor (LIF) and urokinase type-plasminogen activator (u-PA).

## MATERIALS AND METHODS

This study was carried out by using samples of various tissues and fluids as follows. 1) Endometrial tissues were collected during the proliferative and secretory phases of the endometrial cycle by biopsy using Novak curettes; the tissues

---

[a] Supported by grants from the Italian National Council of Research, Nos. 9300660 and 9202504, and from the University of Bologna, No. 930212100.

samples were then fixed in formalin, processed for routine light microscopy and dated according to standard criteria.[8] 2) Uterine fluids, obtained from patients enrolled in the *In Vitro* Fertilization Program, were collected by washing the uterine cavity with 3 ml of Human Tubal Fluid (HTF, Irvine Scientific, Santa Ana, CA) with sterile polyethylene intrauterine catheters (Laboratoire CCD, France) at the beginning of the therapeutic protocol (t0) and at ovulation (t1). 3) Trophoblastic tissues were obtained from induced and spontaneous abortions (6–9 weeks) and processed as endometrial samples. 4) Follicular and seminal fluids. 5) Fertilization gamete culture media of patients enrolled in the *In Vitro* Fertilization Program. The patients, all of whom gave their informed consent, had not received any hormonal treatment (including oral contraceptives) and had not used an intrauterine device for at least 6 months.

The *endometrial* and *trophoblastic tissues* were processed for immunohistochemical detection of TGF $\beta1$ and u-PA, respectively. The specimens were fixed in 10% buffered formalin, embedded in paraffin and cut into sections about 5 $\mu$m thick. Tissue sections were dewaxed in xylene and dehydrated in graded alcohol. An ABC-phosphatase standard method was applied using rabbit polyclonal anti-human TGF $\beta1$ (Celtrix Laboratories, Inc., California) diluted 1 : 60 on endometrial tissue and anti-human u-PA (Chemicon, UK) at a concentration of 1 $\mu$g/ml on trophoblastic tissue, as primary antibody and incubated for 30 minutes at room temperature. The secondary antiserum was IgG anti-rabbit goat phosphatase (Vector Laboratories) on endometrial tissue and IgG anti-mouse (Sigma) on trophoblastic tissue. The reaction was revealed by Tetratotized new fuchsin. The slides were then rinsed in water before dehydration in ethanol and xylene and mounted as usual.

*Uterine fluids* were analyzed by immunodot blot analysis for TGF $\beta1$ detection, while the *follicular* and *seminal* fluids and *fertilization gamete culture media* (before and after change-over) were examined by immunodot blot for u-PA detection and by ELISA for LIF detection. The samples were stored at $-70°C$ and thawed immediately before use. Dot blots were produced on cellulose nitrate membranes using a dot blot manifold (Bio-Rad Bio Dot apparatus). Dot blot analysis was performed with a TGF $\beta1$ detection kit (Becton Dickinson Labware, USA) using a purified anti-human TGF $\beta1$ IgG (turkey) as primary antibody. Four $\mu$g/ml of this antibody were incubated by rocking for 2 hours at room temperature. After washing, the membrane was incubated by rocking for 1 hour in 0.8 $\mu$g/ml anti-turkey IgG alkaline phosphatase conjugate. Color development was obtained by NBT (nitro blue tetrazolium chloride) and BCIP (5-bromo-4-chloro-3-indolyl phosphate) reagents.

Uterine fluids were evaluated for LIF detection by ELISA using Quantikine TM Human-LIF Immunoassay (R&D System, Minneapolis, MN).

## RESULTS

### Transforming Growth Factor β1 (TGF β1)

The endometrial samples evaluated immunohistochemically showed changes in expression of TGF $\beta1$ during the normal menstrual cycle, both in epithelial and stromal cells. During the proliferative period differences were observed between the early, mid and late phases (FIG. 1). Initially, a positive immunoreaction for TGF $\beta1$ was evident only in the cytoplasm of epithelial glandular cells with residual secretory changes. The stroma showed scattered positive cells in areas of degrada-

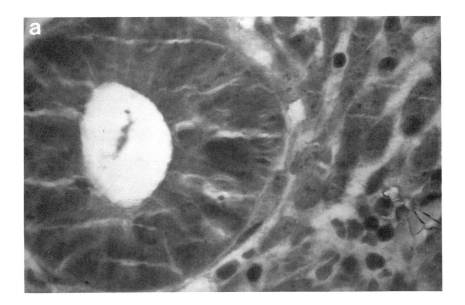

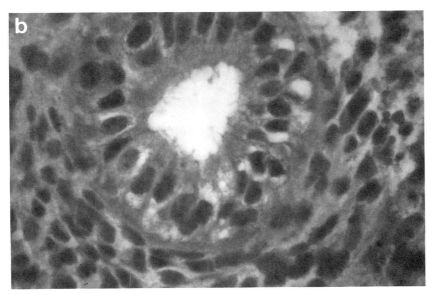

**FIGURE 1.** Immunohistochemical revelation of TGF β1 in endometrial tissue during the normal cycle. **(a)** Early proliferative phase: residual positivity in the cytoplasm of epithelial glandular cells with residual secretory changes. The stroma showed scattered positive cells. **(b)** Late secretory phase: only the glandular epithelial cells showed irregularly distributed positivity. **(c)** Late secretive phase: epithelial and stromal cells showed a strong diffuse positivity.

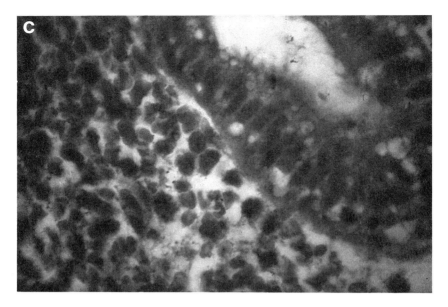

**FIGURE 1** (*Continued*).

tion of the fibrous interstitial reticulum. During the mid and late proliferative phases the positivity increased both in glandular epithelium and in stromal cells. In the secretory phase a decrease in positivity was evident at the early stage, but during the mid and late secretory phases a gradual increase was found. Initially, only the glandular epithelial cells were positive and the stromal cells showed irregularly distributed positivity. In the late phase both the glandular and surface epithelium showed a strong, diffuse reaction; the cytoplasm of the stromal decidualized cells was also strongly positive (FIG. 1a, b, c).

The immunodot blot analysis of the endometrial fluids collected during the therapeutic protocol utilized in the IVF program, at the beginning (t0) and at ovulation (t1), showed the presence of TGF $\beta$1 in all samples examined. There was a quantitative difference between the uterine secretions collected at time t0 and at time t1. The range of TGF $\beta$1 was 0–200 ng/ml in the first group, and 200–2500 ng/ml in the second group. The statistically significant increase in TGF $\beta$1 in group t1 versus group t0 was assessed by Student paired $t$ test ($p < 0.01$). These results performed on 32 cases confirmed previous findings[9] (FIG. 2).

### *Leukemia Inhibitory Factor (LIF)*

The same specimens were processed by ELISA to evaluate the presence of LIF in the endometrial fluids. The presence of this factor was demonstrated only in 2 samples out of 10 collected at the beginning of the therapeutic protocol (t0) with concentrations ranging from 60 to 90 pc/ml. The uterine fluids collected at ovulation (t1) were all negative at the immunoenzymatic dosage (FIG. 3).

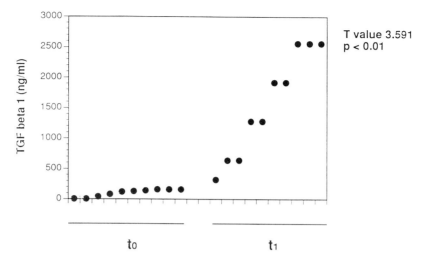

**FIGURE 2.** Immunodot blot analysis of endometrial fluids for TGF $\beta$1. t0: beginning of therapeutic protocol; t1: time of ovulation.

### Urokinase Type-Plasminogen Activator (u-PA)

No immunoreactive u-PA was detected in the follicular fluid samples tested in our study, but the same test for u-PA was positive in all seminal fluid samples examined (FIG. 4).

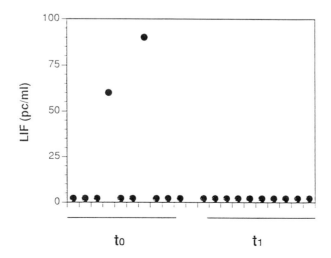

**FIGURE 3.** Immunoenzymatic dosage of endometrial fluids for LIF.

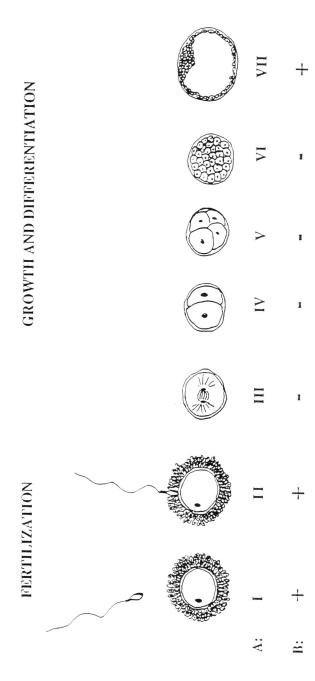

**FIGURE 4.** The presence of u-PA changes during the different steps of oocytes fertilization and embryo growth and differentiation. A: steps of development; B: immunoreaction of u-PA.

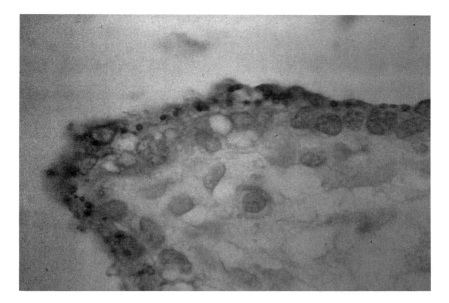

**FIGURE 5.** The expression of u-PA in trophoblastic tissue demonstrated by immunohistochemistry technique.

Fertilization gamete culture media were positive for u-PA in the samples collected before change-over, but became negative after change over.

The samples of trophoblastic tissues tested immunohistochemically showed the presence of urokinase type-plasminogen activator in all tissues (FIG. 5). We found different levels of expression of the proteolytic enzyme in tissues obtained from spontaneous or induced abortions (6–9 weeks). In the first case an irregular positivity was found, while in the second the positivity was more continuous and evident.

## CONCLUSION

The role of uterine fluid in modulating embryo growth and differentiation as well as implantation is not completely clear. Transforming growth factor $\beta 1$, LIF and u-PA may participate in the control of the maternal-embryonic interaction at the time of implantation.

TGF $\beta 1$ is a polypeptide involved in a variety of important physiologic and pathophysiologic processes. It stimulates the growth of some mesenchymal cell types and inhibits the growth of epithelial cell types.[10-11] TGF $\beta 1$ is widely present in different tissues where it stimulates cellular differentiation,[12] promotes the production of extracellular matrix protein[13] and acts as a chemotactic agent.[14] The biological effects of TGF $\beta 1$ on cell proliferation, extracellular matrix formation, differentiation, cell migration, proteolysis and angiogenesis suggest that it may be involved in embryonic development;[15] it controls the proliferation and proteolytic activity of trophoblastic cells, inducing differentiation of the cytotrophoblast in syncytia.[16] Furthermore, TGF $\beta$1 also seems to influence the immunological response by inhibiting a) the growth of T cells, b) the production of immunoglobulin by B cells and c) the cytoxicity of natural killer cells.[17-19]

In the present study TGF $\beta$1 expression at different degrees of intensity was detected during the endometrial cycle. Its immunodetection was particularly evident from days +4 until +7 after the LH surge. The evidence of an increase in the luminal fluid content of TGF $\beta$1 after the induction of ovulation may reflect its relation to ovarian steroid production. At the stage of implantation, TGF $\beta$1 may enhance extracellular matrix production in embryo-maternal interactions through its promotion of procollagen synthesis. It may also affect u-PA activity or PAI activity depending on the amount of these enzymes produced by the embryos at the blastocyst stage. A recent study shows that TGF $\beta$1 also modulates the maternal/embryonic immune response[17-19] and abnormal TGF $\beta$1 production may impair the maternal immunoreaction to embryonic paternal antigens. Embryo invasiveness could be enhanced or reduced according to the cellular patrimony. Inadequate production of TGF $\beta$1 by the human endometrial tissue might be responsible for implantation failure in the early stage of pregnancy or for recurrent abortion.

The presence of TGF $\beta$1 in endometrial fluids may also be important for embryonic growth before adhesion to the predecidualized endometrium. The development of the fertilized oocytes and their growth would seem to be controlled by the endometrial secretion. LIF is a glycoprotein that has multiple effects on various *in vitro* culture systems.[20-21] These include the regulation of the differentiation and proliferation of certain hematopoietic cell lines,[22-24] bone remodeling,[25-26] the inhibition of embryonic stem cell differentiation *in vitro*[27-28] and others. In the mouse system, LIF is synthesized in extraembryonic tissue and may therefore regulate embryonic tissues during development.[29] It is expressed at low levels in many different tissues, but the highest concentration is evident in the uterine endometrial glands specifically on the fourth day of pregnancy.[30] This suggests that one of LIF's principal functions *in vivo* may be to regulate blastocyst growth and implantation. Recent study demonstrated that LIF has a strong relationship with embryo implantation in the mouse. In the present study, the ELISA detection of LIF in the luminal fluid does not prove endometrial production but in 20% of cases it was present in the luminal fluids at a low concentration (range 60 to 90 pc/ml). Probably, the secretion of LIF is correlated with the circulating levels of steroid hormones. LIF removal was not replaced after 8-10 days of ovulation induction. We cannot yet reach any conclusion regarding the role of this factor in humans but the evaluation of endometrial LIF production and its use in embryonic culture should be a matter of further research.

The u-PA is a proteolytic enzyme synthesized and secreted by many cell types such as transformed cells,[31] activated macrophages[32] and stimulated ovarian granulosa cells.[33] The u-PA converts the abundant extracellular zymogen plasminogen into plasmin, an active protease that, directly or indirectly, can promote degradation of all components of the extracellular matrix. Its expression is under the control of hormonal type mediators, the nature of which depends on the cell population considered.[34]

Urokinase is thought to play a central role in regulating extracellular proteolysis in a variety of normal and pathological processes involving tissue destruction and cell migration, such as inflammatory reactions and invasive growth of trophoblast and cancer cells.[35] For this reason we believe that urokinase is involved in the tissue destruction that accompanies the migration of the embryo through the basement membrane underlying the luminal epithelium of the endometrium. Its importance for fertilization of oocytes has already been demonstrated.[36]

In this study we have analyzed the production of the proteolytic enzyme u-PA in different human compartments related to the fertilization process, embryo development and implantation. Urokinase type-plasminogen activator was detected with different techniques in follicular and seminal fluids and in fertilization culture medium. Its presence in seminal fluid is probably strictly connected with the capability of the spermatozoa to perforate the oocyte membrane during the fertilization step. The results obtained from fertilization culture media collected before the oocyte becomes embryo "in vitro," confirm our supposition about the involvement of u-PA in the fertilization process. The failure to detect u-PA in media collected immediately after fertilization suggests to us a quiescent period of the fertilized oocyte, during which the new embryo is not able to synthesize any protein during the period of cell replication leading to the formation of a blastocyst.

The immunohistochemical detection of u-PA in the trophoblastic tissue obtained from spontaneous and voluntary abortion shows the presence of the proteolytic enzyme also in the cytoplasm of the syncitiotrophoblast. These data suggest that the enzyme is involved also in the mechanisms that regulate the capability of embryonic tissue to invade and penetrate the endometrium until the formation of the placenta, and that this activity is modulated by endometrial factors. The absence or overexpression of this proteolytic activity might cause the failure of the beginning of pregnancy and abnormal trophoblastic activity, respectively.

## REFERENCES

1. FLAMIGNI, C., C. BULLETTI, V. POLLI, P. M. CIOTTI, R. A. PREFETTO, A. GALASSI & E. DI COSMO. 1991. Factors regulating interactions between trophoblast and human endometrium. Ann. N.Y. Acad. Sci. **622:** 176–190.
2. NAVOT, D., ANDERSON, K. DROESCH, R. SCOTT, D. KREINER & Z. ROSENWAKS. 1989. Hormonal manipulation of endometrial maturation. J. Clin. Endocrinol. Metab. **68:** 801–807.
3. NAVOT, D., N. LAUFER, J. KOPOLOVIC, R. RABINOVITZ, A. BERKENFIELD, A. LAWIN, M. GRANAT, E. MARGALIOTH & J. SCHENKER. 1986. Artificially induced endometrial cycles and establishment of pregnancies in the absence of ovaries. N. Engl. J. Med. **314:** 806–811.
4. SHANGOLD, M., A. BERKELEY & J. GRAY. 1983. Both midluteal serum progesterone levels and late luteal endometrial histology should be assessed in all infertile women. Fertil. Steril. **40:** 627–630.
5. ZORN, J. R., L. CEIDARD, C. NESSMAN & M. SEVALE. 1984. Delayed endometrial maturation in women with normal progesterone levels. The disharmonic luteal phase syndrome. Gynecol. Obstet. Invest. **17:** 157–162.
6. BALOSH, J. & J. A. VANRELL. 1987. Corpus luteum insufficiency and fertility: a matter of controversy. Hum. Reprod. **2:** 557–567.
7. LI, T. C., P. DOCKERY & I. D. COOKE. 1991. Endometrial development in the luteal phase of women with various types of infertility: comparison with women of normal fertility. Hum. Reprod. **6:** 325–330.
8. NOYES, R. W., A. T. HERTIG & J. ROCK. 1953. Dating of the endometrial biopsy. Fertil. Steril. **1:** 3–5.
9. BULLETTI, C., V. POLLI, A. GALASSI, R. PARMEGGIANI, P. M. CIOTTI, R. SERACCHIOLI & C. FLAMIGNI. 1993. Transforming growth factor $\beta 1$ in human endometrium. J. Assist. Reprod. Submitted for publication.
10. ROBERTS, A. B., M. A. ANZANO, L. M. WAKEFIELD, N. S. ROCHE, D. F. STERN & M. B. SPORN. 1985. Type beta transforming growth factor: a bifunctional regulator of cellular growth. Proc. Natl. Acad. Sci. USA **82:** 119–123.

11. MOSES, H. L., R. F. TUCKER, E. B. LEOF, R. J. COFFEY, JR., J. HALPER & G. D. SHIPLEY. 1985. Type-beta transforming growth factor is a growth stimulator and a growth inhibitor. *In* Cancer Cell. J. Feramisco, B. Ozanne & C. Stiles, Eds. Vol. 3: 65–71. Cold Spring Harbor Press. New York, NY.
12. KESKI-OJA, J., E. B. LEOF, R. M. LYONS, R. J. COFFEY, JR. & H. L. MOSES. 1987. Transforming growth factor and control of neoplastic cell growth. J. Cell. Biochem. **33**: 95–107.
13. IGNOTZ, R. & J. MASSAGUE. 1986. Transforming growth factor-beta stimulates the expression of fibronectin and collagen and their incorporation into extracellular matrix. J. Biol. Chem. **261**: 4337–4345.
14. POSTLETHWAITE, A. E., J. KESKI-OHA, H. MOSES & A. H. KANG. 1986. Stimulation of the chemotactic migration of human fibroblast by transforming growth factor $\beta$. J. Exp. Med. **165**: 251–256.
15. LALA, P. K. & C. H. GRAHAM. 1990. Mechanisms of trophoblast invasiveness and their control: the role of proteases and protease inhibitors. Cancer Metastasis **9**(4): 369–379.
16. TABIDZADEH, S. 1991. Human endometrium: an active site of cytokine production and action. Endocr. Rev. **12**(3): 273–290.
17. CLARK, D. A., K. C. FLANDERS, D. BANWATT, W. MILLAR-BOOK, J. MANUEL, J. STREDRONSKA-CLARK & B. ROWLEY. 1990. Murine pregnancy decidua produces a unique immunosuppressive molecule related to transforming growth factor $\beta 2$. J. Immunol. **144**: 3008–3014.
18. TAMADA, H., M. T. MCMASTER, K. C. FLANDERS, G. K. ANDREW & S. K. DEY. 1990. Cell type-specific expression of transforming growth factor $\beta 1$ in the mouse uterus during perimplantation period. Mol. Endocrinol. **4**: 965–972.
19. GRAHAM, C. H. & P. K. LALA. 1990. A mechanism of control of trophoblast invasion in situ. J. Cell. Physiol. **148**(2): 228–234.
20. GEARING, D. P., N. M. GOUGH, J. A. KING, D. J. HILTON, N. A. NICOLA, R. J. SIMPSON, E. C. NICE, A. KELSO & D. METCALF. 1987. Molecular cloning and expression of cDNA encoding a murine myeloid leukaemia inhibitory factor (LIF). EMBO J. **6**: 3995–4002.
21. RETHJEN, P. D., S. TOTH, A. WILLES, J. K. HEALTH & A. G. SMITH. 1990. Differentiation inhibiting activities produced in matrix associated and diffusible forms that are generated by alternator promoter usage. Cell **62**: 1105–1114.
22. HILTON, D. J., N. A. NICOLA, N. M. GOUGH & D. METCALF. 1988. Resolution and purification of three distinct factors produced by krebs ascites cells which have differentiation-inducing activity on murine myeloid leukemic cell lines. J. Biol. Chem. **263**: 9238–9243.
23. LEARY, A. G., G. G. WONG, S. C. CLARK, A. G. SMITH & M. OGAWA. 1990. Leukaemia inhibitory factor differentiation-inhibiting activity/human interleukin for DA cells augments proliferation of human hematopoietic stem cells. Blood. **75**: 1960–1966.
24. MOREAU, J. F., D. D. DONALDSON, F. BENNETT, J. WITEK-GIANNOTTI, S. C. CLARK & G. G. WONG. 1988. Leukemia inhibitory factor is identical to the myeloid growth factor human interleukin for DA cells. Nature (London) **336**: 690–692.
25. ABE, E., H. TANAKA, Y. ISHIMI, C. MIGAMA, T. HAYASHI, H. NAGASAWA, M. TOMIDA, Y. YAMAGUCHI, M. HOZUMI & T. SUDA. 1986. Differentiation-inducing factor purified from conditioned medium of mitogen-treated spleen cell cultures stimulates bone resorption. Proc. Natl. Acad. Sci. USA. **83**: 5958–5962.
26. ALLAN, E. H., D. J. HILTON, M. A. BROWN, R. S. EVELY, S. YAMITA, D. METCALF, N. M. GOUGH, K. W. NG, N. A. NICOLA & T. J. MARTIN. 1990. Osteoblast displays receptors for and responses to leukemia-inhibitory factor. J. Cell. Physiol. **145**: 110–119.
27. WILLIAMS, R. L., D. J. HILTON, S. PEASE, T. A. WILSON, C. L. STEWART, D. P. GEARING, E. F. WAGNER, D. METCALF, N. A. NICOLA & N. M. GOUGH. 1988. Myeloid leukemia inhibitory factor maintains the developmental potential of embryonic stem cells. Nature (London) **336**: 684–687.
28. SMITH, A. G., J. K. HEALTH, D. D. DONALDSON, G. G. WONG, J. MOREAU, M. STAHL

& D. ROGERS. 1988. Inhibition of pluripotential embryonic stem cell differentiation by purified polypeptides. Nature (London) **336:** 688–690.
29. CONQUET, F. & P. BRULET. 1990. Developmental expression of myeloid leukemia inhibitory factor gene in preimplantation blastocysts and in extraembryonic tissue of mouse embryos. Mol. Cell. Biol. **10:** 3801–3805.
30. BHATT, H., L. J. BRUNET & C. L. STEWART. 1991. Uterine expression of leukemia inhibitory factor coincides with the onset of blastocyst implantation. Proc. Natl. Acad. Sci. USA **88:** 11408–11412.
31. UNKELESS, J. C., A. TOBIA, L. OSSOWSKI, J. P. QUIGLEY, D. B. RIFKIN & E. REICH. 1973. An enzymatic function associated with transformation of fibroblast oncogenic viruses. I. Chick embryo fibroblast cultures transformed by avian RNA tumor viruses. J. Exp. Med. **137:** 85–111.
32. UNKELESS, J. C., S. GORDON & E. REICH. 1974. Secretion of plasminogen activator by stimulated macrophages. J. Exp. Med. **139:** 834–850.
33. BEERS, W. H., S. STRICKLAND & E. REICH. 1975. Ovarian plasminogen activator: relationship to ovulation and hormonal regulation. Cell **6:** 387–394.
34. BLASI, F., J. D. VASSALLI & K. DANO. 1987. Urokinase type plasminogen activator: proenzyme, receptor, and inhibitors. J. Cell. Biol. **104:** 801–804.
35. OWERS, N. O. & R. J. BLANDAU. 1953. Proteolytic activity of the rat and guinea pig blastocyst *in vitro*. *In* The Biology of the Blastocyst. R. L. Blandau, Ed. 207–223. The University of Chicago Press. Chicago.
36. MILWIDSKY, A., H. KANETI, Z. FINCI, N. LAUFER, A. TSAFRIRI & M. MAYER. 1989. Human follicular fluid protease and antiprotease activities: a suggested correlation with ability of oocytes to undergo *in vitro* fertilization. **52:** 274–280.

# Intravenous Immunoglobulin (IVIG) in the Prevention of Implantation Failures

G. DE PLACIDO, F. ZULLO,[a,c] A. MOLLO, F. CAPPIELLO,
A. NAZZARO, N. COLACURCI, AND G. PALUMBO[b]

*Institute of Obstetrics and Gynecology*
[b]*Department of Biology and Molecular
and Cellular Pathology and CEOS/CNR
"Federico II Medical School"
Via Pansini, 5
80131 Naples, Italy*
and
[c]*Institute of Gynecologic and Pediatric Sciences
Catanzaro Medical School c/o "A. Pugliese" Hospital
Viale Pio X
88100 Cantanzaro, Italy*

## INTRODUCTION

The recent spread of very sensitive β-hCG assays and assisted reproductive technologies has revealed how high the rate of very early and preclinical abortions is.[1,2] This has made clear that implantation is the true limiting factor of human reproduction. Implantation necessarily implies a specific immunologic interaction between the embryo and the mother: many immune modifications have been claimed in recent literature to explain the tolerance of the fetal allograft.[3,4] This immune approach has given a theoretical basis to different therapeutic strategies for recurrent abortions involving either a partner or donor leukocyte active immunization[5,6] or passive immunization by intravenous immunoglobulins (IVIG)[7] to prevent implantation failures.[8]

This work, based on a previous preliminary investigation,[9] aims to verify the effectiveness of IVIG treatment in the prevention of implantation failures in an open randomized comparative study versus placebo and to identify possible parameters predictive of conditions liable to be successfully treated by this protocol.

## MATERIAL AND METHODS

### Patients

The patients were thirty-nine women with: a) two or more very early abortions (less than 8 weeks) or biochemical pregnancies (marked by two consecutive increases in β-hCG levels without USG evidence of gestational sac); and b) three or more failed attempts of embryo transfer after IVF, replacing at least three embryos.

---

[a] Send correspondence to this author.

TABLE 1. Clinical Outcome[a]

|  | Cases | PR | IR | AR |
|---|---|---|---|---|
| Group A | 18 | 6/18 (33.3%) | 8/45 (17.7%) | 1/6 (16.6%) |
| Group B | 21 | 4/21 (19.1%) | 4/61 (6.5%) | 2/5 (40.0%) |

[a] $p < 0.05$ (Fisher's Exact Test).

## Protocol and Study Design

Eighteen patients were randomized in the IVIG treatment group (group A) and 21 in the placebo arm (group B). All patients underwent a superovulation protocol, which included ovarian desensitization by GnRH analogs. Before gonadotropin stimulation, patients received the first administration of 200 ml of immunoglobulin concentrate (20 g, group A) or placebo (group B). A second administration was given when β-hCG was positive and, then, every three weeks up to the 20th week of gestation. Following the treatment all patients were monitored for changes in a) serum profile of immunoglobulins, b) unidirectional "mixed lymphocyte culture" (MFC) (to detect possible blocking factors[5]), and c) trophoblast penetration through a three-dimensional support. The latter test was performed *in vitro* using a specific endometrial primary cell culture, according to a procedure originally described by us, named "double tube microinvasion test" and detailed in Reference 10. In brief, the test consists in matching primary endometrial cell culture (from endometrial biopsies from the previous cycle stimulated in the same way as at the time of implantation), with a choriocarcinoma cell line (JEG-3) in two separate Millipore tubes (5 mm diameter). After 48 hours culture in suspension in Ham F-10 supplemented with 5% FBS to allow cells to adhere to walls and to produce extracellular matrix, the two tubes were put head by head and held together with a cuff. Five days later, a number of trophoblast cells (identified by MoAb PKK1 for cytokeratine) migrated into the endometrium: the entity of this migration and the number of migrated cells was finally measured.

## RESULTS AND DISCUSSION

Clinical outcome in group A (IVIG) and B (placebo) is reported in TABLE 1. It may be seen that while the pregnancy rate (PR) was not statistically significant (33.3 vs 19.1), the implantation rate (IR) in the IVIG group was remarkably higher ($p < 0.05$) as compared to the placebo group (17.7% vs 6.5%). The abortion rate (AR) was 16.6% in group A and 40.0% in the placebo group. At $T_0$ the immunoglobulin serum profile and the one way "mixed lymphocyte culture" (MFC) were not different in patients of both groups; at T1 (*i.e.*, after treatment) "mixed lymphocyte culture" was not significantly modified; the obvious change in the serum immunoglobulin profile was observed in the IVIG group. A good correlation was observed between the "double tube microinvasion test" and the clinical outcome. Only in 3 out of 15 cases tested (4 cases were not assayed because cell cultures were lost), the number of trophoblast cells at 3 mm distance from the interface out of the total number of trophoblast cells at the interface was lower than 5% and, more important, in 2 of these 3 cases an ongoing pregnancy resulted after IVIG treatment. Among the remaining 12 cases, showing a microinvasion greater than 5% at 3 mm, pregnancy was observed only in a single case. These findings suggest that those cases in which the trophoblast invasion during the test with prepared endometrium is defective may be responsive to an immune treatment.

In view of a possible wide application of the "double tube microinvasion test" as a prognostic assay for the use of the intravenous immunoglobulin in the prevention of implantation failures, and considering the high cost of this treatment, it is clear that more studies, either clinically oriented and/or laboratory based, are necessary.

## REFERENCES

1. EDMONDS, D. K., K. S. LINDSAY, J. F. MILLER, E. WILLIAMSON & P. J. WOOD. 1982. Early embryonic mortality in women. Fertil. Steril. **38:** 447–453.
2. WILCOX, A. J. & B. C. WEIBERG. 1988. Incidence of early loss of pregnancy. N. Engl. J. Med. **319:** 189–194.
3. HILL, J. A. 1990. Immunological mechanism of pregnancy maintenance and failure: a critique of theories and therapy. Am. J. Reprod. Immunol. Microbiol. **22:** 33–42.
4. CLARK, D. A. 1988. Host immunoregulatory mechanism and the success of the conceptus fertilized *in vivo* and *in vitro*. *In* Early Pregnancy Loss: Mechanism and Treatment. R. W. Beard & F. Sharp, Eds. 125. RCOG. London.
5. UNANDER, A. M. & A. LINDHOLM. 1986. Transfusion of leukocyte-rich erythrocyte concentrates; a successful treatment in selected cases of habitual abortions. Am. J. Obstet. Gynecol. **154:** 516.
6. BEER, A. E. 1983. "Immunopathologic factors contributing to recurrent spontaneous abortion in humans. Am. J. Reprod. Immunol. **4:** 182.
7. MUELLER-ECKHARDT, G., O. HEINE, J. NEPPERT, W. KUNZEL & C. MUELLER-ECKHARDT. 1989. Treatment of recurrent spontaneous abortion (RSA) by intravenous immunoglobulin (IVIG): a pilot study. J. Reprod. Immunol. (Suppl.), July 4th. International Congress of Reproductive Immunology; Abstract book, p. 113.
8. MOWBRAY, J. F. 1989. Immunization with paternal cells in treatment of very early recurrent abortions. J. Reprod. Immunol. (Suppl.) **23:** 1–214.
9. DE PLACIDO, G., F. ZULLO, N. COLACURCI, D. PERRONE, A. NAZZARO, F. PAOLILLO & U. MONTEMAGNO. 1991. Immunological treatment of implantation failure. Ann. N.Y. Acad. Sci. **622:** 291.
10. NAZZARO, A., N. COLACURCI, F. ZULLO, M. GALASSO, I. STRINA & G. DE PLACIDO. 1991. Manipulation of human first trimester trophoblast and choriocarcinoma cell invasion of decidua and foetal skin *in vitro*. New Trends Gynaecol. Obstet. **7:** 000.

# Immunologically Mediated Abortion (IMA)

## A Minireview

E. GIACOMUCCI, C. BULLETTI, V. POLLI,
AND C. FLAMIGNI

*Reproductive Medicine Unit*
*Department of Obstetrics and Gynecology*
*University of Bologna*
*Via Massarenti 13*
*40138 Bologna, Italy*

### INTRODUCTION

Roughly 22% of all clinical pregnancies evolve into "spontaneous abortions."[1] The causes of spontaneous abortion have been determined in under 60% of the total and comprise genetic, infectious, hormonal and immunological factors.[2] In some cases the immune tolerance mechanism may be impaired and the fetus immunologically rejected (IMA = immunologically mediated abortion).[3] The frequency of recurrent abortion among pregnant women is about 0.4–0.8%.[4] The risk of recurrent abortion increases with the number of past abortions: after one abortion the risk is 24%; after two consecutive abortions it is 26%; after three abortions, 32%.[1]

### BASIC ASPECT

During preimplantation and up to the end of implantation the *cell-mediated immune mechanism* (potential alloimmune etiologies) is responsible for early abortion. This mechanism involves immunocompetent endometrial granulated lymphocytes (eGL), already present before decidualization, and their production of soluble factors or cytokines.[5] Some studies have shown that efficient functioning and an adequate number of decidual cells are required to maintain the semiallogenic fetus (50% exogenous antigens), and pregnancy has been likened to a straightforward natural allograft.[6] Once the implantation process is over, after blastocyst penetration of the stroma and the decidual reaction of uterine tissue, IMA could be caused by a *humoral mechanism*[7] (antipaternal cytoxic antibodies or autoantibodies etiology) or by the production of paternal anti-MHC antibodies, or even by an autoimmune disorder leading to the production of autoantibodies (antiphospholipid antibodies, antinuclear antibodies or polyclonal B cell activation).[2] The diagnostic work-up adopted to select IMA patients is crucial and includes primary (karyotype of both partners, toxo-test, hysterosalpingography, endometrial biopsy, thyroid function tests, serum hPRL, luteal phase dating)[8] and secondary (full hemochromocytometric test, search for LE cells (or Hargraves cells), lupus anticoagulant, anticardiolipin, antinuclear antibodies, rheumatoid factor, blood complement, VDRL (venereal disease research laboratory)[9] investigations. Therapeutical approaches vary depending on the presence of autoimmune disorders. If autoimmune disorders are demonstrated, therapies with different combinations of corticosteroids, aspirin and heparin or intravenous immunoglobulin are used.[10] When there is not this evidence, therapy with paternal or donor peripheral blood mononuclear cells should be used.[11]

## REFERENCES

1. HILL, J. A. & D. J. ANDERSON. 1990. Arch. Immunol. Ther. Exp. **38:** 11–119.
2. DUDLEY, D. J. & D. W. BRANCH. 1989. Clin. Obstet. Gynecol. **32**(3): 520.
3. REDMAN, C. W. 1990. Res. Immunol. **141**(2): 169–175.
4. STRAY-PETERSEN, B. & S. STRAY-PETERSEN. 1984. Am. J. Obstet. Gynecol. **148:** 140.
5. BULMER, J. N., M. LONGFELLOW & A. RITSON. 1991. Ann. N.Y. Acad. Sci.: **622:** 57–68.
6. VOISIN, G. A. 1987. *In* Colloques INSERM. G. Chaouat, Ed. 3. INSERM Pubbl. Paris.
7. SCOTT, J. R., N. S. ROTE & D. W. BRANCH. 1987. Obstet. Gynecol. **70:** 645.
8. XU, L., V. CHANG, A. MURPHY, J. A. ROCK, M. DAMEWOOD, W. SCHLAFF & H. A. ZACUR. 1990. Am. J. Obstet. Gynecol. **163:** 1493–1497.
9. MAIER, D. B. & A. PARKE. 1989. Fertil. Steril. **51**(2): 280–285.
10. ORVIETO, R., A. ACHIRON, Z. BEU-RAFAEL & R. ACHIRON. 1991. Fertil. Steril. **56**(6): 1013–1020.
11. BEER, A. E., J. F. QUEBBEMAN, J. W. I. AYERS & R. F. HAINES. 1981. Am. J. Obstet. Gynecol. **141:** 987.

# Regulation of Endometrial Differentiation by Synthetic Steroids *in Vitro*

L. KIESEL AND M. MAPPES

*Department of Obstetrics and Gynecology*
*University Women's Hospital Tübingen*
*Schleichstraße 4*
*W-72076 Tübingen, Germany*

## INTRODUCTION

During the monthly cycle physiological steroids regulate the proliferation and differentiation of the endometrium. With increasing estradiol concentrations in the serum during the proliferative phase of the cycle the endometrium develops a high mitotic activity on the epithelial and stromal cells. When the secretory phase is reached, estradiol concentrations decrease and progesterone secretion is enhanced. This induces the abandonment of mitosis activity of epithelial and stromal cells. At this time period secretory changes of the glandular epithelium occur and the decidualization of the stromal cells starts. This differentiation of the stromal cells is followed by the secretion of low concentrations of prolactin during the late secretory phase of the cycle.[1,2] Prolactin of endometrial origin is identical with prolactin secreted in the lactotrope cells of the pituitary gland in terms of its biochemistry, immunology and amino acid sequence.[3,4] *In vitro* experiments showed that endometrial prolactin secretion is stimulated by progesterone and inhibited by estradiol, paralleled by respective responses on decidualization.[5-8] Prolactin has been regarded, therefore, as an indicator for the differentiation of the endometrium.

Nowadays synthetic steroids are used for contraception or as valuable tools in therapy of hormonal disorders. The advantages of synthetic steroids include a higher bond to the receptors as well as a higher half-life before decomposition. Since many pathways of synthetic steroids are still not well understood, investigations are made to comprehend the effects of synthetic steroids on proliferation and differentiation of endometrial cells in *in vitro* cultures.

### In vitro *Influence of Physiological Steroids on Endometrial Cell Cultures*

Cyclic changes of the endometrium have been correlated with periodic alterations in serum concentrations of estrogens and progestins. The actions of these sex steroids are thought to be mediated, at least partly, by the local production of various growth factors found in the endometrium. In order to investigate the steroidal influence by physiologic and synthetic steroids and/or growth factors on the modulation of synthesis, secretion and functional changes of the endometrium, an *in vitro* cell model for long-term experiments was developed.

## Cell Culture

Endometrial tissue for premenopausal women undergoing a hysterectomy for benign conditions was dissociated into single cell solutions enzymatically and seeded on culture dishes without separation of epithelial and stromal cells. After 4 days of preculturing (day −4 to −1) with DMEM/F12 + 10% fetal calf serum (FCS) to induce an optimal adhesion on the culture dishes, the medium was replaced by DMEM/F12 without phenol red + insulin-transferrin-selenite (ITS) in order to minimize the nondefined influence of steroids and growth factors contained in the FCS. Starting the experiments on day 0 by medium shift, estradiol (10 nM), progesterone (100 nM) or the combination estradiol + progesterone (10 nM + 100 nM) was added. Until day 27 the medium was changed every third day and steroids were substituted with every medium change. The medium was collected and frozen at −20°C until the concentration of prolactin, a marker for cell differentiation, was determined by an enzymatic immunofluorescent assay (EIA). Proliferation rate of cells was assessed every third day during the experimental period by crystal-violet-staining and photometric evaluation, as well as cell counting by hemocytometer (Thoma-chamber).

## Proliferation of Endometrial Cell Cultures under Different Culture Conditions

Fetal calf serum containing steroids and growth factors evokes a dose-dependent increase of cell proliferation until confluence is attained (results not shown). Phenol red, an added indicator in the medium, has estrogen-like activity.[9] In presence of 10% FCS no effects based on phenol red could be observed.

When FCS was replaced by ITS the cell proliferation was decreased due to lack of steroids and growth factors, without the loss of cell viability. Endometrial cells cultured in DMEM/F12 without phenol red exhibited a longer proliferation phase up to day 18, while the cultures incubated with DMEM/F12 containing phenol red achieved the proliferation maximum on day 12 (FIG. 1).

Modest differences caused by phenol red were observed in cultures incubated with DMEM/F12 + ITS. This confirms the results of Berthois et al.[9] that phenol red has a weak estrogen capacity, for the cultures incubated with 10% FCS in the cell groups with and without phenol red exhibited no differences, which were probably covered by steroids and growth factors contained in FCS.

After 12 days of incubating phase with and without steroids in DMEM/F12 without phenol red, the first differences in cell proliferation were observed. Proliferation of endometrial cell cultures by substitution of estradiol alone revealed no difference from the control groups (inhibition by 8%). The substitution of progesterone alone enhanced cell proliferation without significance by 26% on day 27 only. The combination of estrogen and progesterone enhanced cell proliferation on days 12, 18 and 27 by 5%, 6% and 44%, respectively (FIG. 2).

Hammond et al.[10] examined enriched endometrial stromal cells in culture and could not induce the proliferation by adding estradiol ($10^{-10} - 10^{-8}$ mol/l), too. By subculturing the cells, the proliferation potency decreased constantly.[10] Chegini et al.[11] achieved our results more specifically, for in these experiments estradiol *or* progesterone (1 μM) had no effect on proliferation, while estradiol *and* progesterone (1 μM) enhanced the cell numbers in low amounts.[11] The proliferative effect of progesterone was observed on endometrial, stromal cells by Irwin et al.[12] who published the hypothesis that endometrial, epithelial cells stimulate by paracrine pathways the proliferation and differentiation of stromal cells. Our experi-

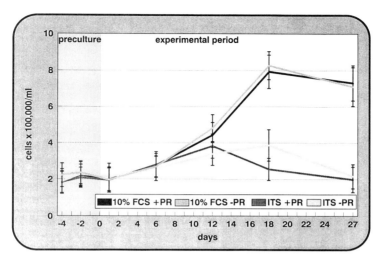

**FIGURE 1.** Effects of 10% fetal calf serum (FCS) and insulin-transferrin-selenite (ITS) on cell proliferation in DMEM/F12 with and without phenol red. +PR: with phenol red, −PR: without phenol red.

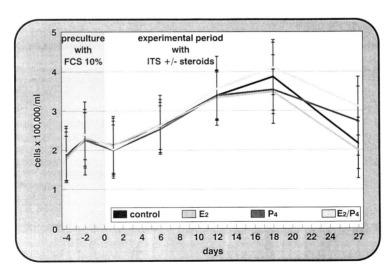

**FIGURE 2.** Effects of added physiological steroids on endometrial long-term cell cultures. $E_2$: estradiol (10 nM), $P_4$: progesterone (100 nM), $E_2/P_4$: combination of estradiol (10 nM) and progesterone (100 nM).

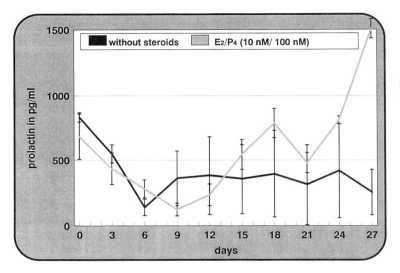

**FIGURE 3.** Influence of steroids on prolactin secretion in long-term endometrial cell cultures. $E_2/P_4$: combination of estradiol (10 nM) and progesterone (100 nM).

ments investigated cell cultures containing epithelial cells as well as stromal cells. For the steroidal effects being observed in these cultures (FIG. 2), the suggestion is made that cellular interactions between epithelial and stromal cells may be regulated and enhanced additionally by other factors—especially growth factors.

### Differentiation of Endometrial Cell Cultures under Steroidal Influence

Prolactin is secreted by endometrial, stromal cells during the luteal phase of the monthly cycle and serves as a marker for differentiation.[2] Endometrial prolactin is identical in biochemistry and immunology to the prolactin secreted by the pituitary gland.[3-7] Prolactin secretion is induced *in vitro* by application of progesterone and is related to the expression of estrogen and progesterone receptors.[8-11]

Endometrial cell cultures incubated with DMEM/F12 + ITS without steroids exhibited a decrease of prolactin secretion between day 6 and 9. This decrease appeared in all cultures and may be a retarded effect of the 10% FCS added during the preculture phase. In cultures incubated with DMEM/F12 + ITS without steroids, prolactin secretion did not stimulate until day 27. In contrast, in cell cultures stimulated with estradiol and progesterone prolactin secretion increased after the typical minimum on day 9, up to tenfold on day 27 (FIG. 3).

### In Vitro *Influence of Growth Factors on Endometrial Cell Cultures*

The influence of physiological steroids added to cell cultures on epithelial and stromal endometrial cells was modest. The suggestion that perhaps growth factors modulate the effect of steroids on proliferation and differentiation of endometrial

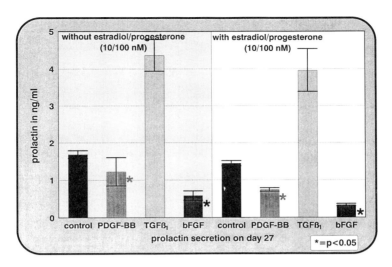

**FIGURE 4.** Influence of growth factors on proliferation of endometrial cell cultures. PDGF (2 ng/ml), TGF$\beta_1$ (1 ng/ml) or bFGF (1 ng/ml) were substituted every third day.

cells led to the investigation of the influence of growth factors on these *in vitro* cell cultures. The same cultures were chosen, and every third day platelet-derived growth factor BB (PDGF-BB, 2 ng/ml), transforming growth factor $\beta_1$ (TGF$\beta_1$, 1 ng/ml) or basic fibroblast growth factor (bFGF, 1 ng/ml) were added to the medium with or without estradiol/progesterone (10 nM/100 nM). During the experimental period of 27 days every third day the proliferation potency and the grade of differentiation by prolactin secretion were analyzed.

### *Effects of Growth Factors on Proliferation in Endometrial Cell Cultures*

The proliferation of endometrial cell cultures was influenced by growth factors. PDGF-BB enhanced the proliferation rate on day 27 by 28% without steroid application and by 24% with steroid substitution. TGF$\beta_1$ inhibited the proliferation by 57% and 53% without and with steroid conditions, respectively, and bFGF inhibited proliferation on day 27 by 12% without steroid supplement, but enhanced modestly by 5% with added steroids (FIG. 4).

The effect of PDGF-BB was inhibited by steroids with 23%. TGF$\beta_1$ had 13% lower effect on proliferation under steroid supplement and bFGF exhibited with 6% the lowest effects. The addition of bFGF to the cultures revealed no significant effect on proliferation in the presence or absence of steroids under conditions investigated.

Other groups examined the influence of PDGF in short-term experiments (24–72 h) on the proliferation of endometrial, stromal cells. PDGF in combination with FCS had an enhanced effect. Estradiol ($10^{-8} - 10^{-10}$ M) and PDGF increased the proliferation more, but only additively and not synergistically.[12,16] PDGF-AB was detected in stromal cells during the whole cycle and the enhancing effect on the proliferation was achieved. PDGF-BB has a higher biological effectiveness, but the receptor-$\beta$ is reduced during the luteal phase. Steroids had no influence.[11] Our results confirm with the stimulating effect on proliferation, but the influence of steroids was modest inhibiting, in contrast to the results of other investigators.

TGF$\beta_{1+3}$ was detected in stromal cells and TGF$\beta_1$ was observed inhibiting DNA-synthesis in epithelial cells, but enhancing the synthesis in stromal cells. Estradiol ($10^{-8}$ M) inhibited DNA-synthesis by 40% in epithelial cells and estradiol in combination with TGF$\beta_1$ had no effect on epithelial cells.[17] Other groups observed an inhibition of proliferation on stromal endometrial cells.

FGF a + b was analyzed by detecting the mRNA with PCR in stromal cells.[18] The receptors for aFGF and bFGF were demonstrated by PCR in stromal cells after 1, 2 and 3 weeks of culturing.[19] Several groups observed an increase in proliferation in stromal cells and no influence of steroids.[10,12,20] Our results exhibit a decrease without steroid supplement and an increase with steroid-culturing, but in a very modest effect. Maybe bFGF plays a role in the interaction between epithelial and stromal cells.

### *Differentiation of Endometrial Cell Cultures under the Supplementation with Growth Factors*

The differentiation of endometrial cell cultures was even more influenced by growth factors than was observed regarding their proliferation. PDGF-BB without added steroids inhibited prolacting secretion by 27% on day 27, and with steroid supplementation the decrease of prolactin concentrations in the medium achieved by 50%. TGF$\beta_1$ enhanced prolactin secretion without steroids by 158% and with application of steroids the secretion increased to 174% on day 27. The effects of

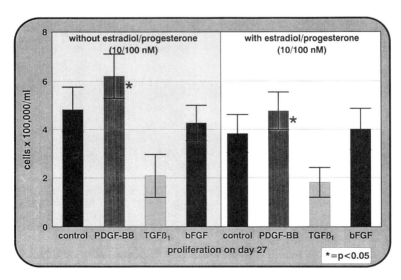

**FIGURE 5.** Influence of growth factors on prolactin secretion as a marker for differentiation of endometrial cell cultures cultured without and with steroids. *: significant change as compared to the column to the *left*.

TGF$\beta_1$ started on day 18. Basic FGF in contrast inhibited the prolactin secretion to 66% and 77%, of control values without and with steroid substitution, respectively.

The differences of prolactin concentration in the medium were higher in cultures treated with estradiol/progesterone in comparison to the control groups cultured without growth factors. Secretion rates in control groups treated without and with steroids were different, lower in cultures with steroid supplementation by 14%. PDGF-BB and bFGF had a lower prolactin production by 40% and 43%, respectively, and TGF$\beta_1$ with 9% was not influenced by steroids (FIG. 5).

The effect of PDGF on differentiation has not yet been examined. Magoffin et al.[21] analyzed an increased differentiation potency and production of progesterone under treatment of TGF$\beta$,[21] and Irwin et al.[12] observed a decreased prolactin secretion under the treatment of bFGF without effects of steroids. Also, products of differentiation like laminin and fibronectin were decreased by culturing endometrial stromal cells with bFGF without steroids.[12]

These data partially confirm our investigations and suggest that steroids and growth factors modulate the proliferation and differentiation of endometrial cells in a complex fashion.

## REFERENCES

1. HEFFNER, L. J., D. A. IDDENDEN & C. R. LYTTLE. 1986. Electrophoretic analyses of secreted human endometrial proteins: identification and characterization of luteal phase prolactin. J. Clin. Endocrinol. Metab. **62:** 1288–1291.
2. RANDOLPH, J. F., JR., H. PEEGEL, R. ANSBACHER & K. M. J. MENON. 1990. In vitro induction of prolactin production and aromatase activity by gonadal steroids exclusively in the stroma of separated proliferative human endometrium. J. Obstet. Gynecol. **162:** 1109–1114.
3. HEALY, D. L. 1984. The clinical significance of endometrial prolactin. Aust. N. Z. J. Obstet. Gynecol. **5:** 95–105.
4. HUANG, J. R., L. TSENG, P. BISHOF & O. A. JÄNNE. 1987. Regulation of prolactin production by progestin, estrogen and relaxin in human endometrial stromal cells. Endocrinology **121:** 2011–2017.
5. DALY, D. C., I. A. MASLAR & D. H. RIDDICK. 1983. Prolactin production during in vitro decidualisation of proliferative endometrium. Am. J. Obstet. Gynecol. **145:** 672–678.
6. BRAVERMAN, M. B., A. BAGNI, D. DE ZIEGLER, I. DEN & E. GURPIDE. 1984. Isolation of prolactin-producing cells from first and second trimester decidua. J. Clin. Endocrinol. Metab. **58:** 521–526.
7. MASLAR, I. A., S. POWER, P. CRADDOCK & R. ANSBACHER. 1986. Decidual prolactin production by organ cultures of human endometrium: effects of continuous and intermittent progesterone treatment. Biol. Reprod. **34:** 741–750.
8. MASLAR, I. A. & R. ANSBACHER. 1986. Effects of progesterone on decidual prolactin production by organ cultures of human endometrium. Endocrinology **118:** 2102–2108.
9. BERTHOIS, Y., J. A. KATZENELLENBOGEN & B. S. KATZENELLENBOGEN. 1986. Phenol red in tissue culture media is a weak estrogen: implications concerning the study of estrogen-responsive cells in culture. Proc. Natl. Acad. Sci. USA **83:** 2496–2500.
10. HAMMOND, M. G., S.-T. OH, J. ANNERS, E. S. SURREY & J. HALME. 1993. The effect of growth factors on the proliferation of human endometrial stromal cells in culture. Am. J. Obstet. Gynecol. **168:** 1131–1138.
11. CHEGINI, N. & R. S. WILLIAMS. 1992. Immunocytochemical localization of transforming growth factors (TGFs) TGF-$\alpha$ and TGF-$\beta$ in human ovarian tissues. J. Clin. Endocrinol. Metab. **74:** 973–980.
12. IRWIN, J. C., W. H. UTIAN & R. L. ECKERT. 1991. Sex steroids and growth factors differentially regulate the growth and differentiation of cultured human endometrial stromal cells. Endocrinology **129**(5): 2385–2392.

13. MASLAR, I. A. & D. H. RIDDICK. 1979. Prolactin production by human endometrium during the normal menstrual cycle. Am. J. Obstet. Gynecol. **135:** 751–754.
14. LOCKWOOD, C. J., Y. NEMERSON, S. GULLER, G. KRIKUN, M. ALVAREZ, V. HAUSKNECHT, E. GURPIDE & F. SCHATZ. 1993. Progestational regulation of human endometrial stromal cell tissue factor expression during decidualization. J. Clin. Endocrinol. Metab. **76:** 231–236.
15. WU, W.-X., J. BROOKS, M. R. MILLAR, W. L. LEDGER, A. F. GLASIER & A. S. MCNEILLY. 1993. Immunolocalization of oestrogen and progesterone receptors in the human decidua in relation to prolactin production. Hum. Reprod. **8**(7): 1129–1135.
16. SURREY, E. S. & J. HALME. 1991. Effect of platelet-derived growth factor on endometrial stromal cell proliferation *in vitro:* a model for endometriosis? Fertil. Steril. **56:** 672–679.
17. MARSHBURN, P. B., A. M. ARICI, M. L. CASEY, C. H. GREEN & I. GREEN. 1993. Expression of TGF$\beta$ mRNA and the modulation of DNA synthesis by TGF$\beta_1$ in human endometrial cells. Soc. Gynecol. Invest. **S31:** 84.
18. RAJPUT-WILLIAMS, J., D. S. C. JONES, J. P. SCHOFIELD, M. LINDSAY & S. K. SMITH. 1991. Demonstration of expression of acidic and basic fibroblast growth factors in human endometrium. J. Reprod. Fert. **71:** 41.
19. CHOI, Y. M., M. D. HORNSTEIN & J. YEH. 1993. Gene expression of basic fibroblast growth factor and basic fibroblast growth factor receptor in the cultured human endometrial stromal cells. J. Reprod. Fert. **206:** 171.
20. GOSPODAROWICZ, D. 1989. Fibroblast growth factor: involvement in early embryonic development and ovarian function. Semin. Reprod. Endocrinol. **7:** 21–39.
21. MAGOFFIN, D. A., B. GANCEDO & G. F. ERICKSON. 1989. Transforming growth factor-$\beta$ promotes differentiation of ovarian theca-interstitial cells but inhibits androgen production. Endocrinology **125:** 1951–1958.

# Interaction between Steroid Hormones and Endometrial Opioids[a]

ACHILLE GRAVANIS,[b] ANTONIS MAKRIGIANNAKIS,
CHRISTOS STOURNARAS, AND
ANDREW N. MARGIORIS

*Departments of Pharmacology, Clinical Chemistry*
*and Biochemistry*
*Medical School*
*University of Crete*
*Stavrakia, Iraklion 71110, Greece*

## INTRODUCTION

The opioids β-endorphin and dynorphins have been detected not only in the central nervous system but also in nonneuronal tissues. β-Endorphin derives from the posttranslational modification of the proopiomelanocortin (POMC) molecule. The POMC mRNA is 1.2 kilobases (kb) long and the POMC polypeptide contains only one opioid, the β-endorphin, which exhibits preferential affinity toward the μ and ε opioid receptors, μ being the original morphine receptor.[1,2] The dynorphins derive from the prodynorphin (PDYN) molecule. The PDYN mRNA is about 2.4 kb long. Its translational product PDYN, a 234-amino acid long polypeptide, contains the sequences of α-, β-neoendorphin and that of dynorphins. The dynorphins are potent κ-opioid agonists. Their molecular weight ranges from 2 to 8 kilodaltons (kd). The 2-kd form is the dynorphin A, the 4-kd is the big dynorphin containing the sequences of dynorphin A and dynorphin B, and the 8-kd form contains the sequences of α-neoendorphin, dynorphin A and dynorphin B.[3,4] In the reproductive tract, the POMC transcript and its opioid product β-endorphin are detectable in testes,[5,6] ovaries,[7,8] and endometrium.[9-11] The PDYN transcript and its products are also detectable in the reproductive tract including the uterus.[12,13]

The Ishikawa cells, a permanent cell line deriving from a human endometrial adenocarcinoma, have been found to be relatively well differentiated human endometrium epithelial cells and, thus, they are a good *in vitro* model for the study of the effects of steroid hormones on human epithelial endometrium.[14,15] The aim of the present work was to find out if these cells synthesize and secrete β-endorphin and dynorphins. If this was true, then they could be used for the study of the effects of steroidal and nonsteroidal hormones on endometrial opioids since, as we have seen, normal endometrium produces these opioids. We have found that the Ishikawa cells express the genes coding for the EOP precursors and that they secrete their opioid peptide products. Following these results, the effect of various steroidal hormones was tested on the secretion of β-endorphin and dynorphins

---

[a] This work was supported by a grant from the Greek General Secretariat for Research and Technology (#104D89) to A.G.
[b] Corresponding author.

from the cultured Ishikawa cells. In addition, we also tested the effect of LHRH, since it is the major regulator of anterior pituitary gonadotroph dynorphins.

## MATERIALS AND METHODS

### Cell Cultures

The Ishikawa cells were established as a permanent cell line from a relatively well differentiated endometrial adenocarcinoma.[14] The cells were left to grow for six days in a culture medium composed of Dulbecco's Modified Eagle's Medium (Flow Labs, Irvine, UK), 10 mM L-glutamine, 15 mM HEPES, 100 U/mL penicillin, 0.1 mg/mL streptomycin, and 15% fetal calf serum. Culture media were changed every 48 hours, up to 6 consecutive days. The plates were kept in a $CO_2$ incubator (Forma Scientific) at 5% $CO_2$ and 37°C. On the seventh day, the culture media were replaced by test media (i.e., chemically defined) composed of HAMF12/MEM (Flow Labs) supplemented with 0.1% defatted human serum albumin, 0.2% glucose, 10 mM L-glutamine, 15 mM HEPES and 1% antibiotic-antimycotic solution (Flow Labs) to a final concentration of 100 U/ml penicillin, 100 µg/ml streptomycin and 0.25 µg/ml fungizone. Cells from high density cultures were seeded into 75-cm$^2$ flasks ($10^6$ cells/flask) in medium containing different steroids or 4-hydroxytamoxifen (TAM) diluted in ethanol and different peptides diluted in medium containing 0.1% BSA. For accuracy, ethanol or BSA was added in the control media at a final concentration of 0.1%. For the measurement of protein content and IR-$\beta$-endorphin or IR-dynorphin levels, cells were harvested in HBSS containing 0.05% EDTA (Flow Labs).

### Radioimmunoassays for $\beta$-Endorphin and Dynorphin

Peptides in the culture media and cellular homogenates were concentrated by a C-18 reverse phase column (Sep-Pak, Waters Associates, Milford, MA). Briefly, culture media and cellular homogenates were acidified by 10 volumes of 0.1N HCl and centrifuged at 10.000 rpm for 10 min. The supernatants were extracted by activated Sep-Pak cartridges, washed with 20 ml 0.1N HCl, eluted with 3 ml acetonitrile 80–0.01% HCl, then dried under vacuum (Speed-Vac). The recovery of synthetic $\beta$-endorphin or dynorphin added to representative aliquots was more than 90%. The IR-$\beta$-endorphin content of the above Sep-Pak concentrates was measured by a solid-phase, two-site immunoradiometric assay (Nichols Labs, Irvine, CA) using an antiserum raised against human $\beta$-endorphin.[17] The antiserum exhibited a 16% cross-reaction with $\beta$-lipotropin. The sensitivity of the assay was 14 pg/tube. The intraassay coefficient of variation was 4.1% and the interassay was 7.1%. Additionally, the IR-dynorphin content of the Sep-Rak concentrates was measured by radioimmunoassay using an antiserum raised against synthetic porcine dynorphin$_{(1-13)}$, which is identical to human dynorphin$_{(1-13)}$.[18,19] The antiserum cross-reacts with human dynorphin$_{(1-13)}$ and dynorphin A. It exhibits no cross-reaction with synthetic human $\beta$-endorphin, $\alpha$-neoendorphin, or met- or leuenkephalin. The sensitivity of the assay was 1–2 pg/tube. Results were expressed as pg of IR-$\beta$-endorphin or IR-dynorphin per mg of total cellular protein determined on whole cellular homogenate by the Bradford method[20] using bovine serum albumin as standard.

## Gel Filtration Chromatography

Pooled test medium from Ishikawa cell cultures was centrifuged at 10.000 × g for 10 min and the supernatant was extracted by a C-18 reverse phase column (Sep-Pak), reconstituted in 0.5 ml 10% formic acid containing 0.5% defatted bovine serum albumin and 6 M urea and chromatographed on a Sephadex G-50 column (0.9 × 60 cm, 40 ml bed volume) at a flow rate of 1.5 ml/h. The 1-ml fractions collected were dried under vacuum and reconstituted for radioimmunoassay. The G-50 column was calibrated with blue dextran, human β-lipotropin, human β-endorphin, dynorphin$_{(1-13)}$ and big dynorphin.

## Northern Blot Analysis

Ishikawa cells, and hypothalami, pituitaries and testes from adult male Sprague-Dawley rats were pooled, frozen immediately in liquid nitrogen, and their total RNA was extracted by the guanidine thiocyanate method.[21] Following size-fractionation of the RNAs (50 μg/lane) by electrophoresis through a 1.5%-agarose gel containing 6% formaldehyde and 2 μg/dl of ethidium bromide, the RNAs were viewed under UV to assess their integrity and then they were blotted to a Gene-Screen nylon filter (New England Nuclear, Boston, MA). The filter was prehybridized and hybridized as per Ref. 21. A synthetic 42-mer oligonucleotide, directed against bases 1–42 of the rat POMC mRNA (this area of mRNA is almost identical in both humans and rats, i.e., only two bases are different)[1,22] and a 48-mer oligonucleotide against bases 36–83 of the rat PDYN mRNA (this area of mRNA is identical in both humans and rats)[3] were used as probes. The probes were labeled at the 3' end with (α-$^{32}$P) deoxyadenocine triphosphate (800 Ci/mmole, Amersham, Arlington, IL) and terminal deoxynucleotidyl transferase (BRL, Bethesda, MD) to a specific activity of about 10$^8$ dpm/mg, as per Ref. 21. Blots were washed in 0.2 × SSC, 0.1% SDS for 30 min at 60°C. Autoradiography using Kodak XR film took place at −70°C in the presence of intensifying screens. The approximate size of POMC and PDYN mRNAs was determined relative to 18S and 28S rRNAs.

## Statistical Analysis

To evaluate the dose-response curves we compared the pre- and posttreatment levels of opioid peptides for each dose of steroids, and LHRH concentration tested (mean of IR-β-endorphin and IR-dynorphin in the media ± SEM). The statistical analysis was performed by the one way analysis of variance (ANOVA) and by the unpaired Student $t$ test.

## RESULTS

### Size of the IR-Peptides

The bulk of IR-β-endorphin in the test media exhibited the apparent molecular weight of authentic β-endorphin (FIG. 1), while most of IR-dynorphin that of the

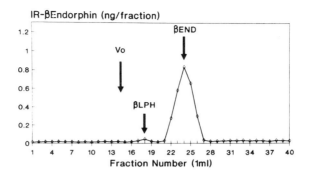

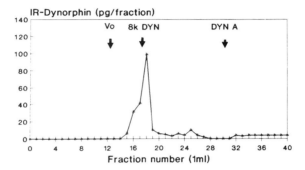

**FIGURE 1.** Sephadex G-50 gel filtration chromatography of Ishikawa cell culture media. One-ml fractions were collected. The *arrows* indicate the void volume (Vo) and the elution positions of human β-lipotropin (β-LPH), synthetic human β-endorphin (β-END), 8-kd dynorphin (8k DYN) and 2-kd dynorphin A (DYN A).

8-kd form of dynorphins; small quantities of a 4-kd material (big dynorphin) was also detectable (FIG. 1).

## Size of the Hybridizing RNAs

FIGURE 2A depicts the Northern blot analysis of RNAs extracted from Ishikawa cells and from rat anterior pituitary and testis. The blot was hybridized with the POMC probe. The size of the hybridizing RNA extracted from the Ishikawa cells (lane 1) was 1.2 kb long and, thus, it appears to be similar or identical to the POMC mRNA present in anterior pituitary (lane 3) but different, in size, to that present in testicular tissue which exhibited, as expected, an approximate size of 0.9 kb (lane 2).

FIGURE 2B depicts the Northern blot analysis of RNAs extracted as per FIGURE 2A. The blot was hybridized with the PDYN probe. The size of hybridizing RNA from the Ishikawa cells was about 2.4 kb long (lane 3), which makes it similar or identical to the PDYN mRNA present in rat pituitary and hypothalamus (lanes 1 and 2).

### Basal and Depolarization-Induced IR-Dynorphin Secretion

IR-dynorphin was detectable in the test media from the Ishikawa cells. Its concentration in the media of 2- and 4-day cultures were 87 ± 9 and 83 ± 7 pg per mg of protein per two days (mean ± SEM, n = 6) respectively (see below, Fig. 4). At day 6, the concentration of IR-dynorphin in the media declined to 44 ± 2 pg per mg of protein. This phenomenon has been already described for $\beta$-endorphin secretion as well as for the estrogen receptor levels and the DNA polymerase $\alpha$ activity, and it takes place when the cell number reaches plateaux; this appears to be a characteristic of Ishikawa cell culture dynamics and has been documented previously.[15,16,22]

Following depolarization in the presence of 54 mM of KCl for 30 and 60 minutes, the secretion of IR-dynorphin increased from 2 ± 0.1 to 55 ± 3 and to 95 ± 4 pg per mg of protein per 30 min, respectively (FIG. 3). The difference in the concentration of IR-dynorphin between basal and KCl-induced depolarization was highly significant by ANOVA test ($p < 0.001$, n = 6).

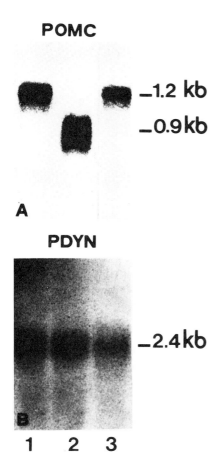

**FIGURE 2.** Northern blot analysis of Ishikawa cells' total RNA. **(A)** Hybridization of the blot with the POMC probe (*lane 1:* Ishikawa cells, *lane 2:* rat testes, *lane 3:* rat pituitary). **(B)** Hybridization with the PDYN probe (*lane 1:* rat pituitary, *lane 2:* rat hypothalamus, *lane 3:* Ishikawa cells).

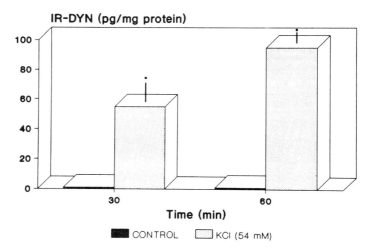

**FIGURE 3.** KCl-induced depolarization of Ishikawa cells. Cells were exposed to 54 mM of KCl for 30 and 60 min and the concentration of IR-dynorphin was measured as described in Materials and Methods. (*) signifies difference of each point from the control ($p < 0.001$).

## Effect of Steroid Hormones

The cells were exposed for 2, 4 and 6 days to different steroid hormones, then the levels of IR-$\beta$-endorphin and IR-dynorphin were measured in the culture media, as described in Materials and Methods. Estradiol, dexamethasone and the antiprogestin-antiglucocorticoid RU486 diminished the release of $\beta$-endorphin from Ishikawa cells in a time-dependent manner, *i.e.*, the maximal effect of these steroids was observed after 4 days of culture. FIGURE 4A depicts the dose response of $\beta$-endorphin secretion from Ishikawa cells exposed for 4 days to estradiol, tamoxifen, dexamethasone and RU486. The maximal inhibitory effect on IR-$\beta$-endorphin secretion of all three steroids tested was observed at 10 nM, after which it plateaued. The antiestrogen tamoxifen exhibited a slight and not statistically significant agonistic effect, *i.e.*, it decreased the secretion of IR-$\beta$-endorphin, only at high concentrations (1 $\mu$M). Progesterone and dihydrotestosterone did not alter the secretion of IR-$\beta$-endorphin. However, all these steroids and the RU486 did not affect the secretion of IR-dynorphin (data summarized in TABLE 1).

## Effect of LHRH

Ishikawa cells were incubated for 2, 4 and 6 days with 100 nM of LHRH. As shown in FIGURE 5, LHRH increased the release of IR-dynorphin in a time-dependent manner, the maximal effect having been observed after 4 days (from $83 \pm 3$ to $200 \pm 34$ pg/mg of protein, $p < 0.001$, n = 6). The stimulatory effect of LHRH on dynorphin secretion was dose-dependent (FIG. 4B). However, LHRH had no affect on the secretion of $\beta$-endorphin (TABLE 1).

## DISCUSSION

The findings described in this study show that the POMC- and the PDYN-derived families of EOP are synthesized by the relatively well differentiated human endometrium epithelial cell-derived Ishikawa cell line. These findings are in agreement with data deriving from normal mammalian endometrial tissues (including human) indicating that EOP are produced by this type of cells.[9-11] In the Ishikawa cells, the POMC and PDYN transcripts as well as their opioid peptide products were all detectable. The POMC transcript appears to be similar or identical, in size, to its anterior pituitary counterpart, *i.e.*, 1.2 kb long and different than that

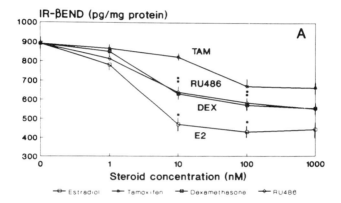

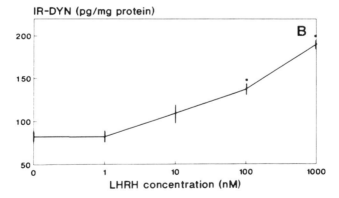

**FIGURE 4.** (**A**) Dose-response curve of IR-β-endorphin release following exposure to each steroid hormone studied. Ishikawa cells were cultured in the presence of $E_2$, TAM, RU486 and DEX (at the indicated concentrations) for 4 days, then IR-β-endorphin levels were measured in the test media. (**B**) Dose-response curve of IR-dynorphin release for LHRH. Ishikawa cells were incubated for 4 days with the indicated concentrations of LHRH, then IR-dynorphin levels were measured in the test media. Results are expressed as pg of IR-peptide per mg of protein (mean ± SEM, n: 6). (*) signifies difference of each point from the control ($p < 0.001$).

**TABLE 1.** Effect of Steroid and Peptide Hormones on Opioid Peptide Secretion from Ishikawa Human Endometrial Cells in Culture

| Hormone | β-Endorphin | Dynorphin |
|---|---|---|
| 17β-Estradiol | decreases | NE[a] |
| Progesterone | NE | NE |
| RU486 | decreases | NE |
| Dexamethasone | decreases | NE |
| Dihydrotestosterone | NE | NE |
| LHRH | NE | increases |
| Oxytocin | NE | NE |

[a] NE: no effect.

present in rat testis. Indeed, in the rodent reproductive tissues, and in the human placenta, the detectable POMC transcript is shorter than that in the central nervous system by about 300 nucleotides.[2,23,24] The physiological significance of the POMC mRNA polymorphism remains to be determined. However, as far as the Ishikawa cells are concerned, this does not appear to be a problem, since their POMC transcript seems to be no different from that present in pituitary. Similarly, the size of the Ishikawa cell PDYN mRNA is apparently similar or identical to that present in both the hypothalamus and anterior pituitary gonadotrophs.

The role(s) that the endometrial opioids play within the uterine cavity is still largely unknown. Clues regarding their physiological function may derive from the study of the regulation of endometrial EOP biosynthesis and secretion. In this regard, we have found that the regulation of the secretion of these opioids by the

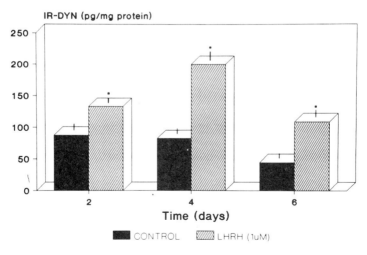

**FIGURE 5.** Time-course of LHRH effect on IR-dynorphin release. Ishikawa cells were cultured for 2, 4 and 6 days with 100 nM of LHRH and the levels of IR-dynorphin were measured in the test media. Results are expressed as pg of IR-peptide per mg of protein (mean ± SEM, n: 6). (*) signifies difference of each point from the control ($p < 0.001$).

Ishikawa cells is opioid type-specific, *i.e.*, it is distinct for each family of opioids. Specifically, estradiol and dexamethasone decreased the secretion of β-endorphin from these cells without affecting the secretion of dynorphins. On the other hand, LHRH which regulates the secretion of anterior pituitary dynorphins, localized only in the gonadotrophs, also increased the secretion of IR-dynorphin while it did not affect β-endorphin. Indeed, the regulation of endometrial opioids appears to have similarities to that in hypothalamus and anterior pituitary. Indeed, it is known that (a) estrogens diminish the secretion of β-endorphin and the levels of POMC mRNA in rat hypothalamus,[25-27] and that (b) LHRH increases the secretion of pituitary dynorphins.[28]

The finding that the regulation of endometrial opioids is different between each type of opioid, *i.e.*, that the POMC- and the PDYN-derived opioids are regulated in a type-specific manner, may indicate that each family of endometrial opioids may be involved in quite different physiological pathways within the uterus. Furthermore, preliminary data from our laboratory have shown that the potent μ-type of opioid receptors antagonist increases, in a dose dependent fashion, the secretion of dynorphins from Ishikawa cells. Since naloxone has been shown to exert a similar effect on guinea-pig ileum dynorphins[29] our findings may suggest a local interaction between two separate endometrial opioid-dependent pathways.

In general, it is postulated that the opioids present in most peripheral tissues may exert local (paracrine or autocrine) effects taking part in the regulation of their microenvironment. In the case of uterus, this argument becomes even more possible since it has been shown that multiple opioid receptors are present in this tissue.[30] Interestingly, β-endorphin appears to increase the concentration of estrogen receptors in uterine epithelial cells thus enhancing the sensitivity of endometrium to estrogens.[31] Apart from their effects on the endometrium, endometrial opioids may also affect the myometrium, since it is known that they exert an inhibitory-relaxant effect on smooth muscle preparations.[32] It is thus possible that uterine opioids may participate in the regulation of myometrial contractility necessary for an efficient movement of the ovum into the tubes and the transport of sperm across the uterine cavity.

It is now known that opioid peptides inhibit cell proliferation in a number of different tissues. Recent findings attribute a suppressive effect of opioids in neural tumors. EOP have been found to inhibit the growth of neuroblastoma and retina cells.[33] As far as Ishikawa cells are concerned, we have shown that estrogens inhibit the release of β-endorphin while at the same time stimulate their proliferation.[14] Thus, the effect of estrogens on cell proliferation may be partially due to their suppression of the production of local opioids thus removing an endogenous brake of endometrial cell proliferation.

Finally, a number of recent findings implicate EOP in the regulation of the immune response. Indeed, uterine opioids may participate, along with corticoids and cytokines,[34] in the regulation of local immune events taking place early in pregnancy, some of which may be associated with the implantation of the fertilized egg into the endometrium.

## SUMMARY

The opioids β-endorphin and the dynorphins belong to two separate families of endogenous opioid peptides (EOP). They are produced not only in the central nervous system but also in nonneural tissues where, as it appears, they act locally via paracrine mechanisms. These opioids have been shown to be produced at multiple sites along the mammalian reproductive tract including the intrauterine cavity. The aim of the present work was to find out if the well differentiated human endometrial cell line of Ishikawa, which has been shown to be a good *in vitro* model for the study of the effects of steroid hormones on human epithelial endometrium, expresses these two EOP. Northern blot hybridization of RNA from these cells showed the presence of a 1.2-kb POMC and a 2.4-kb PDYN transcript. Radioimmunoassay and gel filtration chromatography characterization of the immunoreactive (IR) opioid peptides present in the culture media showed the presence of IR-$\beta$-endorphin and IR-dynorphins. The apparent molecular weight of IR-$\beta$-endorphin was that of authentic $\beta$-endorphin while the bulk of the IR-dynorphin had an apparent molecular weight of 8 kd. The secretion of both opioids could be increased by KCl-induced depolarization. Estrogen and glucocorticoids decreased, in a dose- and time-dependent manner, the secretion of $\beta$-endorphin from the Ishikawa cells while progesterone and dihydrotestosterone did not have a statistically significant effect. The antiprogestin-antiglucocorticoid RU486 acted as an agonist, *i.e.*, it diminished $\beta$-endorphin secretion possibly via glucocorticoid receptors. On the other hand, the secretion of dynorphins was not affected by any of the steroids tested while LHRH, the inducer of gonadotropins and anterior pituitary dynorphins secretion, provoked a time- and dose-dependent increase of their secretion without affecting that of $\beta$-endorphin. These data suggest that the regulation of endometrial opioids production is type-specific. Thus, it is possible that each type of endometrial opioid participates in different local homeostatic loops and exerts distinct paracrine effects.

## REFERENCES

1. DROUIN, J., M. CHAMBERLAND, J. CHARRON, L. JEANNOTTE & M. NEMER. 1985. Structure of the rat proopiomelanocortin (POMC) gene. FEBS Lett. **193:** 54–58.
2. LACAZE-MASMONTEIL, T., Y. DE KEYZER, J. P. LUTTON, A. KAHN & X. BERTAGNA. 1987. Characterization of proopiomelanocortin transcripts in human nonpituitary tissues. Proc. Natl. Acad. Sci. USA **84:** 7261–7265.
3. DOUGLAS, J., C. MCMURRAY, J. GARRETT, J. ADELMAN & L. CALAVETTA. 1989. Characterization of the rat prodynorphin gene. Mol. Endocrinol. **3:** 2970–2078.
4. HOSIKAWA, S., T. TAKAI, M. TOYOSATO, H. TAKAHASHI, M. NODA, H. KAKIDANI, T. KUDO, T. HIROSE, S. INAYAMA, H. HAYASHIDA, T. MIYATA & S. NUMA. 1983. Isolation and structural organization of human proenkephalin B gene. Nature **306:** 611–615.
5. SHARP, B., A. E. PEKARY, N. V. MEYER & J. M. HERSHMAN. 1980. Beta-endorphin in male rat reproductive organs. Biochem. Biophys. Res. Commun. **95:** 618–622.
6. MARGIORIS, A., A. LIOTTA, H. VAUDRY, C. BARDIN & D. KRIEGER. 1983. Characterization of immunoreactive proopiomelanocortin-related peptides in rat testis. Endocrinology **113:** 663–668.
7. LIM, A. T., S. LOLAIT, J. W. BARLOW, S. O. WAI, I. ZOIS, B. H. TOH & J. W. FUNDER. 1983. Immunoreactive $\beta$-endorphin in sheep ovary. Nature **303:** 709–711.
8. SHAHA, C., A. MARGIORIS, A. LIOTTA, D. KRIEGER & C. W. BARDIN. 1984. Demonstration of immunoreactive $\beta$-endorphin and $\gamma$3-melanocyte stimulating hormone-related peptides in the ovaries of neonatal, cycling and pregnant mice. Endocrinology **115:** 378–382.
9. WAHLSTROM, T., T. LAATIKAINEN, K. SALMINEN & J. LEPPALUOTO. 1985. Immunoreactive $\beta$-endorphin is demonstrable in the secretory but not in the proliferative endometrium. Life Sci. **36:** 987–991.
10. PETRAGLIA, F., F. FACCHINETTI, K. M'FUTA, M. RUSPA, J. J. BONAVERA, F. GARDIFLI

& A. R. GENAZANNI. 1986. Endogenous opioid peptides in uterine fluid. Fertil. Steril. **46:** 247–251.
11. LI, WI, C. L. CHEN, P. J. HANSEN & F. W. BAZER. 1987. Beta-endorphin in uterine secretions of pseudopregnant and ovariectomized ovarian steroid-treated gilts. Endocrinology **121:** 1111–1116.
12. DOUGLAS, J., B. COX, B. QUINN, O. CIVELLI & E. HERBERT. 1987. Expression of the prodynorphin gene in male and female mammalian reproductive tissues. Endocrinology **120:** 707–713.
13. MARGIORIS, A., G. KOUKOULIS, M. GRINO & G. CHROUSOS. 1989. In vitro perifused rat tests secrete $\beta$-endorphin and dynorphin: their effect on testosterone secretion. Biol. Reprod. **40:** 776–784.
14. HOLINKA, C., H. HATA, H. KURAMOTO & E. GURPIDE. 1986. Responses to estradiol in a human endometrial adenocarcinoma cell line (Ishikawa cells). J. Steroid Biochem. **24:** 85–91.
15. GRAVANIS, A. & E. GURPIDE. 1986. Effects of estradiol on DNA polymerase $\alpha$ activity in a human endometrial adenocarcinoma cell line (Ishikawa cells). J. Clin. Endocrinol. Metab. **63:** 356–359.
16. HOLINKA, C., H. HATA, A. GRAVANIS, H. KURAMOTO & E. GURPIDE. 1986. Effects of estradiol on proliferation of endometrial adenocarcinoma cells (Ishikawa line). J. Steroid Biochem. **25:** 781–788.
17. ODELL, W. D., R. HORTON, M. ROSENBLATT & M. R. PANDIAN. 1984. The Use of ACTH, Beta-Endorphin and Lipotropin Assays in the Diagnosis of Endocrine Disorders. Nichols Institute Reference Laboratories Manual. Nichols Institute. CA.
18. SUDA, T., T. TOZAWA, S. TACHIBANA, H. DEMURA, K. SHIZUME, A. SASAKI, T. MOURI & Y. MIURA. 1983. Multiple forms of immunoreactive dynorphin in human pituitary and pheochromocytoma. Life Sci. **32:** 865–870.
19. MARGIORIS, A., E. MARKOGIANNAKIS, A. MAKRIGIANNAKIS & A. GRAVANIS. 1992. PC12 rat pheochromocytoma cells synthesize dynorphin. Its secretion is modulated by nicotine and nerve growth factor. Endocrinology **131:** 703–709.
20. BRADFORD, M. 1976. A rapid and sensitive method for the quantitation of protein utilising the principle of protein-dye binding. Anal. Biochem. **72:** 248–254.
21. MANIATIS, T., E. F. FRITSCH & J. SAMBROOK. 1989. Molecular Cloning: a Laboratory Manual. Cold Spring Harbor Laboratory. Cold Spring Harbor, NY.
22. MAKRIGIANNAKIS, A., A. MARGIORIS, E. MARKOGIANNAKIS, C. STOURNARAS & A. GRAVANIS. 1992. Steroid hormones regulate the release of immunoreactive $\beta$-endorphin from the Ishikawa human endometrial cell line. J. Clin. Endocrinol. Metab. **75:** 584–589.
23. CHING-LING, C. & M. MADIGAN. 1987. Regulation of testicular proopiomelanocortin gene in testes. Endocrinology **121:** 590–596.
24. JIN, D., K. MUFFLY, W. OKULICZ & D. KIRPATRICK. 1988. Estrous cycle- and pregnancy-related differences in expression of the proenkephalin and proopiomelanocortin genes in the ovary and uterus. Endocrinology **122:** 1466–1471.
25. WARDLAW, S. L., P. WANG & A. FRANTZ. 1985. Regulation of $\beta$-endorphin and ACTH in brain by estradiol. Life Sci. **37:** 1941–1947.
26. WILCOX, O. & J. ROBERTS. 1985. Estrogen decreases rat hypothalamic proopiomelanocortin messenger ribonucleic acid levels. Endocrinology **117:** 2392–2396.
27. ROBERTS, J., M. BUDARF, J. BAXTER & E. HERBERT. 1979. Selective reduction of pro ACTH/endorphin proteins and mRNA from glucocorticoids in pituitary tumor cells. Biochemistry **18:** 4907–4911.
28. KNEPEL, W., M. SCHWANINGER & K. D. DOHLER. 1985. Corelease of dynorphin-like immunoreactivity, LH and FSH from rat adenohypophysis in vitro. Endocrinology **177:** 481–487.
29. SCHULZ, R., K. METZNER, T. DANDEKAR & C. GRAMSCH. 1986. Opiates induce long term increases in prodynorphin-derived peptide levels in the guinea-pig myenteric plexus. Naunyn-Schmiedebergs Arch. Pharmacol. **333:** 381–386.
30. BARALDI, M., G. GIARRE, M. SANTI, F. FACCHINETTI, F. PETRAGLIA & A. R. GENAZZANI. 1985. Pregnancy-related changes of opioid receptors identified in rat uterine membranes by $^3$H-naloxone binding. Peptides **6:** 971–975.

31. VERTES, M., S. PAMER & J. GARAI. 1986. On the mechanism of opioid-oestradiol interactions. J. Steroid Biochem. **24:** 235–239.
32. PATERSON, S. J., L. E. ROBSON & H. W. KOSTERLITZ. 1984. Opioid receptors. *In* The Peptides. S. Udenfriend & J. Meinhofer, Eds. 147–161. Academic Press. Orlando, FL.
33. ZAGON, IS & P. MCLAUGHLIN. 1987. Endogenous opioid systems regulate cell proliferation. Brain Res. **412:** 68–72.
34. TABIBZADEH, S. S., U. SANTANAM & P. B. SEHGAL. 1989. Cytokine-induced production of IFN-$\beta$2/IL-6 by freshly explanted human endometrial stromal cells: modulation by estradiol-17$\beta$. J. Immunol. **142:** 3134–3139.

# Hormonal Contraception

## Current Status and Future Perspectives

CHRISTIAN F. HOLINKA

*R. W. Johnson Pharmaceutical Research Institute
Raritan, New Jersey 08869*

## INTRODUCTION

The innovative concept of hormonal contraception was pioneered in the 1950s by Gregory Pincus.[1] This area has since been the focus of intensive research, and contraceptive products have undergone extensive post-marketing surveillance parallelled by few other products in pharmaceutical development. A major chemical breakthrough prior to the work of Pincus occurred in the late 1930s, when it was discovered that the addition of an ethinyl group to estradiol in the 17 position yielded an orally active potent estrogen, ethinyl estradiol, which became the most frequently used estrogen in oral contraceptives. Similarly, the quest for an orally active progestogen led to the synthesis, in the early 1950s, of the first 19-nortestosterone-derived specific progestogen with minimal residual androgenic activity.[2]

Oral contraceptives (OCs) were first approved in 1960 for unrestricted use in the U.S. Though initially accepted as highly effective, safe, easy to use and inexpensive, OCs fell into disrepute a few years after their introduction. There was an increasing awareness of a number of negative aspects, including thromboembolic events, adverse metabolic effects, gastrointestinal symptoms, and intermenstrual bleeding associated with high rates of noncompliance and discontinuation. Subsequent clinical efficacy and safety studies led to the gradual reduction of estrogen and progestogen to levels of about one fourth of the early formulations for estrogen and nearly one tenth for progestogens,[3] as illustrated in FIGURE 1. In addition, epidemiologic studies have identified risk factors which allow to exclude individuals at risk from contraceptive use. As a result, hormonal contraception is now considered to have a highly favorable benefit/risk profile.[3] Nevertheless, the need for new contraceptive methods, especially in the U.S., has been emphasized.[4,5] Ongoing research faces the challenge to further reduce metabolic side effects and improve cycle control. At the same time, the availability of new contraceptive methods will broaden the range of choices and thus is likely to enhance motivation and compliance in contraceptive users.

### *Contraception as a Means of Fertility Control*

The rate of increase in the world population is staggering. In the first century of our time, the global population was estimated to be less than 300 million. It took 1,500 years to double it. The first billion was reached in the early 19th century, the second billion by 1927. Thereafter, the global population doubled to four billion in less than 50 years. The fifth billion was reached in 1987, and the sixth is projected for 1997–1998.[6] During the present decade more than 90 million people will be added to this globe each year. FIGURE 2 illustrates the projected increases in the population of different regions of the world from 1990 to 2015. Ninety-four percent of the increase in the world population will be contributed by developing countries. Developed countries, including the former Soviet Union, are expected to grow by about 10% from 1.2 to 1.3 billion. In contrast, Subsaharan Africa is expected to double its population to one billion inhabitants.[7]

The number of contraceptive users in developing countries is expected to increase from 381 million in 1990 to 567 million in 2000.[7] To maintain the world population within the projected framework shown in FIGURE 2, substantial supplies

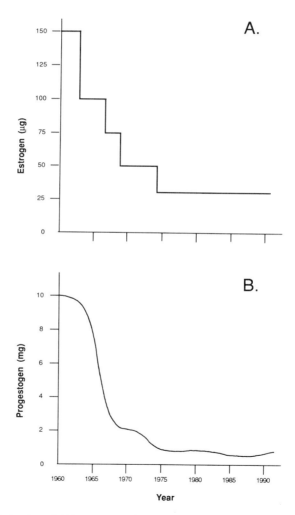

**FIGURE 1.** Reduction of **(A)** estrogen and **(B)** progestogen content in oral contraceptives since their first introduction for clinical use. (From Mishell.[3] Reprinted by permission from the *International Journal of Fertility*.)

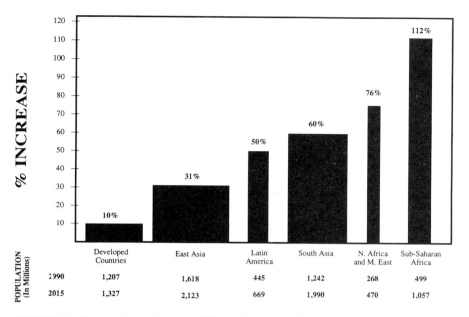

**FIGURE 2.** The world population in 1990 and its expected increase by 2015. The *width* of each bar is proportional to the population in 1990, the *height* is proportional to the percent increase in population by 2015. (Adapted from Segal.[7])

of contraceptives will have to be made available at affordable cost to individuals in developing countries. New and improved contraceptive methods can be expected to contribute substantially to the control of the world population.

## Contraception and Women's Health

Contraception has a substantial impact on women's health, broadly defined in the constitution of the World Health Organization as a state of complete physical, mental and social well-being. It has been emphasized that the health benefits of contraception should be regarded in the framework of this broad definition,[8] in which health is not merely the absense of disease. For many women, a state of mental and social well-being includes the option to balance the time and frequency of childbearing, if at all, against educational, career and other personal choices.

Although maternal and fetal deaths are relatively rare in developed countries, their rates are substantial in developing countries. According to a recent estimate by the World Health Organization, 500,000 women die each year from complications of pregnancy and childbirth, and an estimated 125,000 to 170,000 lose their lives from unsafe abortion practices.[9] Statistics for developing countries from the World Fertility Survey provide striking evidence in favor of control of childbearing patterns, as made possible by contraception. For example, short intervals between childbirth increase the risk of infant mortality by about 60%. Infants born to teenage mothers in developing countries have a 25% greater risk of death than

TABLE 1. Noncontraceptive Health Benefits of Oral Contraceptives[a]

| |
|---|
| Antiestrogenic |
| ↓ Endometrial cancer |
| ↓ Uterine fibroids |
| ↓ Menorrhagia |
| ↓ Benign breast disease |
| ↓ Anemia |
| Ovulation inhibition |
| ↓ Ovarian cancer |
| ↓ Functional ovarian cysts |
| ↓ Dysmenorrhea |
| Other |
| ↓ Ectopic pregnancy |
| ↓ Salpingitis |
| ↓ Bone loss |

[a] Modified from Mishell.[3]

those born to mothers who are 25 to 35 years old.[10] Among the developed countries, teenage pregnancy is highest in the United States,[11] with concomitant health risks to both mother and newborn, many of whom are unwanted. Those statistics and others provide a strong rationale for the use of contraception not merely for population control but for reasons related to health and the psychological and social well-being of both mother and child.

## *Noncontraceptive Health Benefits of Contraception*

The noncontraceptive health benefits of OCs are summarized in TABLE 1. Those benefits must be evaluated in light of the increased risk of cervical neoplasia when OCs are used for five years and longer.[14] Among OC users in the U.S., an estimated 1,600 per 100,000 individuals avoid hospitalization due to beneficial effects other than fertility control.[11] One of the most important noncontraceptive benefits of OCs is the reduction in ovarian cancer, the fourth leading cause of death in U.S. women, which causes more deaths than any other cancer of the female reproductive system.[12] Several studies have demonstrated a decrease in ovarian cancer risk in users vs nonusers.[13] The reduction in risk is about 40% in short-term OC users and is further increased to about 80% in long-term users.[14] A risk reduction is apparent even after a period of pill use as short as one-half year, and the risk reduction continues for at least 15 years after discontinuation of oral contraception.[11]

As with ovarian cancer, there is convincing evidence of a risk reduction in endometrial cancer in OC users, amounting to about 50% in women who use OCs for at least one year. The protection can last for 10 years or longer after discontinuation of OC.[14] Among the other noncontraceptive benefits of OCs are the protection against benign breast disease, uterine fibroids, pelvic inflammatory disease, and the prevention of ectopic pregnancies, the latter as a result of ovulation inhibition. It has been estimated that 139 cases of hospitalization for ectopic pregnancy are avoided annually per 100,000 OC users.[11]

## Contraceptive Hormones

Early combination OCs contained 150 μg estrogen and nearly 10 mg progestogen (FIG. 1), doses which now are considered extremely high. As a result, it became apparent only a few years after the introduction of OCs in the early 1960s that their use was associated with an increased incidence of thromboembolic events,[3] but it was not until 1970 that the estrogen component of OCs was identified as the major dose-dependent risk factor.[15] As a consequence, the estrogen doses have since been reduced to levels as low as 20 to 35 μg ethinyl estradiol. These doses, which represent the lowest consistent with contraceptive efficacy,[3] are now considered very safe for most healthy, nonsmoking women of reproductive age. In addition, new potent progestogens with few androgenic side effects[16,17] have recently become available in the U.S. Current research efforts are therefore focussed not so much on the development of new hormonally active steroids as on new methods of delivery, such as the vaginal ring, and implantable and injectable contraceptives.

## Methods of Hormonal Contraception

While male and female voluntary sterilization rank first among contraceptive methods worldwide, followed by the intrauterine device,[7] hormonal contraceptive methods are used by large numbers of individuals, especially in developed countries. Although the pill is the leading mode of hormonal contraception, a number of nonoral contraceptive methods are currently being developed or improved. Their advantage lies in the avoidance of first-pass effects on the liver. Moreover, implantable devices ensure maximal compliance—a critical issue, since it is known that a large number of pregnancies occur in oral contraceptive users due to missed pills. Among methods under current development are the vaginal ring, containing either estrogen and progestogen combined, or progestogen only.[18] As an alternative to the vaginal ring, vaginally applied pills containing estrogen-progestogen are being developed.[19] Implantable progestogen-only devices and progestogen-only injectables ensure a reliable form of contraception with excellent compliance, although unpredictable vaginal bleeding and spotting constitute a drawback. Current research efforts are also directed at biodegradable implants.[20] Progestogen-containing intrauterine devices are either available or under development, but their hormonal levels in serum are generally not high enough to act systemically on the hypothalamus and pituitary. Like nonhormonal IUDs, they act by inducing a local foreign body reaction in the endometrium,[19] resulting in phagocytosis of sperm and interference with immunologic tolerance that leads to impaired implantation. In addition, the progestogen acts directly on the endometrium to produce an exhausted secretory phase unfavorable to implantation.[22] Antiprogestogens are also being developed as contragestational agents.[23,24] Finally, contraceptive research is focused on immunologic interference with the hypothalamic-pituitary-gonadal axis both in females and males, an area of inquiry that may spawn yet unforeseen methods of molecular modulation of the mechanisms of sperm-ovum interactions with resultant inhibition of implantation.[25]

## REFERENCES

1. PINCUS, G., J. ROCK, C. R. GARCIA, E. RICE-WRAY, M. PANIAGUA, I. RODRIGUEZ &

R. PEDRAS. 1958. Fertility control with oral medication. Am. J. Obstet. Gynecol. **75:** 1333–1346.
2. SPEROFF, L., R. H. GLASS & N. G. KASE. 1989. Steroid contraception. *In* Clinical Gynecologic Endocrinology. 461–498. Williams & Wilkins. Baltimore.
3. MISHELL, D. R. 1992. Oral contraception: past, present, and future perspectives. Int. J. Fertil. **37**(Suppl. 1): 7–18.
4. TRUSSELL, J. & K. KOST. 1987. Contraceptive failure in the United States: a critical review of the literature. Stud. Fam. Plann. **18:** 237–283.
5. MASTROIANNI, L., P. J. DONALDSON & T. T. KANE. 1990. Development of contraceptives—obstacles and opportunities. N. Engl. J. Med. **322:** 482–484.
6. DICZFALUSY, E. 1992. Contraceptive prevalence, reproductive health, and international morality. Am. J. Obstet Gynecol. **166:** 1037–1043.
7. SEGAL, S. J. 1993. Trends in population and contraception. Ann. Med. **25:** 51–56.
8. FATHALLA, M. F. 1993. Contraception and women's health. Br. Med. Bull. **49:** 245–251.
9. World Health Organization. Division of Family Health, 1990. Abortion: a tabulation of available data on the frequency and mortality of unsafe abortion. WHO/MCH/90.14. Geneva: World Health Organization.
10. HOBCRAFT, J. 1987. Does family planning save children's lives? A background paper to: International Conference on Better Health for Women and Children Through Family Planning, Nairobi, Kenya, October 5–9. The Population Council. New York.
11. DERMAN, R. J. 1992. An overview of the noncontraceptive benefits and risks of oral contraception. Int. J. Fertil. **37**(Suppl. 1): 19–26.
12. American Cancer Society. 1992. Cancer Facts and Figures.
13. MISHELL, D. R. 1989. Contraception. N. Engl. J. Med. **320:** 777–787.
14. MISHELL, D. R. 1990. Endometrial and ovarian cancer in OCs. J. Reprod. Med. **35**(Suppl. 4): 469–481.
15. INMAN, W. H. W., M. P. VESSEY, B. WESTERHOLM *et al.* 1970. Thromboembolic disease and the steroidal content of oral contraceptives: a report to the Committee on Safety of Drugs. Br. Med. J. **2:** 203–209.
16. RUNNEBAUM, B. & T. RABE. 1987. New progestogens in oral contraceptives. Am. J. Obstet. Gynecol. **157:** 1059–1063.
17. REBAR, R. W. & K. ZESERSON. 1991. Characteristics of the new progestogens in combination oral contraceptives. Contraception **44:** 1–10.
18. PASQUALE, S. A. 1992. Future directions in contraception. Curr. Opin. Obstet. Gynecol. **4:** 531–535.
19. COUTINO, E. M. 1988. Vaginal pills: systemic contraception induced by vaginal administration of contraceptive pills. *In* Contraception Research for Today and the Nineties. G. P. Talwar, Ed. 67–79. Springer-Verlag. New York.
20. CULLINS, V. E. 1992. Injectable and implantable contraceptives. Curr. Opin. Obstet. Gynecol. **4:** 536–543.
21. MOYER, D. L. & D. R. MISHELL. 1971. Reactions of human endometrium to the intrauterine foreign body. II. Long-term effects on the endometrial histology and cytology. Am. J. Obstet. Gynecol. **111:** 66–80.
22. GINSBURG, K. A. & K. S. MOGHISSI. 1988. Alternate delivery systems for contraceptive progestogens. Fertil. Steril. **49**(Suppl.): 16–30.
23. BAULIEU, E-E. 1988. Antiprogestin Ru 486: a contragestive agent. *In* Contraception Research for Today and the Nineties. G. P. Talwar, Ed. 49–66. Springer-Verlag. New York.
24. SPITZ, I. M. & C. W. BARDIN. 1993. Clinical applications of the antiprogestin RU 486. Endocrinologist **3:** 58–66.
25. LINCOLN, D. W. 1993. Contraception for the year 2020. Br. Med. J. **49:** 222–236.

# Morphological Aspects of Human Endometrium during Hormone Replacement Therapy

LUIGI DE CECCO,[a] DANIELA GERBALDO,
PAOLO CRISTOFORONI, ANTONELLA FERRAIOLO,
VALENTINO REMORGIDA, PATRIZIA BARACCHINI,[b]
AND EZIO FULCHERI[b]

*Department of Obstetrics and Gynecology*
*and*
[b]*Institute of Pathological Anatomy and Histology*
*University of Genoa*
*16132 Genoa, Italy*

## INTRODUCTION

The multiple benefits of hormonal replacement therapy (HRT) in postmenopausal women are well known,[1-3] but it is recognized that the use of cyclic progestogen is necessary to prevent estrogen-related endometrial hyperplasia and, in the long term, the development of adenocarcinoma.[4,5] The follow-up and, in more detail, the endometrial sampling of women on HRT is an important and controversial issue. Many physicians sample the endometrium before initiating the treatment, although genital atrophy and cervical stenosis in postmenopausal women may sometimes preclude this approach. Unanimity on follow-up schedule for HRT patients is far from being reached. Most authors consider irregular bleeding as the uterine symptom requiring endometrial evaluation in the postmenopausal woman receiving combined treatments.[6,7] Quite often, however, blind endometrial biopsies may not be technically adequate, and do not allow the pathologist to express a definitive diagnosis.[8,9] Hysteroscopy may help identify pathologic findings missed by endometrial biopsy and/or reassure that a negative biopsy is the result of an atrophic mucosa.[10] More recently, an increasing amount of data has been reported about HRT-induced endometrial changes, but the multiple variables involved (different hormonal formulations, timing and method of biopsy, length of follow-up, etc.) make very difficult the critical evaluation of endometrial response in this group of patients.[11-14]

The aim of this study was to evaluate the endometrial response to different formulations of HRT, focusing on the morphological aspects by employing hysteroscopy and direct-vision biopsy to properly define the histological patterns.

---

[a] Address correspondence to: Prof. Luigi de Cecco, Istituto di Ginecologia e Ostetricia, Padiglione 1, Ospedale San Martino, Viale Benedetto XV, 10 16132 Genova, Italy.

Meaningful data on endometrial response may lead to a proper definition of minimal follow-up for this growing group of patients.

## MATERIAL AND METHODS

This retrospective study is based on data collected from April 1987 to December 1992 at the Department of Obstetrics and Gynecology of the University of Genoa and taken from protocols of a climacteric surveillance project under ethical approval. Seventy-seven postmenopausal women, without risk factors for breast and endometrial cancer, were examined. None had experienced any spontaneous menstrual bleeding within the previous six months or recieved any treatment during the three months preceding the study. All women were complaining of climacteric symptoms.

Clinical data regarding the subjects under investigation are as follows: mean age 49.1 years (range, 44 to 58), average years since last menstruation 1.9 (range, 1 to 5), body mass index (BMI) $< 0.25$.

All patients had a pretreatment hysteroscopy with direct biopsy for morphological and histological evaluation of the endometrium and then were randomly divided into five groups.

Thirty-eight women were randomized to cyclic estrogen-administration treatments: 16 (group A) had oral conjugated equine estrogens 0.625 mg daily, while 22 women (group B) had transdermal patches (TTS) delivering 0.05 mg of $17\beta$-estradiol per day. Both treatments, lasting six months, 21 days a cycle, were balanced by adding medroxyprogesterone acetate (MPA) 10 mg/day from day 10 to day 21 of estrogen administration.

Thirty-nine patients were randomized to the therapeutic protocols including continuous estrogen administration. All patients had $E_2$-TTS 50 $\mu$g patches applied continuously, but three different progestogens were used in balancing estrogens: 12 women (group C) received MPA 10 mg/day for 14 days every 4 weeks; 15 women (group D) had transdermic nor-ethisterone acetate (NETA) 0.25 mg added to the last 14 $E_2$ patches each cycle; 12 patients (group E) balanced the continuous supply of estrogen with a vaginal cream delivering 100 mg/day of micronized progesterone (VP).

After 6 months of therapy, all patients underwent hysteroscopic and histological evaluation (at day 8 to 12 of progestogen's addiction).

Eighty-seven postmenopausal patients, observed with hysteroscopy and histology after removal of asymptomatic endocervical polyps, represented the study control group.

Hysteroscopy was standardized by using the Chorionscope (Karl Storz GmbH, Tattlingen, Germany) with Hopkins telescope for direct-vision biopsy (forward-oblique telescope: diameter 3 mm; chorionscope sheath: $3.7 \times 5$ mm with instrument channel 5 Fr) which is easily used in these patients, frequently showing stenosis or substenosis of the cervical canal.

Hysteroscopically, the following parameters were considered: pattern of endometrial surface, endometrial thickness and presence of associated lesions such as submucous leiomyomas.[10,15]

Direct biopsies were performed randomly in flat endometrium (fundus), whereas target biopsies were taken in hyperplastic or hypervascular areas or in presence of glandular openings. Serial sections of 10% formalin buffered-fixed and paraffin-embedded material were stained with hematoxylin and eosin and PAS methods.

All specimens were blindly examined by two observers and the endometrium conventionally classified as insufficient tissue for diagnosis, atrophic, proliferative, secretive (the latter two either within a functional or a dysfunctional context) and hyperplastic. Hyperplasia was subclassified into simplex (SH), complex (CH) and atypical (AH).[16-19]

## RESULTS

We performed pre-recruitment hysteroscopic examination of all women included in the study protocols. Hysteroscopy was performed again after six months of therapy, and direct biopsies were taken on both occasions. We noticed some peculiar hysteroscopical patterns related to the morphological response of postmenopausal endometrium following hormone replacement therapy.

Multifocality seemed to be the most typical pattern observed at hysteroscopy, and this finding was confirmed by histology. Histologically, it may be described as a diffuse atrophic endometrium with focal, minimal proliferative, secretory, as well as hyperplastic areas. The proliferative pattern observed at hysteroscopy was morphologically similar to that observed in early follicular phase (1–2 mm of thickness). However, the secretive pattern was quite different from the one present in physiologic cycles. Hysteroscopically, the endometrium appears thinner than the corresponding functional endometrium and often irregular; histologically it is characterized by short glands showing a secretory pattern within an oedematous and vascularized stroma.

At hysteroscopy, the observed hyperplastic patterns, always with a low risk appearance, were focal, irregularly distributed, and not restricted to the uterine fundus; sometimes they could be identified as prominent glands within an atrophic context. No widespread or high risk hyperplastic pattern was found. Histologically the hyperplastic patterns, usually similar to those observed during the functional cycles, often presented stromal abnormalities resembling those found in dysfunctional endometria.

TABLE 1 shows the histological reports of the 77 women divided into the five studied groups. TABLE 2 gives the histology of the 87 controls. Statistical analysis did not show any significant difference between basal endometrial status of the patients and control group. The histological reports of the target biopsies obtained after six months of HRT are presented in TABLE 3. Overall, 53.2% of the biopsies showed an atrophic endometrium, while 16.9% were secretive.

As a matter of fact, a large amount (38%) of the 6-month biopsies were diagnosed as "mixed endometrium," being constituted by various areas of functional endometrium (both proliferative and secretive) within a diffuse atrophic context.

TABLE 1. Hormone Replacement Therapy: Basal Histologic Report

| Endometrium | Group | | | | | Total |
| --- | --- | --- | --- | --- | --- | --- |
| | A | B | C | D | E | |
| Atrophic | 13 (81.2%) | 18 (81.8%) | 9 (75.0%) | 12 (80.0%) | 10 (83.3%) | 62 (80.5%) |
| Proliferative | 2 (12.5%) | 3 (13.6%) | 3 (25.0%) | 2 (13.3%) | 2 (16.7%) | 12 (15.6%) |
| Hyperplastic | 1 (6.2%) | 1 (4.5%) | 0 | 1 (6.7%) | 0 | 3 (3.9%) |
| Secretive | 0 | 0 | 0 | 0 | 0 | 0 |
| Total | 16 | 22 | 12 | 15 | 12 | 77 (100.0%) |

TABLE 2. Control Group. Histologic Report

| Endometrium | | |
|---|---|---|
| Atrophic | 72 | (82.8%) |
| Proliferative | 11 | (12.6%) |
| Hyperplastic | 4 | (4.6%) |
| Secretive | 0 | (0%) |
| Total | 87 | (100%) |

However, we classified these findings on the basis of their prevalent histological pattern. Thus, an atrophic endometrium with mild signs of proliferation was described as dysfunctional mixed endometrium with proliferative aspects and reported here as proliferative.

No complex or atypical hyperplasia was found in these patients. Also, we never received a pathologist's report accounting for insufficient material for diagnosis: this shows that a good endometrial specimen including stroma and glands without distortion can always be accomplished on the basis of direct vision biopsy.

Statistical analysis on the data was performed, first looking at the overall results of HRT as compared to controls. The occurrence of atrophic endometrium was consistently lower ($p < 0.001$, chi square 16.6) in the treated patients as compared to those untreated. Significant differences, even if small, were noticed for SH endometrium, hyperplasia being more common within the treated patients ($p < 0.05$). No difference was found regarding the occurrence of proliferative endometrium, or when the "risky" endometria (proliferative plus SH) were considered together. We did not analyze the frequency of secretive endometrium, because it was never found within the control group.

A second step was to consider the differences between cyclic and continuous estrogen treatments. We noticed a significant difference between cyclic and continuous protocols, 18 out of 38 (47.4%) versus 23 out of 39 (59.0%), respectively, in inducing atrophic endometrium ($p < 0.01$). No difference was found regarding the occurrence of proliferative as well as hyperplastic endometrium within the various study groups, while the finding of secretive endometrium was more common in the cyclic protocols ($p < 0.01$).

## DISCUSSION

Progestins have been evaluated for more than twenty years as inhibitors of the expected estrogen-related hyperplasia in postmenopausal patients on estrogen

TABLE 3. Hormone Replacement Therapy: Endometrial Histology after 6 Months of Therapy

| Endometrium | Group | | | | | Total |
|---|---|---|---|---|---|---|
| | A | B | C | D | E | |
| Atrophic | 7 (43.7%) | 11 (50.0%) | 8 (66.6%) | 10 (66.6%) | 5 (41.7%) | 41 (53.2%) |
| Proliferative | 1 (6.2%) | 4 (18.2%) | 2 (16.7%) | 3 (20.0%) | 1 (8.3%) | 11 (14.3%) |
| Hyperplastic | 3 (18.7%) | 4 (18.2%) | 1 (8.3%) | 2 (13.3%) | 2 (16.6%) | 12 (15.6%) |
| Secretive | 4 (25.0%) | 4 (18.2%) | 1 (8.3%) | 1 (6.7%) | 3 (25.0%) | 13 (16.9%) |
| Total | 16 | 22 | 12 | 15 | 12 | 77 (100.0%) |

replacement therapy (ERT). They have been demonstrated in controlled clinical studies to be effective in the prevention of endometrial hyperplasia associated with the administration of continuous as well as cyclic estrogen therapy.[5,20]

Whitehead and co-workers[21] have provided a biochemical explanation for the effects of progestogens on the estrogen-primed endometrium. They showed a progestin-induced decrease in DNA synthesis and mitotic activity of endometrial samples taken from estrogen-treated postmenopausal women. Six days of progestogen administration were sufficient to increase up to a hyperphysiologic level the activity of estradiol and isocitric dehydrogenase, previously lowered by the estrogen therapy. The knowledge of the biochemical mechanisms involved in the secretory histological changes are of importance in the choice of the appropriate time for biopsying. We performed all the hysteroscopic-guided biopsies between day 8 and day 12 of progestogen administration.

A body of biochemical and morphological data supports the difference in endometrial response observed in patients undergoing hormone replacement therapy.

In greater detail, occurrence of hyperplastic patterns were variously reported by different authors. Varma et al. studied 398 menopausal women receiving HRT. They did not record hyperplasia in patients receiving a progestogen for more than 10 days.[12] Gelflan and Ferenczy reported 4% of simplex hyperplasia occurred in women receiving progestin-balanced estrogen administrations.[14] Whitehead et al. reported 3–4% of endometrial hyperplasia occurred in patients receiving estrogen formulations with the addition of a progestogen for 7 days per month.[22] More recently, Fraser, Whitehead and co-authors reported on 197 endometrial samples

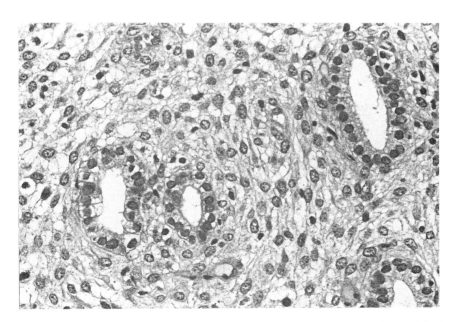

**FIGURE 1.** Atrophic endometrium with minimal secretive pattern of the glands (HE, 250×).

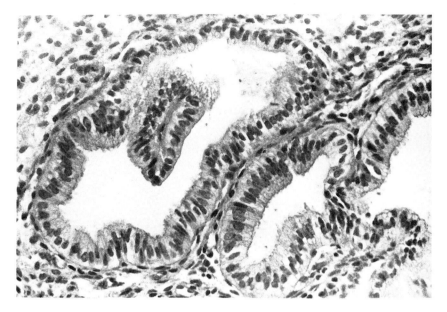

**FIGURE 2.** Predominant secretive pattern with focal signs of simple hyperplasia (HE, 250×).

from patients who had been on combined therapy for 6 months to 7 years. Only four cases showed histological abnormalities, all being atypical hyperplasia.[23]

Our findings sensibly differ from most reports. We recorded an occurrence of simplex hyperplasia after 6 months of HRT as high as 15.5%. Various considerations may explain this observed discordance. First, most of the published case series refer to samples obtained by blind endometrial biopsy.[24] We previously stressed the common hysteroscopic finding of multifocality, with minimal functional areas within a diffuse atrophic endometrium. Obviously, the direct-vision biopsies were focalized on these areas, easily missed by blind biopsy. Moreover, with target biopsy, tissue sampling is always sufficient for diagnosis, thus eliminating the "insufficient tissue for diagnosis" frequently found in the other studies (more than 24% in the study by Archer *et al.*, up to 50% reported by Varma *et al.*, whereas other investigators included inadequate samples in the "normal endometrium" group).[9,12] As a matter of fact, a study published by Hawthorn *et al.* in 1991 used hysteroscopy-directed biopsies to evaluate endometrial status in some of the 15 women on continuous combined HRT;[25] they did not record endometrial abnormalities. However, the biopsies were performed on women with a minimum duration of therapy of 3 years (mean 3.9 years): our findings refer to endometrial aspect after the first 6 months of therapy, and many authors reported a reversion of hyperplasia to atrophic endometrium with the prosecution of combined HRT. Also, the histologic report of dysfunctional atrophic endometrium with mild signs of hyperplasia has been considered as hyperplasia in this study. This may partially explain the lack of concordance with the occurrence of proliferative endometrium, significantly lower in our study than in other reports.[24]

As overall data, mixed endometrial patterns were predominant at the histologic observation; pure proliferative or secretive endometria were rarely found (FIG. 1). When pure functional endometria were recorded, they constantly presented a discordant stroma, showing a typical pattern of dysfunctionality. The observed patterns of simplex hyperplasia can be included in the same histological context.

It may be of interest to remark that in our experience a secretive endometrial pattern should not be considered as a target for HRT patients. The observed pure secretive patterns were quite scarce, cyclic CEE plus MPA treatment being the most effective in inducing them. In the large majority of cases, secretive patterns were included in a context of mixed endometrium, and sometimes areas of hyperplasia were found included within a predominantly secretive endometrial pattern (FIG. 2).

In conclusion, we did not record many differences in endometrial morphology as a consequence of different hormonal formulations. If the continuous protocols were more effective than the cyclic one in obtaining atrophic endometria after six months of therapy and cyclic regimens showed a stronger secretory impact, the complex of histological observations previously reported must be remembered.

## REFERENCES

1. MILLER-BASS, K. & E. ADASHI. Current status and future prospects of transdermal estrogen replacement therapy. 1990. Fertil. Steril. **53:** 961–974.
2. HARLAP, S. 1992. The benefits and risks of hormone replacement therapy: an epidemiologic overview. Am. J. Obstet. Gynecol. **166:** 1986–1992.
3. HENDERSON, B. E., A. PAGANINI-HILL & R. K. ROSS. 1988. Estrogen replacement therapy and protection from acute myocardial infarction. Am. J. Obstet. Gynecol. **159:** 312–317.
4. STUDD, J. W. W. & M. H. THOM. 1981. Oestrogen and endometrial cancer. *In* Progress in Obstetrics and Gynaecology. J. W. W. Studd, Ed. Vol. 1: 182–198. Churchill-Livingstone. Edinburgh.
5. GAMBRELL, R. D., C. A. BAGNELL & R. B. GREENBLATT. 1983. Role of estrogens and progesterone in the etiology and the prevention of the endometrial cancer: review. Am. J. Obstet. Gynecol. **146:** 696–707.
6. CHAMBERS, J. T. & S. K. CHAMBERS. 1992. Endometrial sampling: When? Where? Why? With what? Clin. Obstet. Gynecol. **35:** 28–39.
7. WHITEHEAD, M. I., T. C. HILLARD & D. CROOK. The role and use of progestogens. Obstet. Gynecol. **75**(Suppl. 4): 15–17.
8. KOVACS, G. T. & H. G. BURGER. 1988. Endometrial sampling for women on perimenopausal hormone replacement therapy. Maturitas **10:** 259–262.
9. ARCHER, D. F., K. MCINTYRE-SELTMAN, W. W. WILBORN, E. A. DOWLING, F. CONE, G. W. CREASY & M. E. KAFRISSEN. 1991. Endometrial morphology in asymptomatic postmenopausal women. Am. J. Obstet. Gynecol. **165:** 317–322.
10. DE CECCO, L., D. GERBALDO, E. FULCHERI, A. FERRAIOLO, P. BARACCINI, L. BERNARDINI & G. PESCETTO. 1992. Endometrial response in sequential cyclic therapy assessed with associated hysteroscopy and histology. Maturitas **15:** 199–208.
11. PATERSON, M. E. L, J. WADE-EVANS, D. W. STURDEE *et al.* 1989. Endometrial disease after treatment with estrogens and progestogens in the climacteric. Br. Med. J. **1:** 822–827.
12. VARMA, T. R. 1985. Effect of long-term therapy with estrogen and progesterone on the endometrium of postmenopausal women. Acta Obstet. Gynecol. Scand. **64:** 41–48.
13. WHITEHEAD, M. I., P. T. TOWNSEND, J. PRISE-DAVIES, T. A. RYDER, G. LANE, N. C. SIDDLE & R. J. KING. 1982. Effects of various types and dosages of progestogens on postmenopausal endometrium. J. Reprod. Med. **27:** 539–548.
14. GELFAND, M. M. & A. FERENCZY. 1989. A prospective 1-year study of estrogen and

progestin in postmenopausal women: effects on endometrium. Obstet. Gynecol. **74:** 398–402.
15. HAMOU, J. 1991. Hysteroscopy and Mycrohysteroscopy. A Text and Atlas. Appleton & Lange. San Mateo, CA.
16. DALLENBACH-HELLWEG, G. & H. POULSEN. 1985. Atlas of Endometrial Histopathology. Munksgaard Ed. Copenhagen.
17. HENDRICKSON, M. R. & R. L. KEMPSON. 1987. Endometrial hyperplasia, metaplasia and carcinoma. *In* Obstetrical and Gynaecological Pathology. H. Fox, Ed. 354–365. Churchill-Livingstone. London.
18. MORE, I. A. 1987. The normal human endometrium. *In* Obstetrical and Gynaecological Pathology. H. Fox, Ed. 302–315. Churchill-Livingstone. London.
19. BUCKLEY, C. H. & H. FOX. 1989. Biopsy Pathology of the Endometrium. Chapman and Hall Medical. London.
20. DALLENBACH-HELLWEG, G. 1981. Iatrogenic changes of the endometrium. *In* Histopathology of the Endometrium. G. Dallenbach-Hellweg, Ed. 216–256. Springer-Verlag. Berlin.
21. WHITEHEAD, M. I., P. T. TOWNSEND, J. PRISE-DAVIES, T. A. RYDER, G. LANE, N. C. SIDDLE & R. J. KING. 1982. Actions of progestins on the morphology and biochemistry of the endometrium of postmenopausal women receiving low dose therapy. Am. J. Obstet. Gynecol. **142:** 791–795.
22. WHITEHEAD, M. I., R. J. B. KING, J. McQUEEN *et al.* 1979. Endometrial histology and biochemistry in climacteric women during estrogen and estrogen-progestogen therapy. J. R. Soc. Med. **72:** 322–328.
23. FRASER, D., M. I. WHITEHEAD, J. ENDACOTT, J. MORTON & T. A. RYDER & J. PRYSE-DAVIES. 1989. Are fixed-dose oestrogen/progestogen combinations ideal for all HRT users? Br. J. Obstet. Gynaecol. **96:** 776–782.
24. CREASY, G. W., M. E. KAFRISSEN & D. UPMALIS. 1992. Review of the endometrial effects of estrogens and progestins. Obstet. Gynecol. Surv. **47:** 654–678.
25. HAWTHORN, R. J., K. SPOWART, D. WALSH & D. M. HART. 1991. The endometrial status of women on long-term continuous combined hormone replacement therapy. Br. J. Obstet. Gynaecol. **98:** 939–942.

# Aspects of Hormone Replacement Therapy

CHRISTIAN F. HOLINKA

*R. W. Johnson Pharmaceutical Research Institute*
*Raritan, New Jersey 08869*

Hormone replacement therapy (HRT) occupies a unique place in preventive medicine. Its effectiveness has been widely demonstrated and its benefits translate into large numbers of saved lives and increased levels of well-being. It is well established that the decline in circulating estrogen at menopause and its virtual absence thereafter are associated with thermoregulatory disturbances, genital atrophy and bone loss. In addition, estrogen deficiency correlates with a substantial increase in cardiovascular disease (CVD). Since estrogen replacement therapy (ERT) prevents or reduces those deficits, it has been proposed that ERT should be considered for all women.[1] However, unopposed estrogen therapy increases the risk of endometrial cancer, an adverse event that is prevented by adjunctive progestogen treatment. Yet there is concern that adjunctive progestogen may attenuate the beneficial effects of estrogen.[2] The benefit of protection against endometrial cancer, a disease which numerically affects relatively few individuals and has a relatively good prognosis, must therefore be balanced against the risk of attenuating the protective effect of estrogen against heart disease, which affects large numbers of individuals and is the leading cause of death in postmenopausal women. While the efficacy of adjunctive progestogen to protect against endometrial cancer remains undisputed, it is essential that the lowest effective dose be given to minimize the potential attenuation of the beneficial effects of estrogen. The following presents a short review of the rationale for ERT and discusses factors relevant to the identification in clinical trials of the lowest adjunctive progestogen dose to protect against endometrial cancer.

## *Vasomotor Symptoms*

Vasomotor symptoms (hot flushes, hot flashes) occur in nearly 85% of women as a result of declining estrogen levels and persist in most individuals for at least one year. An estimated 25% of women receive medical care because of severe symptomatology. When untreated, the symptoms subside with time, and most women do not require ERT for longer than 3 to 5 years to treat vasomotor symptoms, but symptoms may continue beyond that period in some individuals.[3] Clinical trials to establish statistically significant treatment effects should be placebo-controlled and double-blind to dissect the placebo contribution to the amelioration of vasomotor symptoms from the drug effect. Typical response patterns to ERT are illustrated in FIGURE 1. Though variable, the maximum response to treatment, evaluated by the subjective experience of hot flushes, occurs after about four weeks.[4] The symptoms recur swiftly after discontinuation of treatment and may rise above pretreatment levels. As shown in FIGURE 1, a double-blind crossover from placebo to treatment three months after initiation of estrogen therapy

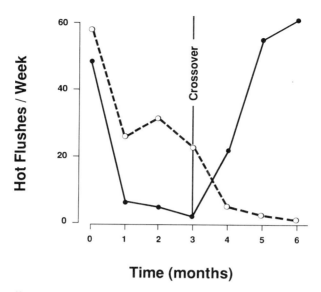

**FIGURE 1.** Effect of estrogen therapy on postmenopausal vasomotor symptoms. The frequency of hot flushes decreased swiftly to levels significantly below placebo in this double-blind study. The symptoms returned to frequencies above those at baseline when placebo was substituted for active treatment three months after start of therapy, while the placebo group became virtually symptom-free after crossover to active treatment. (From Coope et al.[5] Reprinted by permission from the *British Medical Journal*.)

rapidly diminished the incidence of hot flushes in the placebo group, whereas the symptoms rose above baseline when the actively treated group received placebo.[5]

### Genital Atrophy

Vaginal epithelial cells are exquisitely sensitive to hormonal changes. In the absence of inflammation and progestogens, the vaginal epithelium becomes essentially an index of estrogenic activity.[6] Specifically, estrogen promotes cellular growth and maturation, as evidenced in a shift in the desquamated cell population from the immature (parabasal) to the mature (superficial) type. Accordingly, the percentage of superficial cells, and the ratio of superficial/parabasal cells, increase from the early to the late follicular phase of the menstrual cycle. At the postmenopausal state of estrogen deficiency, mostly parabasal cells are present. After ERT, both the percentage of superficial cells and the ratio superficial/parabasal cells increase significantly, as shown in FIGURE 2.[7] The shift from immature to mature cells (the maturation index) is evaluated in clinial trials as the endpoint of estrogen efficacy in the treatment of genital atrophy.

### Psychological Symptoms and Quality of Life

Studies designed to evaluate specific effects of ERT on psychological symptoms need to dissect primary effects of estrogen on those symptoms from secondary effects that are a consequence of favorable physiologic changes, such as reductions in vasomotor symptoms and insomnia. Although it was initially assumed that psychological symptoms associated with the menopause were not effectively treated by hormones,[8] it now appears that ERT may improve psychological symptoms, and possibly memory, independent of its beneficial physiologic effects.[9,10] A study in asymptomatic postmenopausal women, *i.e.*, psychologically well adjusted individuals without subjective complaints of hot flushes, found that estrogen im-

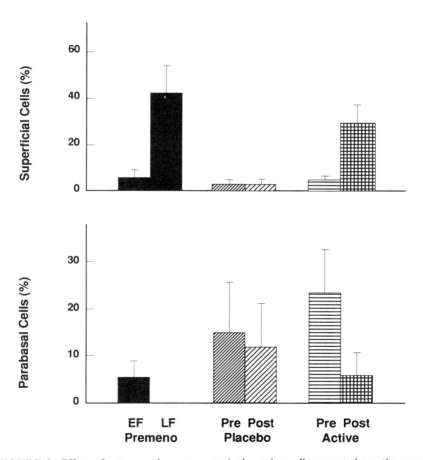

**FIGURE 2.** Effect of estrogen therapy on vaginal cytology. Represented are the mean percentages of immature (parabasal) and mature (superficial) desquamated epithelial cells after three weeks of transdermal ERT at levels resulting in circulating 17$\beta$-estradiol concentrations of about 70 pg/mL. Mature cells, expressed as percentage of total cells, were virtually absent at pretreatment and in the placebo group, but increased significantly in response to ERT, with a corresponding decrease in immature (parabasal) cells. Premenopausal data, given for comparison, show a significant rise in mature cells from the early to the late follicular phase in response to rising estrogen levels. (From Laufer *et al.*[7] Reprinted by permission from the *American Journal of Obstetrics and Gynecology*.)

proved psychological functions and therefore the overall quality of life.[11] Another study also concluded that ERT effectively improved the quality of life.[12]

## Prevention and Treatment of Osteoporosis

Estrogen replacement therapy is the treatment of choice for the prevention of postmenopausal osteoporosis,[13] a disorder which affects between 15 and 20 million individuals in the U.S. and 75 million in Europe, Japan and the U.S. combined.[14] Osteoporosis, therefore, has major consequences regarding the well-being of affected individuals and health care costs. It causes more than 1.3 million fractures annually in the U.S. alone, and its impact on public health can be expected to increase as the world population is aging.[13] The total annual health care cost for fractures in the U.S. is about 6 billion dollars.[15]

Estrogen replacement therapy is highly effective in the prevention of bone loss, as evidenced by the maintenance of bone mineral density (BMD), and fracture rate reduction in postmenopausal women receiving ERT.[14,16] Epidemiologic data indicate a reduction of Colles' fractures by about 50%, and of vertebral fractures up to 90% when ERT is started perimenopausally and is given for at least five years.[14]

While early ERT is advisable, bone loss can be prevented even when treatment is started at a later period, as illustrated in FIGURE 3. In this placebo-controlled, double-blind, 10-year follow-up study, ERT was given to ovariectomized individuals shortly following ovariectomy, or was started three years or six years after ovariectomy. All three groups showed significantly greater metacarpal bone mineral density (BMD) compared to untreated individuals, but the maximal effect was observed when treatment was started early.[17] Several recent reports also suggest that ERT is effective not only in the prevention but in the treatment of osteoporosis. Both oral[18,19] and transdermal[20] administration of estrogen increased bone mass significantly. The addition of a progestogen does not appear to impair the positive effects of estrogen and there is evidence that some progestogens may be bone active by themselves,[21] or add to the effects of estrogen,[22] possibly also in premenopausal women during the menstrual cycle.[23] When administered in large doses in the absence of estrogen, progestogen (10 mg/day norethindrone) was found to increase BMD.[24] Progestogen-only treatment of women at early menopause resulted in less rapid decreases in spinal BMD when compared to placebo,[25] but did not prevent bone loss in any way comparable to ERT.

## ERT and Protection against Cardiovascular Disease

Cardiovascular disease is the major cause of death in postmenopausal women (FIG. 4), and postmenopausal estrogen depletion clearly correlates with the rise in CVD (FIG. 5). Since 1970, over 30 epidemiologic studies have evaluated the incidence of CVD in relation to noncontraceptive estrogen use.[26,27] Most of those studies found a significant decrease in the risk for CVD in users when compared to non-users. Several metaanalyses have estimated the relative risk in estrogen users to be between 0.55 and 0.65.[26–28] Protection against mortality and morbidity from heart disease has major implications for public health, since CVD is the leading cause of death in postmenopausal women, ahead of cancer and other diseases. In the U.S., the mortality from heart disease of women 55 years or older was 488,000 in 1990.[29] A 50-year-old white woman has an estimated 46% life time probability of developing heart disease and a 31% probability of dying from it,[26]

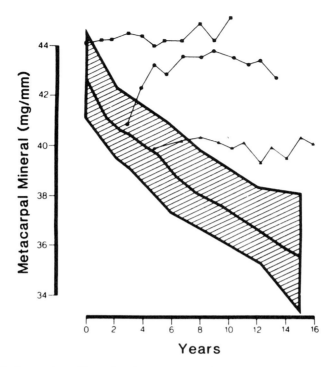

**FIGURE 3.** Prevention of bone loss by estrogen replacement therapy. Women received estrogen shortly after ovariectomy, or three or six years after ovariectomy and were followed up for ten years. Estrogen replacement prevented bone loss in all three groups, but was most effective when started early. The *hatched area* represents the placebo (mean ± S.D.). (From Lindsay.[17] Reprinted by permission from Raven Press.)

and more women will die from CVD, if they are affected by it, than from any other disease.[30]

It is evident from those statistics that the protective effect of ERT against CVD translates into a large reduction in mortality. Based on changes in the relative risks for various diseases as a consequence of ERT (TABLE 1), the total number of lives saved has been calculated to be 5,561/100,000. The reduction in mortality from CVD was calculated to account for over 5,250 of the 5,561 lives saved, that is, 94% of the reduction in death rates in estrogen users is due to the 50% reduction in the risk of CVD.[31,32] Based on the major beneficial impact of ERT on CVD reduction, it has been suggested that, with mortality as an endpoint, CVD should be the primary indication for ERT.[30]

The mechanism underlying the cardioprotective action of estrogen are not fully understood. Estrogens affect the lipid/lipoprotein profiles beneficially by increasing HDL by about 10% and significantly reducing LDL.[26] Nevertheless, the cardioprotective effect appears to be substantially mediated by factors other than favorable lipid profiles.[30] This is borne out by observations in humans,[33] and by data from monkeys fed on an atherogenic diet high in cholesterol.[34] In the

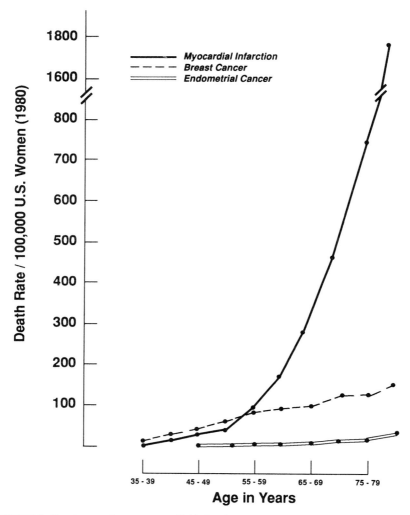

**FIGURE 4.** Death rates due to myocardial infarction, breast cancer and endometrial cancer in U.S. women. (Data from National Center for Health Statistics.)

latter study, monkeys given oral ethinyl estradiol and dl-norgestrel exhibited atherosclerosis to a lesser extent (smaller plaque size) than did the control group, suggesting that the potent estrogenic action of ethinyl estradiol inhibited coronary artery atherosclerosis despite the pronounced progestogen-related lowering of HDL, and despite the high fat diet.

In addition to favorable lipid profiles, a number of other mechanisms have been implicated in mediating the cardioprotective effect of ERT. These include changes in vasoactive substances such as prostaglandins, calcitonin gene-related peptide and endothelial relaxing factors (reviewed in Ref. 35). Both estrogen and progestogen receptors have been demonstrated in blood vessels,[36] and their presence suggests that ovarian steroids may directly act on the vasculature. This hypothesis is supported by reports that the vascular resistance of the uterine arteries is significantly reduced in response to transdermal estradiol, both in premenopausal women with ovarian failure,[37] and in postmenopausal women.[38] Several parameters of aortic blood flow were also favorably influenced by ERT and it was concluded from the data of the study that estrogens increased both the cardiac stroke volume and the flow acceleration.[39] Finally, a significant decrease in resistance to blood flow was demonstrated in the cerebral circulation of postmenopausal women in response to transdermal ERT. This effect was apparent when ERT was given soon after the menopause or many years thereafter.[40]

Although favorable lipid/lipoprotein profiles correlate only partly with cardioprotection, there is nevertheless concern that adjunctive progestogen may attenuate the cardioprotective effects of ERT,[2,41] because some progestogens in large doses are known to affect the lipid and lipoprotein profiles adversely. Therefore, the minimum dose required for endometrial protection should be prescribed,[2] and needs to be identified in clinical trials.

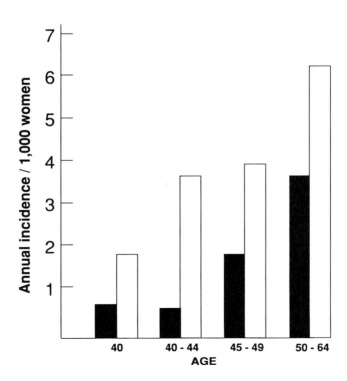

**FIGURE 5.** The incidence of cardiovascular disease relative to estrogen deficiency. The *closed bars* represent premenopausal women, the *open bars* postmenopausal women. (From Lobo.[32] Reprinted by permission from *Obstetrics and Gynecology*.)

TABLE 1. Estimated Changes in Mortality Induced by Estrogen Replacement Therapy[a] in Women Ages 50–75 Years[b]

| Condition | Relative Risk | Cumulative Change in Mortality/100,000 |
|---|---|---|
| Osteoporotic fractures | 0.4 | −563 |
| Gallbladder disease | 1.5 | +2 |
| Endometrial cancer | 2.0 | +63 |
| Breast cancer | 1.1 | +187 |
| Ischemic heart disease | 0.5 | −5250 |
| | | Net change − 5561 |
| | | Net % change − 41% |

[a] 0.625 mg/day.
[b] From Lobo.[32] Reprinted by permission from *Obstetrics and Gynecology*.

## Adjunctive Progestogen

There is substantial evidence that the benefits of ERT are offset by an increased incidence in endometrial cancer,[42] and that adjunctive progestogen fully protects against estrogen-induced endometrial carcinoma.[43,44] However, an evaluation of the overall benefit/risk of adjunctive progestogen must account for the potential adverse effects of some progestogens on lipid/lipoprotein profiles and, as a consequence, a possible impairment of the cardioprotective effect of estrogen by adjunctive progestogen therapy.[2,45,46]

The overwhelming importance of CVD as a public health issue is illustrated by death rates. The mortality from heart disease of women 55 years or older in the U.S. was 488,000 in 1990, the last year for which data are available.[29] By comparison, the expected mortality from endometrial cancer for 1992 is 5,600.[47] Moreover, the survival rates of women with estrogen-related endometrial cancer are higher than those of non-users diagnosed with the same disease.[48,49]

## Estrogen-Dependent and Estrogen-Independent Endometrial Carcinoma

The favorable survival profile of individuals with estrogen-related endometrial cancer may be in part attributable to better medical care of women receiving ERT, but also reflects the characteristic biological properties of estrogen-related endometrial cancers. In this context it is relevant to distinguish estrogen-dependent endometrial cancer, that is, the type of cancer to be prevented by adjunctive progestogen, from estrogen-independent carcinoma. Estrogen-dependent cancers are usually less invasive and morphologically and biochemically better differentiated than estrogen-independent cancers. Morphologically they often represent grade 1 cancers that are characterized by the presence of progesterone receptors.[50–52] The presence of receptors, in turn, suggests that these cancers have retained responsiveness to estrogen, since the progesterone receptor is an estrogen-induced protein. Moreover, progesterone receptors, when present at certain levels in endometrial cancer tissues, appear to be functional, as indicated by secretory changes in response to progestogen both *in vivo*[53] and *in vitro*.[54]

In contrast, a distinct type of endometrial adenocarcinoma appears to be estrogen-independent and not associated with hyperplasia (reviewed in Ref. 55). This type of cancer lacks the biochemical markers indicative of estrogen action, such as progesterone receptors,[56] occurs at a later age, and is less well differentiated and more invasive than the hyperplasia-associated type.[55]

Since the correlation of estrogen-induced endometrial hyperplasia and its progression to cancer was first proposed in the late 1940s,[57] seventeen of 19 case control studies have shown significant increases in the risk of endometrial cancer with unopposed estrogen treatment.[45] The pooled estimates of changes in relative risk from studies in long-term estrogen users (>8 years) compared to never-users was 8.22,[26] an estimate that may be high because it includes high-dose users. Two studies provide data on endometrial cancer risk in women who took 0.625 mg conjugated equine estrogens for at least five years. Those studies show risk ratios of 4.8 and 4.3.[58,59] Another study reported increases in relative risk from 2.1 after 3–5 years of estrogen use to 3.5 after 6 years of use.[60] Importantly, the increased risk persists for many years after discontinuation of treatment.[41]

A long-term study has evaluated the rates of progression of different types of hyperplasia to endometrial adenocarcinoma. This study found that cytologic atypia correlates most closely with progression to cancer. Only about 2% of hyperplasia without cytologic atypia progressed to carcinoma, regardless of architectural complexity of the lesion, whereas approximately 23% of atypical hyperplasias advanced to cancer.[61]

## Clinical Study Design to Evaluate Adjunctive Progestogen Effects

The quantitative identification of the lowest effective dose of adjunctive progestogen represents a major challenge to clinical studies. The assumption underlying such studies is that estrogen-dependent endometrial adenocarcinoma passes through the intermediate state of hyperplasia,[42,57,61,62] and that the protection against hyperplasia by adjunctive progestogen confirms its efficacy in protecting against endometrial cancer. Hyperplasia is therefore considered the principal efficacy endpoint in clinical studies designed to identify the lowest effective dose of adjunctive progestogen.

Since the incidence of hyperplasia depends on estrogen dose and on the duration of treatment, clinical studies need to be conducted over an extended period, usually one year. A meaningful estimate of subject numbers needs to be based on the incidence of hyperplasia in the reference group treated with unopposed estrogen. One study reported a hyperplasia incidence of 2.4 per 100 woman-months at low dose (0.625 mg) and 4.7 at high dose (1.25 mg) of unopposed CCE given for one year.[63] Another study using 0.625 mg CEE for one year found similar incidence rates and detected no difference between cyclic (1 week drug free in a 4-week cycle) and continuous administration of estrogen.[64]

The critical issue in the design of Phase II progestogen dose-ranging studies relates to the possible difference between progestogen doses required to transform proliferative to secretory endometrium, and progestogen doses required to protect against hyperplasia. Since both parameters are progestogen-regulated, in theory one may study one endpoint as a surrogate for the other, provided their regulation required comparable progestogen doses. In that case, secretory changes in the endometrium would be studied preferentially, since these studies are shorter and require fewer subjects than those designed to examine hyperplasia as the primary efficacy parameter. However, it has been proposed that full secretory changes may not be necessary to protect against hyperplasia so long as an estrogen/progestogen ratio is achieved that decreases mitotic activity.[65,66]

TABLE 2. Oral Progestogen Dosage (mg) Required to Produce Secretory Changes in Postmenopausal Women[a]

| Progestogen | Nuclear Estrogen Receptor (REN) | Estradiol Dehydrogenase | Morphological Changes | Consensus |
|---|---|---|---|---|
| Norethindrone | <0.35 | <0.35 | 0.35 | 0.35 |
| dl-Norgestrel | 0.15 | <0.025 | 0.075 | 0.075 |
| MPA | <2.5 | <2.5 | >10.0 | 5.0 |
| Progesterone | 200 | 250 | >310 | 200 |

[a] Modified from King et al.[68]

Moreover, clinical as well as biochemical studies suggest that the progestogen doses required to protect against hyperplasia may be lower than those needed for secretory transformation. For example, it was found that treatment with 5 mg and 10 mg MPA/day achieved full secretory transformation in only 65% or 72% of tissues, respectively.[41] Similarly, 10 mg MPA produced secretory transformation in only 61% of tissues in another study.[67] Nevertheless, it is generally agreed that 10 mg or 5 mg of MPA (and possibly even lower doses) adequately protect against hyperplasia.

The postulate that progestogen doses to protect against hyperplasia may differ from those to produce secretory changes is further strengthened by biochemical studies using different progestogens,[68] as summarized in TABLE 2. As evident from this table, the progestogen doses to produce secretory endometrium are higher than those required for biochemical changes. Of special interest in this context is the suppressive effect of progestogens on the levels of nuclear estradiol receptor at doses lower than those required for secretory changes. Consistent with the findings summarized in TABLE 2 are those of other investigators who also showed that the reduction of estrogen receptor was achieved at lower progestogen doses than those required for the induction of homogeneous secretory changes.[65]

Steroid hormone receptors are an essential link in the sequence of molecular events that cause genomic alterations of target cells in response to hormone exposure. It is therefore likely that a reduction in estrogen receptor levels, as achieved by progestogen doses lower than those required for full secretory changes, closely correlates with reduced responsiveness to estrogen, and therefore with protection against estrogen-dependent endometrial cancer. Further experimental work in support of this biologically important and clinically relevant postulate is needed.

## SUMMARY

The most important benefit of ERT may well be its cardioprotective effect. But unopposed estrogen therapy also carries the risk of inducing endometrial cancer. A compelling body of evidence indicates that adjunctive progestogen protects effectively against estrogen-induced endometrial adenocarcinoma, and that progestogen therapy is effective in the treatment of hyperplasia in most women who have taken unopposed estrogen. Yet there is concern that adjunctive progestogen may attenuate the cardioprotective effects of estrogen. It is therefore agreed that adjunctive progestogen therapy is not indicated for hysterectomized women, and should be given at the lowest effective dose to non-hysterectomized women. Phase II dose-ranging clinical trials using secretory transformation as an efficacy endpoint to estimate protective effects of different doses of progestogen against endometrial hyperplasia/adenocarcinoma are complicated by the possibility that the doses protecting against hyperplasia may differ from those producing secretory changes. Further work is needed to identify one or several progestogen-regulated markers that most closely correlate with protection against estrogen-induced endometrial cancer.

## REFERENCES

1. MISHELL, D. R. 1989. Estrogen replacement therapy: an overview. Am. J. Obstet. Gynecol. **161:** 1825–1827.
2. WHITEHEAD, M. & R. A. LOBO. 1988. Progestagen use in postmenopausal women. Lancet **2:** 1243–1244.
3. NOTELOVITZ, M. 1989. Estrogen replacement therapy: indications, contraindications, and agent selection. Am. J. Obstet. Gynecol. **161:** 1832–1841.
4. HAAS, S., B. WALSH, S. EVANS, M. KRACHE, V. RAVNIKAR & I. SCHIFF. 1988. The effect of transdermal estradiol on hormone and metabolic dynamics over a six-week period. Obstet. Gynecol. **71:** 671–676.
5. COOPE, J., J. M. THOMPSON & L. POLLER. 1975. Effects of 'natural oestrogen' replacement therapy on menopausal symptoms and blood clotting. Br. Med. J. **4:** 139–143.
6. REBAR, R. W. 1991. Practical evaluation of hormonal status. In Reproductive Endocrinology. S. S. C. Yen & R. B. Jaffe, Eds. 830–886. W. B. Saunders. Philadelphia.
7. LAUFER, L. R., J. L. DEFAZIO, J. K. H. LU, D. R. MELDRUM, P. EGGENA, M. P. SAMBHI, J. M. HERSHMAN & H. L. JUDD. 1983. Estrogen replacement therapy by transdermal estradiol administration. Am. J. Obstet. Gynecol. **146:** 533–540.
8. BUNGARY, G. T., M. P. VESSEY & C. K. MCPHERSON. 1980. Study of symptoms in middle life with special reference to the menopause. Br. Med. J. **281:** 181–183.
9. SHERWIN, B. B. & M. M. GELFANT. 1985. Sex steroids and affect in the surgical menopause: a double-blind cross-over study. Psychoneuroendocrinology **10:** 325–335.
10. SHERWIN, B. B. 1988. Affective changes with estrogen and androgen replacement therapy in surgically menopausal women. J. Affective Disord. **14:** 177–187.
11. DITKOFF, E. C., W. G. CRARY, M. CRISTO & R. A. LOBO. 1991. Estrogen improves psychological functions in asymptomatic postmenopausal women. Obstet. Gynecol. **78:** 991–995.
12. WIKLUND, I., J. KARLBERG & L.-A. MATTSSON. 1993. Quality of life of postmenopausal women on a regimen of transdermal estradiol therapy: a double-blind placebo-controlled study. Am. J. Obstet. Gynecol. **168:** 824–830.
13. SESSION, D. R., A. C. KELLY & R. JEWELEWICZ. 1993. Current concepts in estrogen replacement therapy in the menopause. Fertil. Steril. **59:** 277–284.
14. ANONYMOUS. 1991. Consensus development conference: prophylaxis and treatment of osteoporosis. Am. J. Med. **90:** 107–110.
15. GENANT, H. K., D. J. BAYLINK & J. C. GALLAGHER. 1989. Estrogens in the prevention of osteoporosis in postmenopausal women. Am. J. Obstet. Gynecol. **161:** 1842–1846.
16. WEISS, N. S., C. L. URE, J. H. BALLARD, A. R. WILLIAMS & J. R. DALING. 1980. Decreased risk of fractures of the hip and lower forearm with postmenopausal use of estrogen. N. Engl. J. Med. **303:** 1195–1198.
17. LINDSAY, R. 1988. Sex steroids in the pathogenesis and prevention of osteoporosis. In Osteoporosis. B. L. Riggs & L. J. Melton, Eds. 333–358. Raven Press. New York.
18. CHRISTIANSEN, C. & B. J. RIIS. 1990. 17$\beta$-estradiol and continuous norethisterone: a unique treatment for established osteoporosis in elderly. J. Clin. Endocrinol. Metab. **71:** 836–841.

19. LINDSAY, R. & J. F. TOHME. 1990. Estrogen treatment of patients with established postmenopausal osteoporosis. Obstet. Gynecol. **76:** 290–295.
20. LUFKIN, E. G., H. W. WAHNER, W. M. O'FALLON, S. F. HODGSON, M. A. KOTOWICZ, A. W. LANE, H. L. JUDD, R. H. CAPLAN & B. L. RIGGS. 1992. Treatment of postmenopausal osteoporosis with transdermal estrogen. Ann. Int. Med. **117:** 1–9.
21. PRIOR, J. C. 1990. Progesterone as a bone-trophic hormone. Endocr. Rev. **11:** 386–398.
22. CHRISTIANSEN, C., B. J. RIIS, L. NILAS, P. RODBRO & L. DEFTOS. 1985. Uncoupling of bone formation and resorption by combined oestrogen and progestagen therapy in postmenopausal osteoporosis. Lancet **2:** 800–801.
23. PRIOR, J. C. 1989. Trabecular bone loss is associated with abnormal luteal phase length: endogenous progesterone deficiency may be a risk factor for osteoporosis. Int. Proc. J. **1:** 70–73.
24. ABDALLA, H. I., D. M. HART, R. LINDSAY, I. LEGGATE & A. HOOKE. 1985. Prevention of bone loss in postmenopausal women by norethisterone. Obstet. Gynecol. **66:** 789–792.
25. TREMOLLIERES, F., J. M. POUILLES & C. RIBOT. 1993. Effect of long-term administration of progestogen on post-menopausal bone loss: result of a two-year, controlled randomized study. Clin. Endocrinol. **38:** 627–631.
26. GRADY, D., S. M. RUBIN, D. B. PETITTI, C. S. FOX, D. BLACK, B. ETTINGER, V. L. ERNSTER & S. R. CUMMINGS. 1992. Hormone therapy to prevent disease and prolong life in postmenopausal women. Ann. Int. Med. **117:** 1016–1041.
27. STAMPFER, M. J. & S. D. BECHTEL. 1992. Estrogen: what protection against heart disease? Contemp. Obstet. Gynecol. **4:** 13–30.
28. BUSH, T. L. 1990. Noncontraceptive estrogen use and risk of cardiovascular disease: an overview and critique of the literature. *In* The Menopause. Biological and Clinical Consequences of Ovarian Failure: Evolution and Management. S. G. Korenman, Ed. Norwell. Serono Symposia. 211–223.
29. The American Heart Association. 1993. Heart and Stroke Facts Statistics.
30. LOBO, R. A. 1990. Estrogen and cardiovascular disease. Ann. N.Y. Acad. Sci. **592:** 286–294.
31. HENDERSON, B. E., R. K. ROSS, A. PAGANINI-HILL & T. M. MACK. 1986. Estrogen use and cardiovascular disease. Am. J. Obstet. Gynecol. **154:** 1181–1186.
32. LOBO, R. A. 1990. Cardiovascular implications of estrogen replacement therapy. Obstet. Gynecol. **75:** 18S–25S.
33. BUSH, T. L., E. BARRETT-CONNOR, L. D. COWAN, M. H. CRIQUI, R. B. WALLACE, C. M. SUCHINDRAN *et al.* 1987. Cardiovascular mortality and noncontraceptive use of estrogen in women. Results from the Lipid Research Clinics program follow-up study. Circulation **75:** 1102–1109.
34. ADAMS, MM. R., T. B. CLARKSON, D. R. KORITNIK & H. A. NASH. 1987. Contraceptive steroids and coronary artery arteriosclerosis in *Cynomolgus macaques*. Fertil. Steril. **47:** 1010–1018.
35. SARREL, P. M. 1990. Ovarian hormones and the circulation. Maturitas **12:** 287–298.
36. PERROT-APPLANAT, M., M. T. GROYER-PICART, E. GARCIA, F. LORENZO & E. MILGROM. 1988. Immunocytochemical demonstration of estrogen and progesterone receptors in muscle cells of uterine arteries in rabbits and humans. Endocrinology **123:** 1511,
37. DE ZIEGLER, D., R. BESSIS & R. FRYDMAN. 1991. Vascular resistance of uterine arteries: physiological effects of estradiol and progesterone. Fertil. Steril. **55:** 775–779.
38. HILLARD, T. C., T. B. CRAYFORD, T. H. BOURNE, W. P. COLLINS, M. I. WHITEHEAD & S. CAMPBELL. 1992. Differential effects of transdermal estradiol and sequential progestogens on impedance to flow within the uterine arteries of postmenopausal women. Fertil. Steril. **58:** 959–963.
39. PINES, A., E. Z. FISMAN, Y. LEVO, M. AVERBUCH, A. LIDOR, Y. DRORY, A. FINKELSTEIN, M. HETMAN-PERI, M. MOSHKOWITZ, E. BEN-ARI & D. AYALON. 1991. The effects of hormone replacement therapy in normal postmenopausal women: measurements of Doppler-derived parameters of aortic flow. Am. J. Obstet. Gynecol. **164:** 806–812.

40. GANGAR, K. F., S. VYAS, M. WHITEHEAD, D. CROOK, H. MEIRE & S. CAMPBELL. 1991. Pulsatility index in internal carotid artery in relation to transdermal oestradiol and time since menopause. Lancet **338:** 839–842.
41. WHITEHEAD, M. I. & T. C. HILLARD. 1990. The role and use of progestogens. Obstet. Gynecol. **75:** 59S–76S.
42. GUSBERG, S. B. 1976. The individual at risk for endometrial cancer. Am. J. Obstet. Gynecol. **126:** 535–542.
43. GAMBRELL, R. D. 1986. Prevention of endometrial cancer with progestogens. Maturitas **8:** 159–168.
44. PERSSON, I., H.-O. ADAMI, L. BERGKVIST, A. LINDGREN, B. PETTERSSON, R. HOOVER & C. SCHAIRER. 1989. Risk of endometrial cancer after treatment with oestrogens alone or in conjunction with progestogens: results of a prospective study. Br. Med. J. **298:** 147–151.
45. LOBO, R. A. 1992. The role of progestins in hormone replacement therapy. Am. J. Obstet. Gynecol. **166:** 1997–2004.
46. HENDERSON, B. E., M. C. PIKE, R. K. ROSS, T. M. MACK & R. A. LOBO. 1988. Re-evaluating the role of progestogen therapy after the menopause. Fertil. Steril. **49:** 9S–15S.
47. American Cancer Society. 1992. Cancer Facts and Figures.
48. COLLINS, J., A. DONNER, L. N. ALLEN & O. ADAMS. 1980. Oestrogen use and survival in endometrial cancer. Lancet **1:** 961–964.
49. CHU, J., A. I. SCHWEID & N. S. WEISS. 1982. Survival among women with endometrial cancer: a comparison of estrogen users and nonusers. Am. J. Obstet. Gynecol. **143:** 569–573.
50. SYRJALA, P., K. KONTULA, O. JANNE & R. VIHKO. 1978. Steroid receptors in normal and neoplastic human uterine tissue. *In* Endometrial Cancer. M. G. Brush & R. J. B. King, Eds. 242–251. Balliere Tindall. London.
51. MCCARTHY, J. S., T. K. BARTON, B. F. FETTER, W. T. CREASMAN & K. S. MCCARTHY, SR. 1979. Correlation of estrogen and progesterone receptors with histologic differentiation in endometrial adenocarcinoma. Am. J. Pathol. **96:** 171–183.
52. POLLOW, K., M. SCHMIDT-GOLLWITZER & B. POLLOW. 1980. Progesterone and estradiol binding proteins from normal endometrium and endometrial carcinoma: a comparative study. *In* Steroid Receptors and Hormone-Dependent Neoplasia. J. L. Wittliff & O. Dapunt, Eds. 69–94. Masson Publishing U.S.A. New York.
53. HOLINKA, C. F., L. DELIGDISCH, G. DEPPE & E. GURPIDE. 1982. Evaluation of *in vivo* and *in vitro* responses of endometrial adenocarcinoma to progestins. *In* Hormones and Cancer. W. W. Leavitt, Ed. 365–376. Plenum Publishing. New York.
54. HOLINKA, C. F., L. DELIGDISCH & E. GURPIDE. 1984. Histological evaluation of *in vitro* responses of endometrial adenocarcinoma to progestins and their relation to progesterone receptor levels. Cancer Res. **44:** 293–296.
55. DELIGDISCH, L. & C. F. HOLINKA. 1987. Endometrial carcinoma: two diseases? Cancer Detect. Prevent. **10:** 237–246.
56. DELIGDISCH, L. & C. F. HOLINKA. 1986. Progesterone receptors in two groups of endometrial carcinoma. Cancer **57:** 1385–1388.
57. GUSBERG, S. B. 1947. Precursors of corpus carcinoma: estrogens and adenomatous hyperplasia. Am. J. Obstet. Gynecol. **54:** 905–927.
58. MACK, T. M., M. C. PIKE, B. E. HENDERSON, R. I. PFEFFER, V. R. GERKINS & M. ARTHUR. 1976. Estrogens and endometrial cancer in a retirement community. N. Engl. J. Med. **294:** 1262–1267.
59. BURING, J. E., C. J. BAIN & R. L. EHRMANN. 1986. Conjugated estrogen use and risk of endometrial cancer. Am. J. Epidemiol. **124:** 434–441.
60. RUBIN, G. L., H. B. PETERSON, N. C. LEE, E. F. MAES, P. A. WINGO & S. BECKER. 1990. Estrogen replacement therapy and the risk of endometrial cancer: remaining controversies. Am. J. Obstet. Gynecol. **162:** 148–154.
61. KURMAN, R. J., P. F. KAMINSKI & H. J. NORRIS. 1985. The behavior of endometrial hyperplasia. A long-term study of 'untreated' hyperplasia in 170 patients. Cancer **56:** 403–412.

62. GUSBERG, S. B. & A. L. KAPLAN. 1963. Precursors of corpus cancer IV. Adenomatous hyperplasia as stage 0 carcinoma of the endometrium. Am. J. Obstet. Gynecol. **87:** 662–678.
63. GELFANT, M. M. & A. FERENCZY. 1989. A prospective 1-year study of estrogen and progestin in postmenopausal women: effects on the endometrium. Obstet. Gynecol. **74:** 398–402.
64. SCHIFF, I., S. H. KOMAROV, D. CRAMER, D. TULCHINSKY & K. J. RYAN. 1982. Endometrial hyperplasia in women on cyclic or continuous estrogen regimen. Fertil. Steril. **37:** 79–82.
65. GIBBONS, W. E., D. L. MOYER, R. A. LOBO, S. ROY & D. R. MISHELL. 1986. Biochemical and histological effects of sequential estrogen/progestin therapy on the endometrium of postmenopausal women. Am. J. Obstet. Gynecol. **154:** 456–461.
66. MOYER, D. L., B. DE LIGNIERES, P. DRIGUEZ & J. P. PEZ. 1993. Prevention of endometrial hyperplasia by progesterone during long-term estradiol replacement: influence of bleeding pattern and secretory changes. Fertil. Steril. **59:** 992–997.
67. WREN, B. G. 1989. Dose related response of the endometrium to Provera: interim summary results. Int. Proc. J. **1:** 163–164.
68. KING, R. J. B. & M. I. WHITEHEAD. 1986. Assessment of the potency of orally administered progestins in women. Fertil. Steril. **46:** 1062–1066.

# *In Vitro* Bioassays for Drugs with Dual Estrogenic and Progestagenic Activities

LESZEK MARKIEWICZ AND ERLIO GURPIDE

*Mount Sinai School of Medicine (CUNY)*
*Department of Obstetrics, Gynecology*
*and Reproductive Science*
*New York, New York 10029*

## INTRODUCTION

An *in vitro* system based on the estrogen-specific enhancement of alkaline phosphatase (AP) activity in human endometrial adenocarcinoma cells of the Ishikawa line[1] was developed and applied to the measurement of *estrogenic* activities of various steroidal estrogens,[2] isoflavones and other phytoestrogens,[3] as well as to the evaluation of intrinsic estrogenic activities of many progestins commonly used for hormonal therapy.[4] More recently, we developed a similar assay to measure *progestagenic* activities using cells of the human breast cancer line T47D, in which AP is specifically stimulated by progestins.[5] These two methods provide a simple, efficient and inexpensive system to evaluate estrogenic and progestagenic activities of synthetic compounds, natural products and biologic fluids. They are also of special interest in the measurement of relative estrogenic/progestagenic potencies in compounds possessing both activities, as is the case in many of the progestins used as contraceptives and in hormonal replacement therapy for postmenopausal symptoms.

In addition to the specific bioassays with cells of the Ishikawa-Var I and T47D lines, we have developed and applied other *in vitro* systems to obtain qualitative as well as quantitative information on the estrogenic and progestagenic effects of test compounds on human endometrial tissue.[6] One of these systems is based on the previously reported stimulatory effects of estrogens on prostaglandin $F_{2\alpha}$ ($PGF_{2\alpha}$) production by *secretory endometrium*.[7,8] The same tissue allows the *in vitro* evaluation of progestagenic (estrogen antagonistic) activities by measuring the inhibitory effect of a test compound on the action of a fixed amount of $E_2$ added to the culture medium.[6] Fragments of *proliferative endometrium* can be used to evaluate progestagenic activities in test compounds on the basis of a concentration-dependent reduction in $PGF_{2\alpha}$ output[6] and by measuring increases in estradiol 17β-dehydrogenase activity ($E_2DH$).[9] Furthermore, clear evidence of *in vitro* progestagenic effects can be documented histologically by the appearance of subnuclear glandular accumulation of glycogen in proliferative endometrium exposed to a test compound under organ culture conditions.[6,10]

## EXPERIMENTAL DESIGNS

### In Vitro *Bioassays for Hormonal and Antihormonal Activities Using Human Cell Lines*

Cells from either the Ishikawa-Var I or the T47D lines are equally distributed and allowed to attach in microtiter plates of 96 wells. Samples and reference compounds are tested at various concentrations (a column of 8 wells for each concentration) using appropriate blanks. After exposure to the test compound for 3 days the cells are washed and covered with a solution of p-nitrophenyl phosphate to determine the induced AP activity by measuring colorimetrically at different intervals the rate of p-nitrophenol formation.[4] Values obtained from the plate reader are used to generate sigmoidal concentration-response functions allowing the estimation of maximal responses, $EC_{50}$ values and "slope factor" values[11] characterizing those activities.

Accurate relative maximal responses (relative "efficacies") are obtained by including in the same multiwell plate various test compounds as well as standards such as estradiol ($E_2$) or diethylstilbestrol (DES) for estrogens and progesterone (P) or medroxyprogesterone acetate (MPA) for progestins, each at appropriately high concentrations. The tests for maximal response are of particular interest as they establish whether a compound acts as a full or a partial agonist, a distinction of considerable mechanistic and pharmacologic importance.

Antiestrogenic or antiprogestagenic activities can be evaluated in the same system by measuring effects of the antagonist at various concentrations on the actions of a standard agonist at a fixed concentration. These experiments reveal whether the antagonist can completely inhibit the action of the standard by acting as "pure" antagonist or is itself a partial agonist. They also allow the estimation of $IC_{50}$ values and further characterization of the response function.

### In Vitro *Bioassays with Fragments of Human Endometrium*

In contrast to the effects of AP to estrogens in Ishikawa Var-I cells and to progestins in T47D cells, the specific responses of a target tissue to drugs with dual estrogenic and progestagenic activities cannot be predicted since these compounds may affect a particular response either antagonistically or cooperatively. In order to evaluate the net effects of such drugs on a target tissue expressing both estrogen receptor (ER) and progesterone receptor (PR), we have developed and applied *in vitro* systems utilizing fragments of either proliferative or secretory human endometrium in organ culture and measuring $PGF_{2\alpha}$ output, which is enhanced by estrogens and reduced by progestins.[7,8] Evaluation of effects on $E_2DH$ activity and glycogen accumulation in proliferative endometrium under organ culture conditions serve to demonstrate progestagenic effects of a drug possessing dual activities since progestagens enhance the activity of $E_2DH$ and provoke accumulation of glycogen, while estrogens do not affect these effects.

## METHODS

### *Assays for Estrogenic and Antiestrogenic Activities Based on the Stimulation of AP Activity in Ishikawa-Var I Cells*

The human Ishikawa cell line, established by Nishida *et al.*[12] and made available to us by Dr. H. Kuramoto, Kitasato University, Kanagawa-Ken, Japan, was derived from a well differentiated endometrial adenocarcinoma. A variant of this cell line (Ishikawa-Var I) is unresponsive to $E_2$ regarding proliferation but sensitive to the stimulatory effect of estrogens on AP activity. The *in vitro* bioassay for estrogenic actions based on the stimulation of AP activity in these cells has been described elsewhere.[4] In brief, the cells are maintained in phenol red-free Ham's F12 and Dulbecco's Modified Eagle's medium, supplemented with 5% bovine calf serum (CS) pretreated with dextran-coated charcoal. The cells are seeded in 96-well flat bottom Microtest III tissue culture plates at a density of 25,000 cells/well. After addition of test compounds, the cells are incubated for 72 h at 37°C in a humidified atmosphere of 5% $CO_2$-95% air. At the end of the incubation period, growth medium is removed and the plates are rinsed with phosphate-buffered saline and placed on ice. An ice-cold solution consisting of 5 mM $p$-nitrophenyl phosphate, 0.24 mM $MgCl_2$ and 1 mM diethanolamine (pH 9.8) is added to each well and $p$-nitrophenol formation at room temperature is monitored periodically, from 15 to 60 min, at 405 nm using a plate reader to determine AP activity. Concentrations corresponding to half the maximal increase in AP activity ($EC_{50}$) are calculated graphically and by computer-assisted analysis using a KaleidaGraph software.

### *Assays for Progestagenic and Antiprogestagenic Activities Based on the Stimulation of AP Activity in T47D Cells*

The *in vitro* assays for progestagenic and antiprogestagenic activities are based on the progestin-specific stimulation of AP activity in T47D cells,[13] kindly provided by Dr. L. J. Murphy, Department of Physiology, University of Manitoba, Winnipeg, Manitoba, Canada. The cells are maintained in Dulbecco's Modified Eagle's medium supplemented with penicillin 100 U/L, streptomycin 100 µg/L and 10% fetal bovine serum. Twenty-four h before the start of an experiment the serum in the medium is replaced by CS pretreated with dextran-coated charcoal. The cells are distributed in a multiwell culture plate at a density of 50,000 cells/well and exposed to test compounds at various concentrations for 72 h to evaluate their effects on AP activity.[5] This method is similar to the *in vitro* bioassay for estrogenic and antiestrogenic activities based on the stimulation of AP in Ishikawa-Var I cells.

### *Estrogenic/Progestagenic Effects Evaluated with Human Endometrial Fragments under Organ Culture Conditions*

Specimens of histologically normal endometrium are obtained from uteri of patients undergoing hysterectomy for reasons other than endometrial neoplasia, following procedures approved by our Institutional Research Committee. Under a laminar flow hood, the tissue in sterile minimum essential medium containing 1% of an antibiotic-antimycotic mixture is trimmed, washed with Hank's Balanced Salt Solution and cut into small fragments (approx. 1 mm³). Randomized fragments are fixed in formalin for histologic dating according to Noyes *et al.*[14]

### *Evaluation of $PGF_{2\alpha}$ Production by Human Endometrium in Organ Culture*

In order to study the *in vitro* effects of estrogens and progestins on proliferative or secretory endometrium, tissue fragments are placed, as previously described,[6] on lens paper resting on stainless steel grids in various 6 cm diameter polystyrene culture dishes containing 3.5 ml of Ham's F10 medium. The dishes, each holding 4–10 mg of tissue, are kept in an incubator at 37°C in a humidified atmosphere of

5% $CO_2$-95% air. After a 24 h "settling period," the medium is replaced by medium containing the test compounds, alone or in combination; control dishes contained 0.1% ethanol. Incubations are carried out in parallel for another 24 h. The medium from each dish is collected and centrifuged at the end of the incubation period, storing the supernatants at $-70°C$ for $PGF_{2\alpha}$ radioimmunoassay performed on duplicate aliquots and 2 dilutions of unextracted culture medium, as previously described.[8] Tissue from each dish is recovered, washed thoroughly, homogenized and analyzed for protein content, using the method of Lowry et al.[15]

### Evaluation of Progestagenic Activity by Measuring $E_2DH$ Activity

In order to measure hormonal effects on intracellular $E_2DH$ activity, fragments of proliferative endometrium resting on lens paper over a stainless steel grid in 6 cm culture dishes (15–20 mg/dish) are incubated for 2–3 days in media containing test compounds or vehicle, changing medium every 24 h. At the end of the incubation period, the tissue is collected and stored at $-70°C$. Estradiol 17$\beta$-dehydrogenase activity is measured by using a radiometric method previously reported.[9] The reaction mixture consists of an 800-g supernatant of tissue homogenate in 50 mM Tris buffer, pH 8.0, containing about 0.8 mg protein/ml, 18 $\mu$M [$^3$H]$E_2$ (SA approx. 500 dpm/pmol) and 1.4 mM $NAD^+$. The reaction is carried out at 37°C and aliquots, taken at different time intervals between 2 and 8 min, are added to methanol containing [$^{14}$C] estrone ($E_1$) indicator to evaluate losses and a mixture of $E_1$ and $E_2$ carriers (500 $\mu$g each). After centrifugation and evaporation of the supernatants to dryness, the residues are subjected to TLC using silica gel plates to isolate $E_1$. Amounts of [$^3$H]$E_1$ formed are calculated from $^3$H/$^{14}$C ratios in eluted $E_1$ and rates of conversion of $E_2$ to $E_1$ are estimated from the slopes of regression lines corresponding to plots of amounts of $E_1$ formed as a function of incubation times. Enzymatic activities are expressed as nmol $E_1$ formed per mg protein per hour.

### Histologic Evaluation of Glycogen Accumulation

Progestin-induced glycogen accumulation is evaluated histologically by incubating tissue fragments of proliferative endometrium for 72 h in Ham's F10-10% CS containing test compounds or vehicle. Intracellular accumulation of glycogen accumulation is visualized by hematoxylin-eosin staining, as described elsewhere.[6]

### Statistics

Statistical significance of differences between means were estimated by paired Student's $t$ test.

## RESULTS

### Evaluation of Estrogenic and Antiestrogenic Activities

FIGURE 1 shows a representative response curve obtained by stimulation of AP activity in Ishikawa-Var I cells with DES at various concentrations. The

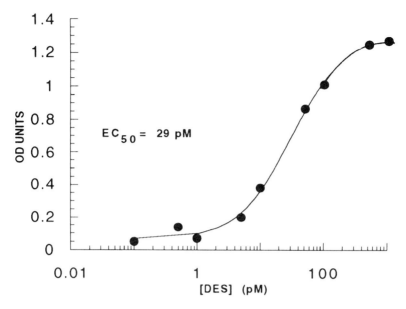

**FIGURE 1.** Concentration dependence of DES effects on AP expression in Ishikawa-Var I cells.

maximal response elicited by this drug (a full agonist) was already achieved at 1 nM concentration and the average $EC_{50}$ value was $28 \pm 12$ pM (n = 8). The concentration-response function was further characterized by a "slope factor" of $1.1 \pm 0.69$.

FIGURE 2 shows that the estrogenic effect of $E_2$ at 1 nM concentration on AP activity can be antagonized by OHTam (panel A) and fully inhibited by the "pure" antiestrogen ICI 164,384 (panel B). This example illustrates the usefulness of the assay in the evaluation of inhibitory effects of antiestrogens allowing their characterization as full or partial antagonistics and the estimation of $IC_{50}$ values.

The *in vitro* bioassay with Ishikawa cells can as well be used for the evaluation of estrogenic activities in drugs with dual estrogenic and progestagenic activities, as previously reported.[4] FIGURE 3 shows estrogenic effects of ORG OD14 (Livial, Organon bv, Oss, The Netherlands) on AP activity and antiestrogenic effects of ICI 164,384 and OHTam, measured in parallel on the same plate. The stimulatory effect of ORG OD14 at 1 $\mu$M concentration in inhibited by equimolar concentration of ICI 164,384 to control values, while OHTam brings down AP activity to the level elicited by OHTam alone at the same concentration. These results indicate that in drugs with dual activities their estrogenic action in Ishikawa cells is ER mediated and is not neutralized by their progestagenic component.

## *Evaluation of Progestagenic and Antiprogestagenic Activities*

FIGURE 4 shows a representative concentration-response curve obtained by stimulation of AP activity with MPA in T47D cells. In a series of 18 experiments

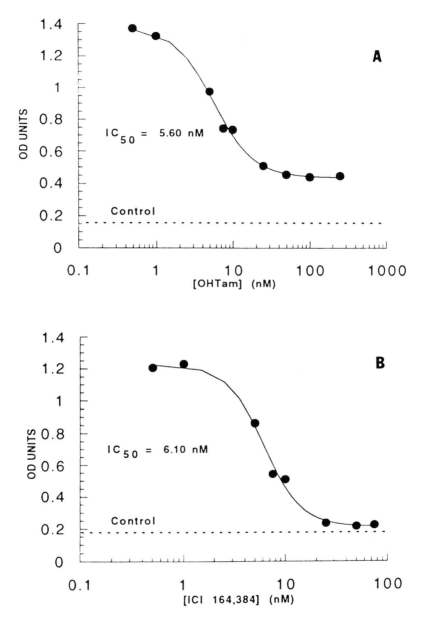

**FIGURE 2.** Concentration dependence of inhibitory effects of **(A)** OHTam and **(B)** ICI 164,384 on AP induction by $E_2$ (1 nM) in Ishikawa-Var I cells.

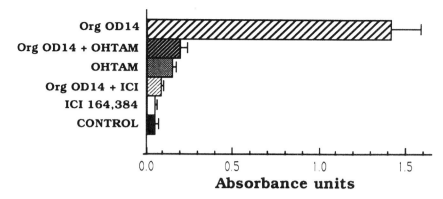

**FIGURE 3.** Antiestrogenic effects of OHTam and ICI 164,384 (1 μM) on ORG OD14 (1 μM) stimulation of AP in Ishikawa cells.

the average value for maximal activity under the assay conditions (MPA is a full agonist) was already achieved at a 1 nM concentration. The $EC_{50}$ value for MPA was $150 \pm 27$ pM and the "slope factor" was found to be $2.8 \pm 1.02$.

FIGURE 5 shows concentration-dependent antagonistic effects of RU 486 (Mifepristone, Roussel-UCLAF, Romainville, France) (panel A) and ZK 98299 (Onapristone, Schering AG, Berlin, Germany) (panel B) on AP activity stimulated

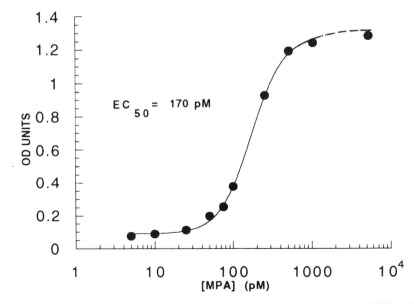

**FIGURE 4.** Concentration dependence of MPA effects on AP expression in T47D cells.

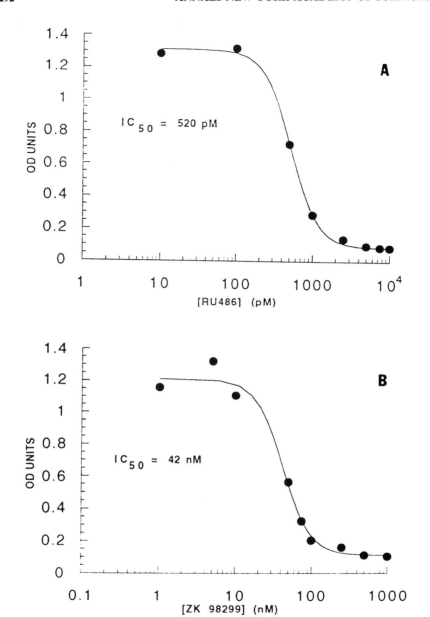

**FIGURE 5.** Concentration dependence of inhibitory effects of **(A)** RU 486 and **(B)** ZK 98299 on induction of AP by MPA (1 nM) in T47D cells.

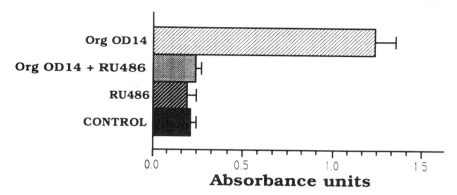

**FIGURE 6.** Antiprogestagenic effects of RU 486 (10 nM) on ORG OD14 (10 nM) stimulation of AP activity in T47D cells.

by MPA at 1 nM concentration. Such inhibition is consistent with PR-mediated AP responses in this system. Antagonistic potency of the two "pure" antiprogestins were evaluated by comparing their $IC_{50}$ values: the antiprogestagenic potency of RU 486 ($IC_{50} = 0.52$ nM) is about 80 times greater than the potency of ZK 98299 ($IC_{50} = 42$ nM) under these experimental conditions.

FIGURE 6 illustrates the progestagenic effect of ORG OD14 at the concentration of 10 nM, sufficient to elicit maximal stimulation of AP in T47D cells, and the complete inhibition of this effect by the antiprogestagenic RU 486 at equimolar concentration.

### *Evaluation of Effects of Compounds with Dual Estrogenic and Progestagenic Activities on Endometrial Explants*

FIGURE 7 illustrates effects of ORG OD14 and R2323 (Gestrinone, Roussel-UCLAF) on $PGF_{2\alpha}$ production by *proliferative endometrium* under organ culture

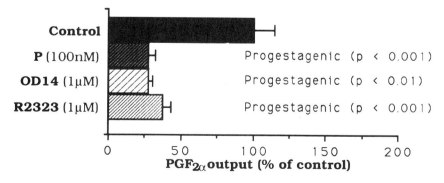

**FIGURE 7.** Progestagenic (inhibitory) effects of P, ORG OD14 and R2323 on basal output of $PGF_{2\alpha}$ by fragments of proliferative endometrium under organ culture conditions in a 24-h incubation period.

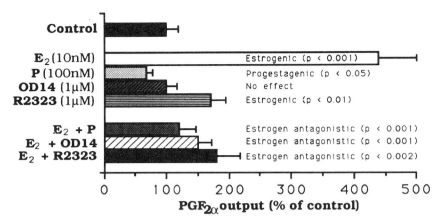

**FIGURE 8.** Estrogenic, progestagenic and estrogen-antagonistic effects of $E_2$, P, ORG OD14 and R2323, alone and in combination, on $PGF_{2\alpha}$ output by fragments of secretory endometrium under organ culture conditions in a 24-h incubation period.

conditions. Basal output of $PGF_{2\alpha}$, which is higher in proliferative than in secretory endometrium, was significantly decreased after 24 h exposure to 0.1 $\mu$M P; a similar effect was produced by ORG OD14 or R2323 at 1 $\mu$M concentration.

FIGURE 8 shows that $E_2$ increases, and P decreases, $PGF_{2\alpha}$ output by fragments of *secretory endometrium*. Tested in parallel, ORG OD14 at 1 $\mu$M concentration did not affect $PGF_{2\alpha}$ output, suggesting that the intrinsic estrogenic activity of this compound is counterbalanced by its progestagenic (fully agonistic) activity on this response. In contrast, R2323 (a partial progestagenic agonist) was weakly but significantly ($p < 0.01$) estrogenic under the same experimental conditions. FIGURE 8 also shows estrogen-antagonistic effects, usually associated with progestagenic activity, as demonstrated by mixing $E_2$ at 10 nM concentration with P in 10-fold molar excess and with ORG OD14 or R2323 in 100-fold molar excess.

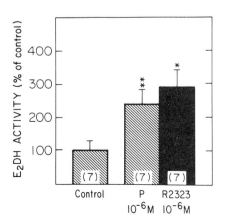

**FIGURE 9.** Stimulation of $E_2DH$ by P and R2323 in fragments of proliferative endometrium under organ culture conditions in a 72-h incubation period.

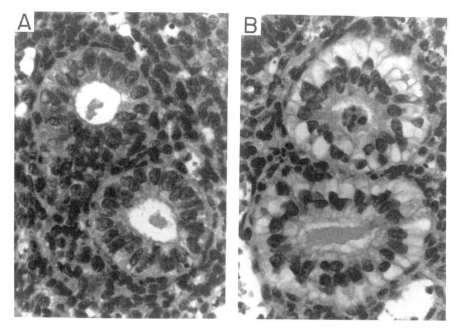

**FIGURE 10.** Subnuclear glycogen accumulation in proliferative endometrium after 72 h in culture medium **(A)** alone or **(B)** in the presence of 1 $\mu$M R2323.

These compounds counteracted the stimulatory effect of $E_2$ on $PGF_{2\alpha}$ output by secretory endometrium (FIG. 8).

Also as examples of the applicability of these methods, FIGURE 9 shows stimulatory effects of R2323 on concentration of $E_2DH$ and FIGURE 10 further documents the progestagenic activity of this compound by presenting histologic evidence of its inductive effect on glycogen accumulation in proliferative endometrium under organ culture conditions.

## DISCUSSION

The cells used for the *in vitro* bioassays described in this report are derived from well-differentiated tumors of human target tissues (endometrium and breast) responsive to estrogens and progestins. They offer a realistic model to evaluate potencies of the tested compounds at the target tissue since in addition to acting through activation of receptors, as suggested by the inhibitory actions of antiestrogens and antiprogestins, these cells express enzymes involved in steroid metabolism. Furthermore, the specificity of the AP activity response to estrogens in endometrial Ishikawa cells and to progestins in T47D breast cells make these assays suitable for the evaluation of relative estrogenic and progestagenic activities coexisting in some compounds, a topic of considerable pharmacologic interest since it has been suggested that the potential estrogenic activity of these drugs may stimulate human breast cancer cell proliferation.[16]

Additional information on net effects on responses that are affected by both types of hormonal activities may be obtained *in vitro* by using endometrial tissue endowed with both ER and PR, as illustrated by differences in the effects of some of the compounds used in the present study. The net actions elicited by a drug activating ER and PR simultaneously may represent the result of cooperative or inhibitory interactions. For instance, progestins lower ER levels reducing the estrogenic effects whereas estrogens increase PR levels enhancing the progestagenic effects.

Quantitative studies using the bioassays utilizing Ishikawa-Var I and T47D cells have yielded information on characteristics of compounds with dual estrogenic and progestagenic potential activities for various drugs used in hormone replacement therapy. A recent report on those studies[5] includes data on relative maximal activities ("efficacy") and $EC_{50}$ values corresponding to each of those activities.

Measurements of maximal effects elicited by different compounds tested in parallel experiments allowed their classification as full or as partial agonists. $EC_{50}$ values were estimated from concentration-response functions and served to determine relative potencies of full agonists. Similar assays were applied to the evaluation of antiestrogenic and antiprogestagenic activities by measuring $IC_{50}$ values for pure antagonists. Partial agonists were found to act as inhibitors when present in large excess in mixtures with full agonists, an effect that can be explained as resulting from competition for receptor binding.[5]

## REFERENCES

1. HOLINKA, C. F., H. HATA, H. KURAMOTO & E. GURPIDE. 1986. Effects of steroid hormones and antisteroids on alkaline phosphatase activity in human endometrial cancer cells (Ishikawa line). Cancer Res. **46:** 2771–2774.
2. LITTLEFIELD, B. A., E. GURPIDE, L. MARKIEWICZ, B. MCKINLY & R. B. HOCHBERG. 1990. A simple and sensitive microtiter plate estrogen bioassay based on stimulation of alkaline phosphatase in Ishikawa cells: estrogenic action of $\Delta^5$ adrenal steroids. Endocrinology **127:** 2757–2762.
3. MARKIEWICZ, L., J. GAREY, H. ADLERCREUTZ & E. GURPIDE. 1993. *In vitro* bioassays of non-steroidal phytoestrogens. J. Steroid Biochem. Mol. Biol. **45:** 399–405.
4. MARKIEWICZ, L., R. B. HOCHBERG & E. GURPIDE. 1992. Intrinsic estrogenicity of some progestagenic drugs. J. Steroid Biochem. Mol. Biol. **41:** 53–58.
5. MARKIEWICZ, L. & E. GURPIDE. 1994. Estrogenic and progestagenic activities coexisting in steroidal drugs: quantitative evaluation by *in vitro* bioassays with human cells. J. Steroid Biochem. Mol. Biol. **48:** 89–94.
6. MARKIEWICZ, L. & E. GURPIDE. 1990. *In vitro* evaluation of estrogenic, estrogen antagonistic and progestagenic effects of a steroidal drug (Org OD-14) and its metabolites on human endometrium. J. Steroid Biochem. Mol. Biol. **35:** 535–541.
7. ABEL, M. H. & D. T. BAIRD. 1980. The effect of 17β-estradiol and progesterone on prostaglandin production by endometrium maintained in organ culture. Endocrinology **106:** 1599–1606.
8. SCHATZ, F., L. MARKIEWICZ, P. BARG & E. GURPIDE. 1985. *In vitro* effects of ovarian steroids on prostaglandin $F_{2\alpha}$ output by human endometrium and endometrial epithelial cells. J. Clin. Endocrinol. Metab. **61:** 361–367.
9. TSENG, L. & E. GURPIDE. 1975. Induction of human endometrial estradiol dehydrogenase by progestins. Endocrinology **97:** 825.
10. KOHORN, E. I. & R. TCHAO. 1969. Conversion of proliferative endometrium to secretory endometrium by progesterone in organ culture. J. Endocrinol. **45:** 401–405.
11. DE LEAN, A., P. J. MUNSON & D. RODBARD. 1978. Simultaneous analysis of families

of sigmoidal curves: application to bioassay, radioligand assay, and physiological dose-response curves. Am. J. Physiol. **235**(2): E97–E102.
12. NISHIDA, M., K. KASAHARA, M. KANEKO & H. IWASAKI. 1985. Establishment of a new human endometrial adenocarcinoma cell line, Ishikawa cells, containing estrogen and progesterone receptors. Acta Obstet. Gynaec. Jap. **37:** 1103–1111.
13. DI LORENZO, A. ALBERTINI & D. ZAVA. 1991. Progestin regulation of alkaline phosphatase in the human breast cancer cell line T47D. Cancer Res. **51:** 4470–4475.
14. NOYES, R. W., A. T. HERTIG & J. ROCK. 1950. Dating the endometrial biopsy. Fert. Steril. **1:** 3–25.
15. LOWRY, O. H., N. J. ROSENBROUGH, A. L. FARR & R. J. RANDALL. 1951. Protein measurement with the Folin-phenol reagent. J. Biol. Chem. **193:** 266.
16. JENG, M.-H., C. J. PARKER & V. C. JORDAN. 1992. Estrogenic potential of progestins in oral contraceptives to stimulate human breast cancer cell proliferation. Cancer Res. **52:** 6539–6546.

# Epidermal Growth Factor Receptor Expression and Endometrial Cancer Histotypes[a]

VALERIO M. JASONNI,[b] DONATELLA SANTINI,[c]
ANDREA AMADORI,[b] CLAUDIO CECCARELLI,[c]
AND SILVIA NALDI[b]

[b]Department of Obstetrics and Gynecology
[c]Department of Pathology
University of Bologna
S. Orsola General Hospital
Via Massarenti, 13
40123 Bologna, Italy

## INTRODUCTION

It is generally accepted that growth factors (GF) and growth factor receptors (GF-R) are implicated in control of normal and neoplastic cells' growth. The epidermal growth factor receptor (EGF-R) is an early constituent of the developing uterus.[1] Since the EGF-R is detectable in the female genital tract earlier than the oestrogen receptor (ER)[2] and these endometrial ER-deficient cells are responsive to oestrogen mitogenic signalling,[3] epidermal growth factor (EGF) and/or EGF-R might be involved in transducing oestrogen stimulus. On the other hand, oestrogens are able to induce the EGF-R synthesis in uterine tissues.[4] The endometrial EGF-R increases during the follicular phase and decreases in the late luteal[5,6] indicating the stimulatory effects of oestrogens and the inhibiting action of progesterone. These interrelationships between ovarian hormones and EGF-R appear to suggest an important role of this growth factor receptor in the endometrial growth control. However, the role of EGF-R in endometrial cancer is not well understood. While EGF-R was related to the endometrial cancer invasiveness or prognosis by some Authors,[7] others were unable to find any relationship with histological grade, extent of miometrial invasion and prognosis.[8-10] Endometrial cancer presents various histotypes that were rarely considered in the studies reported in literature. Therefore, we attempted to investigate the EGF-R expression related to the histotype of endometrial cancer.

## EXPERIMENTS

The samples of 34 consecutive cases of primary endometrial carcinoma surgically treated by hysterectomy at the Reproductive Medicine Unit were

---

[a] We are very grateful to the Associazione per lo Studio delle Terapie Ormonali (A.S.T.O.) and to the Istituto Oncologico Romagnolo (I.O.R.).

selected from the files of the Department of Pathology, S. Orsola Hospital, University of Bologna. From each case one to four paraffin-embedded blocks containing the more significative neoplastic areas were selected for histological and immunohistochemical evaluation. The patients' histories of parity, hormone therapy, and endocrine or metabolic disorders were collected. Data regarding the clinical and pathological stage according to FIGO system were recorded. For routine histological diagnosis serial sections from each block were obtained and stained according to: hematoxilin eosin, periodic acid shiff (p.a.s.) with and without diastase digestion, alcian blue, mucicarmine and tricrome-Masson methods. The tumors were histologically classified and graded as currently recommended by the International Society of Gynaecological Pathology.[11] Neoplasms containing more than one type of histological differentiation were always specified and finally classified under their major component (50%). In our review the endometrial carcinomas with at least 5% of squamous differentiation were recorded separately and in accordance with the literature[12] classified as adenocarcinomas with squamous (SQ) differentiation. In our study we also maintained the further definition of adenoacanthoma (AA), when the neoplasia contained squamous elements that were benign; adenosquamous (AS) carcinoma when the neoplastic tissue contained clear malignant keratinizing and nonkeratinizing cytological features admixed with the glandular tissue and infiltrating the stroma in an evident invasive fashion. Moreover, a vascular invasion consisting of malignant squamous carcinomatous elements was also considered as a further important finding to reinforce the diagnosis of AS carcinoma. Tumors were staged according to FIGO system.[13]

## METHODOLOGY

From each formalin-fixed paraffin embedded selected block four micron serial sections were cut and collected on poly-L-lysine precoated slides (two sections to each slide) and allowed to dry overnight at 37°C. Sections were then processed according to a streptavidin-biotin-peroxidase complex (SABC) method.

Sections were dewaxed, brought to absolute ethanol and then immersed in a methanol/$H_2O_2$/0.3% solution for 20' to abolish endogenous peroxidase's activity. Sections were then washed and incubated in a moist chamber with the following reagents: normal horse serum diluted 1:500 specific monoclonal antibody at proper dilution (overnight); anti-mouse Ig biotinylated antibody 1:500 (Vector Laboratories, Burlingame, CA); streptavidin-biotin-peroxidase complex 1:250 (BIOSPA, Milan, Italy). The immunological reaction was evidentiated by using a 3,3'-diaminobenzidine tetrahydrochloride/$H_2O_2$/0.03% solution in PBS. Sections were counterstained with Harry's haematoxylin, dehydrated and mounted in Eukitt (O. Kindler GmbH, Freiburg, Germany). Negative controls were performed for each case by omitting primary antibody in one of the sections for slide. We used monoclonal anti-EGF-R antibody (clone C11) diluted 1:12,000 (Cambridge Research Biochemical Ltd, Gadbook Park Northwitch, Cheshire, UK).

The evaluation of EGF-R positivity was semiquantitative and based on immunostaining density and distribution. The reaction was characterized as: absent (− −); only rare stained elements (+/−); weak (+) almost <10% immunostained cells; moderate (++) >10% immunostained cells; strong (+++) >50% of positive elements.

TABLE 1. Histological Features and EGF-R Expression in Endometrial Cancer (34 Cases)[a]

| Histotypes | No. Cases | EGF-R ( ) = No. Cases |
|---|---|---|
| AE | 5 | − (4) |
|    |   | +/− (1) |
| AA | 9 | − (1) |
|    |   | +/− (2) |
|    |   | + (4) |
|    |   | ++ (1) |
|    |   | +++ (1) |
| AS | 14 | − (11) |
|    |    | +/− (1) |
|    |    | + (1) |
|    |    | ++ (1) |
| SP | 4 | − (4) |
| M  | 2 | − (2) |

[a] AE = classical endometrioid adenocarcinoma; AA = endometrial adenocarcinoma with benign squamous metaplasia (adenoacanthoma); AS = adenosquamous adenocarcinoma; SP = serous papillary adenocarcinoma; M = mucinous adenocarcinoma; − = absent; +/− = only rare stained elements; + = weak positivity ($<10\%$); ++ = moderate positivity ($>10\%$, $<50\%$); +++ = strong positivity ($>50\%$).

## RESULTS

Of the 34 cases of invasive endometrial carcinoma considered in this study, 5 were histologically classified as classical endometrioid adenocarcinoma (EA, 2 grade I and 3 grade II according to WHO), 2 were of mucinous (M) type, 4 were classified as serous papillary (SP) type with intermixed clear cell areas, and 23 were endometrial carcinoma with SQ cell differentiation. This latter group included 9 adenocarcinomas with benign SQ metaplasia (or AA) and 14 AS carcinomas. The EGF-R expression related to the endometrial cancer histotypes is reported in TABLE 1. Positive staining with anti-EGF-R antibody was recognized in 8 out of 9 AA and in 3 out of 14 AS carcinomas, respectively. Classical EA as well as M and SP endometrial carcinomas were mainly unreactive by using anti-EGF-R antibody showing only weak traces of immunostaining in a negligible number of cells. The immunohistochemical evidentiation of EGF-R showed marked heterogeneity in the cellular staining pattern. Mainly, the general pattern of cellular immunoreactivity was cytoplasmic with a granular accumulation toward the secretory surface or with a cell membrane accentuation. Among the positive cases, only 2 AA and 1 AS showed a minority of elements immunostained by anti-EGF-R antibody, all other cases showed a more diffuse EGF-R positivity, ranging from weak (+) 4 AA and 1 AS respectively; to moderate (++) 1 AA and 1 AS; to strong (+++) 1 AA only. EGF-R immunoreactivity was mainly confined to the neoplastic areas exhibiting a SQ cell differentiation irrespective of their mature or immature metaplastic appearance (FIG. 1). In particular, no apparent difference in the positive immunoreaction was evident between basal-reserve-like cells and epithelial spinous layers within SQ metaplastic component. However, spinous cells presented more often a diffuse cytoplasmic EGF-R positivity while the basal-reserve-like elements showed a granular cytoplasmic expression. In five of the

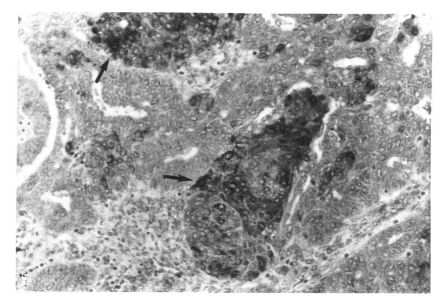

**FIGURE 1.** EGF-R in endometrial carcinoma (adenoacanthoma type). The immunoreactivity is mainly confined to the areas with SQ differentiation (*arrows*). (SABC method, 300×.)

latter cases a positive immunoreaction was also present in part of the neoplastic glandular areas (FIG. 2), indistinguishable by morphology from the remaining unstained glandular tissue.

Positive staining for anti-EGF-R antibody was not significantly associated to clinico-pathological parameters such as tumor size, miometrial invasion, histological grade, vascular neoplastic involvement and tumor stage.

## DISCUSSION

Studies on the expression of EGF-R in endometrial carcinoma led to conflicting results[7-10,14-16] and, further, rarely indicate the degree of growth factors assays in relation to the histomorphologic patterns of the tumor. In fact, little histological information is included in the previous studies being the only morphological constant reference regarding tumor grade.[10,14] In addition, the majority of these investigations reported the assessment of a receptor assay[9,10] using extracted or homogenized tissues. Thus it is impossible with these procedures to correlate the expression of different growth factors with the carcinomatous and/or benign patterns with confidence. Further, endometrial carcinoma rarely shows a single and "pure" histotype. More frequently it shows a variety of histological differentiations as well as entraps benign or malignant squamous areas. This study was initiated to compare the immunohistochemical distribution of EGF-R with the different morphological patterns in a series of conventional sections of formalin-fixed, paraffin-embedded endometrial carcinoma.

EGF-R staining was observed in endometrial cancer with squamous (SQ) differentiation and particularly in those with benign squamous metaplasia, the so-called adenoacanthoma (AA). These results may in part explain the variable expression of the EGF-R in endometrial cancer reported in the literature.[7-10] It has been demonstrated that the EGF-R is differently expressed according to the type of cell, from nothing with lymphoid cells to a high of 250.000 per cell with keratinocytes.[17-19] Furthermore, the EGF-R is the only mitogenic signal required "*in vitro*" by keratinocytes.[20,21] EGF-R expression in a series of malignancies has been highlighted only in squamous tumors[22] as well as in squamous tumors of the female genital tract.[16,23] Analysis of DNA revealed that the amplification of the gene encoding the EGF-R is frequently observed and is related to EGF-R mRNA amounts in cells. These results strongly suggest that EGF-R over-expression is an important step in the transformation of squamous cells.

The EGF-R is a normal constituent of regulatory mechanisms in endometrial cells. It is upregulated by oestrogens and is involved in transducing oestrogen signals to endometrial cells. On the other hand, the EGF-R shows a mitogenic effect on endometrial cells in the absence of oestrogens.[24] However, as malignant transformation progresses, cells loose their normal control mechanisms as steroid hormones, growth factors and their own receptors. Therefore, the EGF-R might not be required for proliferation of malignant cells. Nevertheless, the EGF-R could be an important step in the malignant transformation of squamous tumor.[19] In the present study the EGF-R was detected in endometrial cancer with SQ differentiation, especially in AA. In this latter group the EGF-R was observed prevalently in SQ components. The pattern of immunoreactivity for the EGF-R has been

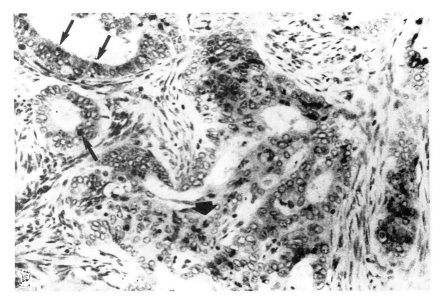

**FIGURE 2.** Endometrial adenoacanthoma showing EGF-R staining both in SQ (*wide arrow*) and glandular (*slender arrows*) areas (SABC method, 300×.)

consistent with those reported in the literature: cell surface granular expression as described for the A431 epidermoid carcinoma cell line,[25] diffuse cytoplasmatic staining probably due to receptor production and internalization of the receptor complex.[26]

The EGF-R is known to influence cellular differentiation in epidermal keratinocytes and should not only be considered involved in a mitogenic mechanism.[19] Specific EGF-R distribution within benign SQ areas of our cases of AA should be prevalently related to the processes of differentiation. However, in some cases EGF-R immunostaining was also present in some glandular areas indistinguishable by morphology from the remaining unstained adenocarcinomatous tissue. It is difficult to explain these observations but it seems reasonable to suppose that EGF-R expression might be related to a different step of cellular differentiation and transformation that is not detectable by morphology. Altogether these observations are in agreement with the above-mentioned relation between EGF-R expression and cellular differentiation. In conclusion, our data indicate that the antigenic determinant recognized by anti-EGF-R antibody OM-11-951 clone C11 was preferentially expressed by the endometrial adenocarcinoma with benign SQ differentiation. The use of different antibodies, precedures, differences in tissue processing and sampling may explain the divergent results[7-10,14] reported in literature.

The remarkable specific association of EGF-R expression and adenocarcinoma with SQ metaplasia seems to suggest a specific involvement of the EGF-R as revealed by this antibody in tumor differentiation with a preferential expression in SQ areas. The present study is the first report clearly demonstrating that EGF-R expression in endometrial cancer is related to the histomorphological type.

## SUMMARY

Epidermal growth factor receptor (EGF-R) has been implicated in the growth of endometrial cancer. In the present study, immunostaining of EGF-R was investigated in different endometrial cancer histotypes. For this purpose 34 surgical samples of primary endometrial carcinoma were studied using monoclonal anti-EGF-R antibody. The endometrial carcinomas were classified according to the International Society of Gynaecological Pathology (I.S.G.P.). EGF-R expression was observed in: 1 of 5 classical endometrioid adenocarcinomas (AE), in 8 of 9 endometrial adenocarcinomas with benign squamous metaplasia (AA), and in 3 of 14 adenosquamous adenocarcinomas (AS). In mucinous (M) and serous papillary adenocarcinoma (SP) EGF-R immunostaining was not observed. The EGF-R positivity was observed in endometrial cancer with squamous (SQ) differentiation, especially in those with benign SQ metaplasia. These results suggest that EGF-R immunostaining is related to the endometrial cancer histotype regardless of the tumor grade or extent of miometrial invasion.

## REFERENCES

1. Bossert, N. L., K. G. Nelson, K. A. Ross, T. Takahashi & J. A. McLachlan. 1990. Epidermal growth factor binding and receptor distribution in the mouse reproductive tract during development. Dev. Biol. **142:** 75–85.
2. Yamashita, S., R. R. Newbold, J. A. McLachlan & K. S. Korach. 1989. Developmental pattern of estrogen receptor expression in female mouse genital tracts. Endocrinology **125:** 2888–2896.

3. YAMASHITA, S., R. R. NEWBOLD, J. A. MCLACHLAN & K. S. KORACH. 1990. The role of the estrogen receptor in uterine epithelial proliferation and cytodifferentiation in neonatal mice. Endocrinology **127:** 2456–2463.
4. MUKKU, V. R. & G. M. STANCEL. 1985. Regulation of epidermal growth factor receptor by estrogen. J. Biol. Chem. **260:** 9820–9824.
5. TAKETANI, Y. & M. MIZUNO. 1988. Cyclic changes in epidermal growth factor receptor in human endometrium during menstrual cycle. Endocrinol. Jpn. **35:** 19–25.
6. JASONNI, V. M., C. BULLETTI, M. BALDUCCI, S. NALDI, G. MARTINELLI, A. GALASSI *et al.* 1991. The effect of progestin on factors influencing growth and invasion of endometrial carcinoma. Ann. N.Y. Acad. Sci. **622:** 463–468.
7. BATTAGLIA, F., G. SCAMBIA, P. B. PANICI *et al.* 1989. Epidermal growth factor receptor expression in gynecological malignancies. Gynecol. Obstet. Invest. **27:** 42–44.
8. BERCHUCK, A., A. P. SOISSON, G. J. OLT *et al.* 1989. Epidermal growth factor receptor expression in normal and malignant endometrium. Am. J. Obstet. Gynecol. **161:** 1247–1252.
9. LEAKE, R., L. CARR & F. RINALDI. 1991. Autocrine and paracrine effects in the endometrium. Ann. N.Y. Acad. Sci. **622:** 145–148.
10. REYNOLDS, R. K., F. TALAVERA, J. A. ROBERTS, M. P. HOPKINS & K. M. J. MENON. 1990. Characterization of epidermal growth factor receptor in normal and neoplastic human endometrium. Cancer **66:** 1967–1974.
11. ZAINO, R. S. *et al.* 1991. The significance of squamous differentiation in endometrial carcinoma. Cancer **68:** 2293–2302.
12. SILVEBERG, S. G. & R. J. KURMORE. 1992. Atlas of Tumor Pathology: Tumors of the Uterine Corpus and Gestational Trophoblastic Diseases. J. Rosai, Ed. Third Series Fascicle 3 AFIP. 47–89.
13. Anonymous. 1989. Announcements. FIGO Stages. 1988 revision. Gynecol. Oncol. **35:** 125–127.
14. NYHOLM, H. C. J., A. L. NIELSEN & B. OTTESEN. 1993. Expression of epidermal growth factor receptors in human endometrial carcinoma. Int. J. Gynecol. Pathol. **12:** 241–245.
15. BAUKNECHT, T., M. KOHLER, I. JANZ & A. PFLEIDERER. 1989. The occurrence of epidermal growth factor receptors and the characterization of EGF-like factors in human ovarian, endometrial, cervical and breast cancer. J. Cancer Res. Clin. Oncol. **115:** 193–199.
16. KORC, M., C. A. HAUSSLER & N. S. TROOKMAN. 1987. Divergent effects of epidermal growth factor and transforming growth factors on a human endometrial carcinoma cell line. Cancer Res. **47:** 4909–4914.
17. COWLEY, G., J. A. SMITH, B. GUSTERSON, F. HENDLER & B. OZANNE. 1984. The amount of EGF receptor is elevated on squamous cell carcinoma. *In* Cancer Cell. The Transformed Phenotype. Vol. 1: 5–10. Cold Spring Harbor Laboratory. Cold Spring Harbor, NY.
18. COWLEY, G. P., J. A. SMITH & B. A. GUSTERSON. 1986. Increased EGF receptor on human squamous carcinoma cell lines. Br. J. Cancer **53:** 223–229.
19. OZANNE, B., A. SCHUM, C. S. RICHARDS *et al.* 1985. Evidence from increased EGF receptor in epidermal malignancies. Growth Factors and Transformation. *In* Cancer Cells. Vol. 3: 41–49. Cold Spring Harbor Laboratory. Cold Spring Harbor, NY.
20. TSAO, M. C., B. J. WALTHALL & R. G. HAM. 1982. Clonal growth of normal human epidermal keratinocytes in a defined medium. J. Cell. Physiol. **110:** 219–229.
21. WILLE, J. J., M. R. PITTELKOW, G. D. SHIPLEY & R. E. SCOTT. 1984. Integrated control of growth and differentiation of normal human prokeratinocytes cultured in serum free medium: cloned analyses, growth kinetics and cell surface studies. J. Cell. Physiol. **121:** 31–44.
22. OZANNE, B. & C. S. RICHARDS. 1986. Over-expression of the EGF receptor is a hallmark of squamous cell carcinomas. J. Pathol. **149:** 9–14.
23. HENDLER, F. J. & B. W. OZANNE. 1984. Human squamous cell lung cancers express increased epidermal growth factor receptors. J. Clin. Invest. **74:** 647–651.
24. MCLACHLAN, J. A., K. G. NELSON, T. TAKAHASHI, N. L. BOSSERT, R. R. NEWBOLD

& K. S. KORACH. 1991. Estrogens and growth factors in the development, growth and function of the female reproductive tract. *In* Growth Factors in Reproduction. David W. Schomberg, Ed. Springer Verlag, Inc. New York.
25. WATERFIELD, M., L. MAYES, P. STROOBANT, P. BENNET, S. YOUNG, P. GOODFELLOW, P. BANTING & OZANNE B. 1982. A monoclonal antibody to the human epidermal growth factor receptor. J. Cell. Biochem. **20:** 149–161.
26. GUSTERSON, B., G. COWLEY, H. SMITH & O. BRADFORD. 1984. Cellular localization of epidermal growth factor receptor. Cell Biol. Int. Rep. **8:** 649–658.

# Clinical Response of Abnormal Endometrial Growth to Hormonal Treatment

E. LÓPEZ DE LA OSA GONZÁLEZ

*Department of Obstetrics and Gynecology*
*Universidad Complutense*
*Hospital Universitario San Carlos*
*28040 Madrid, Spain*

## INTRODUCTION

For more than three decades endometrial hyperplasia and advanced stages of adenocarcinoma have been known to respond to hormonal treatment. Initially, only empirical clinical data supported our understanding of the facts, and this knowledge widened as we advanced in deciphering the intricate network of signals responsible for the sequence of events in the different cell populations of this complex and peculiar tissue.

After the positive results with natural progesterone, progestins took over and made the core of our clinical results. A brief, confusing and somewhat frustrating experience derived from certain expectations with the use of antiestrogenic drugs, probably helped to fuel efforts that evolved into a broader vision beyond the too simplistic estrogen/progesterone balance theory.

Recently, consistent with the rationale of the estrogen blockade, the use of Gn-RH agonists was advocated. Little information is available on this matter, and preliminary information of an ongoing clinico-pathological study is presented here.

### *Progesterone and Progestins*

Since the early observation by Kelley and Baker in 1960 that progesterone treatment in patients with metastatic endometrial cancer showed clinical remissions, further focusing on this therapeutical possibility, and the results obtained,[1] established progestins as a form of treatment for advanced endometrial cancer. Later on, a better knowledge of the biology of this tumor, the understanding of the role of steroid hormone receptors and the definition of prognostic factors including histopathologic tumor grade, data on ploidy and the content of steroid receptors, allowed the recognition of different tumor types also responding differently to hormonal treatment.

The inclusion of radioimmunoanalytical procedures as a common clinical practice offered better knowledge of the foreseeable response of every individual patient, as did also some clinial tests based on the measurement of biochemical intracellular profiles such as the differences in the estradiol-17$\beta$ dehydrogenase or isocitric dehydrogenase activities.[2,3]

There is general agreement on the concept that the presence of progesterone receptors is necessary to elicit a response to progestin treatment, as proved in the different clinical studies reviewed by Kauppila.[4]

Progesterone initially, and later progestins because of their higher potency, lack of side effects and easier route of administration, have been a treatment of choice for simple to severe endometrial hyperplasia, provided there were no atypia, due to the different intracellular mechanisms of action of such a hormone (activation of the estradiol dehydrogenase enzyme system, reduction of available estrogen receptor sites, inhibition of DNA synthesis), which ultimately would induce a regression of the hyperplastic changes.[5]

Medroxyprogesterone acetate has also been shown to exert regressive changes on well differentiated endometrial adenocarcinoma, although these regressive changes are more easily induced on well differentiated tumors with high levels of progesterone receptors.[6] These findings, however, should not modify the common first indication of surgery for this type of tumor, hormonal treatment remaining an adjuvant possibility.

The morphological changes observed in the hyperplastic endometria under the effect of progestins show similarities with an early secretory phase, absence of mitosis, monostratified arrangement of the nuclei in the glandular layer and a general image of inactive epithelium, together with deciduoid changes in the stromal cells.

The regressive effect is not so consistent on the adenocarcinoma, as seen in those cases where hyperplastic changes coexist with areas of carcinoma and the tumoral features remain with little modification, isolated among a secretory-like pattern of the regressed hyperplastic tissue.[7]

## *Effect of Tamoxifen*

Mention has to be made of the effect of Tamoxifen on the endometrium for a proper understanding of hormonal actions. However, in this particular case it is rather the converse effect that has been found. After the good results obtained with the treatment of Tamoxifen as adjuvant in the therapy of breast cancer, there was a rationale for a similar application in patients with endometrial cancer, and though there were initial data in this direction, important information derived from a trial in Stockholm, which showed a significant increase of primary endometrial cancers among patients receiving Tamoxifen.[8] Treatment with Tamoxifen is generally given to patients as adjuvant therapy for breast cancer, and has been correlated with different forms of endometrial abnormal growth from endometrial hyperplasia to adenocarcinoma, as is also shown in two recent reports.[9,10] Further studies both at the clinical and biochemical levels have proved a stimulatory effect of Tamoxifen on the endometrial epithelium of an estrogen-like sort. Furthermore, a stimulatory effect of Tamoxifen on endometrial cancer cells (Ishikawa cell line) in culture could be shown.[11]

Most patients receiving this form of adjuvant treatment do not develop this particular type of endometrial response, showing atrophic patterns with occasional proliferation. However, the unpredictability of the malignant development under this therapy requires some form of monitoring that should be done in the form of regular endometrial biopsies, as suggested by Gusberg.[12]

## *Gn-RH Analogs*

The effectiveness of the use of this new family of synthetic hormonal agents in the treatment of a large array of conditions where steroid hormones, and specifically estradiol, have to be downregulated, suggested its application in the case of abnormal endometrial growth. A rationale similar to the one considered for the use of progestins impedes the primary and only hormonal approach to treatment in the case of endometrial cancer. Very little information regarding the experience with this type of medication is available. A recent report presents some interesting results in a group of 17 patients with recurrent and progestogen-resistant endometrial cancer.[13] Six patients responded and one showed complete response. Five patients were still in remission 7 to 30 months after the treatment. Two patients maintained the disease in stable condition, and 8 died of progression of the tumor.

Our experience is based on a group of 30 patients showing different degrees of endometrial hyperplasia, without atypia, to be treated for six months with triptorelin 3.75 mg in monthly depot injections. Thus far only some of the patients have completed the treatment regimen. The morphology of the endometrial biopsies shows a pattern comparable to a mid-proliferative phase, with straight glands whose epithelium shows a monolayer nuclear arrangement, with absence of vacuolar formations. The stroma is devoid of mitosis and presents a peculiar fibroblastoid pattern. The ultrastructural image with transmission electron microscopy shows a substantial reduction in the number of cell organelles, strongly altered mytochondrial images and a high content in collagen.

The important morphological changes observed in hyperplastic endometria under the effect of long-term treatment with Gn-RH analogs, in conjunction with the fact that a significant number of clinical remissions have been obtained in endometrial adenocarcinomas not responding to progesterone treatment, suggest the possibility of a direct effect on the abnormal epithelial cell and its intrinsic metabolic features. An important issue to establish with this tissue is the possible, direct or indirect, effect of the Gn-RH analog on the different growth factors so far identified as controlling the development of the epithelial endometrial cell.

## SUMMARY

The diverse types of abnormal endometrial tissue growth have received different forms of treatment, with a particular emphasis on the use of hormonal agents. Hyperplastic endometria have benefited from progesterone or progestin therapies, with good results. Endometrial cancer is a disease with a major indication for surgical treatment. However, advanced clinical stages have been shown to improve as a result of different medical treatments. This presentation reviews the literature on this subject, includes some considerations on the role of some antiestrogens as endometrial tumor promoters in certain patients undergoing adjuvant therapy, and discusses the possibilities of Gn-RH analogs, one of the recent proposals in the treatment of adenocarcinoms and endometrial hyperplasia, including morphological observations of an investigation currently in progress in our department.

## REFERENCES

1. KELLEY, R. M. & W. H. BAKER. 1965. The role of progesterone in human endometrial cancer. Cancer Res. **25:** 1190–1192.
2. TSENG, L. & E. GURPIDE. 1974. Estradiol and 20α dihydroprogesterone dehydrogenase activities in human endometrium during the menstrual cycle. Endocrinology **94:** 419–423.

3. LANE, G. & R. J. B. KING. 1989. The histochemistry of oestradiol 17β and isocitric dehydrogenases in endometrial carcinoma. J. Steroid Biochem. **33:** 853–858.
4. KAUPPILA, A. 1989. Oestrogen and progestin receptors as prognostic indicators in endometrial cancer. Acta Oncol. **28:** 561–566.
5. JOHN, H. A., J. S. CORNES, W. D. JACKSON & P. BYE. 1974. Effect of a systemically administered progesterone on the istopathology of endometrial carcinoma. J. Obstet. Gynaecol. Br. Commonw. **8:** 786–790.
6. DELIGDISCH, L. & C. F. HOLINKA. 1986. Progesterone receptors in two groups of endometrial adenocarcinoma. Cancer **57:** 1385–1388.
7. DELIGDISCH, L. 1993. Effects of hormone therapy on the endometrium. Mod. Pathol. **6:** 94–106.
8. FORNANDER, T., L. E. RUTQVIST, B. CEDERMARK, U. GLAS, A. MATTSON, J. D. SILVERSWARD, L. SKOOG, A. SOMELL, T. THEVE, N. WILKING, J. ASKERGREN & M. L. HJOLMAR. 1989. Adjuvant tamoxifen in early breast cancer: occurrence of new primary cancers. Lancet **1:** 117–120.
9. MALFETANO, J. H. 1990. Tamoxifen associated endometrial carcinoma in postmenopausal breast cancer patients. Gynecol. Oncol. **39:** 82–86.
10. SEGNA, R. A., P. R. DOTTINO, L. DELIGDISCH & C. J. COHEN. 1992. Tamoxifen and endometrial neoplasia: a report of eleven cases. Mt. Sinai J. Med. **59:** 416–418.
11. ANZAI, Y., C. F. HOLINKA, H. KURAMOTO & E. GURPIDE. 1989. Stimulatory effects of 4-hydroxytamoxifen on proliferation of human endometrial adenocarcinoma cells (Ishikawa line). Cancer Res. **49:** 2362–2365.
12. GUSBERG, S. B. 1990. Tamoxifen for breast cancer: associated endometrial cancer. Cancer **65:** 1463–1464.
13. GALLAGHER, C. J., R. T. D. OLIVER, D. H. ORAM, C. G. FOWLER, P. R. BLAKE, B. S. MANTELL, M. L. SLEVIN & H. F. HOPE-STONE. 1991. A new treatment for endometrial cancer with gonadotrophin releasing-hormone analog. Br. J. Obstet. Gynaecol. **98:** 1037–1041.

# Tamoxifen and Endometrial Cancer

P. SISMONDI, N. BIGLIA, E. VOLPI, M. GIAI,
AND T. DE GRANDIS

*Institute of Gynecology and Obstetrics*
*Department of Gynecological Oncology*
*University of Turin*
*Via Ventimiglia, 3*
*10126 Turin, Italy*

## INTRODUCTION

Breast cancer represents 30% of all cancers in women and causes about 20% of all cancer deaths, second only to lung cancer.[1] Since the beginning of the 1980s breast cancer incidence has increased approximately 3% per year in the Western world, and it is predicted that cancer will overtake cardiovascular disease as the major cause of death by the early twenty-first century.

Tamoxifen (TAM) is the endocrine treatment of choice for selected patients with all stages of breast cancer, and there are plans to evaluate its use as a preventive treatment in healthy women at high risk for breast tumor.[2,3]

TAM has an estrogen-like influence on the skeletal and cardiovascular systems resulting in decreases in both postmenopausal bone loss[4,5] and low-density lipoprotein levels;[6,7] these effects determine a reduction in the incidence of osteoporosis[8] and coronary heart disease.[9] The positive benefits that may accrue from the estrogen-like actions of TAM on bone and lipids could act as a double-edged sword and could possibly facilitate the promotion of endometrial cancers. In the United States this neoplasia represents 6% of cancer incidence and 2.3% of cancer deaths, compared with 31.5% and 18.4% respectively for breast cancer. As therapeutic use of TAM has extended to 5 years and beyond, and as clinical trials begin to assess the effectiveness of TAM as a preventive treatment, concern about possible long-term adverse effects is justified.[10,11]

The balance of benefits versus risks and unfavorable consequences of long-term treatment have to be considered.

## ADJUVANT THERAPY FOR BREAST CANCER PATIENTS

In a recent overview analysis of 133 randomized clinical trials involving 70,000 women treated with adjuvant therapy, TAM has proved to be effective in the treatment of breast cancer.[12] During the first 5 years of TAM there was an estimated 8.3% increase in recurrence-free survival; in addition, TAM increased the time between recurrence and death, producing a 3.6% decrease in mortality at 5 years, increasing to 6.2% at 10 years. This suggests that TAM produces a survival advantage beyond the point at which it is no longer providing benefit in preventing recurrence.

The proportional reduction in annual risk is 25% for recurrence-free survival and 17% for overall survival.

The proportional risk reductions are similar for node-negative and node-positive women, so the absolute risk reduction is greater among node-positive women.

TABLE 1. Cumulative Frequency of Controlateral Breast Cancers in Clinical Trials of Adjuvant Tamoxifen Therapy Compared with Placebo or Observation in Women with Early-Stage Breast Cancer[a]

| Clinical Trials | Patients Treated with TAM | | Controls | |
|---|---|---|---|---|
| | No. Patients | No. Cancers (%) | No. Patients | No. Cancers (%) |
| NATO[17] | 564 | 15 (2.6%) | 567 | 17 (3%) |
| Scottish[18] | 661 | 9 (1.4%) | 651 | 12 (1.8%) |
| Stockholm[19] | 931 | 18 (1.9%) | 915 | 32 (3.5%) |
| Copenhagen[20] | 164 | 3 (1.8%) | 153 | 4 (2.6%) |
| Toronto-Edmonton[21] | 198 | 3 (1.5%) | 202 | 3 (1.5%) |
| ECOG 1178[22] | 91 | 1 (1.1%) | 90 | 3 (3.3%) |
| NSABP B-14[23] | 1419 | 23 (1.6%) | 1428 | 32 (2.2%) |
| CRC[32] | 947 | 7 (0.7%) | 965 | 18 (1.9%) |
| Total | 4975 | 79 (1.6%) | 4971 | 121 (2.4%) |

[a] Based on Nayfield.[50]

The estrogen receptor (ER) content of breast tumors represents an excellent marker for prognosis during TAM treatment; however, TAM has produced a response also in 10% of patients with ER-negative tumors.

The overview analysis indicated that doses of more than 20 mg/day do not provide advantages, while duration of treatment correlates positively with benefit; in fact experimental studies have shown that TAM is a cytostatic rather than a cytotoxic drug and this type of action requires a prolonged treatment.

## CHEMOPREVENTION FOR HIGH-RISK BREAST CANCER WOMEN

There is a wealth of biological and clinical information to encourage the use of TAM as a chemopreventive agent.

In the laboratory, TAM prevents the initiation of rat mammary tumors with carcinogens[13,14] and long-term therapy suppresses the development of the disease if the drug is administered after initiation.[15,16] In breast cancer patients the risk of a carcinoma of the controlateral breast is increased 3 times compared to the general population; the incidence has been estimated at 8 per 1000 annually.

The tumoristatic activity of TAM should impede the growth of undetected hormone-responsive controlateral breast cancers. Laboratory data were confirmed by several clinical trials which showed a statistically significant reduction of about 40% of second primary breast carcinoma in patients receiving adjuvant TAM (TABLE 1).[17-24]

## ENDOMETRIAL CANCER IN TAMOXIFEN-TREATED PATIENTS

TAM has been found to stimulate the growth of endometrial cancer in the laboratory;[25-27] in the athymic mouse model, ER-positive endometrial tumors can be stimulated to grow in the presence of TAM.

The antiestrogenic property of TAM is related to its capacity to occupy the ER in endometrial target cells; in postmenopausal women with little estradiol available, TAM can readily act estrogenically by that receptor action.[28]

Uncontrolled case series of endometrial cancers were reported among women receiving TAM (TABLE 2);[29-49] TABLE 3[17-23] reviews the rates of endometrial cancer in several clinical trials. The cumulative frequency of endometrial cancer in all women receiving TAM is 0.5% versus 0.1% in the control group.[50] When the higher-dose Stockholm trial[19] (40 mg/day) is excluded, the differences in frequency in the 6 trials using 20 mg/day are not as dramatic: 0.3% (9/3097 TAM-treated patients) compared with 0.1% (4/3091 control subjects). These results include those of the two large Scottish trials[18] and of the National Surgical Adjuvant Breast and Bowel Project,[23] in which the lower dose of TAM has been administered continuously for at least 5 years. The TAM-associated increase in risk of endometrial cancer is similar in magnitude to that associated with postmenopausal estrogen replacement therapy.

A retrospective, population-based study using the Northern Alberta Breast Cancer Registry shows no increased risk of uterine cancer with TAM use. Thirty-one cases of endometrial cancer were found in 10,075 women who were diagnosed as having a breast cancer from 1953 to 1988; 3 cases were reported in the group treated with TAM (1874 pts, 0.16%) and 28 cases were observed in the group without TAM (8201 cases, 0.29%).[51]

Not all authors agree about an increased incidence of endometrial cancer during TAM. Symptoms of uterine cancer in postmenopause (vaginal bleeding and vaginal discharge) are similar to those induced by long-term TAM treatment. It is possible that TAM will result in a higher detection rate of latent endometrial carcinoma, determining an artificially increased correlation between TAM and endometrial cancer.[10,45] Moreover, it is important to consider that several cases present a too short delay between the beginning of TAM treatment and the diagnosis of endometrial cancer and that, in the major part of the studies, the pretreatment condition of uterine cavity is not verified. It is possible in several cases that TAM has only stimulated the occurrence of a preexisting endometrial tumor.

TABLE 2. Tamoxifen and Endometrial Cancer—Case Reports

| Author | No. Cases | Dosage (mg) | Duration (Months) |
|---|---|---|---|
| Killackey[29] | 3 | 20 | 7–14 |
| Pons[30] | 1 | 30 | 10 |
| Hardell[31] | 11 | 40 | 12–120 |
| Fornander[32] | 13 | 40 | 24–60 |
| Dauplat[33] | 2 | 20–30 | 18–24 |
| Mathew[34] | 5 | 20 | 50–96 |
| Malfetano[35] | 7 | 20 | 18–48 |
| Atlante[36] | 4 | 40–60 | 24–60 |
| Neven[37] | 1 | 20 | 36 |
| Rodier[38] | 1 | 40 | 8 |
| Segna[39] | 11 | 10–20 | 5–84 |
| Uziely[40] | 2 | n.r. | >24 |
| Osborne[41] | 4 | n.r. | 12 |
| O'Neill[42] | 1 | 20 | 60 |
| Mignotte[43] | 20 | 20 | 29–102 |
| Deprest[44] | 1 | 40 | 96 |
| Le Bouedec[45] | 4 | 20–30 | 3–30 |
| Spinelli[46] | 3 | 20 | 24–60 |
| Palacios[47] | 1 | 20 | 104 |
| Teshima[48] | 4 | 20–40 | 24–96 |
| Samelis[49] | 1 | 20–40 | 24–156 |

TABLE 3. Cumulative Frequency of Uterine Cancers in Clinical Trials of Adjuvant Tamoxifen Therapy Compared with Placebo or Observation in Women with Early-Stage Breast Cancer[a]

| Clinical Trials | Patients Treated with TAM | | Controls | |
|---|---|---|---|---|
| | No. Patients | No. Cancers (%) | No. Patients | No. Cancers (%) |
| NATO[17] (20 mg/day) | 564 | 0 (0%) | 567 | 0 (0%) |
| Scottish[18] (20 mg/day) | 661 | 4 (0.6%) | 651 | 2 (0.3%) |
| Stockholm[19] (40 mg/day) | 931 | 13 (1.4%) | 915 | 2 (0.2%) |
| Copenhagen[20] (20 mg/day) | 164 | 2 (1.2%) | 153 | 0 (0%) |
| Toronto-Edmonton[21] (20 mg/day) | 198 | 0 (0%) | 202 | 1 (0.5%) |
| ECOG 1178[22] (20 mg/day) | 91 | 1 (1.1%) | 90 | 1 (1.1%) |
| NSABP B-14[23] (20 mg/day) | 1419 | 2 (0.1%) | 1428 | 0 (0%) |
| Total | 4028 | 22 (0.5%) | 4006 | 6 (0.1%) |
| Total 20 mg/day | 3097 | 9 (0.3%) | 3091 | 4 (0.1%) |

[a] Based on Nayfield.[50]

## Gynecological Surveillance

### Vaginal Cytodiagnosis

An indication about the estrogenic activity of TAM on the uterus may be derived from vaginal cytodiagnosis. The maturity index (MI) of postmenopausal patients often shows evidence of the estrogenic effect of TAM, with an increase of intermediate cells and superficial cells compared with control patients;[48,52] however, no correlation was found between dose and duration of TAM and the degree of cellular response.

Endocervical smears of these patients also showed a higher proportion of cells with hyperplastic nuclei, while no association with the development of atypical cells was observed.[53]

### Transvaginal Ultrasound

Since the endometrium can easily be visualized by transvaginal ultrasound (TVS), this method has been suggested as a means of following patients receiving TAM.

In postmenopausal women the endometrial sonogram generally appears as a thin linear echo. In case of endometrial hyperplasia ultrasound shows a well defined, thick and highly reflective layer occupying the whole endometrial cavity and surrounded by a symmetrical poorly reflective zone. An irregular, thickened, highly reflective area of endometrial lining with loss of the surrounding symmetrical area of low amplitude echoes is suspicious for endometrial carcinoma.[54,55]

Sonographic uterine findings of postmenopausal patients treated with TAM are frequently abnormal (TABLE 4).[53,56–59] The sonographic imagines include: thick, hyperechoic, homogeneous tissue; hyperechoic tissue with multiple small cystic spaces, heterogeneous tissue with small cystic spaces; solid heterogeneous tissue and polyps. Because different pathologic findings frequently coexist, sonography is of limited use in the diagnosis of specific abnormalities.[58]

Long-term treatment with TAM has an estrogenic effect on the postmenopausal uterus: compared with the control group, TAM-treated patients had a thicker endometrium, a larger uterine volume and an increased occurrence of polyps as determined by TVS.

A correlation between echographic endometrial patterns and histology in postmenopausal women not receiving TAM has been demonstrated by several authors. In a recent study performed on 120 postmenopausal patients with abnormal vaginal bleeding, 98 women had endometrial thickness less than 5 mm; histologic examination revealed atrophic endometrium in 76 cases and insufficient tissue in the other 22 cases. In 22 patients endometrial thickness was greater than 5 mm and hystology revealed 10 cases of hyperplastic endometrium, 8 endometrial cancers and 4 polyps.[55]

On the contrary, in women receiving TAM a correlation between the endometrial width, as measured by TVS, and the histological finding is often absent. In a study performed on 71 asymptomatic postmenopausal patients treated with TAM, among the 71 patients with thicker endometrium (6–46 mm), 50 (69%) yielded no endometrial tissue at biopsy, 17 (23.6%) demonstrated a normal proliferative endometrium, 3 (4%) had an endometrial polyp and 1 (1.4%) had hyperplastic endometrium.[59]

In the study of Lahti, despite on the ultrasound image of thicker endometrium in TAM-treated patients, hysteroscopic examination showed an atrophic endometrium in 28% of the cases in the TAM group compared with 87% of the control subjects; an increased occurrence of precancerous lesions in association with TAM treatment was not observed.[56]

All women treated with TAM presenting with a sonogram suggestive of endometrial neoplasia should undergo biopsy; however, the definitive diagnosis could be less alarming.

*Endometrial Sampling*

Most endometrial biopsies of postmenopausal patients treated with TAM show inactive and atrophic endometrium with occasional proliferative features; however, hyperplastic endometrial changes are also reported (TABLE 5).[57,59,60]

TABLE 4. Vaginal Ultrasound Findings in TAM-Treated and Control Postmenopausal Women

| Author | Dose (mg) | Duration (Months) | Endometrial Thickness (mm) | |
|---|---|---|---|---|
| | | | Cases | Controls |
| Lahti[56] | 20–40 | 30 | 10.4 | 4.2 |
| Uzan[57] | 20 | 12 | 5 before TAM 7 after TAM | |
| Hulka[58] | | | 22 (8–38) | |
| Rayter[53] | n.r. | >36 | 8.9 | 7.8 |
| Cohen[59] | 20–30 | 6–96 | 6–46 | |
| Sismondi | 20–30 | 1–120 | 9 (2–46) | 4 (1–12) |

TABLE 5. Histologic Endometrial Findings in Postmenopausal TAM-Treated Patients

| Author | Normal/Absent | Atrophic | Proliferative | Hyperplastic | Carcinoma |
|---|---|---|---|---|---|
| Cohen[59] | 50 (69.4%) | | 17 (23%) | 1 (1.4%) | 1 (1.4%) |
| Gal[24] | | | | 7/38 (18%) | |
| Uzan[57] [a] | 3/8 (37.7%) | | | 5/8 (63.3%) | |
| Sismondi[b] | 2/29 (6.8%) | 16/29 (55%) | 2/29 (6.8%) | 3/29 (10.3%) | 1/29 (3.4%) |

[a] Endometrial thickness >8 mm.
[b] Symptomatic patients or endometrial thickness >5 mm.

In the study of Gal 18% of the postmenopausal breast cancer women showed endometrial hyperplasia after 12 months of TAM 20 mg/day; 11 patients were examined before and during treatment, and in 3/11 (27%) endometrial hyperplasia was found while on therapy.[60]

De Muylder found that the rate of endometrial hyperplasia appears to be related to the cumulative dose of TAM; the latency period between TAM exposure and endometrial hyperplasia was at least 15 months, and 24 months on average; on the contrary, nearly half the polyps were detected after less than 1 year.[61]

It is unclear why some postmenopausal women respond to TAM with a proliferative endometrium, whereas others respond with endometrial atrophy. In a recent study an association was found between the absence of ER/PR in breast cancer tissue and a lack of endometrial abnormalities in curettage specimens of patients treated with TAM. All women with endometrial abnormalities were ER positive; however, higher ER or PR concentrations show no correlations with a higher frequency of abnormal abnormalities. It is possible that postmenopausal breast cancer patients are less vulnerable to the development of endometrial modifications in case of negative ER or PR breast tumors.[62]

*Hysteroscopy*

Patients with abnormal uterine ultrasound or vaginal bleeding may be evaluated by hysteroscopy. However, in many cases, TAM-treated patients with abnormal uterine sonogram show an atrophic endometrium with no abnormality at hysteroscopic examination (TABLE 6).[56,61] It is possible that TAM affects myometrium rather than the endometrium; this effect probably represents a direct action of the drug, not mediated by estradiol.[63]

Uzan[57] monitored 35 breast cancer patients treated with TAM 20 mg/day with TVS and endometrial sampling before TAM administration and every 3 months

TABLE 6. Hysteroscopic Findings in Postmenopausal TAM-Treated and Control Patients

| Author | Atrophic/Normal | Polyps | Fibroids | Hyperplasia | Carcinoma |
|---|---|---|---|---|---|
| Lahti[56] | | | | | |
| Cases | 13/47 (28%) | 17/51 (36%) | 8/51 (17%) | 2/51 (4%) | 1/51 (2%) |
| Controls | 42/48 (87%) | 5/52 (10%) | 2/52 (4%) | 1/52 (2%) | 0 (0%) |
| De Muylder[61] | 23/46 (50%) | 13/46 (28.2%) | | 8/46 (17.4%) | 2/46 (4%) |

of therapy; suspicious cases underwent hysteroscopy. The mean total thickness of the endometrium increased from 5 to 7 mm after 12 months of TAM; in 8/35 patients the total thickness increased above normal (>8 mm) and subsequent hysteroscopy showed that 3 had normal endometrium, 3 simple hyperplasia and 1 atypical hyperplasia. An estrogenic action was also seen in the uterine arteries where the blood flow velocity changes were consistent with those described in postmenopausal women receiving estrogen. It is worth noting that this effect was of rapid onset (1–3 months of TAM) and then seemed to stabilize and perhaps even reduce slightly.

### *Prognosis of TAM-Associated Endometrial Cancers*

Endometrial tumors that develop in breast cancer patients treated with TAM are generally diagnosed at an early stage and have a high grade of curability.

However, recently several cases of high grade endometrial cancers or uncommon histological types have been reported in the literature in women receiving TAM. Silva[64] found a higher incidence of clear cell carcinoma and serous carcinoma of the endometrium in patients treated with TAM compared to patients who did not receive TAM and developed uterine cancers. Deligdisch[65] reported 9 cases of endometrial cancers in TAM-treated patients: 2 were poorly differentiated and in 3 cases a deep myometrial invasion was present. In a retrospective review of 53 patients with a history of breast cancer who subsequently developed endometrial cancer, the mean interval between detection of breast and endometrial cancer was 5 years in the TAM group and 12 years in the nontreated group. 67% of patients in the TAM group had poorly differentiated endometrioid carcinomas or carcinomas associated with poor outcome, as compared with 24% in the nontreated group. The author concludes that women receiving TAM who subsequently develop uterine cancer are at risk for high grade endometrial cancer at poor prognosis; TAM-associated uterine cancers may have different bases from those associated with steroidal estrogen treatment.[66]

## OUR EXPERIENCE WITH ENDOMETRIAL SONOGRAPHIC PATTERN IN PATIENTS EXPOSED TO TAMOXIFEN

To evaluate the effect of the therapy with TAM on the endometrium of women already treated for breast carcinoma we scanned 147 patients. A first group had TAM therapy (20–30 mg/day) (95 cases), while the control group never had adjuvant therapy after surgical treatment (52 cases).

The median age of the patients was 61 (range 41–82); no difference was found between the two groups. All but four patients were postmenopausal.

Twenty-eight patients of the first group had vaginal bleeding.

The median time of treatment was 24 months (1–120 months).

Two different ultrasonographic devices were used: a Bruel & Kjaer type 1846 with the 7 MHz probe (type 8538) and Aloka SSD-680 with the 5 MHz probe.

Transvaginal scanning was performed with emptied bladder and the patient lying in anti-Trendelenburg position to let the ovaries be nearer to the vagina.

Endometrial thickness was calculated averaging the two different diameters measured in transverse and longitudinal scanning, excluding the periendometrial halo. Furthermore, the endometrial texture was evaluated, considering the homogeneity of the endometrial pattern, the presence of little anechogenic areas and the presence of fluid in the uterine cavity.

The limit to perform biopsy was 5 mm, at the beginning of our experience, also because no paper about TAM and endometrium was published at that time. In a second phase this limit was increased to 10 mm.

Endometrial biopsy was performed either by dilatation and curettage or more frequently by suction curettage (Securette).

A database was set up and statistical analysis was performed with Epi-Info (Version 5).

## Results

The median endometrial thickness of the TAM group was 9.0 mm (2.0–46.0) versus 4.0 mm (1.0–2.0) of the control group. The difference is significant (Wilcoxon two-sample test $p < 0.0001$).

Forty-eight out of 95 (54.3%) patients in the first group showed an endometrial thickness less than or equal to 10 mm, while only 3 patients in the control group did so.

The endometrium of the patients receiving TAM had a typical sonographic pattern which is characterized by thickening and dishomogeneity with small anechogenic areas of different sizes (1–5 mm), which was diagnosed in 52 out of 95 cases. The dishomogeneity of the endometrial pattern can be shown when the endometrial thickness is under 10 mm (13 cases, 26.4%). In 9 patients in the first group TVS also showed ovarian anechogenic cysts which were considered as functional.

Thirty-four endometrial biopsies were attempted in 147 patients: 29 in the patients receiving TAM and 5 in the control group. In 2 cases biopsy was impossible and the patient was released. The histological results of the biopsies are shown in the TABLE 5.

## CONCLUSIONS

TAM is the endocrine treatment of choice for all stages of breast cancer in both pre and postmenopausal women.

The estrogen-like influence of TAM on the skeletal and cardiovascular systems results in decreases in the incidence of osteoporosis and coronary heart disease, which are major causes of morbidity and mortality in postmenopausal age. TAM also determines a significant decreased rate of controlateral breast cancers, and is probably beneficial over and above the primary actions as antitumor agent.

TAM appears to play a role in increasing the risk of developing endometrial cancer from 0.1% to 0.3–0.5% depending on dosage. The 5-fold excess in endometrial cancer risk reported by the Stockholm trial, which used 40 mg TAM daily, is not confirmed in several trials using 20 mg daily. In the light of the extensive use of this drug, the overall incidence of endometrial cancer is rather modest and is probably of less concern than is the administration of estrogens to healthy postmenopausal women, where no protective effect against breast cancer is observed. Issues on safety are under constant review, but concerns about TAM as a promoter of endometrial cancer in women have not, as yet, proved to be of clinical relevance. Nevertheless, physicians should follow up women receiving TAM with periodic gynecological examination and endometrial sampling of symptomatic cases. The value of TVS remains to be established.

Available data on long-term therapy has shown that this drug is effective and safe; after 4.5 million women-years of experience with TAM, the evidence indicates that the benefits of TAM treatment for breast cancer outweigh its known toxicity.

No patient should be denied adjuvant TAM therapy for breast cancer because of the potential to develop endometrial carcinoma. Metastatic breast cancer is invariably fatal, whereas endometrial cancer is a curable disease.

The situation will continue to be reviewed during the development of the prevention trials in Europe and the USA, but, in the light of the current knowledge, it is probable that TAM may be beneficial also in healthy women at high risk for breast cancer.

## REFERENCES

1. Cancer Facts and Figures 1991. 1991. American Cancer Society, Inc. Atlanta.
2. POWLES, T. J., C. R. TILLYER, A. L. JONES et al. 1992. Prevention of breast cancer with tamoxifen—an update on the Royal Marsden Hospital pilot programme. Eur. J. Cancer **26:** 680–684.
3. JORDAN, V. C. 1990. Tamoxifen for the prevention of breast cancer. In Cancer Prevention. V. T. De Vita, Jr., S. Hellman & S. A. Rosenberg, Eds. 1–12. Lippincott. Philadelphia, PA.
4. TURKEN, S., E. SIRIS, D. SELDIN et al. 1989. Effects of tamoxifen on spinal bone density in women with breast cancer. J. Natl. Cancer Inst. **81:** 1086–1088.
5. LOVE, R. R., R. B. MAZESS, H. S. BARDEN et al. 1992. Effects of tamoxifen on bone mineral density in postmenopausal women with breast cancer. N. Engl. J. Med. **326:** 852–856.
6. LOVE, R. R., P. NEWCOMB, D. A. WEIBE et al. 1990. Effects of tamoxifen therapy on lipid and lipoprotein levels in postmenopausal patients with node-negative breast cancer. J. Natl. Cancer Inst. **82:** 1310–1311.
7. DEWAR, J. A., J. M. HOROBIN, & P. E. PREECE. 1992. Long term effects of tamoxifen on blood lipid values in breast cancer. Br. Med. J. **305:** 225–226.
8. RYAN, W. G., J. WOLTER & J. D. BAGDADE. 1991. Apparent beneficial effects of tamoxifen on bone mineral content in patients with breast cancer: preliminary study. Osteoporosis Int. **2:** 39–41.
9. MCDONALD, C. C. & H. J. STEWART. 1991. Fatal myocardial infarction in the Scottish adjuvant tamoxifen trial. Br. Med. J. **303:** 435–437.
10. CATHERINO, W. H. & V. C. JORDAN. 1993. A risk-benefit assessment of tamoxifen therapy. Drug Safety **8:** 381–397.
11. JORDAN, V. C. 1992. Overview from the international conference on long-term tamoxifen therapy for breast cancer. J. Natl. Cancer Inst. **84**(4): 231–234.
12. Early Breast Cancer Trialists' Collaborative Group. 1992. Systemic treatment of early breast cancer by hormonal, cytotoxic, or immune therapy. Lancet **339:** 1–15.
13. JORDAN, V. C. 1974. Antitumor activity of the antioestrogen ICI 46,474 (tamoxifen) in the dimethylbenzanthracene (DMBA) induced rat mammary carcinoma model. J. Steroid Biochem. **5:** 365.
14. JORDAN, V. C. 1976. Effect of tamoxifen (ICI 46,474) on initiation and growth of DMBA-induced rat mammary carcinomata. Eur. J. Cancer **12:** 419–424.
15. JORDAN, V. C. 1983. Laboratory studies to develop general principles for the adjuvant treatment of breast cancer with antiestrogens: problems and potential for future clinical applications. Breast Cancer Res. Treat. 3(Suppl.): S73–86.
16. JORDAN, V. C., M. K. LABABIDI & S. LANGHAN-FAHEY. 1991. Suppression of mouse mammary tumorigenesis by long term tamoxifen therapy. J. Natl. Cancer Inst. **83:** 492–496.
17. Nolvadex Adjuvant Trial Organization. 1988. Controlled trial of tamoxifen as a single adjuvant agent in the management of early breast cancer. Br. J. Cancer **57:** 608–611.
18. Breast Cancer Trials Committee, Scottish Cancer Trials Office (MRC), Edinburgh.

1987. Adjuvant tamoxifen in the management of operable breast cancer: the Scottish trial. Lancet **2:** 171–175.
19. RUTQVIST, L. E., B. CEDERMARK, U. GLAS et al. 1987. The Stockholm trial on adjuvant tamoxifen in early breast cancer. Breast Cancer Res. Treat. **10:** 255–266.
20. PALSHOF, T., H. T. MOURISDEN, J. L. DAEHNFELDT et al. 1985. Adjuvant endocrine therapy in pre- and postmenopausal women with operable breast cancer. Rev. Endocrine-Related Cancer Suppl. **17:** 43–50.
21. PRITCHARD, K. I., J. W. MEAKIN, N. F. BOYD et al. 1987. Adjuvant tamoxifen in postmenopausal women with axillary node positive breast cancer: an update. In Adjuvant Therapy of Cancer. V. S. E. Salmon, Ed. 391–400. Grune & Stratton. New York, NY.
22. CUMMINGS, F. J., R. GRAY, T. E. DAVIS et al. 1986. Tamoxifen versus placebo: double-blind adjuvant trial in elderly women with stage II breast cancer. In Proceedings of the NIH Consensus Development Conference on Adjuvant Chemotherapy and Endocrine Therapies for Breast Cancer. 119–123. National Institutes of Health. Bethesda, MD.
23. FISHER, B., J. COSTANTINO, C. REDMOND et al. 1989. A randomized clinical trial evaluating tamoxifen in the treatment of patients with node negative breast cancer who have estrogen receptor positive tumors. N. Engl. J. Med. **320:** 479–484.
24. C. R. C. Adjuvant Breast Trial Working Party. 1988. Cyclophosphamide and tamoxifen as adjuvant therapies in the management of breast cancer. Br. J. Cancer **57:** 604–607.
25. GOTTARDIS, M. M., S. P. ROBINSON & V. C. JORDAN. 1988. Estradiol-stimulated growth of MCF-7 tumors implanted in athymic mice. A model to study the tumoristatic action of tamoxifen. J. Steroid Biochem. **30:** 311–314.
26. GOTTARDIS, M. M., M. E. RICCHIO, P. G. SATYASWAROOP & V. C. JORDAN. 1990. Effect of steroidal and non-steroidal antiestrogens on the growth of a tamoxifen-stimulated human endometrial carcinoma (EnCa101) in athymic mice. Cancer Res. **50:** 3189–3192.
27. SATYASWAROOP, P. G., R. J. ZAINO & R. MORTEL. 1984. Estrogen-like effects of tamoxifen on human endometrial carcinoma transplanted into nude mice. Cancer Res. **44:** 4006–4010.
28. GUSBERG, S. B. 1990. Tamoxifen for breast cancer: associated endometrial cancer. Cancer **65:** 1463–1464.
29. KILLACKEY, M. A., T. B. HAKES & V. K. PIERCE. 1985. Endometrial adenocarcinoma in breast cancer patients receiving tamoxifen. Cancer Treat. Rep. **69:** 237–238.
30. PONS, J. Y. & L. RIGONNOT. 1988. Hyperplasie de l'endomètre chez le patientes ménopausées traitées par le tamoxifène pour cancer mammaire. J. Gynécol. Obstét. Biol. Reprod. **17:** 11–20.
31. HARDELL, L. 1988. Tamoxifen as a risk factor for carcinoma of corpus uteri. Lancet **2:** 563.
32. FORNANDER, T., B. CEDERMARK, A. MATTSSON et al. 1989. Adjuvant tamoxifen in early breast cancer: occurrence of new primary cancers. Lancet **1:** 117–120.
33. DAUPLAT, J., G. LE BOUEDEC & J. L. ACHARD. 1990. Adénocarcinome de l'endomètre chez 2 malades prenant du tamoxifène. Presse Méd. **19:** 380–381.
34. MATHEW, A., A. B. CHABON, B. KABAKOW, M. DRUCKER & R. HIRSCHMAN. 1990. Endometrial carcinoma in five patients with breast cancer on tamoxifen therapy. N.Y. State J. Med. **90:** 207–208.
35. MALFETANO, J. H. 1990. Tamoxifen-associated endometrial carcinoma in post-menopausal breast cancer patients. Gynecol. Oncol. **39:** 82–84.
36. ATLANTE, G., M. POZZI, C. VINCENZONI & G. VOCATURO. 1990. Four case reports presenting new acquisitions on the association between breast and endometrial carcinoma. Gynecol. Oncol. **37:** 378–380.
37. NEVEN, P., X. DE MUYLDER, Y. VAN BELLE, G. VANDERICK & E. DE MUYLDER. 1989. Tamoxifen and the uterus and endometrium. Lancet **1:** 375.
38. RODIER, J. F., E. CAMUS, J. C. JANSER, R. RENAUD & D. RODIER. 1990. Tamoxifène et adénocarcinome endomètrial. Bull. Cancer **77:** 1207–1210.
39. SEGNA, R. A., P. R. DOTTINO, L. DELIGDISCH & C. J. COHEN. 1992. Tamoxifen and endometrial cancer. Mt. Sinai J. Med. **59**(5): 416–418.

40. UZIELY, B., D. DOREMBUS, G. BRUFMAN, A. LEWIN, R. CATANE & S. MOR-YOSEF. 1992. The effect of tamoxifen on the endometrium (meeting abstract). Proc. Annu. Meet. Am. Assoc. Cancer Res. **33:** A1678.
41. OSBORNE, C. K. 1991. Intergroup adjuvant studies with chemotherapy without or with tamoxifen (meeting abstract). International Conference on Long-Term Antihormonal Therapy for Breast Cancer. 14. Lake Buena Vista, FL.
42. O'NEILL, E. & W. RODRIGUEZ-MOJICA. 1992. Asymptomatic carcinoma of the endometrium in a patient on adjunctive tamoxifen therapy for carcinoma of the breast. Bol. Asoc. Med. Puerto Rico **84**(2): 74–77.
43. MIGNOTTE, H., A. J. SASCO, C. LASSET, S. SAEZ & M. RIVOIRE. 1992. (Traitement adjuvant de cancer du sein par tamoxifène et cancer de l'endomètre.) Adjuvant therapy by tamoxifen for breast cancer and endometrium carcinoma. Bull. Cancer **79**(10): 969–977.
44. DEPREST, J., P. NEVEN & P. IDE. 1992. An unusual type of endometrial cancer, related to tamoxifen? Eur. J. Obstet. Gynecol. Reprod. Biol. **46**(2–3): 147–150.
45. LE BOUEDEC, G. & J. DAUPLAT. 1992. (Cancer de l'endomètre du aux anti-estrogenes.) Endometrial carcinoma due to anti-estrogen therapy. Rev. Fr. Gynecol. Obstet. **87**(6): 345–348.
46. SPINELLI, G., N. BARDAZZI, A. CITERNESI, M. FONTANAROSA & P. CURRIEL. 1991. Endometrial carcinoma in tamoxifen-treated breast cancer patients. J. Chemother. **3**(4): 267–270.
47. PALACIOS, A., S. PERTUSA, A. MONTOYA & R. MARTINEZ-SAN PEDRO. 1993. (Cancer de mama, tamoxifeno y utero.) Breast cancer, tamoxifen and the uterus. Med. Clin. **100**(12): 479.
48. TESHIMA, H., M. IKENABA, K. YOKOSUKA, K. HASUMI, K. MASUBUCHI, M. YOSHIMOTO, F. KASUMI et al. 1990. Does long-term administration of tamoxifen cause the endometrial adenocarcinoma in breast cancer patients after operation? Igaku No Ayumi **154:** 509–510.
49. SAMELIS, S. F., G. P. STATHOPOULOS, N. A. MALAMUS, E. KONDILI, N. P. MOSCHOPOULOS & P. PAPACOSTAS. 1992. Toxicity of long-term treatment with tamoxifen in breast cancer patients. Ann. Oncol. **3**(Suppl. 5): 78, Abs. 300.
50. NAYFIELD, S. G., J. E. KARP, L. G. FORD, F. A. DORR & B. S. KRAMER. 1991. Potential role of tamoxifen in prevention of breast cancer. J. Natl. Cancer Inst. **83**(20): 1450–1449.
51. CHAMPION, P. E., J. M. NAVHOLTZ, H. JENKINS, G. MACLEAN, S. ALLEN & A. LEES. 1991. Is tamoxifen increasing the risk of uterine malignancy in women treated for breast cancer? Breast Cancer Res. Treat. **19:** 195.
52. EELLS, T. P., H. D. ALPERN, C. GRZYWACZ, R. W. MACMILLAN & J. E. OLSON. 1990. The effect of tamoxifen on squamous maturation in Papanicolau stained cervical smears of postmenopausal women. Cytopathology **1:** 263–268.
53. RAYTER, Z., J. C. GAZET, J. SHEPHERD, P. A. TROTT & W. SVENSON. 1993. Effect of adjuvant tamoxifen on gynaecological cytology. Eur. J. Surg. Oncol. **19:** 101.
54. NASRI, M. N., J. H. SHEPHERD, M. E. SETCHELL, D. G. LOWE & T. CHARD. 1991. The role of vaginal scan in measurement of endometrial thickness in postmenopausal women. Br. J. Obstet. Gynaecol. **98:** 470–475.
55. BOTSIS, D., D. KASSANOS, E. PYRGIOTIS & P. A. ZOURLAS. 1992. Vaginal sonography of the endometrium in postmenopausal women. Clin. Exp. Obstet. Gynaecol. **19**(3): 189–192.
56. LAHTI, E., G. BLANCO, A. KAUPPILA, M. APAJA-SARKKINEN, P. J. TASKINEN & T. LAATIKAINEN. 1993. Endometrial changes in postmenopausal breast cancer patients receiving tamoxifen. Obstet. Gynecol. **81**(5) Part 1: 660–664.
57. UZAN, S., N. PERROT & M. UZAN. 1992. Tamoxifen: vaginosonography and color Doppler assessment of the uterus (letter). Ultrasound Obstet. Gynecol. **2**(4): 306.
58. HULKA, C. A. & D. A. HALL. 1993. Endometrial abnormalities associated with tamoxifen therapy for breast cancer: sonographic and pathological correlation. Am. J. Roentgenol. **160**(4): 809–812.
59. COHEN, I., D. J. D. ROSEN, R. TEPPER, M. CORDOBA, Y. SHAPIRA, M. M. ALTARAS

*et al.* 1993. Ultrasonographic evaluation of the endometrium and correlation with endometrial sampling in postmenopausal patients treated with tamoxifen. J. Ultrasound Med. **12**(5): 275–280.
60. GAL, D., S. KOPEL, M. BASHEVKIN, J. LEBOWICZ, R. LEV & M. L. TANCER. 1991. Oncogenic potential of tamoxifen on endometria of postmenopausal women with breast cancer—preliminary report. Gynaecol. Oncol. **42**(2): 120–123.
61. DE MUYLDER, X., P. NEVEN, M. DE SOMER, Y. VAN BELLE, G. VANDERICK & E. DE MUYLDER. 1991. Endometrial lesions in patients undergoing tamoxifen therapy. Int. J. Gynaecol. Obstet. **36**(2): 127–130.
62. COHEN, I., M. ALTARAS, D. J. D. ROSEN, Y. SHAPIRA, M. CORDOBA, D. YIGAEL *et al.* 1992. Oestrogen and progesterone receptor status in breast cancer and development of endometrial abnormalities (letter). Lancet **340**: 312.
63. ANTEBY, E., S. YAGEL, D. ZACUT, Z. PALTI & D. HOCHNER-CELNIKIER. 1992. False sonographic appearance of endometrial neoplasia in postmenopausal women treated with tamoxifen (letter). Lancet **340:** 433–434.
64. SILVA, E. & C. TORNOS. 1993. Malignant neoplasm of the uterine corpus in patients with breast carcinoma. The effects of tamoxifen. Mod. Pathol. **6**(1): 78A, Abs. 445.
65. DELIGDISCH, L., C. J. COHEN & P. DOTTINO. 1991. Tamoxifen therapy and endometrial neoplasia. Eur. J. Cancer. **27**(Suppl. 2): S127, Abs 755.
66. MAGRIPLES, U., F. NAFTOLIN, P. E. SCHWARTZ & M. L. CARCANGIU. 1993. High-grade endometrial carcinoma in tamoxifen-treated breast cancer patients. J. Clin. Oncol. **11**(2): 485–490.

# Cytokine Regulation of Cellular Proliferation in Endometriosis

NANCY A. KLEIN, GABRIELA M. PÉRGOLA,
RAJESHWAR RAO TEKMAL, IRIS A. MONTOYA,
TAMMY D. DEY, AND ROBERT S. SCHENKEN[a]

*Department of Obstetrics and Gynecology*
*Division of Reproductive Endocrinology and Infertility*
*University of Texas Health Science Center at San Antonio*
*7703 Floyd Curl Drive*
*San Antonio, Texas 78284-7836*

## INTRODUCTION

Leukocytes comprise up to 25% of the cell population in proliferative and secretory endometrial stroma.[1,2] Immunocytochemical studies have shown that the majority of these leukocytes are T cells and macrophages.[1-5] Considerable evidence suggests a paracrine role for resident leukocytes-secreted and cytokines in regulating cell growth and differentiation in normal eutopic endometrium (UE). Cultures of endometrial stromal cells produce interferon gamma (IFNγ),[6] interleukin-1 (IL-1),[7,8] and interleukin-6 (IL-6),[7,9] and endometrial receptors to IFNγ[10] and IL-1[6,11] have been demonstrated by immunocytochemistry. IFNγ decreases BrdU incorporation into cultured endometrial epithelial cells,[12] and it has been suggested that this antiproliferative effect may be related to the decreased proliferative activity found in the basalis layer of UE.[5]

To assess whether resident T cells and macrophages may play a role in regulating cell proliferation of endometriosis, we employed a dual-staining immunohistochemical technique with monoclonal antibodies to Ki67 (proliferation marker) and leukocyte markers, to show that (1) the concentration of leukocytes is significantly greater in ectopic endometrium (EE) than in UE, and (2) the proliferative activity of endometrial stromal and epithelial cells is significantly less in EE than in UE. To assess whether the lower proliferative activity observed in EE may be related to increased numbers of resident leukocytes expressing IFNγ, *in situ* hybridization studies were performed and confirmed an increase in T cells and macrophage IFNγ messenger ribonucleic acid (mRNA) expression in EE. These studies suggest a possible paracrine role for resident leukocytes and IFNγ in regulating cell proliferation in endometriosis.

## MATERIALS AND METHODS

### Tissue Collection

Endometriotic tissue was obtained from women (aged 22–43) undergoing surgery for pelvic pain or infertility in the proliferative phase of the menstrual cycle.

---

[a] Corresponding author.

None of the patients had received recent hormonal therapy. Specimens included biopsies of superficial peritoneal implants, appearing as raised reddish nodules (n = 12); ovarian endometriomas; and superficial ovarian endometriosis (n = 5). Control tissue consisted of proliferative (n = 8) or secretory (n = 13) UE obtained from 17 cycling women (aged 28–45) undergoing diagnostic endometrial aspiration biopsy or hysterectomy for non-endometrial pathology. Tissue was immediately snap-frozen in liquid nitrogen and stored at −70°C until sectioning.

## Histology

Serial 4-μm frozen sections were placed on baked glycine-coated slides, air-dried, and fixed for five minutes in acetone at 4°C. Sections were transferred to tris-buffered saline (TBS; 0.1 M Tris-Cl, 0.15 M NaCl, pH 7.4) prior to routine staining with hematoxylin and eosin for immunocytochemistry. Eutopic endometria were dated histologically according to the criteria of Noyes *et al.*[13]

## Immunocytochemistry

Sections were first stained for the nuclear proliferation marker Ki67, and then for the surface antigen CD45 (leukocyte common antigen; AMAC, Inc., Westbrook, ME), CD3 (T-cell marker; DAKO Corporation, Carpinteria, CA), or CD11c (tissue macrophage marker; DAKO). Briefly, slides were incubated at 37°C with normal horse serum followed by mouse monoclonal antibody to Ki67 (DAKO), biotinylated anti-mouse secondary antibody, and, finally, avidin-biotin peroxidase complex (Vectastain©, catalogue #PK6102; Vector Laboratories, Inc., Burlingame, CA). Slides were then reacted in a mixture of diaminobenzidine (DAB) and hydrogen peroxide, which yielded a brown nuclear reaction product. After washing, the procedure was repeated with the substitution of one of the leukocyte marker antibodies as the primary antibody, and 4-chloro-1-naphthol-$H_2O_2$ as the chromagen, to produce a blue reaction product. Slides were washed in TBS following each step of the sequence. Sections were lightly counterstained with hematoxylin, coverslipped, and examined by light microscopy. Primary antibodies were used at a dilution of 1 : 50, and secondary antibody at 1 : 200. For endometriosis specimens, sections were pre-incubated for 20 minutes with 0.3% hydrogen peroxide in methanol for quenching of endogenous peroxidase activity. Similar quenching of UE specimens did not affect nuclear or membrane staining. Negative controls consisted of substituting TBS or non-immune mouse serum at equivalent protein concentrations for the primary antibody.

Some sections of eutopic (n = 6) and ectopic (n = 6) endometria were incubated for 1 hour at 37°C with a monoclonal antibody to human IFNγ receptor (Genzyme Corporation, Cambridge, MA) diluted 1 : 250 in phosphate buffered saline (PBS) with 1% bovine serum albumin. After washing with TBS, slides were incubated with biotinylated horse anti-mouse secondary antibody at 37°C for 20 minutes, followed by an avidin-biotin peroxidase complex and developed in DAB.

Sections were examined under oil immersion. The proportion of cells staining for each of the antigens was obtained by counting a minimum of 500 cells in the stroma or epithelium or a minimum of 100 cells contained in lymphoid aggregates.

Proportions were compared using an unpaired *t* test and results expressed as mean percentages with standard errors of the mean. Prior to data analysis, a non-linear transformation (arcsine transformation) was performed which resulted in equal detectability of differences between proportions.[14]

### IFN$_\gamma$ Riboprobes and in Situ Hybridization

Immunocytochemistry was performed with monoclonal antibodies to CD45, CD3 or CD11c described above. Sections were than fixed with 4% paraformaldehyde for five minutes and processed for *in situ* hybridization. $^{32}$P-labeled riboprobes were prepared from plasmid containing the Aval-Hinc II 900 bp fragment of the human IFN$\gamma$ complimentary deoxy ribonucleic acid (cDNA) inserted into the pGEM3Z multiple cloning site. Plasmid was linearized with HindIII restriction enzyme and transcribed with T7 RNA polymerase to obtain mRNA-complementary riboprobe (antisense), or plasmid was linearized with EcoR1 and transcribed with SP6 RNA polymerase to obtain mRNA-like (sense) riboprobe using $^{32}$P-CTP (New England Nuclear, Wilmington, DE) and a riboprobe kit (Promega Biotec, Madison, WI) according to the manufacturer's suggestions. Prehybridization and hybridization were carried out as described by Singer *et al.*,[15] Harper *et al.*[16] and Chan *et al.*[17] Briefly, sections were washed with RNAse-free TBS for one hour and with PBS for five minutes. Sections were then treated with acetic anhydride followed by Tris-glycine solution and incubated with prehybridization buffer (50% formamide, 0.3 M NaCl, 20 mM Tris-Cl [pH 8.0], 10% dextran sulfate, 10% mM Na pyrophosphate, 1× Denhardt's solution, 100 $\mu$g/ml yeast tRNA and 100 $\mu$g/ml salmon sperm DNA) for one to two hours at 45°C in a humidified chamber. Hybridization was carried out with the same buffer as above containing 2–3 × 10$^5$ cpm/section of IFN$\gamma$ riboprobe, sense or antisense, for four to six hours. Slides were washed twice for 10 minutes each with 2 × SSC (1 × SSC = 0.15 M NaCl, 0.015 M Na citrate, pH 7.0). Nonhybridized probe was digested with 50 $\mu$g/ml RNAse A in 10 mM Tris-Cl, pH 8.0, 0.3 M NaCl, for 30 minutes at 37°C. The slides were then washed twice for 30 minutes each at 45°C with 50% formamide containing 2 × SSC and rinsed with 2 × SSC. After dehydration in graded ethanol solutions, slides were dipped in NTB-2 emulsion (1:1 dilution; Eastman Kodak Co., Rochester, NY). After exposure for 10–15 days at 4°C, slides were developed with Kodak D-19 developer, fixed with Kodak Rapidfix, and counterstained with hematoxylin.

Sections were examined under oil immersion. The proportions of CD45-, CD3-, and CD11c-positive cells expressing mRNA for IFN$\gamma$ were obtained by counting a minimum of 500 cells in the stroma or epithelium and expressed as a percent of the total. Sections processed for the combination of immunocytochemistry and *in situ* hybridization were compared to sections processed for immunocytochemistry or *in situ* hybridization alone. No significant differences were noted in the proportions and distributions of cells expressing CD antigens and IFN$\gamma$ mRNA. Means were compared using the non-parametric Mann-Whitney U test performed using the computer package, Minitab (Minitab, Inc., State College, PA) on a personal computer. Results are expressed as mean ± standard error of the mean.

## RESULTS

### Histologic Characteristics

Routine histologic staining of UE tissue revealed normal proliferative and secretory endometria with no evidence of endometritis or other endometrial pathology. Examination of EE revealed weakly proliferative glands and stroma with surrounding fibrosis and frequent deposits of hemosiderin.

## *Cell Populations and Proliferative Activity*

Cells labeled with CD45, CD3 or CD11c were identified by their plasma membrane reactivity, and proliferating cells were distinguished by nuclear staining (FIG. 1). Eutopic endometrium contained CD45+ cells scattered throughout the stroma as well as aggregates of these cells found primarily in the basalis adjacent to glands. Many of the scattered cells were closely juxtaposed to the basement membrane of the glandular epithelium. In addition, occasional CD45+ cells were found within the glandular and surface epithelium. Staining with CD3 and CD11c revealed that the majority of the CD45+ cells represented T-cells and macrophages.

Endometriotic tissue contained significantly higher proportions of scattered stromal CD45+, CD3+ and CD11c+ cells as compared with UE in either the proliferative or secretory phase ($p \leq 0.02$, TABLE 1). There were no significant differences between peritoneal implants and endometriomas in the proportions of scattered cells expressing each CD marker. Rare CD45+ cells were found within the endometriotic glandular epithelium. Only occasional implants contained lymphoid aggregates located near the glands.

Sections of normal UE demonstrated variable degrees of proliferative activity in both CD-positive and CD-negative cells, as evidenced by nuclear staining for

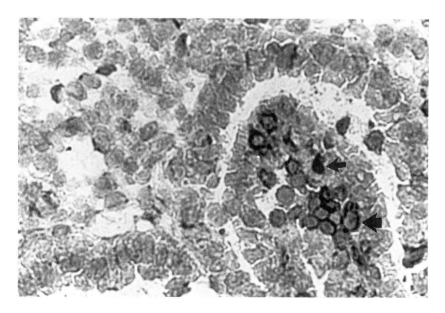

**FIGURE 1.** Photomicrographs of EE stained for CD45 (plasma membrane reactivity; *large arrow*) and Ki67 (nuclear reactivity; *small arrow*) aggregate adjacent to glands. Note minimal proliferative activity in glandular epithelium.

TABLE 1. Proportion of Scattered Stromal Cells Staining for Lymphoid Cell Antigens[a]

| Tissue | % CD45+ | % CD3+ | % CD11c+ |
|---|---|---|---|
| Proliferative endometrium (n = 9) | 7.5 ± 0.8 | 6.4 ± 0.7 | 3.8 ± 0.3 |
| Secretory endometrium (n = 8) | 11.1 ± 1.2 | 5.0 ± 0.6 | 4.5 ± 0.3 |
| Endometriosis (n = 17) | 19.0 ± 1.4[b] | 9.9 ± 0.8[b] | 9.3 ± 1.0[b] |

[a] Data are expressed as mean ± standard errors of the mean.
[b] Different from proliferative and secretory endometrium, $p \leq 0.02$.

Ki67 (FIG. 1). Dual-staining revealed a low level of proliferative activity in leukocytes scattered throughout the stroma as well as in those found in aggregates located near glands. In UE, the proliferative activity of the scattered leukocytes was greatest in the late secretory phase. In EE, proliferative activity was also noted in the scattered leukocyte population. The percentage of the total stromal cell population composed of proliferating CD45+ cells was similar in UE and EE (0.7% ± 0.2 vs 0.6% ± 0.1) although a significantly greater proportion of the CD45-positive cells were proliferating in UE as compared to EE (9.0% ± 2.1 vs 3.1% ± 1.0; $p = 0.005$). The lymphoid aggregates observed in EE rarely contained proliferating cells.

The percentage of Ki67+ glandular epithelial cells in normal endometrium was significantly greater in the proliferative phase than in the secretory phase (5.7% vs 3.3%, respectively; $p = 0.03$). Endometriotic tissue contained glands with only occasional cells staining for Ki67 in proportions consistently less than 1%. In endometrium, proliferative activity of CD-negative stromal cells was greater in the proliferative phase than in the secretory phase (8.3% vs 5.1%, respectively; $p = 0.03$). In all phases of the menstrual cycle, the proportion of endometrial epithelial and stromal cells staining for Ki67 was lower in the basalis compared with the upper functionalis layers. Minimal CD-negative stromal cell/fibroblast proliferative activity was detected in all endometriosis specimens examined (1.4% vs 8.3% for proliferative endometrium, and 5.1% for secretory endometrium; $p < 0.0001$).

All sections stained with TBS or non-immune mouse serum in place of the primary antibody were negative for nuclear or plasma membrane staining. Nonspecific staining of hemosiderin deposits in endometriotic tissue was considerably reduced by quenching with 0.03% hydrogen peroxide in methanol prior to immunostaining.

## $IFN_\gamma$ in Situ Hybridization

Some cells staining positive for the leukocyte cell markers also expressed IFNγ mRNA, demonstrated by a concentration of black silver grains overlying the nucleus and cytoplasm in addition to membrane immunostaining (FIG. 2). Control sections incubated with the IFNγ sense riboprobe did not show concentrated black silver grains over cells. This lack of hybridization with IFNγ mRNA indicates the specificity of the riboprobe used. Concentrations of cells in the stroma staining for leukocyte markers and also expressing IFNγ mRNA are shown in FIGURE 3. The proportion of these dually positive cells was significantly greater in EE than

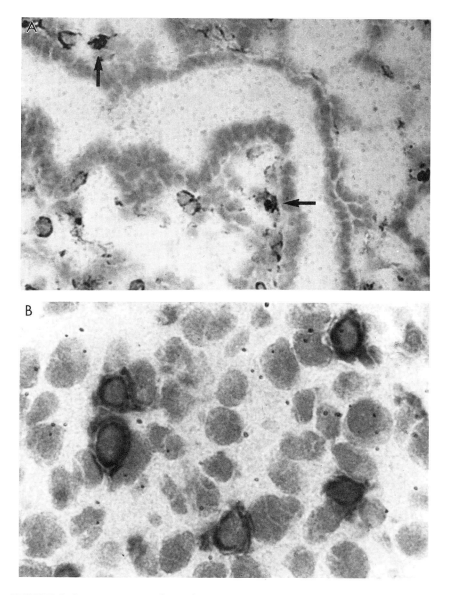

**FIGURE 2.** Late secretory endometrium processed for immunocytochemistry and *in situ* hybridization. **(A)** IFNγ antisense riboprobe (40×); CD45-positive cells also expressing IFNγ mRNA are noted by the *arrows*. **(B)** IFNγ sense riboprobe (100×); scattered nonspecific black silver grains are noted without concentration over cells. (From Klein *et al.*[28] Reprinted by permission from the *American Journal of Reproductive Immunology*.)

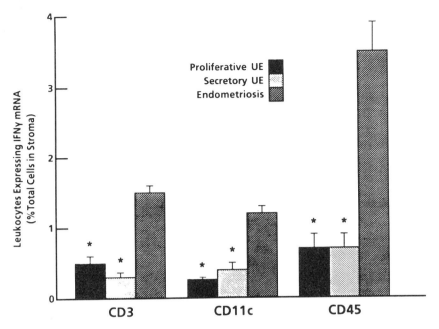

**FIGURE 3.** Percentage of CD45-, CD3-, and CD11c-positive cells expressing IFNγ mRNA in UE and EE, expressed as percent of the total cells in the stroma. *$p < 0.01$. (From Klein et al.[28] Reprinted by permission from the *American Journal of Reproductive Immunology*.)

in either proliferative or secretory UE ($p < 0.05$). In addition, we compared the proportion of each leukocyte type expressing IFNγ mRNA (FIG. 4). IFNγ mRNA was demonstrated in both CD45-positive cells and T cells and in a smaller proportion of macrophages. Expression of IFNγ mRNA by each of these cell types was greater in EE than in either secretory or proliferative UE ($p < 0.05$).

All sections of EE and normal UE immunostained for IFNγ receptor expressed the receptor in glandular epithelial cells. Endothelial cells as well as scattered cells in the stroma were also positive for IFNγ receptor. Serial sections stained with CD11c showed a similar pattern of stromal staining, suggesting that the scattered IFNγ receptor-expressing cells may represent CD11c-positive macrophages.

## DISCUSSION

This study establishes the presence of resident leukocytes in endometriotic tissue. As in UE, the majority of these cells are T cells and macrophages. The presence of leukocytes, both scattered and in aggregates, in normal UE has been well documented.[1–5] The present study demonstrates that scattered T cells (CD3+) and macrophages (CD11c+) in EE are present in higher concentrations than in UE. However, lymphoid aggregates are less common in EE.

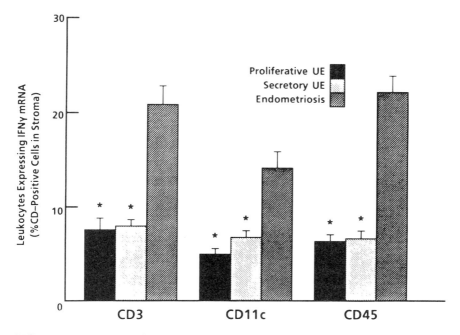

**FIGURE 4.** Percentage of leukocytes expressing IFNγ mRNA in UE and EE expressed as the percent of each leukocyte type. *$p < 0.01$. (From Klein et al.[28] Reprinted by permission from the *American Journal of Reproductive Immunology*.)

Overall, the observed proliferative activity of both glandular and stromal components is significantly lower in EE than in UE. There is evidence suggesting that inhibitory cytokines decrease proliferative activity of endometrial cellular components. IFNγ decreases Brd-U (a thymidine analog) incorporation into cultured endometrial epithelial cells.[12] IL-1β inhibits ³H-thymidine incorporation into cultured endometrial stromal cells.[18] The possibility that resident leukocytes may provide a source of IFNγ activity is supported by the *in vitro* observation that anti-serum to IFNγ[19] inhibits endometrial T-cell-induced HLA-DR expression in endometrial epithelial cells. The larger number of lymphoid cells present in aggregates in the basalis may be involved in the low level of proliferative activity and enhanced HLA-DR expression found in this region. Decreased glandular epithelial proliferative activity in the secretory phase[5,20] may also be functionally correlated with increased numbers and proliferative activity of leukocytes present during the secretory phase.[5,21]

Our findings of IFNγ mRNA and IFNγ receptor expression in both UE and EE further support a paracrine role for IFNγ in these tissues. We observed that leukocyte IFNγ expression is enhanced in EE as compared to UE. This was evidenced by both an increased percentage of leukocytes expressing IFNγ and a greater proportion of both T cells and macrophages demonstrate the IFNγ message. A local antiproliferative effect of IFNγ might contribute to the lower proliferative activity in EE as previously observed by decreased c-myc[22] expression in EE as compared to UE. The low level of expression of IFNγ we observed may be due to transient and intermittent transcription sufficient only to produce effects on a local level.

Our finding of endometrial macrophage expression of IFNγ mRNA has not been described previously. Although T cell production of IFNγ has been extensively studied, IFNγ production has also been demonstrated in macrophages and natural killer (NK) cells. Macrophages isolated from mouse spleen, bone marrow and peritoneum,[23,24] and purified alveolar macrophages from patients with sarcoidosis[25] and normal subjects[26] produce IFNγ in culture. The monoclonal antibody to CD11c may have some cross-reactivity with granulocytes, including NK cells.[27] CD16-positive NK cells account for a very small percentage of endometrial leukocytes[1,3] and are therefore unlikely to account for all of the CD11c-positive, IFNγ-expressing cells. However, a significant population of CD16-negative granulocytes morphologically similar to NK cells has been described in the stroma of UE.[3] The CD11c-positive, IFNγ mRNA-positive cells identified in this study have not been characterized. Further studies are also needed to determine whether the cells that express mRNA or IFNγ are also capable of IFNγ secretion.

In conclusion, we observed that (1) the concentration of scattered LCs is significantly greater in EE than in UE; (2) the proliferative activity of endometrial stromal and epithelial cells is significantly lower in EE than in UE; (3) the proportion of proliferating CD45+ stromal cells is similar in UE and in EE; (4) the overall concentration of T cells and macrophages expressing IFNγ mRNA is greater in EE than in UE; (5) the percentage of each leukocyte type expressing IFNγ mRNA is also greater in EE; and (6) both ectopic and eutopic endometrial glands, as well as scattered cells in the stroma, express IFNγ receptor. We conclude that these findings support a possible paracrine role for resident leukocytes and IFNγ in regulating cell proliferation in endometriosis.

## SUMMARY

**Objective:** This study was designed (1) to characterize the resident leukocyte population in ectopic endometrium (EE), (2) to assess proliferative activity of cellular components in EE, (3) to assess whether resident leukocytes in EE express IFNγ mRNA and (4) to demonstrate endometrial epithelial cell IFNγ receptors in EE.

**Study Design:** Biopsies of EE and normal eutopic endometrium (UE) were studied immunocytochemically using monoclonal antibodies specific for CD45 leukocyte common antigen, CD3 (a T cell marker), CD11c (a macrophage marker), and Ki67 (proliferation marker). Leukocyte types were identified immunocytochemically, followed by *in situ* hybridization to assess expression of IFNγ mRNA. IFNγ receptor expression was assessed by immunocytochemistry.

**Results:** The percentage of scattered stromal cells staining for each CD marker was greater in EE than in UE. The proliferative activity of endometrial stromal cells and epithelial cells was significantly less in EE than in UE. The overall concentration of T cells and macrophages expressing IFNγ mRNA was significantly greater in EE than in UE. The percentage of each leukocyte type expressing IFNγ mRNA was also greater in EE than in UE, and IFNγ receptors were present in glandular epithelium of EE.

**Conclusions:** These findings support a possible paracrine role for resident leukocytes and IFNγ in regulating cell proliferation in endometriosis.

## ACKNOWLEDGMENTS

The authors would like to thank Dr. Jeff Hasdey for providing the plasmid construct containing the IFNγ cDNA. We also wish to thank Ms. Irma Garcia and Ms. Gretta Small for their valuable assistance in the preparation of the manuscript.

## REFERENCES

1. KAMAT, B. R. & P. G. ISAACSON. 1987. The immunocytochemical distribution of leukocytic subpopulations in human endometrium. Am. J. Pathol. **127**: 66–73.
2. MARSHALL, R. J. & D. B. JONES. 1988. An immunohistochemical study of lymphoid tissue in human endometrium. Int. J. Gynecol. Pathol. **7**: 225–235.
3. BULMER, J. N., D. P. LUNNY & S. V. HAGIN. 1988. Immunohistochemical characterization of stromal leukocytes in nonpregnant human endometrium. Am. J. Reprod. Immunol. Microbiol. **17**: 83–90.
4. MORRIS, H., J. EDWARDS, A. TILTMAN & M. EMMS. 1985. Endometrial lymphoid tissue: an immunohistological study. J. Clin. Pathol. **38**: 644–652.
5. TABIBZADEH, S. 1990. Proliferative activity of lymphoid cells in human endometrium throughout the menstrual cycle. J. Clin. Endocrinol. Metab. **70**: 437–443.
6. TABIBZADEH, S. 1991. Cytokine regulation of human endometrial function. Ann. N.Y. Acad. Sci. **622**: 89–98.
7. SEMER, D., K. REISLER, P. C. MACDONALD & M. L. CASEY. 1991. Responsiveness of human endometrial stromal cells to cytokines. Ann. N.Y. Acad. Sci. **622**: 99–110.
8. ROMERO, R., Y. K. WU, D. T. BRODY, E. OYARZUN, G. W. DUFF & S. K. DURUM. 1989. Human decidua: a source of interleukin-1. Obstet. Gynecol. **73**: 31–34.
9. TABIBZADEH, S. S., U. SANTHANAM, P. B. SEHGAL & L. T. MAY. 1989. Cytokine-induced production of IFN-$\beta_2$/IL-6 by freshly explanted human endometrial stromal cells: modulation by estradiol-17$\beta$. J. Immunol. **142**: 3134–3139.
10. TABIBZADEH, S. 1990. Evidence of T-cell activation and potential cytokine action in human endometrium. J. Clin. Endocrinol. Metab. **71**: 645–649.
11. TABIBZADEH, S., K. L. KAFFKA, P. G. SATYASWAROOP & P. L. KLLIAN. 1990. Interleukin-1 (IL-1) regulation of human endometrial function: presence of IL-1 receptor correlates with IL-1 stimulated prostaglandin $E_2$ production. J. Clin. Endocrinol. Metab. **70**: 1000–1006.
12. TABIBZADEH, S. S., P. G. SATYASWAROOP & P. N. RAO. 1988. Antiproliferative effect of interferon-γ in human endometrial epithelial cells *in vitro*: potential local growth modulatory role in endometrium. J. Clin. Endocrinol. Metab. **67**: 131–138.
13. NOYES, R. W. & A. T. HERTIG. 1955. Dating the endometrial biopsy. Fertil. Steril. **1**: 3–25.
14. COHEN, J. 1988. Statistical Power Analysis for the Behavioral Sciences. 2nd edit. Lawrence Erlbaum Associates. Hillsdale, NJ.
15. SINGER, R. H., J. B. LAWRENCE & C. VILLNAVE. 1986. Optimization of *in situ* hybridization using isotopic and non-isotopic detection methods. Bio. Techniques **4**: 230–250.
16. HARPER, M. E., L. M. MASELLE, R. C. GALLO & F. WONG-STAAL. 1986. Detection of lymphocytes expressing human T-lymphotrophic virus type III in lymph nodes and peripheral blood from infected individuals by *in situ* hybridization. Proc. Natl. Acad. Sci. **83**: 772–776.
17. CHAN, S. H., B. PERUSSIA, J. W. GUPTA, M. KOBAYASHI, M. POSPISIL, H. A. YOUNG, S. F. WOLF, D. YOUNG, S. C. CLAVEK & G. TRINCHIERI. 1991. Induction of interferon-γ production by natural killer stimulatory factor: characterization of the responder cells and synergy with other inducers. J. Exp. Med. **173**: 869–879.
18. VAN LE, L., S. T. OH, J. A. ANNERS, C. A. RINHART & J. HALME. 1992. Interleukin-1 inhibits growth of normal human endometrial stromal cells. Obstet. Gynecol. **80**: 405–409.

19. TABIBZADEH, S. S., M. A. GERBER & P. G. SATYASWAROOP. 1986. Induction of HLA-DR antigen expression in endometrial epithelial cells *in vitro* by recombinant γ-interferon. Am. J. Pathol. **125:** 90–96.
20. FERENCZY, A., G. BERTRAND & M. M. GELFAND. 1979. Proliferation kinetics of human endometrium during the normal menstrual cycle. Am. J. Obstet. Gynecol. **133:** 859–867.
21. PACE, D., L. MORRISON & J. N. BULMER. 1989. Proliferative activity in endometrial stromal granulocytes throughout menstrual cycle and early pregnancy. J. Clin. Pathol. **42:** 35–39.
22. SCHENKEN, R. S., J. V. JOHNSON & R. M. RIEHL. 1991. C-myc protooncogene polypeptide expression in endometriosis. Am. J. Obstet. Gynecol. **164:** 1031–1036.
23. NEUMANN, C. & C. SORG. 1977. Immune interferon. I. Production by lymphokine-activated murine macrophages. Eur. J. Immunol. **7:** 719–725.
24. OLSTAD, R., M. DEGRE & R. SELJELID. 1981. Production of immune interferone (type II) in cocultures of mouse peritoneal macrophages and syngeneic tumor cells. Scand. J. Immunol. **13:** 605–608.
25. ROBINSON, B. W. S., T. L. MCLEMORE & R. G. CRYSTAL. 1985. Gamma interferon is spontaneously released by alveolar macrophages and lung T lymphocytes in patients with pulmonary sarcoidosis. J. Clin. Invest. **75:** 1488–1495.
26. NUGENT, K. M., J. GLAZIER, M. M. MONICK & G. W. HUNNINGHAKE. 1985. Stimulated human alveolar macrophages secrete interferon. Am. Rev. Respir. Dis. **131:** 714–718.
27. LANIER, U., M. A. ARNAOUT, R. SCHWARTING, N. L. WARNER & G. D. ROSS. 1985. p150/95, third member of the LFA-1/CR$_3$ polypeptide family identified by anti-leu M5 monoclonal antibody. Eur. J. Immunol. **15:** 713–718.
28. KLEIN, N. A., G. M. PÉRGOLA, R. RAO-TEKMAL, T. D. DEY & R. S. SCHENKEN. 1994. Enhanced expression of resident leukocyte interferon γ mRNA in endometriosis. Am. J. Reprod. Immunol. **30**.

# Deeply Infiltrating Endometriosis Is a Disease Whereas Mild Endometriosis Could Be Considered a Non-Disease

PHILIPPE R. KONINCKX,[a] DIDIER OOSTERLYNCK,
THOMAS D'HOOGHE,[b] AND CHRISTEL MEULEMAN

*Division of Gynecologic Endoscopic Surgery*
*Department of Obstetrics and Gynecology*
*University Hospital Gasthuisberg*
*K. U. Leuven*
*B-3000 Leuven, Belgium*

## INTRODUCTION

Endometriosis was described as a severe pathology necessitating radical surgery at the beginning of this century.[1-2] Defined morphologically as endometrial glands outside the uterine cavity both adenomyosis in the recto-vaginal septum, and chocolate cysts in the ovary were recognized as endometriosis.

Since the introduction of laparoscopy in the late sixties, the awareness that endometriosis is a very frequent disease has progressively increased. Initially typical lesions such as black puckered lesions and cystic ovarian endometriomas, which in their most severe forms were associated with extensive pelvic adhesions were described. In the early eighties, laparoscopic scrutiny led to the recognition of a whole variety of small white vesicles, red vesicles, flame-like lesions, polipoid lesions, and brown lesions as subtle forms of endometriosis.[3-4] Even a normal peritoneum was sometimes found to hide microscopical endometriosis.[5-6] In the late eighties $CO_2$-laser-excision techniques led to the observation that some typical lesions infiltrate deep into the subperitoneal stroma.[7-8] Although unexpected in the beginning, since it is found in women with a normal clinical examination, we rapidly realized that the most severe form of deep endometriosis presented clinically with extensive and painful nodularities in the pouch of Douglas. Now more subtle forms of deep endometriosis are being diagnosed.

Besides a brief review of deeply infiltrating endometriosis as a specific entity of severe endometriosis, an attempt will be made to consider the question whether endometriosis should always be regarded as a pathological condition or whether some forms of endometriosis could be considered a natural condition occurring in all women. In this concept only some forms of endometriosis should be considered pathological. This would not only change the question "Why do some women develop endometriosis?" into "Why does endometriosis develop in some women into a pathological condition?" but it could also stir up new ideas on prevention and treatment of endometriosis.

---

[a] Reprint requests: Prof. Dr. P. R. Koninckx, Department of Obstetrics and Gynecology, University Hospital Gasthuisberg, Herestraat 49, B-3000 Leuven, Belgium.

[b] Present address: Fearing Research Laboratory, Harvard Medical School, SGMB 204, 250 Longwood Avenue, Boston, MA 02115.

## *Definition and Types of Deep Endometriosis*

We defined deeply infiltrating endometriosis as endometriosis which infiltrates deeper than 5 mm under the peritoneum.[7-10] This choice of 5 mm was made because of morphological and epidemiological observations. Morphologically, superficial endometriosis (mostly subtle lesions) is an active disease in some 50% of lesions.[7] Lesions infiltrating only a few mm (mostly typical lesions) have frequently a burnt-out aspect, whereas lesions infiltrating deeper than 5 mm are morphologically the most active lesions. For infiltrating lesions a transition zone between morphologically active and inactive areas is estimated around 5–6 mm of depth. A second argument is derived from the frequency distribution of the depth of infiltration in women with pain and/or infertility, which is clearly biphasic with a nadir at 5–6 mm.[8] Both observations suggest that in the majority of women the endometriotic lesion infiltrates only superficially, and becomes inactive; however, when they infiltrate deeper than 5 mm, the disease becomes more active and aggressive, and develops into a much deeper lesion.

Laparoscopically endometriotic lesions defined as infiltrating deeper than 5 mm from the peritoneal cavity present most frequently as an area with mainly typical but also subtle lesions.[11,12] During excision this lesion which is easily recognized reveals itself as conical shaped becoming progressively smaller in its deeper parts. This lesion, type I, was therefore suggested to be caused by infiltration. Type II lesions are characterized by a small endometriotic lesion, surrounded by a massive bowel retraction. Sometimes at laparoscopy only the retraction is visible and during excision a large endometriotic nodule is revealed to be situated deeply under the bowel, which is retracted over it. In contrast to type I lesions, these lesions thus are characterized mainly by retraction. It is unclear whether type I and type II lesions are different entities or whether these differences are a consequence of the localization of these lesions in the pelvis. Type III lesions are generally laparoscopically small typical lesions, or sometimes even a normal peritoneum, overlying an induration. During excision, a massive spherical and deep lesion becomes apparent. Whereas type I lesions can be found in the uterovesical fold but most frequently in the pouch of Douglas, type III lesions are found exclusively in the pouch of Douglas or on the uterosacral ligaments. For this reason, and because of their morphological aspect type III lesions were suggested to be caused by adenomyosis externa.

The definition of deeply infiltrating endometriosis as endometriosis infiltrating deeper than 5 mm does not rule out that different physiopathological mechanisms could lead to this condition. However, it stresses the concept that once endometriosis is situated deeper than 5 mm under the peritoneum, it becomes a different condition. It is morphologically more active; it starts to grow and forms large nodules with massive pelvic distortion and severe pain.

This concept also emphasizes the differences in physiology between superficial and deep endometriotic lesions. Whereas superficial pelvic endometriosis secrete CA125 and PP14 mainly towards the peritoneal cavity, deep endometriotic nodules secrete CA125 and PP14 mainly towards the blood stream.[13] Similarly it seems logical to postulate that superficial pelvic endometriosis is hormonally influenced mainly by the peritoneal fluid microenvironment, whereas deep endometriosis is mainly influenced by plasma hormone concentrations. A transition zone at a depth of some 5 mm where diffusion from the peritoneal cavity would become less important, seems theoretically acceptable. Deep endometriosis would thus become endometriosis which has escaped from the direct influence of peritoneal fluid (FIG. 1).

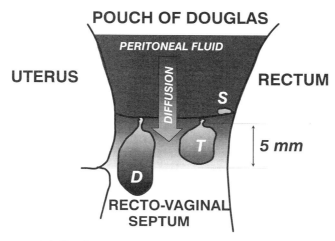

FIGURE 1. Deeply infiltrating endometriosis is defined as endometriosis infiltrating deeper than 5 mm under the pelvic peritoneum (D). It is suggested that subtle (S) and typical (T) lesions are mainly controlled by peritoneal fluid, whereas deep lesions are influenced by plasma hormones. Medical therapy could shrink deep lesions and bring them back under peritoneal fluid control.

## Diagnosis of Deep Endometriosis[11]

*Severe forms of deeply infiltrating endometriosis* are clinically obvious. Extensive nodularities in the pouch of Douglas are felt by bimanual clinical examination. During laparoscopy large areas of pelvic endometriosis presenting as a white plaque with dark brown spots and/or subtle lesions are easily recognized as type I lesions because of the massive induration underneath. Also type II lesions are easily recognized as a small lesion surrounded by bowel retraction and pelvic distorsion. Type III lesions can easily be missed if the laparoscopist is not aware of the nodule felt during the clinical examination, or by palpation during laparoscopy.

*Mild forms of deep endometriosis* on the contrary are easily missed. At clinical examination the endometriosis cannot be felt except during menstruation.[10] Therefore, a routine examination during menstruation is recommended in all women suspected of having deep endometriosis. Sometimes at laparoscopy mild forms of deep endometriosis can only be detected when an induration is felt by palpation under an endometriotic lesion or even when an induration is felt in an otherwise completely normal pouch of Douglas. A preoperative clinical examination preferentially during menstruation can be extremely helpful in recognizing and localizing these lesions.

The extent and depth of both severe and mild forms of deep endometriosis becomes apparent only during excision. Therefore, we recommend that all suspected lesions be excised.[9] During excision the border between endometriosis and normal healthy tissue is scrupulously followed by combining palpation of induration and visual appearance. Since tissue damage and bleeding is minimal using a $CO_2$-laser, preferentially in superpulse mode to avoid carbonization, this is the method of choice to excise deep endometriosis. Scissors give a good feeling of induration and plane of cleavage, but the tissue damage accompanying electrocoagulation, frequently blurs visual inspection. Since depth and lateral spread cannot be judged from the visual appearance, and since deep endometriosis often remains an almost "unexpected" finding during excision, coagulation or vaporization should not be used in any endometriotic lesion which could hide a deeper infiltrating lesion.

Because of the difficulty of making a diagnosis—clinically often unnoticed, laparoscopically sometimes invisible, really apparent only during excision—the clinical usefulness of ultrasound and magnetic resonance imaging (MRI) was investigated. Both techniques failed to detect reliably mild forms of deep endometriosis. Severe endometriosis was seen at MRI but the lateral spread and depth of invasion could not be predicted accurately.[14] CA125 plasma concentrations using a cut off concentration of 25 U/ml was shown to predict deep endometriosis with a sensitivity of 67% and a specificity of 90%.[13] Therefore, CA125 is recommended as a marker to be used in all women suspected of having deep endometriosis. Its clinical utility could become even more important when CA125 concentrations would be assayed during menstruation, or when the ratios between menstrual and follicular concentrations would be used, or when the CA125 concentrations would be used to diagnose type III lesions, which are clinically the most easily missed.

## *Treatment of Deep Endometriosis*

The diagnosis and more specifically the depth of infiltration and the lateral spread of deep endometriosis can only be made during excision. While this is the treatment of choice, our experience over the last five years also shows that the recurrence rate after complete excision is very low. Overall recurrence seems to be less than 10%, and practically speaking in all these women the previous excision could be traced as incomplete. Incomplete excision has been the consequence of inexperience, especially at the beginning of our investigation of deep endometriosis. The proximity of the ureter and the bowel can make a complete excision technically impossible but this has changed with time. Whereas a few years ago we preferred to leave some endometriosis in the bowel wall, we now prefer to perform a complete excision and to suture the bowel endoscopically if necessary. Also the dissection of endometriosis from the ureter is progressively done more completely since ureter lesions and even transsection can be treated endoscopically using a double J.[16-17] Complete excision, for which the $CO_2$-laser is technically the method of choice, thus is the only method for diagnosing and curing deep endometriosis. It is obvious that a complete bowel preparation is mandatory in all women scheduled for excision of deep endometriosis.

Women with deep endometriosis present clinically with pelvic pain or infertility or both.[7-8] Women with pain generally have larger and deeper lesions than women with infertility only: lesions infiltrating deeper than 10 mm almost invariably cause severe pain. The results of complete excision of deep endometriosis in women with pain are excellent, more than 80% of women being and remaining pain free for at least five years, the duration of our actual follow-up period. Also in women with infertility cumulative pregnancy rates of 67% are obtained after six months. Using Cox's multivariate life table analysis, it was demonstrated that in women with a regular cycle, with a normal fertile husband, and without tubal occlusion, when the duration of infertility was taken into account, endometriosis was the main predictor of a subsequent pregnancy. In the group of women with endometriosis, both the presence of deep endometriosis and of cystic ovarian endometriosis emerged as independent variables, whereas mild and moderate endometriosis were no longer significant as predictors.

Medical therapy of endometriosis has repeated been shown to give excellent results in alleviating pain in women with endometriosis.[18,19] Moreover, a large number of women remain pain free for longer periods following medical treatment by danazol, or GnRH agonists. On the other hand, medical treatment has been demonstrated to inactivate endometriosis, not to destroy endometriotic lesions.[20] Knowing that pelvic pain in women with endometriosis without cystic ovarian endometriosis is mainly caused by deep endometriosis, we suggest the following hypothesis. By inactivating endometriosis medical therapy will shrink the endometriotic nodule. If the remaining nodule would become less than 5–6 mm in depth, the endometriotic nodule would again become influenced by substances—hormones diffusing from the peritoneal fluid (FIG. 1). This could explain why many women remain pain free after medical treatment has been stopped. The importance of this concept would be that medical treatment should eventually be given intermittently in order to keep deep endometriosis under the influence of the peritoneal fluid and thus preventing it from further growth and infiltration.

In conclusion, our treatment of deep endometriosis is actually as follows. *Severe deep endometriosis* that is clinically obvious is pretreated with Decapeptyl (3.75 mg/month) or with danazol (400 mg daily) for 3 months. Clinically this makes the endometriotic nodule less vascularized while facilitating dissection. Shrinking of the nodule is anticipated but difficult to prove. *Mild forms of deep endometriosis* that are clinically only suspected are not medically pretreated. On the contrary, some have to undergo laparoscopy during menstruation, since in some women this is the only method of finding and excising deep endometriosis. In women refusing surgery, or with a recurrent disease, medical treatment is given for 6 months to 1 year. If necessary, the same treatment is continued intermittently for periods of 3 months.

## DISCUSSION AND GENERAL CONSIDERATIONS

### *A Model of Endometriosis Which Suggests That Minimal and Mild Endometriosis Is a Natural Condition (FIG. 2)*

Recent observations point to a very high incidence of endometriosis up to 80%—mostly subtle lesions—in women with pain and infertility.[8] Moreover, active remodeling of these lesions has become apparent in the baboon model,[21] whereas repeated laparoscopies suggest that subtle endometriosis is intermittently present in most animals. Since retrograde menstruation seems to be a normal condition occurring in most women we favor the hypothesis that implantation of some endometrial cells, giving rise to subtle lesions, could equally be a natural condition occurring intermittently in almost all women. This concept is consistent with the observation that endometriosis occurs in some 10% of normal fertile women and in some 10% to 20% of normal fertile baboons.[22] We suggest that a few months later, most of these lesions will have disappeared, whereas in some women new lesions at other localizations will be present; similarly some women with endometriosis would thus have become normal whereas others without endometriosis would have subtle lesions. This concept does not rule out that some conditions or influences would favor implantation and that some women would have a higher number and/or frequency of subtle lesions. Women with massive retrograde menstruation or with a LUF syndrome or with lower NK activity[23]

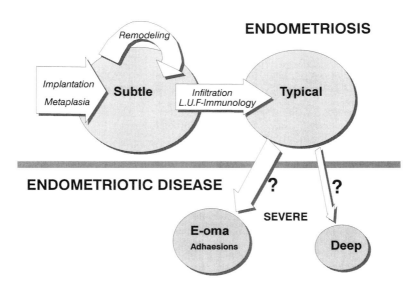

**FIGURE 2.** A model for endometriosis which emphasizes intermittent subtle endometriosis in (almost) all women and active remodeling. Superficial infiltration to burnt out typical lesions is rather frequent but in some women endometriosis develops into an endometriotic disease with severe lesions either cystic ovarian endometriosis or deep endometriosis, or both.

could thus have more implantation sites. Similarly, stress could be important as suggested in women, and since baboons have more and more frequently subtle lesions in captivity than in the wild.[24] Implantation of regurgitated endometrial cells would thus become a random process, which occurs rarely in some women and more frequently in others. At a cross sectional observation this would be reflected by a low or a high incidence of subtle lesions. Most important, however, is that in this concept subtle endometriosis would no longer be considered as a disease, but as a natural condition, only occurring more frequently in some women.

When the normal pelvic clearance mechanisms fail these endometriotic lesions can infiltrate. Our defense mechanisms, however, generally stop and control infiltration which remains superficial and ends as a burnt-out typical lesion. So also for many of these lesions the questions could be asked whether this is a disease, or rather the scar remaining after a healing process. Some of these lesions, however, will further infiltrate and develop into deep lesions.

Considering subtle and some typical lesions, a normal condition would raise the question whether it is useful to treat these lesions as superfluous. Moreover, this concept is consistent with the prevailing clinical observation that these lesions do not cause pain, whereas fertility is not enhanced after medical or surgical treatment.[25,26]

The physiopathological question would thus change from "why do some women develop endometriosis?" into "why does endometriosis become aggressive in some women?" or "why does endometriosis become an endometriotic disease?"

## *Endometriotic Disease: Deep Endometriosis and Ovarian Cystic Endometriosis*

In some women endometriosis becomes aggressive and forms cystic ovarian endometriosis and/or deep endometriosis. These forms will therefore be called endometriotic disease in order to contrast them with subtle lesions and some typical lesions which will be called endometriosis.

Deep endometriosis and cystic ovarian endometriosis are two separate entities of endometriotic disease. They generally do not occur in the same women.[12] Cystic ovarian endometriosis is strongly associated with pelvic adhesions, whereas deep endometriosis is not.[8] Consequently, cystic ovarian endometriosis is classified as stage III or IV of the rAFS classification, whereas deep endometriosis is classified mainly as stages I and II. Both manifestations of the endometriotic disease are statistically found to be independent variables which predict pelvic pain,[8] which predict infertility (paper in preparation), which predict decreased natural killer cell activity in plasma,[27] and which predict increased plasma concentrations of CA125 and PP14.

It is interesting to note that both deep endometriosis and cystic ovarian endometriosis have escaped from the predominant influence of peritoneal fluid (FIG. 1). The former is mainly influenced by plasma concentrations, whereas the latter will probably be influenced to a large extent by ovarian microenvironment with at least much higher steroid hormone concentrations. This model also reemphasizes peritoneal fluid which has a predominant inhibiting role upon the development of endometriotic disease from endometriosis. Future studies will be necessary to determine which factors of this microenvironment—macrophages and natural killer cells, cytokines, angiogenic[28] and growth factors, steroid hormones and specific proteins—are a consequence of the clearing activity of endometriosis, and which factors permit or promote the development of endometriotic disease.

## SUMMARY

Deeply infiltrating endometriosis can be defined as endometriosis infiltrating deeper than 5 mm under the peritoneal surface. Type I is a conical lesion suggested to be caused by infiltration; type II is mainly caused by retraction of the bowel over the lesion; type III is the most severe lesion suggested to be caused by adenomyosis externa. Severe cases are clinically apparent by nodularities in the pouch of Douglas, whereas mild and subtle forms of deep endometriosis are easily missed. Clinical examination during menstruation and scrutiny at laparoscopy for indurations, followed, preferably, by $CO_2$-laser-excision are the key features for diagnosis and treatment. It is importnat to realize that depth of infiltration and lateral spread cannot be evaluated by laparoscopic inspection but only during excision, that CA125 concentration but not ultrasound or nuclear magnetic resonance can be helpful in the diagnosis, and that in the most severe cases medical pretreatment is advocated. Results of excision, as evaluated by disappearance of pain in some 80% of women, by a cumulative pregnancy of some 70% and a low recurrence rate, are excellent.

The peritoneal fluid is thought to play a key role in the physiopathology of deep endometriosis which is considered to be endometriosis which has escaped from the influence of the peritoneal fluid. This concept is clinically important for the medical treatment of endometriosis, which is suggested to shrink deep lesions and to bring them back under peritoneal fluid control.

A model of endometriosis is proposed and discussed. Subtle lesions are considered a natural condition occurring intermittently in all women, whereas we question whether mild endometriosis is a disease. In some women endometriosis has an aggressive behavior and develops into cystic ovarian endometriosis or into deeply infiltrating endometriosis. In this model subtle and mild forms would be called "endometriosis," whereas deep and cystic ovarian forms could be called "endometriotic disease." It is stressed that deep and cystic ovarian endometriosis are two distinct entities, which is important for our understanding of endometriosis, for classification and for treatment of endometriosis.

## ACKNOWLEDGMENTS

Past and present co-workers and co-authors are sincerely thanked for their help and discussions: Dr. Sc. Freddy Cornillie (Centocor Diagnostics Europe, 2018 Antwerpen), Dr. Stephan Demeyere (A. Z. St.-Lucas, 8310 Brugge), Dr. Karine Stukkens (H.-Hartkliniek, 1700 Asse), Dr. Marc Muyldermans (A. Z. Virga Jesse, 3500 Hasselt) and Dr. Jan Deprest (Center for Endoscopic Technologies, 3000 Leuven). Prof. Dan Martin (Memphis, TN), Dr. Chandrit Bambra (Institute of Primate Research, Nairobi, Kenya) and Prof. Markku Seppälä together with Dr. Leena Riittinen (Helsinki University, Finland) are thanked for the opportunity of collaborative studies. The help of Dr. Stefan Lempereur and Dr. Stefaan Wens (Ipsen NV, 9051 Sint-Denijs-Westrem) is greatly appreciated, as well as that of Mrs. Christine Dewit and Mrs. Marie-Josée Vanderheyden in the laboratory, and of Mrs. Marleen Craessaerts as a research nurse. We also thank Mrs. Diane Wolput for her secretarial efficiency.

## REFERENCES

1. SAMPSON, J. A. 1921. Perforating hemorrhagic (chocolate) cysts of the ovary. Their importance and especially their relation to pelvic adenomas of the endometrial type ('adenomyoma' of the uterus, rectovaginal septum, sigmoid, etc.). Arch. Surg. **3:** 245–323.
2. CULLEN, T. S. 1919. The distribution of adenomyomata containing uterine mucosa. Am. J. Obstet. Gynecol. **80:** 130.
3. JANSEN, R. P. S. & P. RUSSELL. 1986. Nonpigmented endometriosis: clinical, laparoscopic and pathologic definition. Am. J. Obstet. Gynecol. **155:** 1154–1159.
4. REDWINE, D. B. 1987. The distribution of endometriosis in the pelvis by age groups and fertility. Fertil. Steril. **47:** 173–175.
5. MARTIN, D. C., G. D. HUBERT, R. VANDER ZWAAG & F. A. EL-ZEKY. 1989. Laparoscopic appearances of peritoneal endometriosis. Fertil. Steril. **51:** 63–67.
6. MURPHY, A. A., D. S. GUZICK & J. A. ROCK. 1989. Letter to the editor. Fertil. Steril. **51:** 1072–1073.
7. CORNILLIE, F. J., D. OOSTERLYNCK, J. M. LAUWERYNS & P. R. KONINCKX. 1990. Deeply infiltrating pelvic endometriosis: histology and clinical significance. Fertil. Steril. **53:** 978–983.
8. KONINCKX, P. R., C. MEULEMAN, S. DEMEYERE, E. LESAFFRE & F. CORNILLIE. 1991. Suggestive evidence that pelvic endometriosis is a progressive disease, whereas deeply infiltrating endometriosis is associated with pelvic pain. Fertil. Steril. **55:** 759–765.
9. KONINCKX, P. R., J. DEPREST, C. MEULEMAN & D. MARTIN. 1993. The method of destruction of endometriosis makes a difference. Letter to the editor. Fertil. Steril. **60:** 202–203.

10. KONINCKX, P. R. 1992. Deeply infiltrating endometriosis. In The Current Status of Endometriosis. I. Brosens & J. Donnez, Eds. 437–446. Parthenon Publ. Group. Carnforth, NY.
11. KONINCKX, P. R. & F. J. CORNILLIE. 1992. Infiltrating endometriosis: infiltration, retraction or adenomyosis externa? In Appearances of Endometriosis. D. Martin, Ed. 9.1–9.8. Gower Med. Publ. London & New York.
12. KONINCKX, P. R. & D. MARTIN. 1992. Deep endometriosis: a consequence of infiltration or retraction or possibly adenomyosis externa? Fertil. Steril. **58**: 924–928.
13. KONINCKX, P. R., L. RIITTINEN, M. SEPPALA & F. J. CORNILLIE. 1992. CA-125 and PP14 concentrations in plasma and peritoneal fluid of women with deeply infiltrating pelvic endometriosis. Fertil. Steril. **57**: 523–530.
14. DEPREST, J., G. MARCHAL & P. R. KONINCKX. 1993. MRI in the diagnosis of deeply infiltrating endometriosis. 22nd Annual Meeting of the American Association of Gynecologic Laparoscopists (AAGL), abstract. San Francisco, Marriott, CA, November 10–14.
15. KONINCKX, P. R., M. MUYLDERMANS, C. MEULEMAN & F. J. CORNILLIE. 1993. CA 125 in the management of endometriosis. Eur. J. Obstet. Gynaecol. Reprod. Biol. **49**: 109–113.
16. NEZHAT, C., F. NEZHAT & B. GREEN. 1992. Laparoscopic treatment of obstructed ureter due to endometriosis by resection and ureteroureterostomy. J. Urol. **148**: 865–868.
17. NEVEN, P., H. VANDEURSEN, L. BAERT & P. R. KONINCKX. 1993. Ureteric injury at laparoscopic surgery: the endoscopic management. Case review. Gynaecol. Endosc. **2**: 45–46.
18. ZORN, J. R., J. MATHIESON, F. RISQUEZ, A. M. COMARU-SCHALLY & A. V. SCHALLY. 1990. Treatment of endometriosis with a delayed release preparation of the agonist D-Trp$^6$-luteinizing hormone-releasing hormone: long-term follow-up in a series of 50 patients. Fertil. Steril. **53**: 401–406.
19. MOGHISSI, K. S. 1993. GnRH agonists in the management of endometriosis. In GnRH Analogues. The State of the Art. B. Lunenfeld & V. Insler, Eds. Vol. 4: 49–53. Parthenon Publishing Group. Lancs, NY.
20. EVERS, J. L. H. 1987. The second look laparoscopy for evaluation of the result of medical treatment of endometriosis should not be performed during ovarian suppression. Fertil. Steril. **47**: 502–504.
21. D'HOOGHE, T. M., C. S. BAMBRA, M. ISAHAKIA & P. R. KONINCKX. 1992. Evolution of spontaneous endometriosis in the baboon (*Papio anubis, Papio cynocephalus*) over a 12 month period. Fertil. Steril. **58**: 409–412.
22. D'HOOGHE, T. M., C. S. BAMBRA, F. J. CORNILLIE, M. ISAHAKIA & P. R. KONINCKX. 1991. Prevalence and laparoscopic appearance of spontaneous endometriosis in the baboon (*Papio anubis, Papio cynocephalus*). Biol. Reprod. **45**: 411–416.
23. OOSTERLYNCK, D., F. J. CORNILLIE, M. WAER, M. VANDEPUTTE & P. R. KONINCKX. 1991. Women with endometriosis show a defect in natural killer activity resulting in a decreased cytotoxicity to autologous endometrium. Fertil. Steril. **56**: 45–51.
24. D'HOOGHE, T. M. et al. 1993. Submitted for publication.
25. SCHENKEN, R. S. & L. R. MALINAK. 1982. Conservative surgery versus expectant management for the infertile patient with mild endometriosis. Fertil. Steril. **37**: 183–186.
26. THOMAS, E. J. & I. D. COOKE. 1987. Successful treatment of asymptomatic endometriosis: does it benefit infertile women? Br. Med. J. **294**: 1117–1119.
27. OOSTERLYNCK, D. J., C. MEULEMAN, M. WAER & P. R. KONINCKX. 1991. The decreased cellular immunity in women with endometriosis is related with the volume and depth of infiltration of endometriosis. Presented at the 47th annual meeting of the AFS, Orlando, FL.
28. OOSTERLYNCK, D. J., C. MEULEMAN, H. SOBIS, M. VANDEPUTTE & P. R. KONINCKX. 1993. Angiogenic activity of peritoneal fluid from women with endometriosis. Fertil. Steril. **59**: 778–782.

# Peritoneal Endometriosis: Two-Dimensional and Three-Dimensional Evaluation of Typical and Subtle Lesions[a]

JACQUES DONNEZ, MICHELLE NISOLLE,
AND FRANÇOISE CASANAS-ROUX

*Infertility Research Unit
Department of Gynecology
Catholic University of Louvain
Cliniques Universitaires St. Luc
Avenue Hippocrate 10
B-1200 Brussels, Belgium*

Endometriosis most commonly affects the pelvic peritoneum close to the ovaries, including the uterosacral ligaments, the ovarian fossa peritoneum, and the peritoneum of the cul-de-sac.

The increased diagnosis of endometriosis at laparoscopy can be explained by the increased experience and ability of the surgeon to detect such subtle lesions. The greatest change has been in the case of "subtle" lesions, which increased from 15% in 1986 to 65% in 1988. The diagnosis of peritoneal endometriosis at the time of laparoscopy is often made by the observation of typically puckered black or bluish lesions. There are, in addition, numerous subtle appearances of peritoneal endometriosis.

These lesions, frequently nonpigmented, were diagnosed as endometriosis following confirmation by biopsy by Jansen and Russell in 1986.

*Typical Lesions*

The typical black peritoneal endometriotic lesion results from tissue bleeding and retention of blood pigment producing brown discoloration of tissue.

Puckered black lesions are a combination of glands, stroma and intraluminal debris.

*Evolution*

The macroscopic appearance of ectopic endometrium is probably dependent upon the longevity of the process. Viable cells may implant and the initial appearance may be an irregularity or discoloration of the peritoneal surface—the earliest sign being hemosiderin staining of the peritoneal surfaces. Initially, these lesions

---

[a] Partially supported by grants from the Fonds de la Recherche Scientifique (Belgique) and from Ipsen Biotech (France).

TABLE 1. Different Appearances of Peritoneal Endometriosis

| |
|---|
| Black |
|     typical puckered black lesion |
| Red |
|     red flamelike lesions (Jansen and Russell, 1986) |
|     glandular excrescences (Jansen, 1986) |
|     petechial peritoneum (Donnez and Nisolle, 1988) |
|     areas of hypervascularization (Donnez and Nisolle, 1988) |
| White |
|     white opacification (Jansen and Russell, 1986) |
|     subovarian adhesions (Jansen, 1986) |
|     yellow-brown peritoneal patches (Jansen, 1986) |
|     circular peritoneal defects (Chatman, 1981) |

may appear hemorrhagic, but menstrual shedding from a viable endometrial implant initiates an inflammatory reaction which provokes a scarification process which, in turn, encloses the implants. The presence of entrapped menstrual debris is responsible for the typical black or bluish appearance. If the inflammatory process obliterates or devascularizes the endometrial cells, eventually this discoloration disappears. A white plaque of old collagen is all that remains of the ectopic implant. Scarring of the peritoneum around endometrial implants is a typical finding. In addition to encapsulating an isolated implant, the scar may deform the surrounding peritoneum or result in the development of adhesions.

## *Subtle Appearances*

Sometimes the subtle endometriotic lesions can be the only lesions seen at laparoscopy. The subtle forms are more common and may be more active than the puckered black lesions (TABLE 1).

The nonpigmented endometriotic peritoneal lesions include essentially the following:

### *Red Lesions*

1) Red flamelike lesions of the peritoneum or red vesicular excrescences more commonly affecting the broad ligament and the uterosacral ligaments. Histologically, red flamelike lesions and vesicular excrescences are due to the presence of active endometriosis surrounded by stroma.

2) Glandular excrescences on the peritoneal surface which in color, translucency and consistency closely resemble the mucosal surface of the endometrium seen at hysteroscopy. Biopsy reveals the presence of numerous endometrial glands.

3) Areas of petechial peritoneum or areas with hypervascularization were diagnosed as endometriosis in our recent study. These lesions resemble the petechial lesions resulting from the manipulation of the peritoneum or from hypervascularization of the peritoneum. They most generally affect the bladder and the broad ligament, and histologically, red blood cells are numerous and endometrial glands are very rare.

*White Lesions*

1) White opacification of the peritoneum which appears as peritoneal scarring or as circumscribed patches, often thickened and sometimes raised. Histologically, white opacified peritoneum is due to the presence of an occasional retroperitoneal glandular structure and scanty stroma surrounded by fibrotic tissue or connective tissue.

2) Subovarian adhesions or adherence between the ovary and the peritoneum of the ovarian fossa, which are distinctive from adhesions characteristic of previous salpingitis or peritonitis. Histologically, connective tissue with sparse endometrial glands was found.

3) Yellow-brown peritoneal patches resembling "café au lait" patches. The histological characteristics are similar to those observed in white opacification, but in the yellow-brown patches the presence of the blood pigment hemosiderin among the stroma cells produces the "café au lait" color.

4) Circular peritoneal defects as described by Chatman. Serial section demonstrates the presence of endometrial glands in more than 50% of cases. Peritoneal endometriosis can thus be found in the visually normal peritoneum of infertile women with or without associated endometriosis.

### *Morphometric Study of Vascularization*

Vascularization of endometriotic implants is probably one of the most important factors of growth and invasion of endometrial glands in other tissue. A stereometric analysis was applied in order to study precisely the vascularization in peritoneal endometriotic foci.

We evaluated histologically the vascularization of typical peritoneal endometriosis and its modifications according to the macroscopic appearance of peritoneal endometriosis.

A 2-D image analysis program set on Vidas computer (Kontron Bildanalyse GmBH, Eching, Germany) was completed by the interactive counting of 262,144 points.

All endometriotic lesions (n = 220) were analyzed field by field using the objective 40× of an Axioskop light microscope (Zeiss, Oberkochen, Germany) and a television camera (Dag-MTI, Michigan City, IN). The histological features were displayed on a television monitor and stored in the memory for processing by the measuring program. The mean of fields analyzed in each case was 13.3 ± 6.7. Histologic structures of interest such as the stroma, the glandular epithelium and lumen, the capillaries and the lymphocytes were drawn moving a cursor. Each different structure was discriminated and grey level images were transferred to binary images. The interactive measurements of the selected parameters (number of structures, area and perimeter of the structures per field) were appended and stored at the end of an existing data base.

Data management and evaluation were checked according to specific search criteria on the Videoplan (Kontron Bildanalyse GmBH, Eching, Germany) and displayed on the television monitor and printed. In all cases, the mitotic index was calculated as previously described (Donnez *et al.* 1992) by counting mitotic figures (prometaphase, metaphase, anaphase, and telophase) for 2000 epithelial cells per biopsy. This is the only method available for women because administration of colchicine or tritiated thymidine is not ethical. The contingency table method, the $\chi^2$ (chisquare) test, the *t* test and the median test were used for statistical analysis.

TABLE 2. Morphometric Study of Stromal Vascularization

|  | Typical Lesions (Black) Group Ia n = 135 | Red Lesions Group Ib n = 35 | White Lesions Group Ic n = 50 | Treated Typical Lesions Group Id n = 45 |
|---|---|---|---|---|
| Number of capillaries/mm$^2$ stroma | 243 | 147 | 206 | 225 |
| Capillary mean surface ($\mu$m$^2$) | 118 ± 84 | 234 ± 192* | 78 ± 43** | 71 ± 40** |
| Capillaries/stroma relative surface (%) | 2.4 | 3.2* | 1.5** | 1.4** |

\* Significantly different from groups Ic and Id.
\*\* Significantly different from group Ia. Modified from Nisolle et al. 1993.

The results concerning the capillaries are shown in TABLE 2. The number of capillaries per mm$^2$ of stroma, their mean surface area and the surface area ratio (capillaries/stroma) were calculated. The mitotic index was calculated in glandular epithelium and its value was 0.1‰ and 0.61‰ respectively in group Ia and group Ib. In group Ic (white lesions), no mitosis was observed. The vascularization of typical peritoneal endometriosis was evaluated in 45 patients after GnRH-agonist therapy.

Our study demonstrated significant differences between the typical (black or bluish) lesion and the "subtle" lesion. Subtle lesions were classified as red lesions (vesicular, red flamelike and glandular excrescences) and as white lesions (white opacification, yellow-brown patches, circular peritoneal defects). When compared to typical lesion data, the vascularization was found to be significantly higher in red lesions and significantly lower in white lesions. This change was due to an increase (red) or a decrease (white) in the volume occupied by the vessels as proved by both the mean capillary surface area and the ratio of capillaries/stroma surface area. This change is more evident in the group of red lesions in which the number of capillaries/mm$^2$ was significantly lower than in the other subgroups.

Thus, in the red lesions, the increased level of vascularization is due to a greater number of larger vessels than in the other groups. In white lesions, there was a great number of smaller vessels although the number of capillaries was higher than in red lesions.

Moreover, the mitotic index was also significantly different in the three groups. Mitotic processes permit the maintenance and the growth of peritoneal endometriosis. The absence of mitosis in white lesions proves their low "activity." According to our data, we suggest that there are probably different types of peritoneal endometriotic lesions, in different stages of development. Red flamelike lesions and glandular excrescences are probably the first stage of early implantation of endometrial glands and stroma.

The growth and aggressiveness of endometrial glands in the stroma has recently been demonstrated by a three-dimensional evaluation (Ito et al. 1990). Indeed, in this group, a higher incidence of glands with ramifications was observed when compared to typical and white lesions. The significantly higher stromal vascularization and epithelial mitotic index could be responsible for the invasion of glands and stroma into the ectopic sites.

Our results demonstrated that there was a significant decrease in the vascularization of the endometriotic foci after GnRH agonist therapy. This change was not due to a reduction in the number of capillaries in the lesion but to a decrease in the area of the vessels. Indeed, in the treated patients (group Id), a predominance of smaller vessels was observed when compared with the untreated patients (group I). This vascularization decrease, observed histologically, was in accordance with the observations made by laparoscopy after hormonal therapy. Vascular effects of the GnRH agonist have also been demonstrated by Doppler on the uterine arteries (Matta *et al.*, 1988). The hypooestradiolemy induced by GnRH-a could also have an effect on the vascular compartment of the endometriotic stroma.

The reduction in the vascularization after hormonal therapy could account for the decrease in the inflammatory reaction observed around the endometriotic foci.

In conclusion, the evaluation of the stromal vascularization permitted the differentiation and classification of the different appearances of peritoneal endometriosis according to their vascularization level. Our study proves that the "activity" of peritoneal endometriosis is related to the vascularity.

## *Three-Dimensional (3-D) Architecture of Endometriosis*

In order to elucidate further biological characteristics of peritoneal endometriotic lesions, for example, how they stereologically develop *in vivo* and how glandular epithelium and stroma are related to the surrounding tissue, a recently advanced stereographic computer-technology was applied for the investigation of three-dimensional (3-D) architectures of peritoneal endometriosis.

## METHODS

All biopsy specimens were fixed in formaldehyde and embedded in paraffin. Six micrometer serial sections were stained with Gomori's trichrome and examined on a blind basis, with a Leitz Orthoplan microscope (Leitz, Wetzlar, Germany).

The histological features of the sections were displayed using an Axioskop microscope (Zeiss, Oberkochen, Germany) through a CCD 72 E camera (Dage-MTI, Michigan City, IN) on a monitor on which two-dimensional (2-D) figures drawn with a digitizer were superimposed using a computer (Vidas, Kontron Bildanalyse GmBH, Eching, Germany). Computer-assisted reconstruction of three-dimensional models was developed with two main aims in mind: (1) to generate a complete multicolored model of a complex structure which can be rotated and viewed from any angle or orientation; (2) to calculate the volumes and surfaces within the 3-D model automatically. The major features of the program include (1) input of serial section data by manual tracing, or automatic contour finding; (2) alignment of sections; (3) editing and reassignment of contours of individual sections; (4) storing contour data in a file; (5) selecting a range of sections and/or a range of elements to be used for reconstruction; (6) reconstructing in a wire frame and/or a solid modelling mode by using parallel projection; (7) rotating reconstruction in the x, y and z plane at variable magnification; (8) viewing inside a model by cutting away part of the reconstruction using an "electronic knife;" (9) calculating surfaces and volumes; (10) plotting reconstruction on a matrix or laser print.

With this program, outlines of glandular structure and endometrial stroma in the serial histological sections were traced by the digitizer, sections were aligned and contour data stored in a file: once all the serial outlines had been digitized and stored, reconstructed (3-D) image models of these *in vivo* structures were displayed on the TV monitor. The 3-D reconstruction could generate a complete multicolored model of the complex structure which could be rotated and viewed from any angle or orientation. Volumes of the reconstructed glandular and stromal structures were obtained by calculation function in the same program. Lumen volume which is the volume attributed to the lumen was also calculated. Ratios of lumen volume/epithelial volume/stromal volume were determined for each specimen. The $\chi^2$ test was used for statistical analysis.

## RESULTS

In 42 women who were undergoing laparoscopy for infertility, peritoneal biopsies of 3 to 5 mm in size were taken from areas of the pelvic peritoneum bearing foci of endometriosis, with a biopsy punch forceps (26–175 DH, Storz, Tuttlingen, Germany). Biopsy was taken from the typical (puckered black) endometriotic implants in all cases.

Group I consisted of 26 women with peritoneal endometriosis who had not previously received any hormonal therapy. All of them underwent laparoscopy during the early luteal phase.

Group II consisted of 17 women who had received a gonadotrophin-releasing hormone agonist (GnRH-a) therapy (Zoladex, ICI, Cambridge, UK) for 12 weeks before biopsy. After a well-known initial stimulation of estradiol (E2) secretion, GnRH-a administration resulted in a postmenopausal E2 secretion range (15 ± 6 pg/ml).

Histologically, all the biopsy specimens showed typical epithelium and stroma of the endometrial type. The reconstructed 3-D image models of the structures in the peritoneal endometriotic lesions were displayed and a pink color was applied for the stroma, a green color for the epithelium and blue color for the lumen.

The 3-D image models were usually indicated as a solid structure; however, models could be displayed as a transparent structure, when they were simultaneously shown with their stromal and epithelial structures.

Stereographically, two types could be easily recognized and classified: (1) The first type is composed of cylinder-like glands without ramifications. The lesion shows a regular distribution of the glandular epithelium in the stromal structure which is also regular (FIG. 1). (2) The second type is composed of glands with ramifications (FIG. 2). Luminal structures are interconnected with one another. Epithelial structures appear like fingers and seem to invade the stroma. The distribution of glandular structures in the stroma is not regular. Many glandular structures formed inside luminal structures whose diameter varied from 22 to 185 $\mu$m.

In all groups, the "external" stromal surface is regular. Like normal uterine epithelial structures, the glandular epithelium has a markedly regular luminal surface. In some cases, the lumen is dilated; in other cases, especially when the ramifications are numerous, the lumen is narrow. The incidence of the first type was 44% in group I and 46% in group II. The incidence of the second type was 56% and 54%, respectively. Volumes of epithelial, stromal and luminal structures were separately measured by computer stereometry and the results are shown in TABLE 3. The stroma/lesion ratio was 62.2% and 51.8% in group I and II, respectively. Although there was a decrease in stroma/lesion ratio in group II, when compared to group I, the difference was not significant. The epithelium/lesion

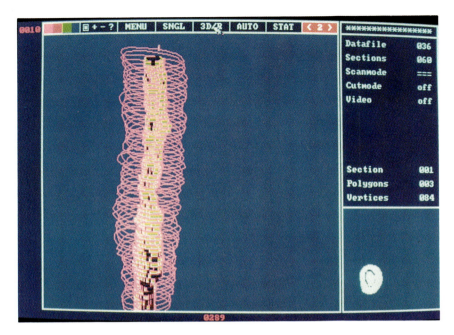

**FIGURE 1.** Cylinder-like gland. Regular distribution of the glandular epithelium in the stroma.

ratio was 19.9% and 14.9%, respectively. The lumen/lesion ratio was 13.2% and 25.2% in groups I and II, respectively. These values were significantly ($p < 0.01$) different.

## COMMENTS

Recently, computer-stereographic studies of skin tissues have been reported describing the advantages of the computer-generated 3-D models of tissue structures. As far as we know, there has been no publication on the topic of endometriosis using computer-graphic mechanical methods of reconstruction.

When compared with the 3-D models demonstrated in other studies, the present 3-D models seemed to be much better and to show more realistic appearances of structures since the structures of the reconstructed models were colored. Furthermore the transparent display of our 3-D models was excellent for the observation of their inside structures. The present study demonstrates that two different types of endometrial peritoneal lesions can be differentiated: (1) a first type without ramification of the glands; (2) a second type in which glands are ramified and connected.

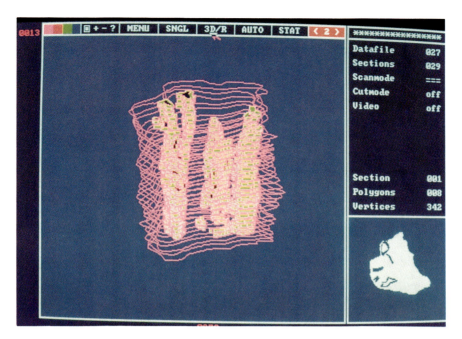

**FIGURE 2.** Glands with ramifications. Luminal structures are interconnected with one another (3-D).

Further studies are needed in order to evaluate if the two different types could be correlated either to the different degree of a "aggressiveness" or to the different appearances of peritoneal endometriosis.

From the present stereographic findings, one may consider that the apparently multifocal occurrence (in 2-D) of glandular epithelium in one lesion is not confirmed by the 3-D study. Indeed, in each peritoneal lesion, epithelial glands are interconnected by luminal structures. Probably, in each peritoneal lesion, epithelial structures occur in a single focus of the stroma and may then gradually develop, elongate and swell forming luminal structures, occasionally with endometrial debris inside. During the expansion, all glands are connected and *no* peripheral epithelial structures become independent by loss of interconnection.

Since each of the peritoneal lesions stereographically reconstructed in the

**TABLE 3.** Stereometry of Volumes of 3-D Structures: Percentage of the Lesion Attributed to the Epithelium, Stroma, or Lumen

| Ratio (%) | Group I<br>n = 26 | Group II<br>n = 16 |
|---|---|---|
| Epithelium/lesion | 19.9% | 14.9% |
| Stroma/lesion | 62.2% | 51.8% |
| Lumen/lesion | 13.2% | 25.2% |

present study was only a part of the peritoneal endometriosis in one patient, it is far too soon to come to any conclusion, but in the future, the 3-D analysis of stereographically reconstructed lesions could contribute to the understanding of the *in vivo* development of endometriosis.

This stereometric study of volumes of 3-D structures revealed the volume distribution in peritoneal endometriosis. The ratios of epithelium, stroma, lumen/ lesion observed in group I and II indicate a stronger effect of the GnRH agonist therapy on the stroma than on the epithelium. This effect could be due to the reduction in stromal vascularization induced by GnRH agonist. The stromal capillary network can also be reconstructed in 3-D. In active lesions, the 3-D evaluation of the capillary network reveals the presence of a great number of larger vessels. After GnRH agonist therapy (as well as in white lesions), the network is composed of smaller vessels.

The present stereographic and stereometric study has shown some new characteristics of peritoneal endometriosis. Further studies will be required to investigate the variations in the 3-D architecture of peritoneal endometriotic lesions among the different appearances of endometriosis in individual patients, among patients of different ages, or among patients having different types of peritoneal endometriosis before and after hormonal therapy.

## REFERENCES

BERGQVIST, A., G. RANNEVIK & J. THORELL. 1981. Estrogen and progesterone cytosol receptor concentration in endometriotic tissue and intrauterine endometrium. Acta Obstet. Gynecol. Scand. **101:** 53–58.

BRAVERMAN, M. S. & I. M. BRAVERMAN. 1986. Three-dimensional reconstructions of objects from serial sections using a microcomputer graphic system. J. Invest. Dermatol. **86:** 290–294.

BROSENS, I., G. VASQUEZ & S. GORDTS. 1984. Scanning electron microscopic study of the pelvic peritoneum in unexplained infertility and endometriosis. Fertil. Steril. **41:** 215.

CHATMAN, D. L. 1981. Pelvic peritoneal defects and endometriosis; Allen-Masters syndrome revisited. Fertil. Steril. **36:** 751.

DONNEZ, J., M. NISOLLE & F. CASANAS-ROUX. 1992. Three-dimensional architectures of peritoneal endometriosis. Fertil. Steril. **57:** 980.

ITO, M., H. YOKOYAMA, K. IKEDA & Y. SAT. 1990. Stereographic analysis of syringomas. Arch. Dermatol. Res. **282:** 17–21.

JANNE, O., A. KAUPPILA & E. KOKKO. 1981. Estrogen and progestin receptors in endometriosis lesions: comparison with endometrial tissue. Am. J. Obstet. Gynecol. **141:** 562–566.

JANSEN, R. P. S. & P. RUSSELL. 1986. Nonpigmented endometriosis: clinical laparoscopic and pathologic definition. Am. J. Obstet. Gynecol. **155:** 1154.

LOX, C. D., L. WORD & M. W. HEINE. 1984. Ultrastructural evaluation of endometriosis. Fertil. Steril. **41:** 755.

MARCHEVSKY, A. M., J. GIL & H. JEANTY. 1987. Computerized interactive morphometry in pathology: current instrumentation and methods. Hum. Pathol. **18:** 320–331.

MARTIN, D. C., G. D. HUBERT, R. VANDER ZWAAG & F. EL-ZEKY. 1989. Laparoscopic appearances of peritoneal endometriosis. Fertil. Steril. **51:** 63.

MATTA, W. H. M., I. STABILLE, R. S. SHAW & S. CAMPBELL. 1988. Doppler assessment of uterine blood flow changes in patients with fibroids receiving the GnRH agonist Buserelin. Fertil. Steril. **49:** 1083.

MURPHY, A. A., W. R. GREEN, D. BOBBIE, Z. C. DE LA CRUZ & J. A. ROCK. 1986. Unsuspected endometriosis documented by scanning electron microscopy in visually normal peritoneum. Fertil. Steril. **46:** 522.

NISOLLE, M., F. CASANAS-ROUX & J. DONNEZ. 1988. Histologic study of ovarian endometriosis after hormonal therapy. Fertil. Steril. **49:** 423.

NISOLLE, M., B. PAINDAVEINE, A. BOURDON, M. BERLIÈRE, F. CASANAS-ROUX & J. DONNEZ. 1990. Histologic study of peritoneal endometriosis in infertile women. Fertil. Steril. **53:** 984–988.

NISOLLE, M., F. CASANAS-ROUX, V. ANAF, J. M. MINE & J. DONNEZ. 1993. Morphometric study of the stromal vascularization in peritoneal endometriosis. Fertil. Steril. **59:** 681.

REDWINE, D. B. 1987. The distribution of endometriosis in the pelvis by age groups and fertility. Fertil. Steril. **47:** 173–175.

RODDICK, J. W., G. CONKEY & E. J. JACOBS. 1960. The hormonal response of endometriotic implants and its relationship to symptomatology. Am. J. Obstet. Gynecol. **79:** 1173–1177.

STRIPLING, M. C., D. C. MARTIN, D. L. CHATMAN, R. VANDER ZWAAG & W. M. POSTON. 1988. Subtle appearances of pelvic endometriosis. Fertil. Steril. **49:** 427.

TAMAYA, T., T. MOTOYAHA & Y. OHONO. 1979. Steroid receptor levels and histology of endometriosis and adenomyosis. Fertil. Steril. **31:** 394–400.

# Epidemiology and Diagnosis of Endometriosis

G. B. MELIS, S. AJOSSA, S. GUERRIERO,
A. M. PAOLETTI, M. ANGIOLUCCI, B. PIRAS,
A. CAFFIERO, AND V. MAIS

*Department of Obstetrics and Gynecology*
*University of Cagliari*
*Cagliari, Italy*

## INTRODUCTION

Endometriosis is defined as the presence of ectopic endometrium with evidence of both cellular activity and progression, with formation of adhesions, or interference with normal reproductive processes.[1] Endometriosis is often associated with infertility, chronic pelvic pain and/or presence of adnexal masses, but typical lesions have also been found in asymptomatic women.[2]

The diagnosis of endometriosis requires direct visualization of the lesions by laparoscopy or laparotomy. For this reason, data on the prevalence of endometriosis in the general population published so far are not conclusive. In fact, only few prospective studies[2-4] have been undertaken, which report a prevalence range of 20–40% in infertile women, 4–65% in patients with chronic pelvic pain, and 1–22% in women submitted to gynecological surgery for other indications.[2]

Considering the high prevalence of the disease Friedman *et al.*[5] have evaluated the reliability of a less invasive diagnostic method, ultrasonography, in all forms of pelvic endometriosis, and demonstrated a possible role only when endometriotic cysts are present. Other authors[6,7] have also analyzed the spectrum of ultrasonographic transabdominal or transvaginal findings of surgically proved endometriomas, but they did not analyze the specificity of these techniques.

Both medical and surgical treatment of endometriosis has greatly improved over the last 20 years,[8] and operative laparoscopy, alone or in combination with medical treatment, has emerged as an indispensable component of modern management of the disease.[9] Therefore, the present study was performed to evaluate the prevalence of pelvic endometriosis in premenopausal women submitted to laparoscopy and/or laparotomy for benign gynecological disease.

In addition, the same subjects were submitted to transvaginal ultrasonography within one week before surgery to evaluate the accuracy of this less invasive technique in differentiating endometriomas from other ovarian cysts.

Finally, the role of operative laparoscopy in the management of endometriosis was evaluated in those patients who underwent laparoscopy for benign ovarian cysts or chronic pelvic pain.

## MATERIALS AND METHODS

All premenopausal nonpregnant women submitted to laparoscopy or laparotomy at the Department of Obstetrics and Gynecology of the University of Cagliari from May 1991 to May 1993 were included in the study (n = 305). The patients, aged 15 to 57 years, underwent surgery for infertility (group 1, n = 59), chronic pelvic pain (group 2, n = 40), benign ovarian cysts (group 3, n = 65), or uterine myomas (group 4, n = 141).

All laparoscopies and laparotomies were carried out by two surgeons only, who recorded their findings on preprinted sheets. During laparoscopies and laparotomies the entire pelvis was systematically inspected. The diagnosis of endometriosis was based on the characteristic visual presentation of the disease. Biopsies were taken when possible. Endometriosis was scored using the Revised American Fertility Society Classification.[10]

All patients were submitted to transvaginal ultrasonography within one week before surgery with a Toshiba Sonolayer–L SAL 77B real time scanner, using a 5 MHz endovaginal mini-convex probe (Toshiba Corporation, Medical System Division, Tokyo, Japan). A second scan was performed if during the first one the ovary was not visualized. All scans were performed by the same physician. After the scan, the physician gave prospective impressions as to the presence of endometriomas if a round-shaped homogeneous hypoechoic "tissue" of low-level echoes was visualized within the ovary. At surgery, all ovarian masses were enucleated from the ovary or removed with the ovary, and all specimens were examined by the same pathologist. To evaluate the role of endovaginal ultrasonography in differentiating endometriomas from other ovarian cysts, the sensitivity, the specificity, the positive and the negative predictive values and the likelihood ratio of a positive (abnormal) test (LR+) and the likelihood ratio of a negative (normal) test (LR−) were calculated for each ovarian cyst visualized during ultrasonographic examinations.[11]

To assess the role of operative laparoscopy in the treatment of endometriosis, only patients undergoing laparoscopy for chronic pelvic pain or benign ovarian cysts were considered (n = 95). When endometriosis was present, the surgeons always tried to treat the disease by operative laparoscopy, shifting to laparotomy only when mandatory. Postoperative residual endometriosis was scored using the Revised American Fertility Society Classification.[10]

## RESULTS

Endometriosis was diagnosed in 76 out of 305 patients (prevalence in the total study population, 24.9%).

In group 1 (infertility), endometriosis was diagnosed in 18 out of 59 patients (30.5%), in group 2 (chronic pelvic pain) in 18 out of 40 patients (45%), in group 3 (benign ovarian cysts) in 28 out of 65 patients (43%), and in group 4 (uterine myomas) in 12 out of 141 patients (8.5%) (FIG. 1).

In group 1, endometriosis was scored as stage I in 10 patients (55.6%), stage II in 2 patients (11.1%), stage III in 4 patients (22.2%) and stage IV in 2 patients (11.1%) (FIG. 1).

In group 2, the stage of endometriosis was I in 9 patients (50%), II in 3 patients (16.7%), III in 3 patients (16.7%) and IV in 3 patients (16.7%) (FIG. 1).

In group 3, endometriosis was scored stage I in 5 patients (17.9%), stage III in 13 patients (46.4%) and stage IV in 10 patients (35.7%) (FIG. 1).

In group 4, endometriosis was scored stage I in 4 patients (33.3%), stage II in 3 patients (25%), stage III in 4 patients (33.3%) and stage IV in 1 patient (8.4%) (FIG. 1).

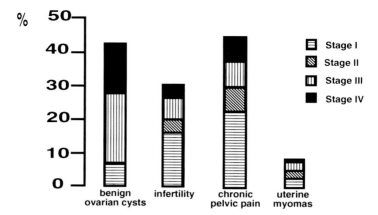

**FIGURE 1.** Prevalence of endometriosis and stages, according to Revised American Fertility Society Classifications, in the four groups of patients.

The distribution of endometriotic lesions in the pelvis is shown in FIGURE 2.

Out of 93 visualized cysts, 31 endometriomas were suspected by endovaginal ultrasonography and 24 were confirmed by pathology. The ultrasonographic findings of the 7 false positive cases (simple cyst, n = 2; hemorrhagic cyst, n = 3; dermoid, n = 1; ovarian fibroid, n = 1) were the same considered as characteristic for endometriomas (FIG. 3).

Conversely, the ultrasonographic diagnosis of nonendometrioma was confirmed by pathology in 57 out of 62 cases (serous cysts, n = 16; simple cysts, n = 14; mucinous cystoadenomas, n = 3; serous cistoadenomas, n = 2; corpora lutea, n = 12; hemorrhagic cysts, n = 5; borderline serous cystoadenoma, n = 1; serous cystoadenocarcinoma, n = 1; teratoma, n = 3). The 5 false negative cases were ovarian masses with anechoic content at ultrasound (FIG. 2).

Therefore, the specificity of endovaginal ultrasonography in differentiating endometriomas from other ovarian masses was 89% with a sensitivity of 83%. The positive and the negative predictive values were 77% and 92%, respectively. The LR+ was 7.5 (good to excellent), and the LR− was 0.19 (good to excellent).[11]

Of the 95 patients who underwent laparoscopy for chronic pelvic pain or benign ovarian cysts 37 had endometriosis. The disease was scored as stage I in 15 patients (40.6%), stage II in 2 patients (5.4%), stage III in 10 patients (27.0%) and stage IV in 10 patients (27.0%). In 29 patients with endometriosis the score was surgically reduced immediately after diagnosis, by operative laparoscopy in 24 cases (82.2%) and by laparotomy in 5 cases only (17.2%) (FIG. 4).

## DISCUSSION

The prevalence of endometriosis in the overall study population was 24.9%, but it was significantly higher in women with infertility, chronic pelvic pain, or benign ovarian cysts than in women with uterine myomas. These findings confirm that the first three indications for surgery are often associated with the presence

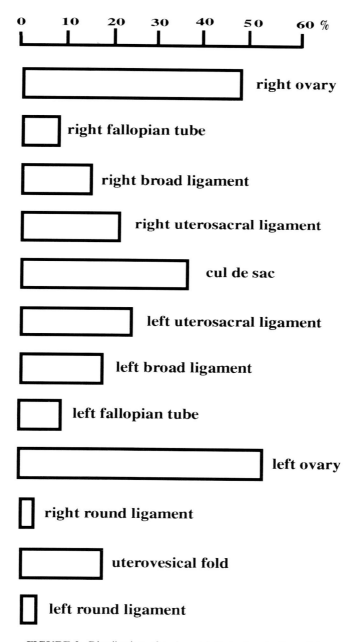

**FIGURE 2.** Distribution of endometriotic lesions in the pelvis.

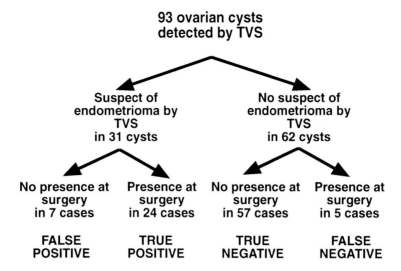

**FIGURE 3.** Flow chart of the role of transvaginal ultrasound in differentiating endometriomas from other ovarian cysts.

of endometriosis.[2] Nevertheless, typical lesions have been found in 8.5% of women with uterine myomas suggesting that endometriosis lesions are not always symptomatic and that "presence of endometriosis" is not a synonym of "disease." Endovaginal ultrasonography showed a high specificity (89%) in differentiating endometriomas from other ovarian masses. This specificity is comparable with the 91% specificity previously reported by other authors for magnetic resonance imaging (MRI).[12] Therefore, the use of MRI is not justified for differentiating benign ovarian masses when endovaginal ultrasonography can be performed, because MRI is a very expensive technique. However, the description of the false positive cases underlines that an ultrasonographic misdiagnosis of endometrioma is possible when the ovarian mass is very small or its content is not clear fluid, as in dermoid or hermorrhagic cysts.

Finally, the present study demonstrates that laparoscopy plays a major role not only in the diagnosis, but also in the surgical treatment of endometriosis. In

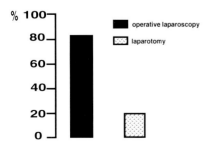

**FIGURE 4.** Percentage of use of laparoscopy or laparotomy in the reduction of score of endometriosis.

fact, in only 5 patients did the surgeons have to shift to laparotomy. In the other cases operative laparoscopy was highly effective in reducing the score or completely removing the lesions during the same procedure started for diagnosis. In addition, laparoscopy determined minimal discomfort for the patients, and minimal damage to the healthy tissue surrounding endometriotic lesions. Therefore, it should be regarded as the technique of choice, especially if reproductive capacity is to be preserved.[9]

## REFERENCES

1. AUDEBERT, A., T. BACKSTROM, D. H. BARLOW, G. BENAGIANO, I. BROSENS, K. BUHLER, J. DONNEZ, J. L. K. EVERS, A. PELLICER, L. METTLER, L. RONNBERG, S. K. SMITH & E. J. THOMAS. 1992. Endometriosis 1991: a discussion document. Hum. Reprod. **7**: 432–435.
2. MAHMOOD, T. A. & A. TEMPLETON. 1991. Prevalence and genesis of endometriosis. Hum. Reprod. **6**: 544–549.
3. MOEN, M. H. 1987. Endometriosis in women at interval sterilization. Acta Obstet. Gynecol. Scand. **66**: 451–454.
4. LIU, D. T. Y. & A. HITCHCOCK. 1986. Endometriosis: its association with retrograde menstruation, dysmenorrhea and tubal pathology. Br. J. Obstet. Gynaecol. **93**: 859–861.
5. FRIEDMAN, H., R. L. VOGELZANG, E. B. MELDENSON, H. L. NEIMAN & M. COHEN. 1985. Endometriosis detection by US with laparoscopic correlation. Radiology **157**: 217–220.
6. ATHEY, P. A. & D. D. DIMENT. 1989. The spectrum of sonographic findings in endometriomas. J. Ultrasound Med. **8**: 487–491.
7. KUPFER, M. C., S. R. SCHWIMER & J. LEBOVIC. 1992. Transvaginal sonographic appearance of endometriomata: spectrum of findings. J. Ultrasound Med. **11**: 129–133.
8. MELIS, G. B., V. MAIS, A. M. PAOLETTI, S. AJOSSA & S. GUERRIERO. 1991. Efficacy and endocrine effects of medical treatment of endometriosis. Ann. N.Y. Acad. Sci. **622**: 275–282.
9. FAYEZ, J. A. & M. F. VOGEL. 1991. Comparison of different treatment methods of endometriomas by laparoscopy. Obstet. Gynecol. **78**: 660–666.
10. The American Fertility Society. 1985. Revised American Fertility Society Classification of Endometriosis. Fertil. Steril. **43**: 351–352.
11. TAYLOR, P. J. & J. A. COLLINS. 1992. The production of spermatozoa and their transport in the male genital tract. *In* Unexplained Infertility. Oxford Medical Publications. 39–68. Oxford University Press. New York.
12. SCOUTT, L. M. & S. M. MCCARTHY. 1991. Imaging of ovarian masses: magnetic resonance imaging. Clin. Obstet. Gynecol. **34**: 443–451.

# The Recurrence of Endometriosis

LUIGI FEDELE, STEFANO BIANCHI,
GIULIANA DI NOLA, MASSIMO CANDIANI,
MAURO BUSACCA, AND MARIO VIGNALI

*II Department of Obstetrics and Gynecology*
*"L. Mangiagalli"*
*University of Milan*
*Via Commenda 12*
*20122 Milan, Italy*

The possibility of endometriosis recurrence after treatment is commonly considered a proof of the difficulty of eradicating the disease and its progressive nature. However, the natural history of endometriosis is unclear and the real rate of recurrence is uncertain. According to both the most accredited pathogenetic theories—implantation and coelomic metaplasia—there may be a state of equilibrium between factors that favor and those that limit the growth of implants with the consequence of static lesions, and an alteration of this equilibrium with the consequence of spread of the disease. Both theories are also compatible with the possibility that after complete elimination of the existing implants the factors that led to the original development of the disease may re-emerge, thus explaining the recurrence.

Only a few of the studies investigating the course of endometriosis have done so prospectively. Repeat laparoscopy performed by Thomas and Cooke[1] on 17 women with minimal and mild endometriosis after 6 months of placebo treatment revealed progression of the lesions in eight of them, improvement in five and total disappearance in four. Progression of nonpigmented lesions to typical pigmented ones was first observed by Janssen and Russel[2] in six patients who underwent two laparoscopies at an interval of 6 to 24 months. The results of two different cross-sectional studies suggest that the nature of endometriosis, at least that of peritoneal disease, is substantially static. In 1987 Redwine[3] reported that the number of pelvic areas involved in the disease does not increase with advancing age. More recently Koninckx *et al.*[4] observed no increase of the total pelvic area involved in endometriosis with an advance in age although the depth of infiltration of the implants was greater and also the incidence of endometriomas. The finding[5] that endometriotic foci are detectable by microscopy in apparently intact peritoneal areas has been confirmed many times. Such foci could progress to form visible and clinically relevant implants.

The currently available data indicate that *ex novo* formation of implants is a relatively infrequent phenomenon whereas lesions appear potentially progressive in about 50% of affected women. Many disease recurrences could represent the evolution of foci not visible at the time of diagnosis and treatment or be due to unrecognized subperitoneal lesions. Another not infrequent cause of recurrence is inadequate, not radical treatment.

## *Recurrence Rates of Endometriosis after Surgical Therapy*

The rates of endometriosis recurrence after surgical treatment vary greatly in the series described in the literature. No prospective study has been performed with the aim of determining the recurrence rate after surgery, and this makes it more difficult to compare the figures reported by the various authors. Other factors that increase the difficulty in interpreting the available data are the considerable differences in follow-up and in disease extension at the first intervention, the fact that a second laparoscopy was not always performed to document any recurrence, and the use of symptoms as a criterion of recurrence.

## Recurrence Rates of Endometriosis after Surgery at Laparotomy

The recurrence rates after conservative surgery for endometriosis at laparotomy (CSEL) reported in the literature vary from 0 to 51%. Bacon's 1949 study[6] of 138 women operated conservatively for endometriosis between 1905 and 1941 included a subgroup requiring further treatment of whom nine (45%) had recurrent disease. In 1953 Meigs[7] evaluated 215 women who had undergone conservative surgery for endometriosis and considered that a second intervention was not necessary in any of them. Ranney[8] performed only one reoperation in 129 women after hysterectomy without salpingo-oophorectomy, but observed recurrence in two of ten women treated conservatively. In Spangler's series[9] the recurrence rate in 105 infertile women after CSEL was 12.8%. The results reported by Andrews and Larsen[10] and Hammond et al.[11] were unfavorable, with recurrence rates of respectively 34% and 51% after combined medical and conservative surgical therapy and 27% and 25% after conservative surgery alone. In 1979 Buttram[12] reported recurrence requiring definitive surgery in six of 138 infertile women. In Punnonen's study,[13] the largest published to date, the frequency of reoperation was 14.6% in the 6- to 10-year follow-up of 903 women treated with CSEL. In Rock's series[14] of 214 infertile women, 29 (13.5%) required reoperation for recurrent endometriosis. In 1983, in what is considered the most important study so far published on the incidence and management of recurrent endometriosis,[15] Wheeler and Malinak observed recurrence in 41 of the 423 patients studied; a revision of the original calculations showed a 5-year cumulative recurrence rate of 19.5%.

## Recurrence Rates of Endometriosis after Laparoscopic Surgery

In 1980 Sulewski et al.[16] reported recurrence in two of 100 infertile women with minimal or mild endometriosis treated by laparoscopic electrocautery. In Reich and McGlynn's study[17] of 71 patients with endometriotic cysts of diameter up to 10 cm treated by laparoscopic surgery, 14 subjects subsequently manifested recurrent endometriosis. Davis[18] on the contrary did not detect any recurrence in 29 women at repeat laparoscopy within 10 weeks of laser vaporization of lesions. Neither did Donnez et al.[19] observe recurrence in eight women with stage II/III endometriosis at a second laparoscopy performed 3 months after the first one. Fayez et al.[20] performed laparoscopic excision on patients with stage I/II endometriosis followed by danazol treatment for six months in 82 women and not in the other 80. Repeat laparoscopy 12 months later in 28 subjects in the former group and 19 in the latter revealed recurrence in seven and three cases, respectively. In Sutton's series,[21] of 181 patients treated by $CO_2$ laser laparoscopy, endometriosis recurrence was detected in 18 of the 33 women who underwent repeat laparoscopy; the new implants were localized at sites different from those previously treated. The same observation was subsequently made by Redwine,[22] who reported a 5-year cumulative recurrence rate of 19% in 359 women with stage I/II endometriosis treated by laparoscopic excision of the implants and followed for a mean period of 2 years. Unlike Wheeler and Malinak,[15] Redwine did not find that the frequency of recurrence rose with length of follow-up, which would confirm the prevalently static nature of the disease. In 1992 Canis et al.[23] observed recurrent endometriomas in four women, probably due to incomplete surgery, in their series of 42 patients with ovarian endometriomas who underwent laparoscopic cystectomy and a repeat laparoscopy 3 to 6 months later.

### Endometriosis Recurrence after Medical Treatment

Unfortunately, after the initial enthusiasm generated by various drugs used to treat endometriosis, it is by now certain that hormonal therapy is unable to eradicate the disease but only able to induce a temporary remission. However, after 6 months' treatment with danazol, gestrinone or a GnRH agonist, a lasting partial remission of symptoms is sometimes obtained and a second treatment unnecessary. The recurrences observed after medical therapy are attributable to the persistence of foci that are only suppressed by pharmacologic hypogonadism.

### Management of Recurrent Endometriosis

A visual and possibly histologic diagnosis of the disease is fundamental in order to correctly program the most appropriate treatment. Symptoms recurrence may in fact be due to other disorders such as pelvic inflammation and adenomyosis. The therapeutic options for the treatment of recurrence are the same as those available for initial treatment of the disease. However, there are differences in the treatment indications. The main aim is to reduce the possibility of further recurrence to a minimum, and recourse to definitive surgery is more frequent in women who have completed their families. To limit the risk of reappearance of pain symptoms in young women as much as possible it is appropriate to perform pelvic denervation, preferably presacral neurectomy, in combination with conservative surgery. In the case of extensive endometriosis and/or suspected subperitoneal lesions access to the pelvic is preferably by laparotomy, as with this technique it is easier to deal with the not infrequent adhesions resulting from the first operation and possibly involving the ureters and rectum. The factors that govern the choice of treatment are as follows, although the presence of associated disorders must also be taken into account:

- the main complaint
- extension of the disease
- the woman's age and desire to conserve menstrual function and/or for future childbearing.

Based on the above criteria we propose the therapeutic algorithm represented in FIGURE 1. The main subdivision is between patients desiring offspring and those with pain symptoms as the main complaint. In patients with stage I/II disease who want children the treatment of choice is operative laparoscopy possibly followed by inclusion in an assisted reproduction program 6 to 12 months later; women over 35 may be included immediately. In the case of infertile women with stage III/IV disease we tend to perform conservative surgery, at laparoscopy or laparotomy, in all those in whom eradication of the disease and restoration of

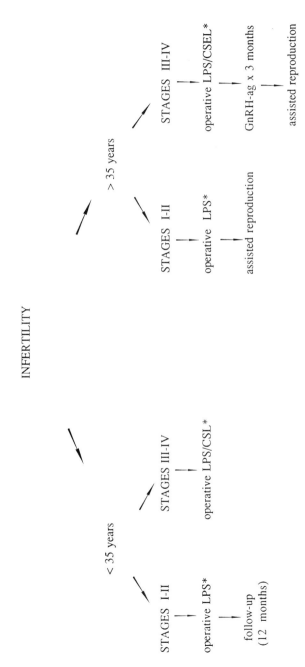

FIGURE 1. Flow chart of recurrent endometriosis therapy for infertility. *Pelvic denervation if midline pelvic pain.

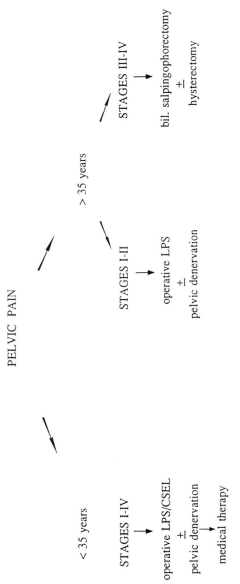

**FIGURE 2.** Flow chart of recurrent endometriosis therapy for pelvic pain.

correct relations between pelvic organs appear possible. This approach seems justified by the results reported by Wheeler and Malinak[15] and Evers,[24] who obtained pregnancy rates of respectively 47% and 38% in 15 and eight women reoperated for endometriosis. Also we have achieved satisfactory results with a pregnancy rate of 28.6% in 42 patients who underwent conservative reoperation for extensive endometriosis.[25] In patients in whom a radical surgery is impossible it is in any case useful to perform surgical maneuvers at laparoscopy that may favor the success of subsequent IVF or GIFT. Assisted reproduction techniques in stage III/IV endometriosis have been successful in only a few cases, but it seems that if the disease is treated first the success rate may be substantially improved.[26] If infertility is present in addition to pain symptoms, pelvic denervation is considered appropriate when the pain is midline.[27] When the dominant symptom is pain (FIG. 2) and the patient is 35 or younger the treatment will consist of conservative surgery at laparoscopy or laparotomy combined with pelvic denervation in case of midline pain. Postoperative medical treatment may be useful in these patients. In women over 35 a conservative operation is indicated only for limited recurrence; in all others definitive surgery is preferable, and must always include bilateral oophorectomy if the ovaries are involved in the disease; the uterus may instead be conserved. This approach is justified on the one hand by the not negligible risk of symptomatic recurrence in women in whom the ovaries are conserved,[28] and on the other hand by the possibility of instituting adequate replacement therapy, as it does not seem able to stimulate the growth of ectopic endometrium.

## REFERENCES

1. THOMAS, E. J. & I. D. COOKE. 1987. Impact of gestrinone on the course of asymptomatic endometriosis. Br. Med. J. **294:** 272–274.
2. JANSEN, R. P. S. & P. RUSSEL. 1986. Nonpigmented endometriosis: clinical, laparoscopic and pathologic definition. Am. J. Obstet. Gynecol. **155:** 1154–1159.
3. REDWINE, D. B. 1987. The distribution of endometriosis in the pelvis by age groups and fertility. Fertil. Steril. **47:** 173–175.
4. KONINCKX, P. R., C. MEULEMAN, S. DEMEYERE, E. LESAFFRE & F. J. CORNILLIE. 1991. Suggestive evidence that pelvic endometriosis is a progressive disease, whereas deeply infiltrating endometriosis is associated with pelvic pain. Fertil. Steril. **55:** 759–765.
5. MURPHY, A. A., W. R. GREEN, D. BOBBIE, Z. C. DE LA CRUZ & J. A. ROCK. 1986. Unsuspected endometriosis documented by scanning electron microscopy in visually normal peritoneum. Fertil. Steril. **46:** 522–413.
6. BACON, W. B. 1949. Results in 138 cases of endometriosis treated by conservative surgery. Am. J. Obstet. Gynecol. **57:** 953–958.
7. MEIGS, J. V. 1953. Endometriosis—etiologic role of marriage and parity; conservative treatment. Obstet. Gynecol. **2:** 46–53.
8. RANNEY, B. 1970. Endometriosis. I. Conservative operations. Am. J. Obstet. Gynecol. **107:** 743–753.
9. SPANGLER, D. B., G. S. JONES & H. W. JONES, JR. 1971. Infertility due to endometriosis. Conservative surgical therapy. Am. J. Obstet. Gynecol. **109:** 850–857.
10. ANDREWS, W. C. & G. D. LARSEN. 1974. Endometriosis treatment with hormonal pseudopregnancy and/or operation. Am. J. Obstet. Gynecol. **118:** 643–651.
11. HAMMOND, C. B., J. A. ROCK & R. T. PARKER. 1976. Conservative treatment of endometriosis: the effects of limited surgery and hormonal pseudopregnancy. Fertil. Steril. **27:** 756–766.
12. BUTTRAM, V. C., JR. 1979. Surgical treatment of endometriosis in the infertile female: a modified approach. Fertil. Steril. **32:** 635–640.

13. PUNNONEN, R., P. KLEMI & V. NIKKANEN. 1980. Recurrent endometriosis. Gynecol. Obstet. Invest. **11:** 307–312.
14. ROCK, J. A., D. S. GUZICK, C. SENGOS, M. SCHWEDITSCH, K. C. SAPP & H. W. JONES, JR. 1981. The conservative surgical treatment of endometriosis: evaluation of pregnancy success with respect to the extent of disease as categorized using contemporary classification systems. Fertil. Steril. **35:** 131–137.
15. WHEELER, J. M. & L. R. MALINAK. 1983. Recurrent endometriosis: incidence, management and prognosis. Am. J. Obstet. Gynecol. **146:** 247–253.
16. SULEWSKI, J. M., F. D. CURCIO, C. BRONITSKY & V. G. STENGER. 1980. The treatment of endometriosis at laparoscopy for infertility. Am. J. Obstet. Gynecol. **188:** 128–132.
17. REICH, H. & F. MCGLYNN. 1986. Treatment of ovarian endometriomas using laparoscopic surgical techniques. J. Reprod. Med. **31:** 577–584.
18. DAVIS, G. D. & R. A. BROOKS. 1988. Excision of pelvic endometriosis with the carbon dioxide laser laparoscope. Obstet. Gynecol. **72:** 816–819.
19. DONNEZ, J. 1987. $CO_2$ laser laparoscopy in infertile women with endometriosis and women with adnexal adhesions. Fertil. Steril. **48:** 390–394.
20. FAYEZ, J. A., L. M. COLLAZO & C. VERNON. 1988. Comparison of different modalities of treatment for minimal and mild endometriosis. Am. J. Obstet. Gynecol. **159:** 927–932.
21. SUTTON, C. 1989. $CO_2$ laser laparoscopy in the treatment of endometriosis. Baillière's Clin. Obstet. Gynecol. **3:** 499–523.
22. REDWINE, D. B. 1991. Conservative laparoscopic excision of endometriosis by sharp dissection: life table analysis of reoperation and persistent or recurrent disease. Fertil. Steril. **56:** 628–634.
23. CANIS, M., G. MAGE, A. VATTIEZ, C. CHAPRON, G. L. POULY & S. BASSIL. 1992. Second-look laparoscopy after laparoscopic cystectomy of large ovarian endometriomas. Fertil. Steril. **58:** 617–619.
24. EVERS, J. L. H., G. A. J. DUNSELMAN, J. A. LAND & P. X. J. M. BOUCKAERT. 1990. Endometriosis: the management of recurrent disease. *In* Endometriosis. R. W. Shaw, Ed. 93–105. Parthenon Publ. Carnforth.
25. CANDIANI, G. B., L. FEDELE, P. VERCELLINI, S. BIANCHI & G. DI NOLA. 1991. Repetitive conservative surgery for recurrence of endometriosis. Obstet. Gynecol. **77:** 421–424.
26. DICKER, D., J. A. GOLDMAN, T. LEVY, D. FELDBERG & J. ASHKENAZI. 1992. The impact of long-term gonadotropin-releasing hormone analogue treatment on preclinical abortions in patients with severe endometriosis undergoing *in vitro* fertilization–embryo transfer. Fertil. Steril. **57:** 597–600.
27. CANDIANI, G. B., L. FEDELE, P. VERCELLINI, S. BIANCHI & G. DI NOLA. 1992. Presacral neurectomy for the treatment of pelvic pain associated with endometriosis: a controlled study. Am. J. Obstet. Gynecol. **167:** 100–103.
28. BUTTRAM, V. C., JR. & J. W. BETTS. 1979. Endometriosis. Curr. Probl. Obstet. Gynecol. **2:** 11–18.

# Parathyroid Hormone and Parathyroid Hormone-Related Protein Stimulate Adenylate Cyclase in Human Endometrial Stromal Cells[a]

M. LINETTE CASEY,[b] AHMET ERK,
AND PAUL C. MACDONALD

*The Cecil H. and Ida Green Center for
Reproductive Biology Sciences
Department of Biochemistry
Department of Obstetrics and Gynecology
The University of Texas Southwestern Medical Center
Dallas, Texas 75235*

## INTRODUCTION

In recent years, there has been appreciable interest in the role of vasoactive proteins in human endometrial function. Endothelin-1 (ET-1), a potent vasoconstrictor, and parathyroid hormone-related protein (PTH-rP), a vasodilator, are produced in human endometrium.[1-3] Evidence also has been presented that the biosynthesis and degradation of ET-1 as well as the biosynthesis of PTH-rP are regulated by ovarian steroid hormones. Specifically, the levels of preproET-1 mRNA in endometrium during late secretory phase and during menses are increased compared with that in the proliferative and early/mid-secretory phases.[1] The specific activity of the metalloproteinase, enkephalinase, which degrades ET-1 and other small, bioactive peptides, is highest at mid-secretory phase of the menstrual cycle when plasma progesterone levels are high. In human endometrial stromal cells in monolayer culture, the specific activity of enkephalinase, the level of enkephalinase protein, and the level of enkephalinase mRNA are increased in response to progestin.[4] On the other hand, estrogen acts in human endometrial stromal cells to increase the levels of PTH-rP mRNA, as well as immunoreactive PTH-rP proteins.[3]

There are other common mechanisms for regulation of the tissue levels of these two vasoactive proteins. Transforming growth factor-$\beta$1 (TGF-$\beta$1) acts to increase the levels of preproET-1 mRNA in endometrial stromal cells[1] as in other cell types.[5] Furthermore, TGF-$\beta$ acts in endometrial stromal cells to decrease the specific activity of enkephalinase, as well as the level of immunoreactive enkephalinase protein.[6] TGF-$\beta$1 also acts in endometrial stromal cells[2] and in other cell types[7] to increase the levels of PTH-rP mRNA and immunoreactive and bioactive PTH-rP protein.

---

[a] This investigation was supported, in part, by USPHS Grant No. 5-P50-HD11149.

[b] Address correspondence to: M. Linette Casey, The Cecil H. and Ida Green Center for Reproductive Biology Sciences, The University of Texas Southwestern Medical Center, 5323 Harry Hines Boulevard, Dallas, TX 75235-9051.

PTH-rP is produced by a number of cell types, both normal and neoplastic, and acts in a wide variety of cells to activate adenylate cyclase.[8] The action(s) of PTH-rP are mediated by way of the PTH/PTH-rP plasma membrane receptor,[8] at least in part, and possibly by way of a unique PTH-rP receptor that does not bind PTH. Fragments of PTH that contain the first 27 amino acids of the protein effect all of the known action of the native protein. PTH is comprised of 84 amino acids, whereas PTH-rP proteins of 139, 141, and 173 amino acids have been deduced from the cDNA. Homology in the amino acid sequences of PTH and PTH-rP is limited to the first 13 amino acids wherein 8 are identical. Interestingly, however, fragments consisting of the first 34 amino acids of either PTH or PTH-rP effect actions *via* the PTH receptor. There is evidence, however, that PTH-rP$_{1-141}$ may act in some systems in a manner different from PTH$_{1-84}$. For example, Abbas *et al.* found that PTH-rP, but not PTH, promoted $Ca^{2+}$ transport in the ovine placenta.[9]

In this study, we evaluated the responsiveness of human endometrial stromal cells in culture to fragments of PTH-rP that are bioactive and known to mimic actions of native PTH-rP and PTH. In particular, we quantified cAMP in the culture medium and in the cells by radioimmunoassay after treatment with various forms of PTH-rP or PTH. The effects of these agents in endometrial stromal cells and in an osteosarcoma cell line, the UMR-106 cells, were compared. The UMR-106 cell line is well-characterized as a PTH and PTH-rP-responsive cell.[10,11] We found that human endometrial stromal cells in monolayer cell culture respond to human PTH$_{1-34}$ and PTH-rP$_{1-34}$ with an increase in cAMP production.

## MATERIALS AND METHODS

### Endometrial Tissue Collection

Endometrial tissue was obtained from uteri of nonpregnant women after hysterectomy, without prior curettage, for reasons other than endometrial disease. The consent form and protocol used for the collection of human tissues was approved by the Institutional Review Board of The University of Texas Southwestern Medical Center.

### Isolation and Culture of Endometrial Stromal Cells

Endometrial stromal cells were prepared as described previously.[1] Endometrial tissue was minced into small pieces ($\sim 1$ mm$^3$), and the minced tissue was incubated at 37°C for 20–30 min in Hanks balanced salt solution that contained Hepes (25 mM), collagenase (1 mg/ml; 134 units/mg), and DNase (0.1 mg/ml; 1950 Kunitz units/ml). The dispersed stromal cells were separated from endometrial glands by filtration through a wire sieve (73 $\mu$m). The stromal cells (in the filtrate) were suspended in Ham F12 : Dulbecco minimal essential medium (F12 : DMEM, 1 : 1, v/v) that contained fetal bovine serum (10%, by volume), penicillin G (100 units/ml), streptomycin sulfate (100 $\mu$g/ml), and amphotericin B (0.25 $\mu$g/ml). The cells were plated in T-75 plastic flasks and maintained in a tissue culture incubator at 37°C in a humidified atmosphere of $CO_2$ (5%) in air until confluent. Then, the cells were passed by standard methods of trypsinization and plated in plastic culture dishes (24-well plates, $\sim 15$ mm diameter wells) at a density of approximately

200,000 cells/well. The culture medium was changed twice weekly until the cells reached confluence.

## UMR-106 Cells in Culture

UMR-106 cells, a rat osteosarcoma cell line, were obtained from The American Type Culture Collection (Rockville Pike, MD). These cells were maintained in Ham F12:Dulbecco minimal essential (F12:DMEM, 1:1, v/v) culture medium that contained fetal bovine serum (10%, v/v) and antibiotics-antimycotics solution (1%, v/v). The cells were passed (1:20 or 1:40) at weekly intervals. Prior to the conduct of experiments, the cells were placed in 24-well plastic plates and allowed to replicate to confluence.

## Treatment of Cells with Test Agents

Confluent, first passage endometrial stromal cells or confluent UMR-106 cells were used for all experiments. After confluence was reached, the cells were treated with serum-free F12:DMEM culture medium that contained bovine serum albumin (0.1%, w/v) for 18–20 h prior to treatment with test agents; studies were conducted with replicates of 3–6 for each experimental condition. The cells were treated with test agents in serum-free F12:DMEM culture medium that contained bovine serum albumin (0.1% w/v) for 2.5–40 min. Thereafter, the culture medium was removed, placed on ice, and stored at $-20°C$ prior to quantification of cAMP (extracellular). Immediately after removing the culture medium, ice-cold aqueous ethanol (65%, v/v; 0.25 ml/well) was added to each well. The cells were placed on ice and fractured by sonication; the sonicate was collected and each well was rinsed with an additional aliquot of ethanol solution (65%). The ethanol solutions were combined, and an aliquot (10%) was taken for determination of cell protein which was quantified (after vacuum evaporation of the solvent) by the method of Lowry et al.[12] Then, the sonicates were centrifuged at $14 \times g$ for 15 min at 4°C. Aliquots of the supernatant were used for quantification of cAMP (intracellular); the solvent was removed by evaporation under vacuum.

## Radioimmunoassay of cAMP

The activation of adenylate cyclase and thence the production of cAMP by UMR-106 and endometrial stromal cells was determined by assessing the cAMP in lysates of cells or in the culture medium. Cyclic AMP was acetylated and quantified by use of radioimmunoassay kits purchased from Amersham Corp. (Arlington Heights, IL) or Advanced Magnetics (Cambridge, MA); [$^{125}$I]cAMP was used as the tracer. All assays were conducted in duplicate; the lower limit of the radioimmunoassays was 1–2 fmol/tube. Intraassay and interassay coefficients of variation were 8% and 14%, respectively.

## Materials

Isobutylmethyl xanthine (IBMX) and forskolin were purchased from Sigma Chemical Corp. (St. Louis, MO). Human $PTH_{1-34}$, $PTH_{1-34}$ amide, $PTH\text{-}rP_{1-34}$,

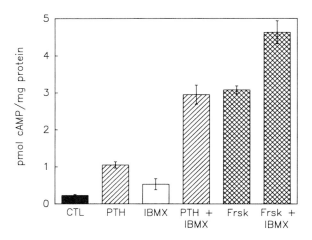

**FIGURE 1.** Cyclic AMP (extracellular) in the culture medium of endometrial stromal cells after treatment for 40 min with test agents. CTL = control; IBMX = isobutylmethyl xanthine (100 $\mu$M); PTH = $PTH_{1-34}$ ($10^{-6}$ M); Frsk = forskolin (10 $\mu$M). The data, normalized to total cell protein, are mean ± SEM for 4 replicates.

$PTH\text{-}rP_{7-34}$, $PTH\text{-}rP_{1-34}$ amide, and $PTH\text{-}rP_{7-34}$ amide, and $PTH\text{-}rP_{7-34}$ ($Asn^{10}$, $Leu^{11}$) amide were purchased from Peptides International (Louisville, KY) or Peninsula Laboratories (Belmont, CA). Culture media were purchased from Irvine Scientific or Grand Island Biological Company.

## RESULTS

Initially, we evaluated the effect of $PTH_{1-34}$ on cAMP production in endometrial stromal cells by determining cAMP in the culture medium after 40 min of incubation. An increase in cAMP was detected in cells treated with $PTH_{1-34}$ ($10^{-6}$ M), compared with that in control cells; and the same was true in cells treated with $PTH_{1-34}$ ($10^{-6}$ M) + IBMX (100 $\mu$M; a phosphodiesterase inhibitor), compared with that in cells treated with IBMX only (FIG. 1). The effect of $PTH_{1-34}$ ($10^{-6}$ M) was not as great as that of forskolin (10 $\mu$M).

The level of cAMP that accumulated after short times (<30 min) of treatment with PTH and PTH-rP was greater in the cells than in the culture medium. Therefore, we chose to quantify cAMP in the cells after 15 min of treatment with test agents; in addition, we used the amide derivatives of PTH and PTH-rP, as the half-life of these is greater than that of the free peptides.

The increase in cAMP production by endometrial stromal cells treated with $PTH\text{-}rP_{1-34}$ amide (FIG. 2), like that in UMR-106 cells (data not shown) was dose-dependent. A maximal response with $PTH\text{-}rP_{1-34}$ amide was attained at concentrations of $10^{-8}$–$10^{-7}$ M. The amount of cAMP that accumulated in the media of

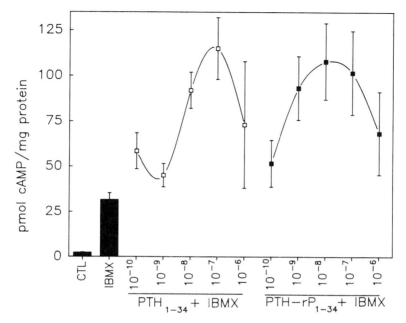

**FIGURE 2.** Cyclic AMP (intracellular) in lysates of endometrial stromal cells after treatment for 15 min with various test agents. CTL = control; IBMX = isobutylmethyl xanthine (100 $\mu$M); PTH$_{1-34}$ or PTH-rP$_{1-34}$ (in various concentrations from $10^{-10}$ to $10^{-6}$ M). The data, normalized to total cell protein, are mean ± SEM for 4 replicates.

UMR cells treated with PTH$_{1-34}$ or PTH-rP$_{1-34}$ free peptides or amide derivatives was much greater (~25–100-fold) than that in endometrial stromal cells.

In endometrial stromal cells or UMR-106 cells treated with PTH$_{7-34}$ amide or PTH-rP$_{7-34}$ amide, cAMP was not increased; in cells treated with either agent together with the shorter peptide, these derivatives, which are considered to be PTH receptor antagonists, did not attenuate the effectiveness of the amide derivatives of PTH$_{1-34}$ or PTH-rP$_{1-34}$ in stimulating cAMP production. Likewise a potent PTH-rP antagonist, [Asn$^{10}$, Leu$^{11}$]-PTH-rP$_{7-34}$ amide at a concentration 100-times that of PTH-rP$_{1-34}$ amide was ineffective in blocking the effectiveness of PTH-rP$_{1-34}$ amide even when cells were preincubated with the antagonist (FIG. 3).

## DISCUSSION

In this study, we found that human endometrial stromal cells responded to treatment with PTH-rP$_{1-34}$ and PTH$_{1-34}$ in a dose-dependent manner by an increase in intra- and extracellular cAMP. The time course of cAMP response (data not shown) in endometrial stromal cells in response to treatment with PTH$_{1-34}$ or PTH-rP$_{1-34}$ was similar to that of UMR-106 cells; but, the magnitude of response was much less. The relatively modest response of human endometrial stromal cells to PTH$_{1-34}$ and PTH-rP$_{1-34}$ is suggestive that PTH-rP produced in these cells is operative in another cell type in the endometrium in a paracrine manner, *e.g.*, vascular smooth muscle, rather than in an autocrine fashion in stromal cells.

The physiological function of PTH-rP synthesized in endometrium is not known. Increased expression of PTH-rP with estrogen treatment of human endometrial stromal cells[3] and in myometrium and nonpregnant rats treated with estrogen[13] are suggestive that hypertrophy and proliferation may be related to an increase in endometrial/myometrial blood flow. Interestingly, PTH-rP mRNA was not detected in rat endometrium/decidua. Previously, we demonstrated that TGF-$\beta$1 acts on endometrial stromal cells in culture to increase the levels of PTH-rP mRNA and the secretion of immunoreactive PTH-rP into the medium.[2] Theide and colleagues also demonstrated that there is transient increase in the level of PTH-rP mRNA in the avian oviduct that is correlated with egg transport during oviposition.[14] Importantly, these investigators also found that PTH-rP mRNA and protein were present principally in the blood-vessel-rich serosal tissue of the oviduct. All of these findings are suggestive that PTH-rP may function to facilitate vascular relaxation and thereby promote blood flow in endometrium and myometrium, which may be associated with cell proliferation in the endometrium and with stretch in the myometrium and oviduct. The finding that PTH-rP$_{1-34}$ is ineffective either in stimulating cAMP production or in attenuating PTH-rP$_{1-34}$

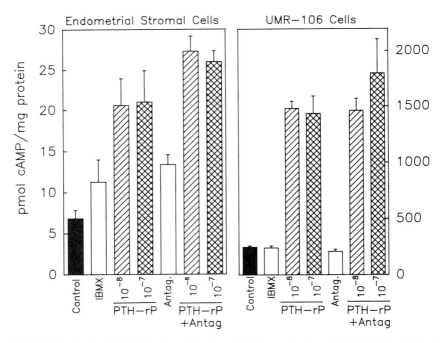

**FIGURE 3.** Cyclic AMP in lysates of endometrial stromal cells and UMR-106 cells (a rat osteosarcoma cell line) after treatment for 15 min with test agents. IBMX = isobutylmethyl xanthine (100 $\mu$M); PTH-rP = PTH-rP$_{1-34}$ amide (at a concentration of $10^{-8}$ or $10^{-7}$ M); Antag. = [Asn$^{10}$, Leu$^{11}$] PTH-rP$_{7-34}$ amide (at a concentration of $10^{-6}$ M). The data, normalized to total cell protein, are mean ± SEM for 3 replicates.

action is suggestive that PTH-rP may be acting through a mechanism other than *via* the PTH receptor.

## ACKNOWLEDGMENTS

We thank Jess Smith and Bobbie Mayhew for skilled technical assistance, Valencia Hoffman for assistance in obtaining tissues, and Kimberly McKinney for expert editorial assistance.

### REFERENCES

1. ECONOMOS, K., P. C. MACDONALD & M. L. CASEY. 1992. Endothelin-1 gene expression and protein biosynthesis in human endometrium: potential modulator of endometrial blood flow. J. Clin. Endocrinol. Metab. **74:** 14–19.
2. CASEY, M. L., M. MIBE, A. ERK & P. C. MACDONALD. 1992. Transforming growth factor-$\beta 1$ stimulation of parathyroid hormone-related protein expression in human uterine cells in culture: mRNA levels and protein secretion. J. Clin. Endocrinol. Metab. **74:** 950–952.
3. CASEY, M. L., M. MIBE & P. C. MACDONALD. 1993. Regulation of parathyroid hormone-related protein gene expression in human endometrial stromal cells in culture. J. Clin. Endocrinol. Metab. **77:** 188–194.
4. CASEY, M. L., J. W. SMITH, K. NAGAI, L. B. HERSH & P. C. MACDONALD. 1991. Progesterone-regulated cyclic modulation of membrane metalloendopeptidase (enkephalinase) in human endometrium. J. Biol. Chem. **266:** 23041–23047.
5. KURIHARA, H., M. YOSHIZUMI, T. SUGIYAMA, F. TAKAKU, M. YANAGISAWA, T. MASAKI, M. HAMAOKI, H. KATO & Y. YAZAKI. 1989. Transforming growth factor-beta stimulates the expression of endothelin mRNA by vascular endothelial cells. Biochem. Biophys. Res. Commun. **159:** 1435–1440.
6. CASEY, M. L., J. W. SMITH, K. NAGAI & P. C. MACDONALD. 1993. Transforming growth factor-$\beta 1$ inhibits enkephalinase (EC 3.4.24.11) gene expression in human endometrial stromal cells and sex skin fibroblasts in culture. J. Clin. Endocrinol. Metab. **77:** 144–150.
7. ALLINSON, E. T. & D. J. DRUCKER. 1992. Parathyroid hormone-like peptide shares features with members of the early response gene family: rapid induction by serum, growth factors, and cycloheximide. Cancer Res. **52:** 3103–3109.
8. MALLETTE, L. E. 1991. The parathyroid polyhormones: new concepts in the spectrum of peptide hormone action. Endocr. Rev. **12:** 110–117.
9. ABBAS, S. K., D. W. PICKARD, C. P. RODDA, J. A. HEATH, R. G. HAMMONDS, W. I. WOOD, I. W. CAPLE, T. J. MARTIN & A. D. CARE. 1989. Stimulation of ovine placental calcium transport by purified natural and recombinant parathyroid hormone-related protein (PTH-rP) preparations. J. Exp. Physiol. **74:** 549–552.
10. PARTRIDGE, N. C., D. ALCORN, V. P. MICHELANGELI, G. RYAN & T. J. MARTIN. 1983. Morphological and biochemical characterization of four clonal osteogenic sarcoma cell lines of rat origin. Cancer Res. **43:** 4308–4314.
11. DIXON, S. J. & J. X. WILSON. 1992. Transforming growth factor-beta stimulates ascorbate transport activity in osteoblastic cells. Endocrinology **130:** 484–489.
12. LOWRY, O. H., N. ROSEBROUGH, A. L. FARR & R. J. RANDALL. 1951. Determination of protein content with the folin-phenol reagent. J. Biol. Chem. **193:** 265–275.
13. THIEDE, M. A., S. C. HARM, D. M. HASSON & R. M. GARDNER. 1991. *In vivo* regulation of PTH-rP messenger ribonucleic acid in the rat uterus by 17$\beta$-estradiol. Endocrinology **128:** 2317–2323.
14. THIEDE, M. A., S. C. HARM, R. L. MCKEE, W. A. GRASSER, L. T. DUONG & R. M. LEACH, JR. 1991. Expression of the parathyroid hormone-related gene in the avian oviduct: potential role as a local modulator of vascular smooth muscle tension and shell gland motility during the egg-laying cycle. Endocrinology **128:** 1956–1958.

# Is Vasopressin Involved as a Local Mediator in the Mechanism of Parturition?

ALESSANDRO MAURI, CARLO TICCONI,
ANNIBALE VOLPE, AND EMILIO PICCIONE[a]

*Department of Gynecology, Obstetrics
and Reproductive Sciences
University of Cagliari
S. Giovanni di Dio Hospital
Via Ospedale 46
09124 Cagliari, Italy*

## INTRODUCTION

Vasopressin is a neurohypophyseal hormone with multiple biological activities. It is a vasoconstricting agent, and as an antidiuretic hormone, it acts on the kidney to increase water retention. Moreover, vasopressin is a potent stimulator of myometrial contractility and is believed to be an important etiological factor in dismenorrhea.[1]

It also has been suggested that vasopressin could play a role in the biomolecular events of preterm and term labor in women.[2] However, the extent of vasopressin involvement in the parturitional process is still largely unknown. Human endometrium and myometrium contain vasopressin receptors, as well as oxytocin receptors.[2,3] During pregnancy, oxytocin receptors in the myometrium sharply increase towards term; conversely, the concentration of myometrial vasopressin receptors is relatively constant with advancing gestation.[4] Nevertheless, vasopressin also could be of importance in stimulating myometrial contractions, since during labor the fetus secretes large amounts of this hormone.[5,6] Vasopressin also could act on the myometrium indirectly by stimulating prostaglandin E2 production by amnion.[7]

Recently, oxytocin gene was found to be expressed in animal and human gestational tissues at term pregnancy.[8] Therefore, it has been suggested that oxytocin could be released by these tissues and that it could act on the uterus not only as an endocrine hormone, but also as a paracrine mediator. Presently, there is no corresponding information on vasopressin.

This study was undertaken to examine the *in vitro* release of vasopressin by human fetal membranes and decidua at term gestation, to verify whether vasopressin is contained in the above tissues and to evaluate whether differences in vasopressin content of these tissues could be detected in relation to term and preterm labor. Vasopressin levels in maternal peripheral, retroplacental and fetal umbilical plasma and in amniotic fluid at term gestation in relation to the presence or the absence of labor were also evaluated.

---

[a] To whom correspondence should be addressed.

## MATERIALS AND METHODS

### Subjects

Seventy-nine healthy women (age range 22 to 37 years) were included in the study. They were divided into three groups: groups 1 and 2 included 74 women with singleton, uncomplicated pregnancy at term who were delivered either vaginally after spontaneous labor (group 1, n = 31) or by elective repeat cesarean section before the onset of labor (group 2, n = 43); group 3 included 5 patients with singleton pregnancy who were delivered vaginally after preterm labor at term 32–35 weeks' gestation.

Gestational age was calculated by the date of the last menstrual period and was confirmed by ultrasonographic examination. Informed consent after full explanation of the purpose of the study was obtained from all patients.

### Retrieval of Biological Fluids

Vasopressin concentration was evaluated in maternal peripheral venous plasma (n = 18), in umbilical arterial and venous plasma (n = 13), in retroplacental plasma (n = 8) and in amniotic fluid (n = 10) from subjects of groups 1 and 2.

Maternal peripheral blood was obtained by antecubital venipuncture at the time of delivery. Umbilical paired arterious and venous blood was obtained immediately after the delivery of the fetus. Retroplacental blood was obtained at the time of delivery by aspirating the space interposed between the partially detached placenta and the uterus with a sterile syringe through the bulging fetal membranes when the placenta emerged either at the hysterotomy site or at the external genitalia. Blood was collected in tubes containing EDTA and centrifuged at 3000 rpm at 4°C for 10 minutes. Plasma was stored at $-20°C$ until vasopressin assay.

Amniotic fluid was obtained during elective cesarean section immediately after the hysterotomy by aspirating the amniotic cavity with a sterile syringe through the intact bulging fetal membranes and during spontaneous labor by transcervical amniocentesis with a cervical dilatation >5 cm before rupture of the membranes. Amniotic fluid was centrifuged at 3000 rpm for 10 minutes at 4°C. The supranatant was collected and stored at $-20°C$ until the assay.

### Incubation Conditions

Reflected fetal membranes with adherent uterine decidua were obtained from 14 women of group 2. They were washed several times in ice-cold sterile saline to remove blood and clots. In six cases, tissues (amnion + chorion + uterine decidua) were immediately processed. In eight cases, amnion was previously peeled away from underlying choriodecidua and then was immediately processed.

All specimens were cut with fine scissors into disks, quantified by wet weight and placed in Petri dishes containing 5 ml of culture medium RPMI 1640 (Gibco, Grand Island, NY) with 10% fetal calf serum, penicillin 100 U/ml and streptomycin 100 $\mu$g/ml. They were incubated for 1 h at 37°C in an atmosphere of 95% $O_2$ and 5% $CO_2$. Culture medium from every experiment was collected, centrifuged at 1800 rpm for 15 minutes to eliminate any cell debris and stored at $-20°C$ until the assay. Tissue viability was checked by the lactic dehydrogenase assay[9] and was found to be 91 ± 3% before and 82 ± 4% after incubation.

## Tissue Processing for Evaluation of Vasopressin Content

The fetal membranes amnion and chorion and the decidua lining the placental plate were collected from six subjects of group 1, five of group 2 and five of group 3. Amnion was peeled away from choriodecidua; the decidua was dissected from the chorion and from the underlying placenta for a 3-mm depth under stereomicroscopic guidance. Two grams of each tissue were minced and rinsed several times in saline. Then, wet specimens were dried by absorbent paper and transferred into 30 × 113-mm polypropylene tubes containing 20 ml of ice-cold 2 N acetic acid and boiled for 10 minutes in a water bath. Tissues were subsequently homogenized and centrifuged at 28000 rpm at 4°C for 15 minutes; the clear supranatant was divided into a series of 16 × 125-mm polypropylene tubes and concentrated under vacuum apparatus (Speed Vac, Savant, Hicksville, NY).

## Vasopressin Extraction and Assay

Samples were resuspended in 0.5 ml of 0.1% trifluoroacetic acid and passed through a Sep Pak C18 cartridge (Waters Associates, Milford, MA) previously washed with 5 ml methanol and 10 ml 0.1% trifluoroacetic acid in water. Vasopressin was eluted with 3 ml of 80 : 20 acetonitrile : water containing 0.1% trifluoroacetic acid. The eluate was concentrated under vacuum and dissolved in buffer for vasopressin assay.

Vasopressin recovery was calculated by adding a known amount of $^{125}$I-vasopressin to samples of tissues and biological fluids and processing these samples as previously reported. The final recovery was approximately 80%.

Vasopressin was measured by radioimmunoassay. The antibody against Arg$^8$-vasopressin was commercially purchased (Arnel, USA) and was characterized by the absence of cross reactivity with oxytocin. $^{125}$I-Arg$^8$-vasopressin was prepared by the chloramine-T method and purified by gel filtration on Sephadex G 25. Arg$^8$-vasopressin (Peninsula Lab., CA) was used as standard. Free and bound $^{125}$I-vasopressin separation was performed by dextrane-coated charcoal. Under our conditions the linear range of the assay was 2.5–50 pg/tube. The intra- and interassay coefficients of variation were 7% and 13%, respectively.

## Statistical Analysis

Data are expressed as means ± SD. Statistical analysis was performed by using Student $t$ test or one-way analysis of variance (ANOVA) followed by Student-Newman-Keuls (SNK) for post-hoc multiple comparisons among groups. Significance was assumed at the $p < 0.05$ level.

# RESULTS

## Vasopressin in Maternal, Umbilical and Retroplacental Plasma and in Amniotic Fluid at Term Gestation in Relation to Labor

Vasopressin concentrations in maternal peripheral venous plasma at term gestation did not change in relation to parturition (FIG. 1). Similarly, the concentrations of vasopressin in retroplacental plasma were not affected by labor (FIG. 2).

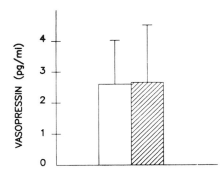

**FIGURE 1.** Vasopressin concentrations in maternal peripheral venous plasma at term gestation in relation to labor. □ = vaginal delivery after spontaneous labor (n = 9); ▨ = cesarean section before the onset of labor (n = 9).

Conversely, vasopressin levels in fetal umbilical artery at term were significantly higher in samples obtained before the onset of labor. The levels of vasopressin in umbilical artery were also higher than in paired venous samples (FIG. 3).

Labor was associated with a marked increase in amniotic fluid concentrations of vasopressin (FIG. 4).

### Vasopressin Release by Fetal Membranes and Uterine Decidua

Explants of human fetal membranes and uterine decidua cultured *in vitro* released vasopressin (TABLE 1). Also isolated amnion released vasopressin. Vasopressin release by amnion tissue, calculated per unit of wet weight, was significantly higher than that by amnion + chorion + uterine decidua (TABLE 1).

### Vasopressin Content of Fetal Membranes and Placental Decidua

Both the placental decidua and the fetal membranes (amnion + chorion) contained relevant amounts of vasopressin. Vasopressin content of placental decidual tissue obtained at term gestation in the absence of labor was significantly higher than that of tissues obtained after labor, both at term and preterm (FIG. 5).

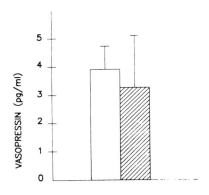

**FIGURE 2.** Vasopressin concentrations in retroplacental plasma at term gestation in relation to labor. □ = vaginal delivery after spontaneous labor (n = 4); ▨ = cesarean section before the onset of labor (n = 4).

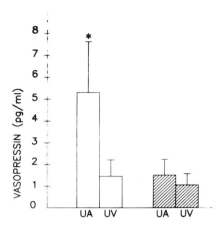

**FIGURE 3.** Vasopressin concentrations in paired samples of fetal arterial and venous umbilical plasma at term gestation in relation to labor. UA = umbilical artery; UV = umbilical vein; ☐ = vaginal delivery after spontaneous labor (n = 7); ▨ = cesarean section before the onset of labor (n = 6). ANOVA: F = 15.09; $p < 0.005$. * Significantly higher ($p < 0.05$) than other means (SNK).

Conversely, vasopressin content of fetal membranes obtained after preterm labor was much higher than that of tissues obtained at term gestation, irrespective of the presence of labor (FIG. 6).

## DISCUSSION

The role of the neurohypophyseal hormone vasopressin in the biomolecular events of labor, both preterm and at term, is still unclear. There is a general

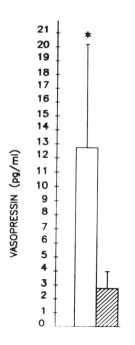

**FIGURE 4.** Vasopressin concentrations in amniotic fluid at term gestation in relation to labor. ☐ = vaginal delivery after spontaneous labor (n = 5); ▨ = cesarean section before the onset of labor (n = 5). * $p < 0.05$.

**TABLE 1.** Vasopressin Release by Explants of Both Fetal Membranes and Uterine Decidua and Isolated Amnion at Term Gestation

|  | Fetal Membranes (Amnion + Chorion + Uterine Decidua) (n = 6) | Amnion (n = 8) |
|---|---|---|
| Vasopressin (pg/g wet wt/1 h) | 3.92 ± 1.61 | 9.36 ± 4.17* |

*$p < 0.05$.

consensus that during labor the maternal peripheral concentrations of vasopressin do not increase.[10] The results of the present study confirm these previously reported observations. Moreover, vasopressin concentrations in retroplacental plasma, obtained from a site close to the myometrium, strictly resemble the concentrations found in maternal peripheral venous plasma and do not change in relation to labor. This finding suggests that maternal blood is a major component of retroplacental blood and further supports the concept that maternal circulating vasopressin is unaffected by the parturitional process.

On the other hand, it has been reported that during labor the fetus produces high amounts of vasopressin.[6] We also found that vasopressin concentrations in fetal umbilical arterial plasma as well as in amniotic fluid are increased after the onset of labor. To explain the high amniotic vasopressin levels during labor, it has been suggested that vasopressin, produced by the fetal posterior pituitary in response to the stressful situation of labor, may diffuse into amniotic fluid, in which little degradation seems to occur.[10] An alternative explanation is that labor might be associated with an increased production of vasopressin by both the fetus and the intrauterine tissues.

Recently, it was reported that mRNA for oxytocin, the other neurohypophyseal hormone besides vasopressin, is present at very high levels in rat and human decidua at term gestation.[8] This observation suggests that oxytocin gene is expressed in intrauterine tissues and that oxytocin could act on the uterus not only as an endocrine hormone, but also as a paracrine mediator. It might also be

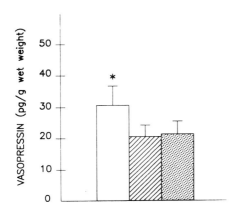

**FIGURE 5.** Vasopressin content of term and preterm placental decidua. □ = term gestation—cesarean section before the onset of labor (n = 5); ▨ = term gestation—vaginal delivery after spontaneous labor (n = 6); ▩ = preterm labor (n = 5). ANOVA: F = 7.55; $p$ = 0.007. * Significantly higher ($p < 0.05$) than other means (SNK).

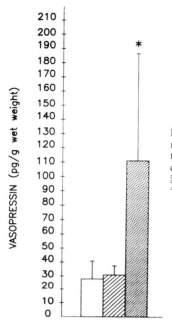

**FIGURE 6.** Vasopressin content of term and preterm fetal membranes. □ = term gestation—cesarean section before the onset of labor (n = 5); ▨ = term gestation—vaginal delivery after spontaneous labor (n = 6); ▦ = preterm labor (n = 4). ANOVA: F = 6.52; $p = 0.01$.
* Significantly higher ($p < 0.05$) than other means (SNK).

suggested that vasopressin could exert a local action within the pregnant uterus during labor.

A major finding of this study is that explants of human fetal membranes and uterine decidua at term gestation release vasopressin and that isolated amnion tissue can release, per unit of wet weight, significantly higher vasopressin than the fetal membranes (amnion + chorion) with attached variable amounts of uterine decidua. Amnion, therefore, could be an important source of vasopressin.

Another major finding of this study is that the fetal membranes amnion and chorion and the placental decidua contain vasopressin and that the pattern of vasopressin content of these tissues markedly changes in different clinical settings. Vasopressin content of the decidua is increased during labor at term; conversely, it remains constant in samples obtained at term but not in labor and in samples obtained after preterm labor. The high vasopressin content of the decidua might reflect a possible, increased local synthesis and release by this tissue during labor at term. On the other hand, vasopressin content of the fetal membranes obtained during preterm labor is much higher than at term, irrespective of the presence or the absence of labor. Again, an increased content might be linked to an increased production.

In summary, the results of this study lead to the following conclusions: 1) during labor, vasopressin levels in intrauterine fluids, with the exception of retroplacental blood, are higher than maternal circulating levels; 2) the fetal membranes and uterine decidua release significant amounts of vasopressin and might be an additional source of vasopressin; 3) the fetal membranes and placental decidua contain vasopressin: vasopressin content of these tissues undergoes changes in different clinical settings, particularly during preterm labor; 4) vasopressin might act in both an endocrine and a paracrine manner in intrauterine tissues during labor.

## ACKNOWLEDGMENTS

We are greatly indebted to Professor Antonio Argiolas, Department of Neurosciences, University of Cagliari, Italy, for useful suggestions.

### REFERENCES

1. STROMBERG, P., M. AKERLUND, M. L. FORSLING & H. KINDAHL. 1983. Involvement of prostaglandins in vasopressin stimulation of the human uterus. Br. J. Obstet. Gynaecol. **90**(4): 332–337.
2. AKERLUND, M. 1993. The role of oxytocin and vasopressin in the initiation of preterm and term labour as well as primary dysmenorrhea. Regul. Pept. **45**: 187–191.
3. MAGGI, M., P. DEL CARLO, G. FANTONI, S. GIANNINI, D. CASPARIS, G. MASSI & M. SERIO. 1990. Human endometrium during pregnancy contains and responds to vasopressin receptors as well as oxytocin receptors. J. Clin. Endocrinol. Metab. **70**(3): 1142–1154.
4. FUCHS, A.-R., F. FUCHS, P. HUSSLEIN, M. J. FERNSTROM & M. S. SOLOFF. 1984. Oxytocin receptors in the human uterus during pregnancy and parturition. Am. J. Obstet. Gynecol. **150**(6): 734–741.
5. HOPPENSTEIN, J. M., F. W. MILTENBERGER & W. H. MORAN, JR. 1968. The increase in blood levels of vasopressin in infants during birth and surgical procedures. Surg. Gynecol. Obstet. **37**: 966–974.
6. CHARD, T., C. N. HUDSON, C. R. W. EDWARDS & N. R. H. BOYD. 1971. Release of oxytocin and vasopressin by the human foetus during labour. Nature **234**: 352–353.
7. MOORE, J. J., G. R. DUBYAK, R. M. MOORE & D. V. KOOY. 1988. Oxytocin activates the inositol-phospholipid-protein kinase C system and stimulates prostaglandin production in human amnion cells. Endocrinology **123**(4): 1771–1777.
8. LEFEBVRE, D. L., A. GIAID, H. BENNETT, R. LARIVIÉRE & H. H. ZINGG. 1992. Oxytocin gene expression in rat uterus. Science **256**: 1553–1555.
9. FARBER, J. L. & E. E. YOUNG. 1981. Accelerated phospholipid degradation in anoxic rat hepatocytes. Arch. Biochem. Biophys. **211**: 312–320.
10. FUCHS, A.-R. & F. FUCHS. 1984. Endocrinology of human parturition: a review. Br. J. Obstet. Gynaecol. **91**(5): 948–967.

# Secretion and Putative Role of Activin and CRF in Human Parturition[a]

FELICE PETRAGLIA,[b] PASQUALE FLORIO,
ANDREA GALLINELLI,
ANTONELLO A. DE MICHEROUX,
ALESSANDRO FERRARI, DAVIDE DE VITA,
LORENZO AGUZZOLI, ALESSANDRO D. GENAZZANI,
AND COSTANTINO DI CARLO[c]

*Department of Obstetrics and Gynecology*
*University of Modena School of Medicine*
*Modena, Italy*
*and*
[c]*Department of Obstetrics and Gynecology*
*University of Naples*
*Naples, Italy*

## INTRODUCTION

The endocrine mechanisms regulating human parturition are not well defined. Several studies have indicated that human placenta has the capacity to produce hormonal substances that may play a fundamental role in the physiology of pregnancy. The capacity of hormonal production in placental cells is critical in providing a favorable uterine environment at implantation, and in regulating growth during pregnancy.[1] Appropriate neuroendocrine signals involved in the initiation of labor, originating from placenta and fetal membranes, have also been suggested.

A good deal of evidence indicates that different local factors participate in the mechanisms regulating myometrial contractile activity. Placental or decidual or amniotic hormonal products may act locally or are released in the maternal circulation or in amniotic fluid. In particular, a new group of molecules has been described in the various intrauterine tissues, the hypothalamic hypophysiotropic hormones: corticotropin-releasing factor (CRF), activin, inhibin, gonadotropin-releasing hormone (GnRH), and somatostatin. They have local action, in some respects comparable to the organization of the hypothalamus-pituitary-target organ axes.[2] A possible role for some of these neuroendocrine factors at parturition has been also suggested by recent investigations.

The end of pregnancy and initiation of labor must be preceded by the ability of the uterus to contract. This last phase of pregnancy may involve a complex set of maternal and fetal factors. As for hormonal changes, it is known that progesterone and estrogen as well as prostaglandins, oxytocin, cortisol, endothelin and sympathomimetic amines may play a role in the events of labor.

Until now attention has been mainly paid to oxytocin. Increased oxytocin release, decreased activity of oxytocinase, and a change in the number of oxytocin

---

[a] This work was supported in part by the Italian National Research Council (CNR) Targeted Project "Prevention and Control Disease Factors," Subproject "Maternal-Infant Diseases," Contract No. 94.00714.PF41.

[b] Address for correspondence: Felice Petraglia, M.D., Department of Obstetrics and Gynecology, University of Modena, Via del Pozzo 71, 41100 Modena, Italy.

receptors in myometrium have been hypothesized. Oxytocin is difficult to measure in peripheral blood and is rapidly metabolized. There is controversy over whether it actually increases in the bloodstream during the course of gestation. Oxytocin interacts with prostaglandin release on muscle contractility.[3] Prostaglandins could act as a trigger for the initiation of labor, but the temporal sequence for this has not yet been established in an animal model.

More evidence for the universal role of prostaglandins in normal delivery is provided by the demonstration that inhibitors of prostaglandin synthesis (aspirin, indomethacin) may postpone the onset of parturition in a wide variety of animal species, including primates and the human, because prostaglandins cause myometrial contractility by acting directly on the cell, presumably by effects on calcium.[4] The action of prostaglandins is influenced by estrogen and progesterone. Several studies have demonstrated that prostaglandin secretion by trophoblast and amnion may be activated by some of the neuroendocrine factors produced by human placenta.[5] In the present paper, evidence of activin and CRF as possible factors involved in human parturition will be reviewed.

### *Activin*

Activin is a typical gonadal homodimeric glycoprotein composed of two beta inhibin subunits: $\beta A$ and $\beta B$. The combination of two $\beta$ subunits gives rise to activin A ($\beta A$ $\beta A$), AB ($\beta A$ $\beta B$), and B ($\beta B$ $\beta B$).[6] These subunits are also expressed in nongonadal tissues.[7]

Human placenta may produce the three forms of activin. Using techniques such as *in situ* hybridization, immunoperoxidase and immunofluorescence, the presence of activin subunits in placental tissues has been shown in early pregnancy, with the more intensive immunostaining detected at term (38-48 weeks).[8,9] Northern blot analysis has shown the expression of $\beta A$ mRNA subunits from early pregnancy, with maximal levels at term gestation.[8]

Also fetal membranes express activin subunit mRNAs and contain immunoreactive activin material,[10] as well as maternal decidua.[11] In fact, human decidua actively produces inhibin subunits with a gestational-related profile, suggesting that decidua may be a further source of activin during pregnancy and emphasizing the endocrine capacity of this tissue.[11] This gestational progressive increase suggests that the production of activin may be related to the progression of pregnancy and/or the increase in potential hormone regulators.

While inhibin levels during pregnancy have been measured during pregnancy in maternal serum as well as in cord blood and amniotic fluid,[12,13] no data are yet available for activin. Using newly developed specific 2-site enzyme-linked immunosorbent assays (ELISA),[14] for the first time we have examined activin A and activin B levels in maternal and cord blood serum and amniotic fluid during gestation, at term and during delivery.[15] The maternal activin A levels in early pregnancy are low and rise significantly by late pregnancy. During early labor they have a further increase, reaching levels similar to those measured during vaginal delivery. In subjects undergoing cesarean section, the levels are significantly lower than those collected during vaginal delivery. Two hours following vaginal or cesarean delivery, maternal activin A serum levels are significantly lower and undetectable 6 hours following parturition. In maternal serum, activin B is largely absent during normal pregnancy. While in the fetal circulation activin A levels are detectable only at delivery, activin B is largely absent in the maternal circulation, but is abundantly present in fetal amniotic fluid and in the cord blood of the fetus prior to birth.[15] This is in agreement with the pattern of activin βA subunit mRNA levels in human trophoblast.[8] The intrauterine origin of the hormone is suggested by the sudden decrease after the delivery of placenta, and by the observation that activin is undetectable in nonpregnant women and within 6 hours postpartum.[15] These findings demonstrate that activins are hormones present in the circulation of the feto-maternal unit. Paracrine or autocrine actions of activin in decidua, amnion and placenta have also been described.[16] Activin is also a potent growth factor, related to the family of TGF-β, and effects of activin on embryogenesis have been shown.[17]

The regulation of placental hormone release is one of the most likely functions of activin.[18] A balancing system between activin and inhibin modulates the gonadotrope function of human placental cells, mimicking the effect that they have on pituitary FSH control. In fact, activin increases progesterone, GnRH and hCG release, while inhibin decreases the release of hCG induced by GnRH, as well as GnRH or progesterone release induced by activin from cultured placental cells.[19]

In addition, activin stimulates prostaglandin $E_2$ release from cultured amnion cells, suggesting another possible role of inhibin and activin in fetal membranes.[10] A complex interaction among hormones, cytokines and growth factors induces the prostanoid synthesis from amniotic cells, and activin may play a role in determining the activation of prostaglandin release going toward term gestation and as a trigger for the initiation of labor. The pattern of circulating activin in biological fluid at the time of labor supports this hypothesis.

### *Corticotropin-Releasing Factor (CRF)*

CRF is a 41-amino acid peptide typically produced by hypothalamic neurons, acting on the release of pituitary POMC-related hormones. Even though brain is the major source of this hormone, in this case human placenta, fetal membranes and decidua produce a CRF with the same chemical and biological neuroendocrine characteristics as its hypothalamic counterpart, suggesting an effect of CRF in gestational tissues.[20-25]

From the seventh week of gestation, intrauterine tissues express CRF mRNA and the levels increase during pregnancy reaching the highest values at term.[23,24] The CRF produced by these tissues is released into maternal circulation, increasing the plasma levels progressively during gestation, having high levels in some physiological and pathological conditions: spontaneous labor and vaginal delivery,[26-29] pre-eclampsia, hypertension and preterm labor.[30-32] Maternal plasma CRF suddenly decrease after placental delivery, indicating that placenta and/or decidua are the major source of CRF in pregnancy. In addition, we evaluated the CRF levels during spontaneous term labor and preterm with or without infection. Plasma CRF levels in women with preterm labor were higher than in pregnant women not in labor. Women in preterm labor without infection who delivered at term showed CRF plasma levels in the same range of values as patients who delivered prematurely and those with infection. These results indicate that the increase of plasma CRF in pregnant women during preterm or term labor occurs independently from infection, suggesting that the mechanism underlying term and preterm parturition are different.[33] In addition, spontaneous term labor and preterm labor leading to preterm delivery are associated with a significant increase of CRF concentration in amniotic fluid, as well as during this occult infection.[34]

More data are available on placental CRF release. *In vitro* experiments show that prostaglandins ($E_2$ and $F_{2\alpha}$), neurotransmitters (noradrenalin, acetylcoline) and neuropeptides (oxytocin, vasopressin, angiotensin II) are active secretagogues for placental CRF, but no changes of CRF effect on ACTH release are produced by oxytocin or vasopressin.[35] In agreement, interleukin-1α (IL-1α)—a peptide mediating immune response—increases the release of CRF from cultured placental cells.[35] The presence of IL-1α in trophoblast and decidua[36,37] suggests that locally produced cytokines modulate placental CRF release, possibly contributing to the increase of plasma CRF and ACTH levels during labor.

Other paracrine and/or autocrine actions have been suggested for placental, decidual and amniotic CRF. In fact, CRF increases the local $PGE_2$ and $PGF_{2\alpha}$ production[25,38] when added to cultures of human placenta, amnion, chorion and decidua. Supporting the hypothesis of a local role of CRF at parturition, recent data indicate that CRF increases the myometrial response to $PGF_{2\alpha}$ *in vitro*.[39] The hypothesis of an immune-endocrine interaction in human parturition is therefore supported by the results obtained in preterm labor.[34,40] Therefore, human intrauterine tissues are the source and the target of CRF.

More recently, the existence of a CRF-binding protein (CRF-BP), a 37-kDa protein of 322 amino acids, has been shown in human plasma:[42] it binds the circulating CRF reducing its biological actions.[43] Human placenta, fetal membranes and maternal decidua express and contain CRF-BP,[44] in the same cells (syncytiotrophoblast) containing ACTH and POMC-related peptides, suggesting that CRF-BP is produced by the target cells of locally producing CRF. CRF-BP plasma levels are high during early pregnancy and drammatically decrease during the third trimester of normal human pregnancy (4–5-fold).[45] Thus, even in presence of increasing CRF plasma levels, the blockade of ACTH releasing activity by CRF-BP may explain the lack of increase of maternal plasma ACTH concentration during pregnancy.

We may hypothesize that local paracrine interactions in intrauterine tissues during labor, when they occur in presence of the major CRF circulating levels in the later phase of pregnancy, CRF-BP levels drop dramatically, not inhibiting the action of CRF on various local targets, like uterine contractility and ACTH and prostaglandin release. Thus, the local increase in CRF may play an important role in reinforcing the mechanism of response to the stress of parturition in both the mother and fetus.

In conclusion, the present paper emphasizes the role of the intrauterine tissues as well as that of the local mechanism in activating the onset of labor and the timing of parturition.

## REFERENCES

1. TULCHINSKY, D. & K. J. RYAN, Eds. 1980. Maternal-Fetal Endocrinology. 9th edit. W. B. Saunders Company. Philadelphia, London, Toronto.
2. PETRAGLIA, F., A. VOLPE, A. R. GENAZZANI, J. RIEVIER, P. E. SAWCHENKO & W. VALE. 1990. Neuroendocrinology of the human placenta. Front. Neuroendocrinol. **11:** 6–37.
3. DYER, R. G. 1988. Oxytocin and parturition—new complications. J. Endocrinol. **116:** 167–168.
4. MITCHELL, M. D. 1991. Current topic: the regulation of placental eicosanoid biosynthesis. Placenta **12:** 557–572.
5. PETRAGLIA, F., M. C. GALASSI, A. C. MANCINI, G. BOTTICELLI, A. VOLPE, G. C. GARUTI & A. SEGRE. 1990. Corticotropin releasing factor, human placenta and parturition. *In* Stress and Related Disorders from Adaptation to Dysfunction. A. R. Genazzani, G. Nappi, F. Petraglia & E. Martignoni, Eds. 373–379. Parthenon Publishing. Casterton Hall, UK.

6. VALE, W., C. RIVIER, A. HSUEH, C. CAMPEN, H. MEUNIER, T. B. NICSAK, J. VAUGHAN, A. CORRIGAN, W. BARDIN, P. SAWCHENKO et al. 1988. Chemical and biological characterization of the inhibin family of protein hormones. Rec. Prog. Horm. Res. **44:** 1–34.
7. MEUNIER, H., C. RIVIER, R. M. EVANS & W. VALE. 1988. Gonadal and extragonadal expression of inhibin $\alpha$, $\beta A$, and $\beta B$ subunits in various tissues predicts diverse functions. Proc. Natl. Acad. Sci. USA **85:** 247–251.
8. PETRAGLIA, F., G. C. GARUTI, L. CALZÀ, V. ROBERTS, L. GIARDINO, A. R. GENAZZANI & W. VALE. 1991. Inhibin subunits in human placenta: localization and messenger ribonucleic acid levels during pregnancy. Am. J. Obstet. Gynecol. **165:** 750–758.
9. RABINOVICI, J., P. C. GOLDSMITH & C. L. LIBRACH. 1992. Localization and regulation of the activin-A dimer in human placental cells. J. Clin. Endocrinol. Metab. **75:** 571–576.
10. PETRAGLIA, F., M. M. ANCESCHI, L. CALZÀ, G. C. GARUTI, P. FUSARO, L. GIARDINO, A. R. GENAZZANI & W. VALE. 1993. Inhibin and activin in human fetal membranes: evidence for an effect on prostaglandin release. J. Clin. Endocrinol. Metab. **77:** 542–547.
11. PETRAGLIA, F., L. CALZÀ, G. C. GARUTI, M. ABRATE, L. GIARDINO, A. R. GENAZZANI, W. VALE & H. MEUNIER. 1990. Presence and synthesis of inhibin subunits in human decidua. J. Clin. Endocrinol. Metab. **71:** 487–492.
12. ABE, Y., Y. HASEGAWA, K. MIYAMOTO et al. 1990. High concentration of plasma immunoreactive inhibin during normal pregnancy in women. J. Clin. Endocrinol. Metab. **71:** 133–137.
13. QU, J., L. VANKREIKEN, C. BRULET & K. THOMAS. 1991. Circulating bioactive inhibin levels during human pregnancy. J. Clin. Endocrinol. Metab. **78:** 862–866.
14. WOODRUFF, T., L. KRUMMEN, D. BALY et al. 1993. Quantitative two site enzyme-linked immunosorbent assays (ELISA) for inhibin A, activin A, and activin B. Hum. Reprod. In press.
15. PETRAGLIA, F., S. GARG, P. FLORIO, M. SADICK, A. GALLINELLI, W. WONG, L. KRUMMEN, G. COMITINI, J. MATHER & T. K. WOODRUFF. 1993. Activin A and activin B measured in maternal serum, cord blood serum, and amniotic fluid during human pregnancy. Endocr. J. **1:** 323–327.
16. PETRAGLIA, F., L. CALZÀ, G. C. GARUTI, B. M. DE RAMUNDO & S. ANGIONI. 1990. New aspects of placental endocrinology. J. Endocrinol. Invest. **13:** 353–371.
17. PETRAGLIA, F., P. SAWCHENKO, A. T. W. LIM, J. RIVIER & W. VALE. 1987. Localization, secretion, and action of inhibin in human placenta. Science **237:** 187–189.
18. YING, S. Y. 1988. Inhibins, activins, and follistatin: gonadal proteins modulating the secretion of follicle-stimulating hormone. Endocr. Rev. **9:** 267–293.
19. PETRAGLIA, F., J. VAUGHAN & W. VALE. 1989. Inhibin and activin modulate the release of gonadotropin-releasing hormone, human chorionic gonadotropin, and progesterone from cultured human placental cells. Proc. Natl. Acad. Sci. USA **86:** 5114–5117.
20. SIJONMAA, O., T. LAATIKAINEN & T. WAHLSTROM. 1988. Corticotropin-releasing factor in human placenta: localization, concentration and release *in vitro*. Placenta **9:** 373–385.
21. SHIBASAKI, T., E. ODAGIRI, K. SHIMUZE & N. LING. 1982. Corticotropin-releasing factor-like activity in human placental extracts. J. Clin. Endocrinol. Metab. **55:** 384–386.
22. GRINO, M., G. P. CHROUSOS & A. N. MARGIORIS. 1987. The corticotropin releasing hormone gene is expressed in human placenta. Biochem. Biophys. Res. Commun. **148:** 1208–1214.
23. FRIM, D. M., R. L. EMANUEL, B. G. ROBINSON, C. M. SMAS, G. K. ADLER & J. A. MAJZOUD. 1988. Characterization and gestational regulation of corticotropin-releasing hormone messenger RNA in human placenta. J. Clin. Invest. **82:** 287–292.
24. PETRAGLIA, F., S. TABANELLI, M. C. GALASSI, G. C. GARUTI, A. C. MANCINI, A. R. GENAZZANI & E. GURPIDE. 1992. Human decidua and *in vitro* decidualized endometrial stromal cells at term contain immunoreactive corticotropin-releasing factor

(CRF) and CRF messenger ribonucleic acid. J. Clin. Endocrinol. Metab. **74:** 1427–1431.
25. JONES, S. A., A. N. BROOKS & J. R. CHALLIS. 1989. Steroids modulate corticotropin-releasing hormone production in human fetal membranes and placenta. J. Endocrinol. Metab. **68:** 825–830.
26. SASAKI, A., O. SHINKAWA, A. N. MARGIORIS, A. S. LIOTTA, S. SATO, O. MURAKAMI, M. GO, Y. SHIMIZU, K. HANEW & K. YOSHINAGA. 1987. Immunoreactive corticotropin-releasing hormone in human plasma during pregnancy, labor, and delivery. J. Clin. Endocrinol. Metab. **64:** 224–229.
27. PETRAGLIA, F., L. GIARDINO, G. COUKOS, L. CALZÀ, W. VALE & A. R. GENAZZANI. 1990. Corticotropin-releasing factor and parturition: plasma and amniotic fluid levels and placental binding sites. Obstet. Gynecol. **75:** 784–789.
28. CAMPBELL, E. A., E. A. LINTON, C. D. WOLFE, P. R. SCRAGGS, M. T. JONES & P. J. LOWRY. 1987. Plasma corticotropin-releasing hormone concentrations during pregnancy and parturition. J. Clin. Endocrinol. Metab. **64:** 1054–1059.
29. GOLAND, R. S., S. L. WARDLAND, R. I. STARK, L. S. BROWN, JR. & A. G. FRANTZ. 1986. High levels of corticotropin-releasing hormone immunoreactivity in maternal and fetal plasma during pregnancy. J. Clin. Endocrinol. Metab. **63:** 1199–1203.
30. WOLF, C. D. A., S. P. PATEL, E. A. LINTON *et al.* 1988. Plasma corticotropin-releasing factor (CRF) in abnormal pregnancy. Br. J. Obstet. Gynaecol. **95:** 1003–1006.
31. KURKI, T., T. LAATIKAINEN, K. SALMINEN-LAPPAILEN & O. YLIKORKALA. 1991. Maternal plasma corticotropin-releasing hormone elevated in preterm labor but uneffected by indomethacin or mylidrin. Br. J. Obstet. Gynaecol. **98:** 685–691.
32. WARREN, W. B., S. L. PATRICK & R. S. GOLAND. 1992. Elevated maternal plasma corticotropin-releasing hormone levels in pregnancies complicated by preterm labor. Am. J. Obstet. Gynecol. **166:** 1198–1207.
33. PETRAGLIA, F., P. FLORIO, L. AGUZZOLI, A. D. GENAZZANI, A. GALLINELLI, A. R. FERRARI & R. ROMERO. 1993. Maternal plasma immunoreactive corticotropin-releasing factor levels in infection-associated term and preterm delivery. Placenta. In press.
34. ROMERO, R., C. BORTOLANI, W. SAPULVEDA, L. AGUZZOLI, D. B. COTTON & F. PETRAGLIA. 1993. Corticotropin-releasing hormone, ACTH and cortisol in term and preterm labor. Abstract. SPO.
35. PETRAGLIA, F., S. SUTTON & W. VALE. 1989. Neurotransmitters and peptides modulate the release of immunoreactive corticotropin-releasing factor from cultured human placental cells. Am. J. Obstet. Gynecol. **160:** 247–251.
36. MAIN, E. K., J. STRIZKI & P. SCHOCHET. 1987. Placental production of immunoregulatory factors: trophoblast is a source of interleukin-1. Trophoblast Res. **2:** 149–152.
37. ROMERO, R., J. K. WU, D. T. BRODY *et al.* Human decidua: a source of interleukin-1. Obstet. Gynecol. **73:** 31–34.
38. JONES, S. A. & J. R. CHALLIS. 1989. Local stimulation of prostaglandin production by corticotropin-releasing hormone in human fetal membranes and placenta. Biochem. Biophys. Res. Commun. **159:** 192–199.
39. BENEDETTO, C., F. PETRAGLIA, L. MAROZIO, L. CHIAROLINI, P. FLORIO, A. R. GENAZZANI & L. MASSOBRIO. 1993. Corticotropin-releasing hormone increases prostaglandin $F_{2\alpha}$ activity on human myometrium *in vitro*. Am. J. Obstet. Gynecol. In press.
40. ROMERO, R., D. T. BRODY, E. OYARZUN, M. MAZOR, J. C. HOBBINS & S. K. DURUM. 1989. Infection and labor. III. Interleukin-1: a signal for the onset of parturition. Am. J. Obstet. Gynecol. **160:** 1117–1123.
41. POTTER, E., D. P. BEHAN, W. H. FISHER, E. A. LINTON, P. J. LOWRY & W. VALE. 1991. cDNA cloning and characterization of the human and rat corticotropin releasing factor-binding proteins. Nature **349:** 423–426.
42. SUDA, T., M. IWASHITA, F. TOZAWA, T. USHIYAMA, N. TOMORI, T. SUMIMOTO, Y. NAKAGAMI, H. DEMURA & K. SHIZUME. Characterization of corticotropin-releasing hormone binding protein in human plasma by chemical cross-linking and its binding during pregnancy. J. Clin. Endocrinol. Metab. **67:** 1278–1283.
43. PETRAGLIA, F., E. POTTER, V. CAMERUN, S. SUTTON, D. P. BEHAN, R. J. WOODS, P. E. SAWCHENKO, P. J. LOWRY & W. VALE. 1993. Corticotropin-releasing factor-

binding protein is produced by human placenta, fetal membranes and maternal decidua. J. Clin. Endocrinol. Metab. **77:** 919–924.
44. LINTON, E. A., A. V. PERKINS, R. J. WOODS, F. EBEN, C. D. A. WOLFE, D. P. BEHAN, E. POTTER, W. VALE & P. J. LOWRY. 1992. Corticotropin releasing hormone-binding protein (CRH-BP): plasma levels decrease during the third trimester of normal human pregnancy. J. Clin. Endocrinol. Metab. **76:** 260–262.

# Antiprogestins in the Induction of Labor

KRISTOF CHWALISZ[a] AND ROBERT E. GARFIELD[b]

*Research Laboratories of Schering AG
Berlin, Germany*

and

[b]*Division of Reproductive Sciences
Department of Obstetrics and Gynecology
The University of Texas, Medical Branch
Galveston, Texas 77550*

## INTRODUCTION

There are maternal or fetal indications for the induction of labor and delivery in approximately 10–15% of term and near-term pregnancies. It is well recognized that the successful induction of labor is largely dependent on the condition of the cervix. If labor induction is performed in the presence of an "unripe" cervix, the duration of labor is prolonged resulting in a high failure rate of induction. As a consequence, there is a significant increase in the overall incidence of instrumental deliveries and cesarean sections as well as a variety of other complications.[1] The introduction of prostaglandins, in particular, vaginally or endocervically administered $PGE_2$, into the clinical routine to soften the cervix before labor induction with oxytocin or intravenous $PGE_2$ has to be considered as a major advance in obstetrics during the last decade. However, prostaglandin use is often associated with side effects and some studies have also reported an increased risk of hyperstimulation of the uterus and higher fetal heart rate abnormalities after local $PGE_2$ application.[1] Moreover, in about one third of women prostaglandins are not effective in inducing cervical ripening. Therefore, there is a need for further advances in cervical ripening and labor induction techniques, especially in terms of increased efficacy and reduced risk in uterine hyperstimulation. The ideal method for the induction of labor should replicate the mechanisms governing spontaneous parturition as closely as possible, *i.e.*, by sequential use of a priming agent with oxytocin. Such a priming treatment should prepare the uterus for labor induction by increasing cervical scores and myometrial responsiveness without stimulating myometrial contractions.

During pregnancy, which is characterized by uterine quiescence, the myometrium is highly unresponsive to uterotonic stimuli and the uterine cervix which is firm and rigid remains closed. Toward the end of pregnancy the myometrium becomes more responsive to uterotonic agents, and cervical ripeness, characterized by changes in the shape and consistency of the cervix, improves. The start

---

[a] Present address: Gynecologic Research, Fertility Control and Hormone Therapy Research, Berlex Laboratories, 300 Fairfield Road, Wayne, NJ 07470-7358.

of this preparatory (conditioning) phase, a precise assessment of which is currently difficult, represents the initiation of parturition. This phase is relatively long in primates (2–3 weeks) and guinea pigs (approx. 10 days), but is short in rats and rabbits (approx. 24 hours). Labor which starts at the end of this phase can be defined as the onset of regular contractions of high amplitude and short duration associated with the dilatation of the uterine cervix and eventually bringing about delivery of the fetus and placenta.

A. Csapo[2] has suggested progesterone as the hormone responsible for the quiescent state of uterine musculature during pregnancy. The level of uterine activity depends on the balance between progesterone and factors promoting uterine contractions. He believes that progesterone withdrawal changes the uterus from an inert state to a highly responsive organ by both increasing uterine responsiveness, due to the lowering of the threshold for excitation to uterotonins, and by inducing the release of "intrinsic uterine stimulants" (i.e., prostaglandins, oxytocin). Csapo has also suggested that progesterone withdrawal results in the release of endogenous stimulants and eventually in the onset of labor. Indeed, in some species such as the rat, rabbit, and sheep ("progesterone-dependent species"), progesterone withdrawal at term, through luteolysis (rat, rabbit) or through the activation of $17\alpha$-hydroxylase by fetal cortisol (sheep), is a signal for parturition. However, in humans and nonhuman primates progesterone does not decline prior to the onset of labor, although experiments with antiprogestins in different species including humans suggest a great similarity in the basic physiological mechanisms for initation of parturition. In guinea pigs and the tree shrew *Tupaja belangeri,* which were our principal models for studying the mechanism of antiprogestin action, the placenta is the source of progesterone during advanced pregnancy with no substantial decline in plasma progesterone levels occurring prior to birth. In guinea pigs, pregnancy is neither interrupted by ovariectomy performed after the luteoplacental shift,[3] nor prolonged by exogenous progesterone.[4]

The synthesis of RU 486 and other progesterone receptor antagonists (antiprogestins) has opened up new therapeutic perspectives and new opportunities to non-invasively investigate the role of progesterone in controlling labor, especially in species showing placental synthesis of progesterone. In this review, we will briefly summarize the animal and clinical studies with antiprogestins, focusing on their mechanism of action in the myometrium and cervix. More extensive reviews of studies on the induction of parturition with antiprogestins and their mechanism of action during advanced pregnancy were published recently.[5–8] These studies show that the labor-inducing activity of antiprogestins is relatively low during early and mid pregnancy but it increases at term. However, antiprogestins enhance myometrial responsiveness to prostaglandins and induce cervical ripening irrespective of the stage of pregnancy. We have called the myometrial and cervical effects of antiprogestins "labor-conditioning effects." The distinction between the labor-conditioning and labor-inducing effects of antiprogestins has helped to change our view of the mechanism for initiation of parturition. Experimental and clinical studies with antiprogestins suggest that the uterus, both the myometrium and the cervix, undergo a conditioning step controlled by progesterone (withdrawal). This step may be common to all species, including humans, although mechanisms controlling the onset of uterine contractions (onset of labor) may vary among species. Antiprogestins will doubtless find broad application in obstetrics as an adjunct to labor and delivery. The potential obstetrical indications for antiprogestins will also be reviewed here.

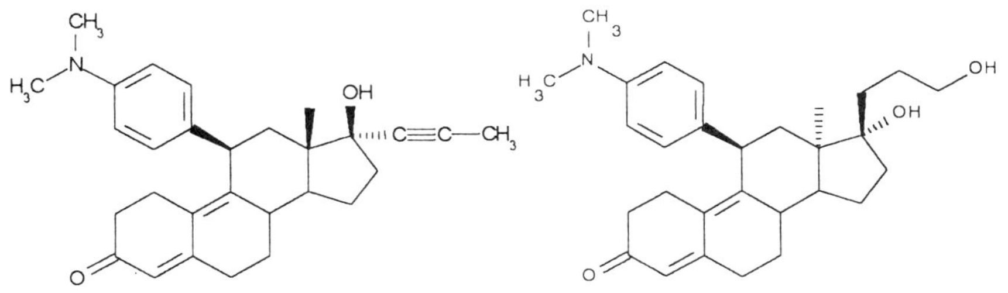

**RU 486 (mifepristone)**              **Onapristone (ZK 98 299)**

**FIGURE 1.** Chemical structures of the antiprogestins RU 486 and onapristone.

## PROGESTERONE ANTAGONISTS

The discovery of the specific progesterone receptor antagonist mifepristone (RU 486) in 1981[9] was a milestone in steroid chemistry and reproductive physiology and medicine. Since this time several new 11β-aryl-substituted steroidal progesterone receptor antagonists with increased antiprogestagenic and reduced antiglucocorticoid activities have been described.[10] FIGURE 1 presents the chemical structure of RU 486 and onapristone (ZK 98 299). Both compounds bind with high affinity to the progesterone and glucocorticoid receptors.[9-11] Compared with RU 486, onapristone has similar antiprogestagenic but reduced antiglucocorticoid activities *in vivo*.[10,11] Both compounds also bind to the androgen receptor and show slight antiandrogenic activity *in vivo*. Neither RU 486 nor onapristone binds to estrogen receptors.

Onapristone is a 13α-configurated (retro) steroid with a different stereochemical structure compared to RU 486, a 13β-configurated antiprogestin.[10] The molecular mechanisms of action of onapristone and RU 486 also seem to vary. RU 486 promotes a dimerization of the progesterone receptor and in its binding to DNA,[12-14] and may, therefore, act as a mixed agonist/antagonist. It has agonistic activity in the endometrium in ovariectomized monkeys[15] and postmenopausal women.[16] On the other hand, onapristone (and some other 13α-configurated antiprogestins) fails to promote the formation of stable receptor dimers and impair the binding of PR-complexes to the progesterone-responsive elements of DNA as evidenced by gel retardation assay.[11,13,18,19] DNA binding is required for activation of transcription, so that onapristone (and some other 13α-antiprogestins) may be regarded as a "pure" progesterone receptor antagonist.[17,13,14] The absence of agonistic activity may explain some special characteristics of onapristone in late-pregnant animals, especially its high labor-inducing activity (see below).

## INDUCTION OF LABOR AND DELIVERY WITH ANTIPROGESTINS: AN OVERVIEW OF ANIMAL AND HUMAN STUDIES

During more advanced stages of pregnancy the myometrium and uterine cervix are major targets for antiprogestins. Labor and delivery depend (a) on the release of endogenous uterotonic agents such as prostaglandins and oxytocin, (b) on high myometrial responsiveness to these stimuli and finally (c) on the state of the cervix. During advanced pregnancy, the occurrence of preterm birth after antiprogestin treatment alone is a parameter predominantly of the labor-inducing activity of these compounds, *i.e.*, their effect on the uterine contractility and perhaps on the release of endogenous uterotonins. However, successful labor contractions may only develop if both myometrium and cervix are prepared for labor and delivery. In some species such as the rat, particularly at preterm, it is difficult to distinguish between the labor-inducing and labor-conditioning effects of antiprogestins on the uterus, because both effects occur almost concurrently. Nevertheless, antiprogestins show predominantly labor-conditioning effects on the uterus in guinea pigs, nonhuman primates and humans *i.e.*, in species with no progesterone withdrawal at term.

## Induction of Parturition Studies in Lower Mammals

In "progesterone-dependent" species such as rats,[20,21] sheep,[24] pigs,[23] and cows,[25] treatment with antiprogestins near term (days 20–21 postcoitum [p.c.]) effectively induces a preterm parturition which is similar to normal parturition at term. In rats, the RU 486 effect can be reversed by the "pure" progestin R5020 (promegestone), indicating that this effect was mediated via the progesterone receptor.[22] In contrast, when given between days 16–18 p.c. neither compound effectively induced parturition, even at high doses, but instead caused bleeding and extremely prolonged deliveries,[20,22] suggesting that the treatment was not effective in inducing uterine contractions. Oxytocin infusion shortened the duration of deliveries in animals primed with onapristone, indicating an increased myometrial responsiveness to oxytocin at this stage of pregnancy.[20] In pigs, a successful labor induction with no adverse effects on the piglets or mothers was reported with the antiprogestin ZK 112 993.[23] RU 486 also induced preterm parturition during late pregnancy in sheep[24] and cattle[25] with no fetal or maternal complications.

In species without progesterone withdrawal at term, such as guinea pigs and *Tupaja belangeri,* the labor-inducing activity is dependent on the stage of pregnancy and the compound used. In guinea pigs treatment with RU 486 and some other 13$\beta$-configurated antiprogestins alone during mid-pregnancy (day 42–43 p.c.; term day 67 ± 3), was not very effective in inducing expulsions, which occurred in only approximately 50% of the animals after a latency of several days.[11] In contrast, onapristone and some other 13$\alpha$-configurated antiprogestins effectively induced preterm parturition on day 61 p.c.[7] These studies show that the efficacy of onapristone alone in inducing labor in guinea pigs increases during the course of pregnancy despite little change in serum progesterone levels. The progestins R5020 (promegestone) and gestodene totally inhibited the labor-inducing activity of onapristone at preterm, a clear indication that this action is mediated by the progesterone receptor.[7] Interestingly, the progesterone synthase inhibitor epostane induced labor neither at mid-pregnancy nor at preterm, but in combination with antiprogestins it acts synergistically in inducing labor and delivery in guinea pigs.[5] The synergistic effect of antiprogestins with epostane was reversed by estrogens and the estrogen precursor androstendione, but not by progesterone, indicating that the increased labor-inducing activity of this combination was predominantly due to the reduced estrogen levels by epostane.[5] Moreover, there was a synergistic effect of tamoxifen and antiprogestins at mid-pregnancy,[5] but not at preterm.[7] Quite surprisingly, estradiol almost totally inhibited spontaneous and onapristone-induced labor in guinea pigs[7,5] and rats (R. E. Garfield, unpublished data). However, a combination of RU 486 and tamoxifen was no more efficient in inducing early abortion in humans than RU 486 alone.[26] In *Tupaja belangeri*, onapristone, RU 486 and epostane had similar effects to those in preterm guinea pigs. Onapristone effectively induced preterm parturition when administered on day 42 p.c. (term: between day 44–46 p.c.), whereas RU 486 had only a marginal effect. Interestingly, epostane (10 mg/animal.day s.c.) did not induce preterm birth despite lowering plasma progesterone levels.[7]

*Effects on Myometrial Responsiveness*

A number of *in vitro*[27] and *in vivo* (see below) studies have clearly shown that antiprogestins increase the myometrial responsiveness to uterotonins, including oxytocin and prostaglandins. An approximately 30-fold increase in uterine responsiveness to both sulprostone ($PGE_2$-analogue)[5,28] and oxytocin[29] was found in mid-pregnant (day 42–43 p.c.) guinea pigs. Normally, at this stage of pregnancy the uterus is insensitive to oxytocin and even very high doses do not effectively induce abortion without antiprogestin priming. Intrauterine pressure recording performed at this stage of pregnancy revealed phasic, labor-like contractions in response to oxytocin in onapristone-primed animals in contrast to tonic reactions in controls. At preterm (day 61 p.c.), when myometrium is becoming sensitive to oxytocin, onapristone additionally increased the myometrial responsiveness to oxytocin (FIG. 2). It was possible to define doses of onapristone and oxytocin which alone did not induce preterm parturition but given sequentially effectively induced preterm birth within a few hours. Onapristone was 10–30 times more effective than RU 486 in increasing myometrial responsiveness to oxytocin in preterm guinea pigs.[29] This myometrial effect is not specific to oxytocin, since both compounds also increased myometrial responsiveness to sulprostone ($PGE_2$-analogue),[5,7] and since there was no increase in myometrial oxytocin receptors in mid-pregnant and preterm guinea pigs.[29]

The efficacy of onapristone in elevating myometrial responsiveness to oxytocin and sulprostone markedly increased during the course of pregnancy. Comparable effects can be obtained with approximately 30-times lower doses of onapristone at preterm (day 61 p.c.) as compared to late pregnancy (day 42–43 p.c.).[7] This is a remarkable effect since there is little difference in serum progesterone levels between these two stages.[7,8] The increasing "sensitivity" of the uterus to antiprogestins during the course of pregnancy indicates that progesterone action also decreases during advanced pregnancy in species displaying no progesterone decrease at term.

*Induction of Parturition with Antiprogestins in Nonhuman Primates*

All studies demonstrate that RU 486 alone, irrespective of the dose and treatment duration, does not successfully induce preterm parturition in cynomolgus[30–32] or rhesus monkeys,[33,34] although it is very effective in combination with oxytocin. Rhesus monkeys treated with RU 486 on approximately day 130 of pregnancy (term = 168 days) were delivered by cesarean section between 48–72 hours after the first treatment because of a lack of any progression of labor.[33] The authors concluded that RU 486 stimulated intense uterine activity (intrauterine pressure;

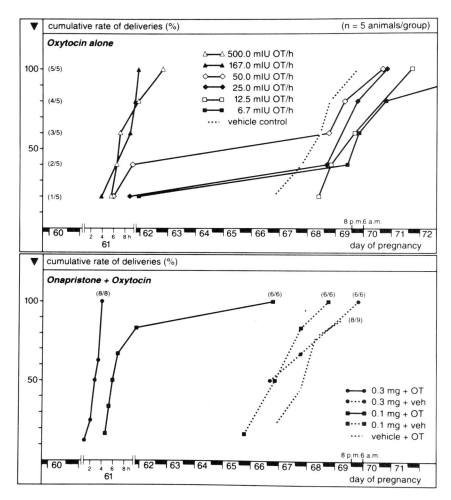

**FIGURE 2.** Induction of preterm parturition with oxytocin (OT) alone (*upper panel*) and after priming with onapristone (*lower panel*). *Upper panel:* oxytocin treatment alone. Oxytocin was given on day 61 p.c. in serial injections of 6.7–500 mU at 1-h intervals (maximum 6 injections) 18 h after vehicle treatment. N = 5/group. Results are presented as cumulative rates of deliveries. *Lower panel.* Oxytocin was given on day 61 p.c. in serial injections of 25.0 mU at 1-h intervals (maximum 6 injections) 18 h after priming with onapristone (0.1–0.3 mg/animal s.c. or vehicle (controls). N = 5–9/group. Results are presented as cumulative rates of deliveries. (Modified from Ref. 43.)

area under the curve), but not cervical ripening. However, the RU 486-induced contractions were irregular, long-lasting and of low amplitude in this study, similar to our observations after both onapristone and RU 486-treatment in guinea pigs.[29] These contractions clearly differ from those seen during spontaneous labor, which are phasic, of short duration and long amplitude and were clearly insufficient to induce deliveries in monkeys. Recently, a study in preterm cynomolgus monkeys (9–17 days before term) evaluated the labor-inducing activity of RU 486 after various doses and regimens.[32] It showed that none of the treatment protocols induced labor or achieved parturition. In this study, RU 486 softened the cervix and increased basal myometrium contractility (transient irritability), irrespective of dose and regimen, but did not induce the characteristic regular uterine contractions required for normal vaginal delivery. Interestingly, epostane treatment of late pregnant rhesus monkeys was effective in inducing parturition without complications.[34] The reason for the contrasting effects of progesterone antagonists and epostane in monkeys is not clear. Epostane is not a specific inhibitor of progesterone secretion, since it also decreased estradiol levels; therefore, its high labor-inducing activity in monkeys may be due to the inhibition of secretion of other steroids.

On the other hand, the sequential treatment with RU 486 and oxytocin 12 hours later was very effective in inducing parturition in cynomolgus monkeys at preterm (day 160 of pregnancy).[31] A manual examination of the cervix prior to oxytocin treatment revealed the ripening effect of RU 486 in terms of an increased dilatation, and a shortening and softening of the cervix. There was no overt toxicity in fetuses, newborns or mothers with RU 486 treatment, which had a stimulatory effect on colostrum and transiently enhanced weight gain in infants, demonstrating that progesterone withdrawal triggers lactogenesis in primates.[31]

## Human Studies with RU 486 during Advanced Pregnancy

It is remarkable that RU 486 alone is fully effective (100%) in preventing or terminating pregnancy only during the perinidatory stage,[35] when the endometrium is the major target for antiprogestins, its efficacy decreasing significantly during the progression of pregnancy. The efficacy of RU 486 in inducing complete abortions, irrespective of dose, is about 80–85% within 10 days after missed menses, about 65% with 56 days of amenorrhea and <40% in the later stages of pregnancy.[36] It can be increased to 95% or more by adding a prostaglandin in pregnant women with amenorrhea of 7 weeks or less.[36] These studies show that myometrial contractions are not entirely activated by RU 486 in women during more advanced stages of pregnancy requiring an added prostaglandin.

### Second-Trimester Pregnancy Termination

Studies which were performed in combination with a prostaglandin (extra-amniotic $PGE_2$, or vaginal gemeprost or 9-meth. $PGE_2$) demonstrated that pretreatment with RU 486 significantly reduced the induction/abortion interval compared to prostaglandin treatment alone, as well as reducing the required dose and related side-effects of a prostaglandin.[37-41] Similar results were reported recently with the orally active $PGE_1$ analogue misoprostol in combination with RU 486.[42] Misoprostol has the potential of becoming the prostaglandin of choice not only for first-trimester terminations[43] but also for second-trimester terminations. Women primed with RU 486 experienced considerably less pain during abortion. RU 486 was more effective than dilapan (an intracervical synthetic tent effectively inducing cervical dilatation) when used in combination with gemeprost to terminate second-trimester pregnancies.[44] The advantage of RU 486 may be due to its additional effect on myometrial responsiveness.

## Intrauterine Fetal Death

Interestingly, RU 486 alone is effective in inducing labor in women with an intrauterine fetal death, therefore, being more successful than in second-trimester abortion in the presence of a living fetus.[45,46] RU 486 (600 mg/day for 2 days), effectively induced labor within 72 h in 63% of patients (17.4% in the placebo group). This indicates that the labor-inducing activity of antiprogestins depends on the presence of a living fetus and/or normal placenta and suggests that the conceptus exerts inhibitory effects on the uterus in humans.

## Induction of Labor at Term

RU 486 (200 mg for two consecutive days) was first used for the induction of labor for medical indications in France by Frydman et al.[47] Women who had not delivered within 4 days were given oxytocin to induce labor. This study primarily evaluated the labor-inducing activity of RU 486, since the interval between priming and labor induction with oxytocin was relatively long. After RU 486, 54% of women had spontaneous labor within 4 days compared with 18% on placebo. The oxytocin consumption was lower after RU 486 treatment in those women who required labor induction, indicating that both uterine cervix and myometrium were prepared for labor and delivery. The rates of cesarean sections and operative vaginal deliveries were comparable in both groups, and neither infants nor women experienced any side effects.[47] In this study, the labor induction rate of 54% after RU 486 alone, although statistically significant, was not high, considering the advanced gestational age of women. However, the efficacy of RU 486 alone to induce labor and delivery increases dramatically in cases of postdate pregnancies (C. Lelaidier, personal communication), which is consistent with our guinea pig studies showing an increasing efficacy of antiprogestins alone during the course of pregnancy (see above). Multicentric, dose-finding studies are currently in progress in France whose aim is to determine the minimal effective labor-inducing dose of RU 486.[48] Although the available data are encouraging and no adverse effects of RU 486 on the fetus or newborn have been reported to date, large-scale studies will be needed to confirm the safety of RU 486 for newborns, since the transplacental passage of RU 486 was demonstrated in monkeys[49] and women.[50]

## EFFECTS OF ANTIPROGESTINS ON UTERINE PROSTAGLANDINS

Although the role of prostaglandins in the initiation of human parturition remains controversial, their increased production and/or release during the active phase of labor may be obligatory for the expulsion of the fetus and placenta. Progesterone is generally believed to exert an inhibitory effect on uterine prostaglandins during the luteal phase of the cycle and pregnancy.[2] However, studies with antiprogestins performed in guinea pigs[5,11,28] and sheep[51] question this view. In guinea pigs, onapristone treatment inhibited luteolysis and decreased PGFM concentrations in peripheral blood, indicating that the release of uterine PGF2α responsible for luteolysis was suppressed.[5,11,28] A similar antiluteolytic effect of RU 486 was described in sheep.[51] These studies indicate that progesterone may not inhibit the production or release of uterine prostaglandins; on the contrary it may even be essential for their production, and may trigger the uterine PGF2α pulses at the end of the luteal phase in guinea pigs and sheep. The downregulation of uterine prostaglandins during human pregnancy may be the function of the embryo and not of progesterone,[51] in a similar way in which the antiluteolytic protein oTP-1 controls uterine prostaglandins during early pregnancy in sheep.[52] In humans, a protein termed gravidin has been suggested to play such a role.[53,54] Gravidin, which inhibits phospholipase $A_2$ activity in a cell-free assay, reduces PGF2α production and arachidonic acid release from human endometrial cells and shares many features of the secretory component of IgA, was shown to be present in human amniotic fluid. The main source of gravidin is chorion, and its production decreases after delivery, so that the uterine prostaglandins may be released from this inhibition near term.[53,54] The concept that progesterone does not downregulate uterine prostaglandins would explain why RU 486 is ineffective without a prostaglandin in inducing first- and second-trimester abortions in humans. In a second-trimester abortion study, there was no significant increase in PGEM or PGFM concentrations in peripheral maternal plasma within 24 h after administering RU 486 (*i.e.*, prior to $PGE_2$ treatment).[39] In addition, indomethacin influenced neither the increase of uterine activity nor the ripening effect of RU 486 during the first-trimester abortions.[55]

Nevertheless these studies do not exclude the possibility of antiprogestins having an influence on prostaglandin metabolism.[56] Indeed, RU 486 reduces the decidual concentration of prostaglandin dehydrogenase (PGDH) *in vivo* during early pregnancy.[55] In humans, PGDH is the main enzyme inactivating prostaglandins, and endometrial PGDH is clearly controlled by progesterone.[55,56] Since RU 486 has to be combined with prostaglandins to achieve expulsions, this mechanism does not entirely compensate for the antiprogestin-induced prostaglandin "deficiency."

## MECHANISM OF ACTION OF ANTIPROGESTINS IN THE MYOMETRIUM

The experimental and human studies reviewed above clearly demonstrate that the principal antiprogestin action in the pregnant uterus is its conditioning effect (*i.e.*, the suspension of the state of extraordinary refractoriness to contraction to a state of preparedness for labor and delivery). These studies also helped to define the role of progesterone during pregnancy, including the control of gap junctions, L-arginine-nitric oxide-cGMP-system, calcium channels and probably other still unknown mechanisms.

### *Effects on Gap Junctions*

Gap junctions are intercellular channels connecting the interiors of two (myometrial) cells, propagation sites, and the basis for synchrony during labor. In all species studied, the onset and progression of labor contractile activity is invariably associated with the presence of large numbers of gap junctions.[58] The increase in gap junctions could be the major mechanism of increased myometrial responsiveness to uterotonins following antiprogestin treatment, and the most important mechanism of antiprogestin action on the pregnant uterus. An enhanced electrical coupling, due to the increased density of gap junctions in the myometrium following treatment with various antiprogestins, was demonstrated in rats[27] and guinea pigs.[29,59] In late-pregnant guinea pigs, a dramatic increase in connexin 43-binding has been found after onapristone treatment (FIG. 3). The results of intrauterine pressure measurements support a role for gap junctions in electrical coupling. Phasic and coordinated responses to oxytocin injections in onapristone-treated guinea pigs indicate that the propagation of electrical events was enhanced by this treatment.[29]

### *Effects on Oxytocin Receptors*

The myometrium of various species, including humans, is most reactive to oxytocin either near or at the time of parturition. This enhanced myometrial responsiveness to oxytocin has been attributed to an increase in myometrial oxytocin receptor concentrations. It has been suggested that the increase in oxytocin receptor concentrations in the myometrium and decidua at term is one of the primary factors leading to the initiation of parturition.[60] However, our studies performed in late-pregnant guinea pigs and clinical studies with RU 486 indicate that progesterone does not control oxytocin receptor synthesis in these species. In pregnant guinea pigs, onapristone dramatically enhanced myometrial responsiveness to oxytocin without increasing the myometrial oxytocin receptor concentrations, whereas the gradual increase in oxytocin receptors was accompanied by rising progesterone levels during pregnancy. These data provide further evidence that a rise in oxytocin receptor concentrations alone may not be the only mechanism for oxytocin to be effective as suggested previously.[60] In early-pregnant women, both RU 486 and epostane[61] enhanced uterine reactivity to prostaglandins, but not to oxytocin,[62] suggesting that myometrial oxytocin receptors did not increase after progesterone withdrawal. On the other hand, RU 486 did increase myometrial oxytocin receptors in pregnant rabbits.[63] In contrast to guinea pigs, nonhuman primates and humans, progesterone withdrawal leads to the onset of labor in rabbits, so that mechanisms regulating myometrial oxytocin receptors may be different in such a "progesterone-dependent" species.

### *Effects on the Nitric Oxide System*

Nitric oxide (NO), synthesized from the amino acid L-arginine by a family of enzymes, the nitric oxide synthases, is involved in controlling the relaxation of various smooth muscles.[64,65] NO actions are mediated by the activation of guanylate cyclase and the consequent increase of cGMP in target cells. Our studies in rats[64,65] and guinea pigs (K. Chwalisz, unpublished data) indicate that the L-arginine-NO-cGMP-system is present in the uterus and may play an important role in uterine relaxation, pregnancy maintenance, fetal perfusion and the regulation of blood pressure. It has been observed in pregnant rats that the ability of L-arginine (nitric oxide substrate) and 8-bromo-cyclic guanosine monophosphate to relax the uterus decreases after progesterone withdrawal, both spontaneously

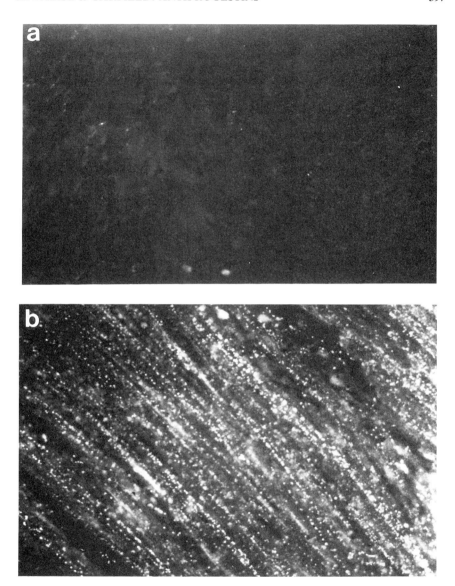

**FIGURE 3.** Effect of onapristone on gap junctions in late pregnant guinea pigs: immunocytochemical staining with antibodies to connexin 43. Light micrograph (1000×) of myometrial tissue **(a)** from a control animal on day 45 p.c. and **(b)** from an animal after two-days' treatment with 10.0 mg onapristone s.c. on day 43–44 p.c. In (a) note the lack of staining as compared to (b). In (b) note the abundance of bright fluorescent spots which represent gap junction. (From Aubeny & Baulieu.[43] Reprinted by permission from *Comptes Rendus de l'Académie des Sciences*.)

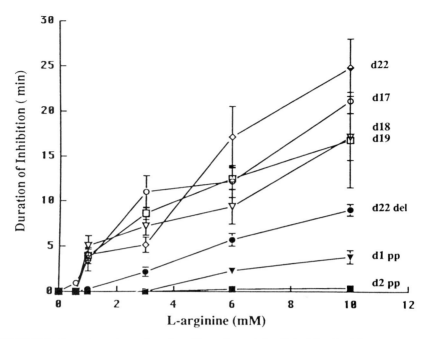

**FIGURE 4.** Dose-dependent relaxation effects of L-arginine (0.1 mM to 10 mM) on spontaneously contracting uterine strips from rats at different stages of gestation, during delivery and postpartum. The tissues were obtained on days 17–22 (d17, d18, d19 and d22) of gestation, on day 22 (d22 del) during spontaneous delivery (1–3 pups delivered), or on 1 (d1pp) and 2 (d2pp) days postpartum. The duration of complete inhibition of spontaneous uterine contractions are dose-dependent. Data are analyzed by repeated measures ANOVA on seven groups. The effects of L-arginine from concentrations of 1 mM are significnatly ($p < 0.01$) decreased during spontaneous delivery at term and postpartum compared to all other times. Each data point represents the mean ± SEM. The total number of strips studied at each time period was 8–16 from 4–6 animals per group.[88]

at term (FIG. 4) and after onapristone treatment (FIG. 5), which strongly suggests that the nitric oxide-dependent relaxation (nitric oxide synthesis and/or the effector system of cGMP) in the uterus is controlled by progesterone.[6,64,65] Therefore, the nitric oxide system may contribute to the maintenance of uterine quiescence during pregnancy, when progesterone levels are elevated, but not during delivery. The decrease in NO production and/or in the cGMP effector system in the uterus may represent an important mechanism for the initiation of parturition.

### Effects on Calcium Channels

Extracellular calcium is required for myometrial cells to contract forcefully and calcium enters muscle cells via specific channels. As action potentials propagate over the uterus (via gap junctions, see above) they depolarize muscle cells and open calcium channels. Two major types of calcium channels are believed to exist: (1) voltage-dependent channels (VDC) responsive to changes in membrane potentials and (2) receptor-operated channels, which open when agonists bind to their receptors. The excitability of the uterus may be dependent on calcium channel density, which may increase during the course of pregnancy in preparation of the uterine muscle for labor. In pregnant rats, the L (long lasting)-type VDC mRNA levels rose 7-fold from day 15 to day 22 p.c. and declined during labor (FIG. 6). The decrease in VDC mRNA during labor indicates a rapid decline in synthesis when the channels are likely to have reached their highest level. Onapristone treatment on day 18 p.c. led to a significant increase in their levels within 8 hours, indicating that progesterone controls the expression of voltage-dependent calcium channels (FIG. 7) in rats.[66]

## CERVICAL EFFECTS OF ANTIPROGESTINS

It is now well established that the ripening of the uterine cervix, which occurs progressively during late pregnancy, is the result of an active biochemical process involving degradative enzymes and changes in the synthesis of extracellular matrix proteins and glycoproteins, immune cells and inflammation mediators (such as

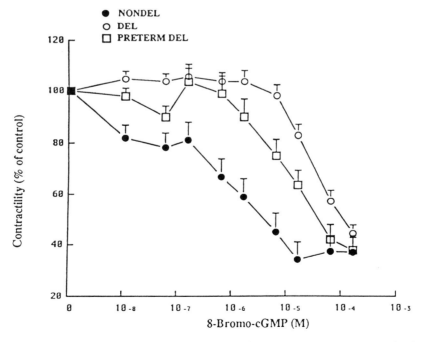

FIGURE 5. 8-Bromo-cGMP dose relaxation curves for uterine tissues from rats delivering spontaneously at term (DEL), preterm after onapristone treatment (PRETERM DEL) on day 18 of gestation. Each point represents means + SEM for 4 strips from each animal, with 4 rats/group.[88]

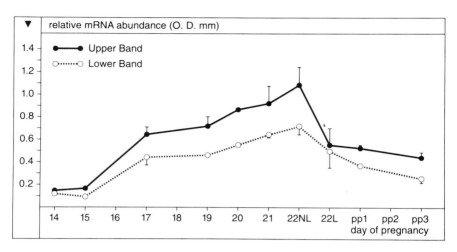

**FIGURE 6.** Gestational changes of calcium channel $\alpha$1-subunit mRNA levels in rat myometrium by RT-PCR. *Upper band:* 372-bp product; *lower band:* 339-bp product. One-way analysis of variance shows significant differences ($p < 0.001$, $p = 0.032$) when comparisons were made among different days of pregnancy (375-bp products, 339-bp products, respectively). At points lacking a standard error bar, the error was smaller than or equal to the size of open or closed circle. (From N. Tezuka, M. Ali, K. Chwalisz & R. E. Garfield, unpublished.)

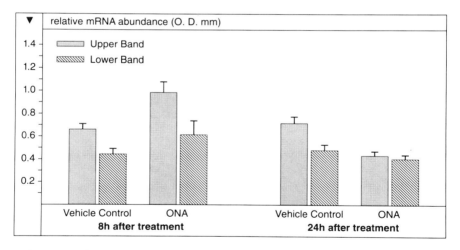

**FIGURE 7.** Effect of onapristone on calcium channel $\alpha$1-subunit mRNA levels in rat myometrium by RT-PCR after onapristone treatment. *Upper band:* 372-bp product; *lower band:* 339-bp product. Rats at day 17 p.c. were injected s.c. with 10 mg of onapristone. The autopsy was performed at 8 and 24 h after treatment. One way analysis of variance shows significant differences ($p < 0.001$) when comparisons are made among different hours after onapristone injection in 372-bp products, not in 339-bp products ($p = 0.0386$). (From N. Tezuka, M. Ali, K. Chwalisz & R. E. Garfield, unpublished.)

cytokines and prostaglandins) and relaxin.[67] However, the exact mechanism which controls, or more importantly which initiates this process is still unknown. Animal and clinical studies with antiprogestins show that progesterone may be the principal factor controlling cervical ripening and its withdrawal may initiate the biochemical cascade leading to a remodelling of the connective tissue of the cervix.

*Animals Studies*

Our biomechanical studies in pregnant rats and guinea pigs showed an increased extensibility and dilatation of the cervix after treatment with different antiprogestins including onapristone and RU 486[11,68] (FIG. 8a). These effects were dose-dependent and were observed long before the onset of labor, indicating that cervical changes precede labor following antiprogestin treatment and are not the result of uterine contractions.[68] In onapristone-treated guinea pigs, electron microscopic examinations revealed a dissolution, splitting up and dissociation of collagen fibers, expansion of the interfibrillar space due to edema as well as highly active fibroblasts with cytoplasmic components typical for secretory cells and polyploid nuclei.[69] This was associated with an infiltration of the polymorphonuclear granulocytes, macrophages and mast cells (FIG. 8b). Similar morphological changes were observed in control animals just before term. The "pure" progesterone agonist promegestone (R5020) fully reversed the onapristone effects on the cervix, so that the observed effects were mediated via the progesterone receptor.[7,68] The results of monkey studies are conflicting. RU 486 induced cervical ripening in preterm (9–17 days before term) cynomolgus monkeys,[31,32] whereas studies in rhesus mon-

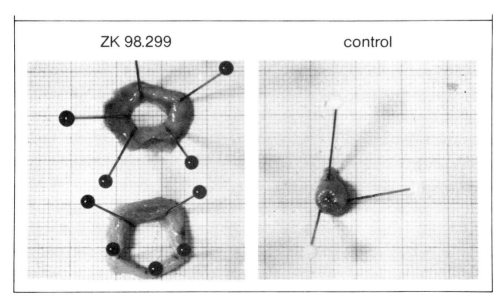

**FIGURE 8a.** Effect of onapristone (3 mg s.c.) on the cervix in pregnant guinea pigs 15 h after treatment on day 59 p.c.

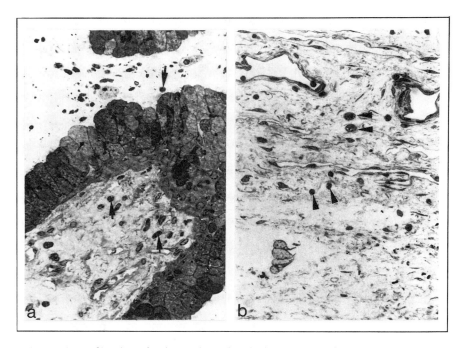

**FIGURE 8b.** Infiltration of polymorphonuclear leukocytes into the guinea pig cervix on day 60 p.c., 15 h after onapristone treatment (1.0 mg s.c.); light micrographs of semi-thin sections. **(a)** The lamina propria of the plica palmata exhibits widely separated collagen fibers as well as many polymorphonuclear leukocytes (*arrows*) which can also be found within the cervical lumen (400×). **(b)** In addition to the widely separated collagen fibers and the increased amount of interfibrillar ground substance, different kinds of free cells (*arrowheads*) can be found (320×). (From Hegele-Hartung *et al.*[69] Reprinted by permission from *Human Reproduction*.)

keys performed during earlier stages of pregnancy (approximately 38 days before term) failed to demonstrate its ripening effect.[33] However, the cervical status was assessed by manual examination in both studies, a method being quite insensitive, and a combined RU 486 plus oxytocin treatment was effective in inducing delivery in cynomolgus monkeys,[45] so that the cervix was prepared for delivery.

### Cervical Ripening with RU 486 in Women

The clinical experience with RU 486 made during different stages of pregnancy and in nonpregnant women is consistent with the results of animal studies, demonstrating (directly or indirectly) its ripening effect on the uterine cervix. The shortening of induction-delivery intervals with RU 486 is clear and indirect evidence of its cervical effect. The ripening effect of RU 486 was objectively assessed by biomechanical and morphological criteria in a number of studies performed during the first trimester,[70-73] and in one study performed during the second trimester of gestation,[38] as well as in nonpregnant women,[74] indicating that pregnancy is not essential. It is still unclear whether the ripening effect of RU 486 is dose-related in women. Further biochemical studies, employing improved assessment methods of cervical dilatation and extensibility are needed to clarify the question of a dose-dependency in terms of the cervical effects of antiprogestins in humans.

### Mechanism of Action of Antiprogestins on the Uterine Cervix

Biochemical and morphological studies performed by us[7,68] and other investigators[75,76] show that an increased collagenolysis takes place within the cervix following antiprogestin treatment in guinea pigs. In term guinea pigs, there was a marked increase in procollagenase, collagenase inhibitory activity, and net procollagenase activity;[75] a rise in serum collagenase levels correlating with the state of the cervix was found in pregnant women.[77] Progesterone inhibited the procollagenase gene expression and blocked the estradiol-induced increase in collagenase production in monolayer cell cultures derived from pregnant guinea pig cervices,[76] and almost totally abolished the release of matrix metalloproteinases, collagenase, and related gelatinases in human endometrial explants, an effect which was antagonized by RU 486.[78] These studies suggest that progesterone may control the collagenase activity in the uterine cervix.

### The Role of Prostaglandins

The available data indicate that antiprogestins do not act on the cervix by means of stimulating endogenous prostaglandin production, since the prostaglandin synthese inhibitors do not inhibit this effect. Our studies show that indomethacine has no effect on the onapristone-induced cervical ripening,[68] whereas it fully inhibits cervical ripening induced with LPS in pregnant guinea pigs.[79] Diclofenac blocked RU 486-induced labor, but did not antagonize its ripening effect on the cervix in pregnant rats.[80] Similarly, naproxen also did not inhibit the effect of RU 486 on the cervix during first-trimester abortion in women.[81]

### The Role of Cytokines

An "inflammatory reaction" seems to be a physiological mechanism of cervical ripening.[82] An infiltration of white blood cells into the cervix occurs in women at term, accompanied by the dissolution of the connective tissue matrix around polymorphonuclear leukocytes, and the presence of activated and degranulated eosinophiles.[83] While a similar reaction occurs in the pregnant guinea pig cervix after onapristone (see above), with no indomethacin effect, we suggested that the enzymatic activity originates from inflammatory cells and chemotactic agents like cytokines (*e.g.*, IL-8, IL-1$\beta$) mediate antiprogestin effects in the cervix.[68] Cytokines are clearly involved in normal parturition during cervical ripening, while uterine cervix explants from pregnant rabbits[84] and pregnant women[85] are capable of producing large amounts of IL-1 and IL-8, respectively. Additionally, progesterone inhibits and RU 486 stimulates IL-8 release in human choriodecidual cells *in vitro*.[86] We recently demonstrated, by means of morphological and biomechanical criteria, the IL-8 and IL-1$\beta$ efficacy in inducing cervical ripening in pregnant guinea pigs after topical administration in gel.[87] Cervical ripening was achieved with both cytokines without inducing labor and was similar to the physiological process at term and to the effects seen after onapristone. Thus, progesterone may act as an immunosuppressor in the cervix and antiprogestin treatment (or spontaneous progesterone withdrawal) may activate the cytokine cascade. IL-8, which induces neutrophil migration into tissues and causes degranulation of the specific granule containing collagenase, may act at the end-point of this cascade during both normal and antiprogestin-induced parturition.

## DISCUSSION AND CONCLUSIONS

The data on antiprogestins in various species reviewed here clearly indicate that progesterone plays an essential role in pregnancy maintenance in all mammals investigated to date, and that antiprogestin treatment results in the initiation of parturition (*i.e.*, transition from quiescence to preparedness of the uterus), although not always in the onset of active labor. Species with physiological progesterone withdrawal at term (rats, rabbits, sheep, pigs and cows) respond to antiprogestins during late pregnancy by a preterm parturition similar to the normal process. Species without progesterone withdrawal prior to parturition (guinea pigs, *Tupaja belangeri*, nonhuman primates and humans) respond by an increase in myometrial responsiveness and cervical ripening, but not always in the induction of preterm birth. In these species, both myometrial responsiveness and the state of the cervix are controlled by progesterone during pregnancy. Indeed, the state of the cervix correlates very well with the myometrial sensitivity to oxytocin, and the manual evaluation of the cervix is a common method used to predict preterm birth in women. These studies also demonstrate that there are striking similarities in the molecular events of parturition, especially in the preparatory process, despite well-known differences in the endocrinology of parturition.

For many years labor has been considered as the transition from inactive muscle to active muscle by adding a uterotonin or withdrawing from tonic inhibition. These models defined neither the uterine stages of labor nor the progesterone action. Studies with antiprogestins in different species, especially those we have carried out on gap junctions, nitric oxide and calcium channels indicate that they may be inappropriate. Based on these studies we proposed that the uterus (myometrium and cervix) undergoes a conditioning (preparatory) step[5-7] which prepares it for labor and delivery, whereas the exogenous or endogenous uterotonic agents may induce uterine contractions (FIG. 9). This perhaps irreversible step of parturition may be initiated by progesterone withdrawal (both progesterone receptor blockade or synthesis inhibition) or by other factors, *e.g.*, cytokines. Indeed, the effects of the cytokines IL-1β, TFNα and IL-8, which play a role in preterm labor associated with infection, are similar to those induced by antiprogestins (*i.e.*, delayed response, little direct effect on myometrium contractions).[88] The active phase of labor may be nonspecific in which almost every uterotonin (oxytocin, PGs, endothelin, etc.) may induce successful contractions and delivery.

However, it has been known for many years that progesterone withdrawal does not occur in women, and no other mechanisms attenuating progesterone action without changes in the peripheral blood have been established to date. Studies with antiprogestins discussed above strongly indicate that such a mechanism must exist in the pregnant human uterus, and identifying this mechanism has to be considered as a fundamental question in obstetrics. In guinea pigs, the efficacy of onapristone in inducing uterine responsiveness to oxytocin and prostaglandins substantially increases during the course of pregnancy, despite

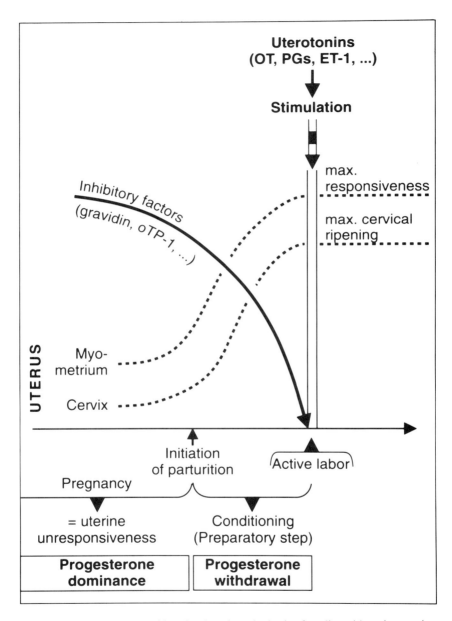

**FIGURE 9.** Model of parturition developed on the basis of studies with antiprogestins.

little change in serum progesterone levels. At preterm, 30-times lower doses of onapristone and a single treatment are required to achieve a similar response to both oxytocin and sulprostone compared to mid-pregnancy (see above). Moreover, the spontaneous increase in both myometrial responsiveness and cervical ripening in guinea pigs (and humans) occurs in the presence of increasing progesterone concentrations in maternal blood. A hypothetical explanation of this phenomenon may be that the target organ sensitivity to progesterone decreases at term (*e.g.*, at receptor or postreceptor levels). Another possibility is that a "natural" antiprogestin, which may be either a steroid or a protein, is secreted in increasing amounts during late pregnancy. Recently, on the basis of *in vitro* experiments, TGF$\beta$ was proposed as a physiological antiprogestin.[89] However, TGF$\beta$ is also steroid-dependent and further studies are needed to establish its role in parturition.

The major mechanism of antiprogestin action on the late pregnant uterus (FIG. 10) may be to induce a synthesis of the gap junction proteins which are essential for the development of phasic and coordinated responses to uterotonins. In addition, antiprogestins also downregulate the L-arginine- nitric oxide-cGMP-system which is partly responsible for uterine relaxation[6,64,65] and may stimulate myometrial calcium channel biosynthesis and thereby increase the excitability of myometrial cells.[66] A second important component of the conditioning effect of antiprogestins is cervical ripening which could be mediated by cytokines (IL-8, IL-1$\beta$, etc.). However, the role of leukotrienes and relaxin in cervical ripening cannot be excluded. The downregulation of the cytokines during pregnancy may be the result of the immunosuppressive action of progesterone.

Mechanism(s) controlling the release of uterotonins, *e.g.*, prostaglandins, oxytocin, endothelin, which eventually trigger the onset of labor (active labor) may not depend on progesterone. These uterotonins may be under tonic inhibition of fetal and/or placental factors during pregnancy (*e.g.*, gravidin, oTP-1-like inhibitors) and may decrease prior to delivery (FIG. 9). This release of endogenous inhibition occurring at term may explain why onapristone alone induces premature birth at preterm, but not during mid-gestation in guinea pigs (see above), and why RU 486 alone induces labor in postterm pregnancies (see above) and in intrauterine fetal death.[46]

Onapristone shows a suitable profile for obstetrical indications. It has a higher labor-inducing activity in both guinea pigs and *Tupaja belangeri* at preterm than RU 486, possibly due to the absence of progesterone-agonistic activity in these species. It is also 10–30 times more effective than RU 486 in inducing myometrial responsiveness and cervical ripening in guinea pigs. Onapristone is a short-acting antiprogestin, its half-life is about 2–4 h in women after oral application (K. Zurth, unpublished data) (the half-life of RU 486 ranges between 24–48 h), and its on-and-off rates to the progesterone receptor are similar to those of progesterone (K. H. Fritzemeier, unpublished data). Onapristone also shows substantially lower antiglucocorticoid activity *in vivo*,[11] although further safety studies of labor induction with onapristone are needed in nonhuman primates.

TABLE 1 presents the potential obstetrical indications for antiprogestins. They may be used as an adjunct to labor and delivery during second-trimester pregnancy termination, in intrauterine fetal death, in the induction of labor at term in the presence of medical indication for pregnancy termination, to treat postterm pregnancies, and perhaps to facilitate parturition. The most exciting indication for antiprogestins seems to be the induction of labor at term in combination with oxytocin. We have shown that both cervical ripening and myometrial responsiveness are induced with antiprogestins without influencing uterine contractions, which is a preferable obstetrical situation. If the uterus (myometrium and cervix)

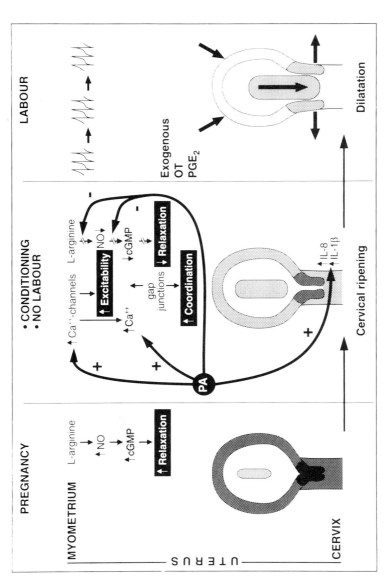

**FIGURE 10.** Mechanisms of action of antiprogestins (AP) on the pregnant uterus during advanced pregnancy. IL, interleukin; OT, oxytocin; $PGE_2$, prostaglandin $E_2$. (From Chwalisz.[8] Reprinted by permission from *Human Reproduction*.)

TABLE 1. Obstetrical Indication of Antiprogestins

| Indication | Additional Treatment | Comment |
|---|---|---|
| 1. Second-trimester abortion | prostaglandins | |
| 2. Intrauterine fetal death | (prostaglandins, oxytocin) | antiprogestins may be effective alone |
| 3. Induction of labor at term because of medical indications | oxytocin | |
| 4. Postterm pregnancy | | antiprogestins may be effective alone |
| 5. Dysfunctional labor (primary dysfunctional labor, secondary arrest of labor) (?) | (oxytocin) | antiprogestins may be effective alone |

is prepared for delivery, sequential oxytocin treatment would permit better control of uterine contractility. The preparation of the myometrium in terms of increased sensitivity to oxytocin or prostaglandins is unique to antiprogestins.

Although no acute or long-term unwanted effects of RU 486 have been reported in women or newborns, and despite encouraging animal data, further studies are needed to establish the safety of RU 486 and other antiprogestins before they can be routinely recommended as an adjunct to labor and delivery with living infants.

## ACKNOWLEDGMENTS

The initial phase of this research was conducted and supported by Dr. Elger and we would like to acknowledge this fruitful collaboration. We are grateful to Dr. S. H. Hasan for hormone determinations and to B. Kosub, Mrs. B. Bragulla, Mrs. H. Altmann, Mrs. G. Bauer, and Mr. S. Althof for their excellent technical assistance in performing experimental studies.

## REFERENCES

1. KEIRSE, M. J. N. 1992. Therapeutic use of prostaglandins. Ballière's Clin. Obstet. Gynecol. **6:** 787–809.
2. CSAPO, A. I. 1981. Force of labour. In Principles and Practice of Obstetrics and Perinatology. L. Iffy & H. A. Kaminetzky, Eds. Vol. 2: 761–799. John Wiley & Sons. New York.
3. ELGER, W. 1979. Pharmacology of parturition and abortion. Anim. Reprod. Sci. **2:** 133–148.
4. PORTER, D. G. 1970. The failure of progesterone to affect myometrial activity in the guinea pig. J. Endocrinol. **46:** 425–434.
5. ELGER, W., K. CHWALISZ, M. FÄHNRICH, S. H. HASAN, D. LAURENT, S. BEIER, E. OTTOW, G. NEEF & R. E. GARFIELD. 1990. Studies on labour-conditioning and labour-inducing effects of antiprogesterones in animal models. In: Uterine Contractility: Mechanisms of Control. R. E. Garfield, Ed. 153–157. Serono Symposia, USA. Norwell, MA.
6. GARFIELD, R. E. & C. YALLAMPALLI. 1993. Control of myometrial contractility and labor. In Basic Mechanisms Controlling Term and Preterm Labor. Ernst Schering Research Foundation Workshop 7. K. Chwalisz & R. E. Garfield, Eds. 1–29. Springer

Verlag. Berlin, Heidelberg, New York, London, Paris, Tokyo, Hong Kong, Barcelona, Budapest.
7. CHWALISZ, K. 1993. Role of progesterone in the control of labor. *In* Basic Mechanisms Controlling Term and Preterm Labor. Ernst Schering Research Foundation Workshop 7. K. Chwalisz & R. E. Garfield, Eds. 97–163. Springer Verlag. Berlin, Heidelberg, New York, London, Paris, Tokyo, Hong Kong, Barcelona, Budapest.
8. CHWALISZ, K. 1994. The use of progesterone antagonists for cervical ripening and as an adjunct to labour and delivery. Hum. Reprod. In press.
9. PHILIBERT, D., M. MOGUILEWSKY, M. MARY, D. LECAQUE, C. TOURNEMINE, J. SECCHI & R. DERAEDT. 1985. Pharmacological profile of RU 486 in animals. *In* The Antiprogesterone Steroid RU 486 and Human Fertility Control. E. E. Baulieu & S. J. Segal, Eds. 49–68. Plenum Press. New York.
10. NEFF, G., S. BEIER, W. ELGER, D. HENDERSON & R. WIECHERT. 1984. New steroids with antiprogestational and antiglucocorticoid activities. Steroids **44**: 349–372.
11. ELGER, W., S. BEIER, K. CHWALISZ, M. FÄHNRICH, S. H. HASAN, D. HENDERSON, G. NEEF & R. ROHDE. 1986. Studies on the mechanism of action of progesterone antagonists. J. Steroid Biochem. **25**: 835–845.
12. MEYER, M. E., A. PORNON, J. JINGWEI, M. T. BOCQUEL, P. CHAMBON & H. GRONEMEYER. 1990. Agonistic and antagonistic activities of RU 486 on the functions of the human progesterone receptor. EMBO J. **12**: 3923–3932.
13. HORWITZ, K. B. 1992. The molecular biology of RU 486. Is there a role for antiprogestins in the treatment of breast cancer? Endocr. Rev. **13**(2): 146–163.
14. GRONEMEYER, H., B. BENHAMOU, M. BERRY, M. T. BOCQUEL, D. GOFFLO, T. GARCIA, T. LEROUGE, D. METZER, M. E. MEYER, L. TORA, A. VERGEZAC & P. CHAMBON. 1992. Mechanism of antihormone action. J. Steroid Biochem. Mol. Biol. **41**: 217–221.
15. KOERING, M. J., D. L. HEALY & G. D. HODGEN. 1986. Morphologic response of endometrium to a progesterone receptor antagonist, RU 486, in monkeys. Fertil. Steril. **45**: 280–287.
16. GRAVANIS, A., G. SCHAISON, M. GEORGE, J. DE BRUX, P. G. SATYASWAROOP, E. E. BAULIEU & P. ROBEL. 1985. Endometrial and pituitary responses to the steroidal antiprogestin RU 486 in postmenopausal women. J. Clin. Endocrinol. Metab. **60**: 156–163.
17. KLEIN-HITPASS, L., A. C. B. CATO, D. HENDERSON & G. U. RYFFEL. 1991. Two types of antiprogestins identified by their differential action in transcriptionally active extracts from T47D cells. Nucleic Acids Res. **19**: 1227–1234.
18. TAKIMOTO, G. S., D. M. TASSET, A. C. EPPERT & K. B. HORWITZ. 1992. Hormone-induced progesterone receptor phosphorylation consists of sequential DNA-dependent stages: analysis with zinc finger mutants and the progesterone antagonist ZK 89 299. Proc. Natl. Acad. Sci. USA **89**: 3050–3054.
19. BECK, C. A., N. L. WEIGEL, N. L. MOYER, S. K. NORDEEN & D. P. EDWARDS. 1993. The progesterone antagonist RU 486 acquires agonistic activity upon stimulation of cAMP signaling pathways. Proc. Natl. Acad. Sci. USA **90**: 441–445.
20. CHWALISZ, K., H. ALTMANN & W. ELGER. 1986. Induction of premature parturition in the rat with antigestagens. Acta Endocrinol. (Suppl.) **111**: 12 (abstract).
21. BOSC, M. J., G. GERMAIN, A. NICOLLE, M. MOUREN, D. PHILIBERT & E. E. BAULIEU. 1987. Control of birth in rats by RU 486, an antiprogesterone compound. J. Reprod. Fertil. **79**: 1–8.
22. GARFIELD, R. E., J. M. GASC & E. E. BAULIEU. 1987. Effect of the antiprogesterone RU 486 on preterm birth in the rat. Am. J. Obstet. Gynecol. **157**: 1281–1285.
23. HÖFIG, A., W. ELGER, K. CHWALISZ, S. H. HASAN, G. NEEF & F. ELLENDORFF. 1988. Induction of parturition in the pig with the antigestagen ZK 112 993. Acta Endocrinol. (Suppl.) **87**: 193.
24. GAZOL, O. S., Y. LI, C. SCHWABE & L. L. ANDERSON. 1993. Attenuation of antepartum relaxin surge and induction of parturition by antiprogesterone RU 486 in sheep. J. Reprod. Fertil. **97**: 233–240.
25. LI, Y., R. PEREZGROVAS, O. S. GAZAL, C. SCHWABE & L. L. ANDERSON. 1991. Antiprogesterone, RU 486, facilitates parturition in cattle. Endocrinology **129**: 765–770.

26. VAN LOOK, P. F. A. & H. VON HERTZEN. 1993. Antiprogestogens: perspectives from a global research program. In Clinical Applications of Mifepristone (RU 486) and Other Antiprogestins. Assessing the Science and Recommending a Research Agenda. M. S. Donaldson, L. Dorflinger, S. S. Brown & L. Z. Benet, Eds. 253–278. National Academy Press. Washington, DC.
27. GARFIELD, R. E. & S. BEIER. 1989. Increased myometrial responsiveness to oxytocin during term and preterm labour. Am. J. Obstet. Gynecol. **161**: 454–461.
28. ELGER, W., M. FÄHNRICH, S. BEIER, SHI SHAO QING & K. CHWALISZ. 1987. Endometrial and myometrial effects of progesterone antagonists in pregnant guinea pigs. Am. J. Obstet. Gynecol. **157**: 1065–1074.
29. CHWALISZ, K., F. FAHRENHOLZ, M. HACKENBERG, R. GARFIELD & W. ELGER. 1991. The progesterone antagonist onapristone increases the effectiveness of oxytocin to produce delivery without changing the myometrial oxytocin receptor concentrations. Am. J. Obstet. Gynecol. **165**(6): 1760–1770.
30. GERMAIN, G., D. PHILIBERT, J. POTTIER, M. MOUREN, E. E. BAULIEU & C. SUREAU. 1985. Effect of the antiprogesterone agent RU 486 on the natural cycle and gestation in intact cynomolgus monkeys. In The Antiprogestin Steroid RU 486 and Human Fertility Control. E. E. Baulieu & S. J. Segal, Eds. 155–167. Plenum Press. New York.
31. WOLF, J. P., M. SINOSICH, T. ANDERSON, A. ULMANN, E. E. BAULIEU & G. D. HODGEN. 1989. Progesterone antagonist (RU 486) for cervical dilatation, labor induction, and delivery in monkeys: effectiveness in combination with oxytocin. Am. J. Obstet. Gynecol. **160**: 45–47.
32. WOLF, J. P., J. SIMON, M. ITSKOVITZ, M. J. SINOSICH, A. ULMANN, E. E. BAULIEU & G. D. HODGEN. 1993. Progesterone antagonist RU 486 accommodates, but does not induce labour and delivery in primates. Hum. Reprod. **8**: 759–763.
33. HALUSKA, G. J., F. Z. STANCZYK, M. J. COOK & M. J. NOVY. 1987. Temporal changes in uterine activity and prostaglandin response to RU 486 in rhesus macaques in late gestation. Am. J. Obstet. Gynecol. **157**: 1487–1495.
34. NOVY, M. J. & G. J. HALUSKA. 1993. New perspectives on estrogen, progesterone. and oxytocin action in primate parturition. In Basic Mechanisms Controlling Term and Preterm Labor. Ernst Schering Research Foundation Workshop 7. K. Chwalisz & R. E. Garfield, Eds. 163–197. Springer Verlag. Berlin, Heidelberg, New York, London, Paris, Tokyo, Hong Kong, Barcelona, Budapest.
35. GLASIER, A., K. J. THONG, M. DEWAR, M. MACKIE & D. T. BAIRD. 1992. Mifepristone (RU 486) compared with high-dose oestrogen and progestostogen for emergency postcoital contraception. N. Engl. J. Med. **327**: 1041–1044.
36. VAN LOOK, P. F. A. & M. BYGDEMAN. 1989. Antiprogestational steroids: a new dimension in human fertility regulation. Oxf. Rev. Reprod. Biol. **11**: 1–60.
37. URQUHART, D. R. & A. A. TEMPLETON. 1990b. The use of mifepristone prior to prostaglandin-induced mid-trimester abortion. Hum. Reprod. **5**: 883–886.
38. FRYDMAN, R., H. FERNANDEZ, J. C. PONS & A. ULMANN. 1988. Mifepristone (RU 486) and late pregnancy termination: a double-blind study of two different doses. Hum. Reprod. **3**: 803–806.
39. HILL, N. C. W., M. SELINGER, J. FERGUSON, A. LÓPEZ BERNAL & I. Z. MACKENZIE. 1990. The physiological and clinical effect of progesterone inhibition with mifepristone (RU 486) in the second trimester. Br. J. Obstet. Gynaecol. **97**: 487–492.
40. RODGER, M. W. & D. BAIRD. 1990. Pretreatment with mifepristone (RU 486) reduces interval between prostaglandin administration and expulsion in second trimester abortion. Br. J. Obstet. Gynaecol. **97**: 41–45.
41. GOTTLIEB, C. & M. BYGDEMAN. 1991. The use of antiprogestin (RU 486) for termination of second trimester pregnancy. Acta Obstet. Gynecol. Scand. **70**: 199–203.
42. EL-RAFAEY, H., K. HINSHOW & A. TEMPLETON. 1993. The abortifacient effect of misoprostol in the second trimester. A randomized comparison with gemeprost in patient pre-treated with mifepristone (RU 486) Hum. Reprod. **8**: 1744–1746.
43. AUBENY, E. & E. E. BAULIEU. 1991. Contragestive activity of RU 486 and oral active prostaglandin combination. Comptes Rendus de l'Académie des Sciences **312**: 539–545.

44. THONG, K. J. & D. T. BAIRD. 1992. A study of gemeprost alone, dilapan or mifepristone in combination with gemeprost for the termination of second trimester pregnancy. Contraception **46:** 11–17.
45. CABROL, D., M. BOUVIER D'YVOIRE, E. MERMET, L. CEDARD, C. SUREAU & E. E. BAULIEU. 1985. Induction of labour with mifepristone after intrauterine fetal death. Lancet **2:** 1019.
46. CABROL, D., C. DUBOIS, H. CRONJE, J. M. GONNET, M. GUILLOT, B. MARIA, J. MOODLEY, J. F. OURY, J. M. THOULON, A. TREISSER, D. ULMANN, S. CORREL & A. ULMANN. 1990. Induction of labour with mifepristone (RU 486) in intrauterine fetal death. Am. J. Obstet. Gynecol. **163:** 540–542.
47. FRYDMAN, R., C. LELAIDIER, C. BATON-SAINT-MLEUX, H. FERNANDEZ, M. VIAL & P. BOURGET. 1992. Labour induction in women at term with mifepristone (RU 486): a double-blind, randomized, placebo-controlled study. Obstet. Gynecol. **80:** 972–975.
48. ULMANN, A. & L. SILVESTRE. 1993. Uses of antiprogestins after 63 days of amenorrhoea. *In* Clinical Applications of Mifepristone (RU 486) and Other Antiprogestins. Assessing the Science and Recommending a Research Agenda. M. S. Donaldson, L. Dorflinger, S. S. Brown & L. Z. Benet, Eds. 174–182. National Academy Press. Washington, DC.
49. WOLF, J. P., C. F. CHILIK, J. ITSKOVITZ, D. WEYMAN, T. L. ANDERSON, A. ULMANN, E. E. BAULIEU & G. D. HODGEN. 1988. Transplacental passage of a progesterone antagonist in monkeys. Am. J. Obstet. Gynecol. **159:** 328–342.
50. HILL, N. C. W., M. SELINGER, J. FERGUSON & I. Z. MACKENZIE. 1991. Transplacental passage of mifepristone and its influence on maternal and fetal steroid concentrations in the second trimester of pregnancy. Hum. Reprod. **6:** 458–462.
51. MORGAN, G. L., R. D. GEISERT, J. P. MCCANN, F. W. BAZER, T. L. OTT, M. A. MIRANDO & M. STEWART. 1993. Failure of luteolysis and extension of interoestrus interval in sheep treated with the progesterone antagonist mifepristone (RU 486). J. Reprod. Fertil. **98**(2): 451–457.
52. BAZER, F. W. 1991. Uterine-conceptus interactions during the peri-implantation period. *In* Cellular Signals Controlling Uterine Function. L. A. Lavia, Ed. 119–137. Plenum Press. New York, London.
53. WILSON, T., G. C. LIGGINS, G. P. AIMER & S. J. M. SKINNER. 1985. Partial purification and characterisation of two compounds from amniotic fluid which inhibit phospholipase activity in human endometrial cells. Biochem. Biophys. Res. Comm. **131**(1): 22–29.
54. WILSON, T., G. C. LIGGINS & L. JOE. 1989. Purification and characterization of a uterine phospholipase inhibitor that loses activity after labor onset in women. Am. J. Obstet. Gynecol. **160:** 602–606.
55. NORMAN, J. E., R. W. KELLY & D. T. BAIRD. 1991. Uterine activity and decidual prostaglandin production in women in early pregnancy in response to mifepristone with or without indomethacin *in vivo*. Hum. Reprod. **6:** 740–744.
56. NORMAN, J. E., W. X. WU, R. W. KELLY, A. F. GLASIER, A. S. MCNEILLY & D. T. BAIRD. 1991. Effects of mifepristone *in vivo* on decidual prostaglandin synthesis and metabolism. Contraception **44**(1): 89–98.
57. CHENG, L., R. W. KELLY, K. J. THONG, R. HUME & D. T. BAIRD. 1993. The effects of mifepristone (RU 486) on prostaglandin dehydrogenase in decidual and chorionic tissue in early pregnancy. Hum. Reprod. **8:** 705–709.
58. GARFIELD, R. E. & E. L. HERTZBERG. 1190. Cell-to-cell coupling in the myometrium: Emil Bozler's prediction. *In* Frontiers in Smooth Muscle Research. N. Sperelakis & J. D. Wood, Eds. 673–681. Wiley-Liss. New York.
59. SAKAI, N., M. G. BLENNERHASSETT & R. E. GARFIELD. 1992. Effects of antiprogesterones on myometrial cell-to-cell coupling in pregnant guinea pigs. Biol. Reprod. **46:** 385–365.
60. FUCHS, A. R., F. FUCHS, P. HUSSLEIN, M. S. SOLOFF & M. FERNSTROM. 1982. Oxytocin receptors and human parturition: a dual role for oxytocin in the initiation of labor. Science **215:** 1396–1398.
61. WEBSTER, M. A., N. S. PHIPPS & M. D. G. GILLMER. 1985. Myometrial activity in

first trimester human pregnancy after epostane therapy: effect of intravenous oxytocin. Br. J. Obstet. Gynaecol. **92:** 957–962.
62. SWAHN, M. L. & M. BYGDEMAN. 1988. The effect of the antiprogestin RU 486 on uterine contractility and sensitivity to prostaglandin and oxytocin. Br. J. Obstet. Gynaecol. **95:** 126–134.
63. JACOBSON, L., R. K. RIEMER, A. C. GOLDFIEN, D. LYKINS, P. K. SIITERI & J. M. ROBERTS. 1987. Rabbit myometrial oxytocin and $\alpha_2$-adrenergic receptors are increased by oestrogen but are differentially regulated by progesterone. Endocrinology **120:** 1184–1189.
64. YALLAMPALLI, C. D. V. M., H. IZUMI, M. M. S. BYAM-SMITH & R. E. GARFIELD. 1994. An L-arginine-nitric oxide-cyclic guanosine monophosphate system exists in the uterus and inhibits contractility during pregnancy. Am. J. Obstet. Gynecol. **170:** 175–185.
65. IZUMI, H., C. YALLAMPALI & R. E. GARFIELD. 1993. Gestational changes in L-arginine-induced relaxation of pregnant rat and human myometrial smooth muscle. Am. J. Obstet. Gynecol. **169:** 1327–1337.
66. TEZUKA, N., M. ALI, K. CHWALISZ & R. E. GARFIELD. 1993. Increased mRNA levels for the L-type $Ca2++$ channels in rat myometrium prior to term and preterm labor. Physiologist **36**(5). APS Conference: Signal Transduction and Gene Regulation, November 17–20, 1993, San Francisco, California (Abstract 5.25).
67. LEPPERT, P. C. 1992. Cervical softening, effacement and dilatation: a complex biochemical cascade. J. Mat. Fet. Med. **1:** 213–223.
68. CHWALISZ, K., C. HEGELE-HARTUNG, R. SCHULZ, SHI SHAO QING, P. T. LOUTON, & W. ELGER. 1991. Progesterone control of cervical ripening—experimental studies with the progesterone antagonists onapristone, lilopristone and mifepristone. *In* The Extracellular Matrix of the Uterus, Cervix and Fetal Membranes: Synthesis, Degradation and Hormonal Regulation. P. Leppert & F. Woessner, Eds. 119–131. Perinatology Press.
69. HEGELE-HARTUNG, C., K. CHWALISZ, H. M. BEIER & W. ELGER. 1989. Ripening of the uterine cervix of the guinea pig after treatment with the progesterone antagonist onapristone (ZK 98 299): an electron microscopic study. Hum. Reprod. **4:** 369–377.
70. DURLOT, F., C. DUBOIS, J. BRUNERIE & FRYDMAN. 1988. Efficacy of progesterone antagonist RU 486 (mifepristone) for pre-operative cervical dilatation during first trimester abortion. Hum. Reprod. **3:** 583–584.
71. RADESTADT, A., N. J. CHRISTENSEN & L. STRÖMBERG. 1988. Induced cervical ripening with mifepristone in first trimester abortion: a double-blind randomized biochemical study. Contraception **38:** 101–112.
72. World Health Organization. 1990. The use of mifepristone (RU 486) for cervical preparation in the first trimester pregnancy termination by vacuum aspiration. Br. J. Obstet. Gynaecol. **97:** 260–266.
73. URQUHART, D. R. & A. A. TEMPLETON. 1990. Mifepristone (RU 486) for cervical priming prior to surgically induced abortion in the late first trimester. Contraception **42:** 191–199.
74. GUPTA, J. K. & N. JOHNSON. 1990. Effect of mifepristone on dilatation of the pregnant and nonpregnant cervix. Lancet **335:** 1238–1240.
75. RAJABI, M., S. SOLOMON & R. POOLE. 1991. Biochemical evidence of collagenase-mediated collagenolysis as a mechanism of cervical dilatation at parturition in the guinea pig. Biol. Reprod. **45:** 764–772.
76. RAJABI, M., S. SOLOMON & R. POOLE. 1991. Hormonal regulation of interstitial collagenase in the uterine cervix of the pregnant guinea pig. Endocrinology **128:** 863–871.
77. GRANSTRÖM, L. M., E. E. GUNVOR, A. MALMSTRÖM, U. ULMSTEN & J. F. WOESSNER. 1992. Serum collagenase levels in relation to the state of the human cervix during pregnancy and labour. Am. J. Obstet. Gynecol. **167:** 1284–1288.
78. MARBAIX, E., J. DONNEZ, P. J. COURRTOY & Y. EECKHOUT. 1992. Progesterone regulates the activity of collagenase and related gelatinases A and B in human endometrial explants. Proc. Natl. Acad. Sci. USA **89:** 11789–11793.
79. BUKOWSKI, R., G. ROTH & K. CHWALISZ. 1994. Lipopolysaccharide (LPS-endotoxin)

induces cervical ripening in pregnant guinea pigs: a process mediated by prostaglandins. Soc. Gynecol. Invest., March 23–26, 1994. Chicago, IL. Scientific Program and Abstracts (abstract).
80. CABROL, D., B. CARBONNE, A. BIENKIEWICZ, E. DALLOT, A. E. ALJ & L. CEDARD. 1991. Induction of labour and cervical maturation using mifepristone (RU 486) in the late pregnant rat. Influence of a cyclooxygenase inhibitor (diclofenac). Prostaglandins **42:** 71–79.
81. RADESTADT, A. & M. BYGDEMAN. 1992. Cervical softening with mifepristone (RU 486) after pretreatment with naproxen. A double-blind randomized study. Contraception **45:** 221–227.
82. LIGGINS, G. C. 1981. Cervical ripening as an inflammatory reaction. *In* The Cervix in Pregnancy and Labour. D. A. Ellwood & A. B. M. Anderson, Eds. 1–19. Churchill Livingstone. Edinburgh.
83. JUNGUEIRA, L. C. U., M. ZUGAIB, G. S. MONTES, O. M. S. TOLEDO, R. M. KRISZTAN & K. M. SHIGIHARA. 1980. Morphologic and histochemical evidence for the occurrence of collagenolysis and for the role of neutrophylic polymorphonuclear leukocytes during cervical dilatation. Am. J. Obstet. Gynecol. **138:** 273.
84. HIRO, D., D. HIORO, Y. OJIMA & Y. MORI. 1988. Spontaneous production of interleukin 1-like factors from pregnant rabbit uterine cervix. Am. J. Obstet. Gynecol. **159:** 261–265.
85. BARCLEY, C. G., J. E. BRENNAND, R. W. KELLY & A. A. CALDER. 1993. Interleukin-8 production by the human cervix. Am. J. Obstet. Gynecol. **169:** 625–632.
86. KELLY, R. W., R. LEASK & A. A. CALDER. 1992. Choriodecidual production of interleukin-8 and the mechanism of parturition. Lancet **339:** 776–777.
87. CHWALISZ, K., P. SCHOLZ, CH. HEGELE-HARTUNG, G. ROTH & R. BUKOWSKI. 1993b. Cervical ripening with interleukin 1$\beta$ (IL-1$\beta$) and tumor necrosis factor-$\alpha$ (TNF-$\alpha$) in pregnant guinea pigs. Soc. Gynecol. Invest. Scientific Program and Abstracts, 40th Annual Meeting, March 31–April 3, 1993. Toronto, Ontario. Abstract S27.
88. BUKOWSKI, R., P. SCHOLZ, S. H. HASAN & K. CHWALISZ. 1993. Induction of preterm parturition with the interleukin 1$\beta$, tumor necrosis factor-$\alpha$ (TNF-$\alpha$) and with LPS in guinea pigs. Soc. Gynecol. Invest. Scientific Program and Abstracts, 40th Annual Meeting, March 31–April 3, 1993. Toronto, Ontario. Abstract S26.
89. CASEY, M. L. & P. C. MACDONALD. 1993. Transforming growth factor-$\beta$ (TGF-$\beta$) acts as a gene-specific antiprogestin. Soc. Gynecol. Invest. Scientific Program and Abstracts, 40th Annual Meeting, March 31–April 3, 1993. Toronto, Ontario. Abstract S2.

# The Preterm Labor Syndrome

ROBERTO ROMERO,[a,c,d] MOSHE MAZOR,[b]
HERNAN MUNOZ,[c] RICARDO GOMEZ,[c]
MAURIZIO GALASSO,[a] AND DAVID M. SHERER

[a]Department of Obstetrics and Gynecology
Wayne State University
Hutzel Hospital
Detroit, Michigan

[b]Soroka Medical Center
Ben-Gurion University
Beer-Sheva, Israel

[c]Perinatology Branch
National Institutes of Child Health
and Human Development
Bethesda, Maryland

## INTRODUCTION

Prematurity is the leading cause of perinatal morbidity and mortality worldwide.[1] It affects 5–10% of births. Preterm neonates have a 120 times higher risk of death than term neonates.[2–4] Survivors are at risk for short-term and long-term morbidity, which includes bronchopulmonary dysplasia, blindness and psychomotor retardation.[5–10] The prevention of premature birth is the single most important challenge to modern obstetrics today. Progress in this area has been hampered by lack of understanding of the basic mechanisms responsible for premature labor and delivery.

The implicit paradigm which has governed the study of preterm parturition is that term and preterm labor are fundamentally the same processes except for the gestational age at which they occur. Indeed, they share a common terminal pathway composed of uterine contractility, cervical dilatation and rupture of membranes.[11] We propose that the fundamental difference between term and preterm labor is that the former results from physiologic activation of the components of the common terminal pathway while preterm labor results from a disease process which extemporaneously activates this common terminal pathway. This article will review the evidence that preterm labor is a pathologic condition caused by multiple etiologies, and hence should be considered a syndrome: the Preterm Labor Syndrome.

### The Common Terminal Pathway of Parturition

We define the common terminal pathway as the anatomical, biochemical, endocrinological, and clinical events which occur both in term and preterm labor.

---

[d] Correspondence: Roberto Romero, M.D., Hutzel Hospital, Department of OB/GYN, 4707 St. Antoine Blvd., Detroit, Michigan 48201.

Broadly conceptualized, the common terminal pathway can be considered to have three main components: uterine contractility, cervical ripening (dilatation and effacement) and decidual/membrane activation. The term decidual/membrane activation refers to the changes occurring in the fetal membranes and decidua which eventually lead to separation of the lower pole of the chorioamniotic membranes from the decidua and ruptured membranes.

## *Uterine Contractility*

Although the myometrial activity occurs throughout pregnancy, labor is characterized by a dramatic change in the pattern of uterine contractility which evolves from "contractures" to "contractions." Nathanielsz et al.[12,13] have defined "contractures" as epochs of myometrial activity lasting several minutes, associated with modest increase in intrauterine pressure and very fragmented bursts of electrical activity in the electromyogram. In contrast, "contractions" are epochs of myometrial activity of short duration, associated with dramatic increases in intrauterine pressure and electromyographic activity.

The switch from a predominant "contracture" pattern to a predominant "contraction" pattern occurs physiologically during normal labor,[14] or can be induced by pathological events such as food withdrawal, infection, and maternal intraabdominal surgery.[15-17]

Of considerable interest is that the switch from the "contracture" to the "contraction" pattern begins at night and that labor is preceded by a progressive nocturnal increase in uterine activity of the "contraction" pattern.[18,19] The circadian nature of this rhythm suggests that uterine activity is under neural control, as neurons are the only cells known to have an independent circadian rhythm.

A role for oxytocin in the control of the switch from contractures to contractions is supported by the observations that oxytocin concentrations in maternal plasma increase following a circadian pattern similar to that of uterine contractility,[18] and administration of an oxytocin antagonist to monkeys obliterates this nocturnal increase in uterine activity.[20-22] The switch from contracture to contraction pattern is a reversible phenomenon. It can be induced by fasting in pregnant sheep and reversed by feeding.[15,23-25] Although existence of a similar phenomenon in humans is less clear, the "Yom Kippur effect" may be considered its equivalent. This term refers to the increased birth rate in Israel immediately after the fasting period of the Yom Kippur holiday.[26]

The appearance of gap junctions, and an increased expression of gap junction protein (connexin 43) have been implicated as the cellular and molecular events responsible for the change from contractions to contractures. Indeed, a great number of a gap junctions develop in myometrium just prior to labor and disappear shortly after delivery.[27-32] A recent study has indicated that gap junction and the expression of connexin 43 in human myometrium formation is similar in term and preterm labor.[33] In summary, an increase in human myometrial contractility is a common feature of both term and preterm labor.

## *Cervical Ripening*

The uterine cervix is essentially a connective tissue organ. Smooth muscle cells account for less than 8% of the distal part of the cervix.[34] The ability of the cervix to retain the conceptus during pregnancy is unlikely to depend upon a traditional muscular sphincteric mechanism. Indeed, perfusion of strips of human cervix with vasopressin, a hormone that stimulates smooth muscle contraction, induces a very modest contractile response in comparison to that of strips from the isthmus and fundus.[35] It is now understood that the normal function of the cervix during pregnancy depends upon the regulation of fibrous connective tissue. This tissue is formed by abundant extracellular matrix which surrounds individual cells. The major macromolecular components of the extracellular matrix are collagen, proteoaminoglycans, elastin, and various glycoproteins, such as fibronectins. Collagen is considered the most important component of the extracellular matrix determining the tensile strength of fibrous connective tissue. Changes in cervical characteristics during pregnancy have been attributed to changes in collagen content and metabolism. Proteoaminoglycans have also been implicated in cervical physiology. The proteoaminoglycan decorin or PG-S2 has a high affinity for collagen, can cover the surface of the collagen fibrils, stabilizing them and promoting the formation of thicker collagen bundles of fibers. In contrast, PG-S1 (byglycan) has no affinity for collagen, and therefore, can disorganize collagen fibrils. The predominant dermatan sulfate proteoglycan in the nonpregnant state is PG-S2 and in the term pregnant state is PG-S1.[36]

The biochemical events which have been implicated in cervical ripening are: 1) a decrease in total collagen content; 2) increase in collagen solubility (probably indicating degradation or newly synthesized weaker collagen) and 3) increase in collagenolytic activity (both collagenase and leukocyte elastase). Contrary to what is generally believed, extracellular matrix turnover in the cervix is very high, and thus, mechanical properties of the cervix can change very quickly.

Uldbjerg et al. have clearly demonstrated the importance of collagen content in cervical dilatation. They found a strong correlation between the collagen content (measured by hydroxyproline determination) of cervical biopsies obtained after delivery and the time required for the cervix to dilate from 2 to 10 cm.[37]

The changes in extracellular matrix components during cervical ripening have been likened to an inflammatory response.[38] Indeed, during cervical ripening there is an influx of inflammatory cells (macrophages, neutrophils, mast cells, eosinophils, etc.) into the cervical stroma. It has been proposed that these cells produce cytokines (i.e., interleukin-1) and other mediators such as prostaglandins which have an effect on extracellular matrix metabolism.[39-41]

The chain of events leading to physiologic cervical ripening has not been completely defined. However, strong evidence supports a role for sex steroid hormones, a concept that has important clinical implications. This evidence includes: 1) intravenous administration of 17 beta estradiol induces cervical ripening;[42] 2) estrogen stimulates collagen degradation *in vitro*;[43] 3) progesterone blocks the estrogen-induced collagenolysis *in vitro*;[43] 4) the administration of progesterone receptor antagonist induces cervical ripening in the first trimester of pregnancy.[44] It is unknown if this effect is mediated through prostaglandins.

Prostaglandins have been widely used to induce cervical ripening prior to induction of labor or abortion. Within hours of administration, $PGE_2$ produces clinical and histologic cervical changes resembling physiologic ripening, which normally develops over several weeks of gestation. The mechanism of action of $PGE_2$ is thought to involve stimulation of collagenolytic activity and synthesis of PG-S1 by cervical tissue.[36]

Cervical changes antecede the onset of labor, are gradual and develop over several weeks.[45] Cervical ripening is not a process unique to term labor, but it also occurs in the context of preterm labor. Wood et al. were the first to report that a short cervix was a risk factor for preterm labor and delivery.[46] This observation has been subsequently confirmed by several investigators.[46-53] The largest study examining the relationship between cervical ripening and the subsequent risk of preterm delivery published to date was conducted in France by Papiernik et al.[47] Serial digital examinations were conducted in 8,303 women of whom 4,430 had a gestational age of less than 37 weeks. Dilatation of the internal os of the cervix was found to be the most important risk factor for the occurrence of preterm delivery. Once dilatation of the internal os occurred, the interval to delivery was similar in patients who subsequently went into either spontaneous term or preterm labor. This observation indicates that cervical ripening is a general feature of human parturition, and it occurs in a similar way in preterm and term parturition.

Although cervical shortening is traditionally considered to be an irreversible change, many anecdotal clinical observations indicate that patients go "backwards." In other words, a shortened, soft and mildly undilated cervix may subsequently become longer, firmer and closed. Similar observations have been demonstrated with pharmacological manipulation in the pregnant ewe. In this animal species, dexamethasone administration induces cervical ripening and uterine contractility. However, it is possible to delay delivery by arresting uterine contractility and reversing cervical compliance by administering large doses of progesterone.[54]

### Decidual/Membrane Activation

We use this term to refer to a complex set of anatomical and biochemical events which lead to separation of the lower pole of the membranes from the decidua of the lower uterine segment and, eventually, the occurrence of spontaneous rupture of membranes.

During pregnancy the chorioamniotic membranes fuse with the decidua. In preparation for delivery, biochemical events take place to allow separation and postpartum expulsion of the membranes. Fibronectins are a family of important extracellular cements. The available evidence indicates that this fibronectin dissolves and can be found in the vagina during both term and preterm parturition, and therefore, it also belongs to this common terminal pathway of parturition.[55-57]

### Activation of the Common Terminal Pathway

The central question in the understanding of preterm labor is whether the signals responsible for the activation of the common terminal pathway are similar in term and preterm labor. Prostaglandins have been considered the key mediators for the onset of labor since they can induce myometrial contractility[58-61] and changes in extracellular matrix metabolism associated with cervical ripening[62-66] and decidua/membrane activation.[67-73]

The evidence traditionally invoked which supports a role for prostaglandins in the initiation of human labor includes: 1) administration of prostaglandins can induce early or late termination of pregnancy (abortion or labor);[67,74-84] 2) treatment with indomethacin or aspirin can delay spontaneous onset of parturition in animals;[85-88] 3) concentrations of prostaglandins in plasma and amniotic fluid increase during labor[89-97] and 4) intraamniotic injection of arachidonic acid induces abortion.[98] Although this reasoning has been accepted for many years, it does not constitute unequivocal evidence for either an obligatory or a causal role of prostaglandins in the mechanisms responsible for the initiation of labor. For example, prostaglandins' ability to induce abortion or labor when administered in pharmacological doses is not evidence that they participate in the mechanisms of normal parturition.

Recently, the role of prostaglandins in the onset of labor has been challenged by a set of observations demonstrating that prostaglandin concentrations in amniotic fluid do not increase "early" but "late" during the course of spontaneous labor at term.[99,100] These data have been interpreted as indicating that prostaglandins do not participate in the initiation of human labor and that their accumulation in amniotic fluid is the consequence of labor.[99,100]

Previous observations reporting an increase in amniotic fluid prostaglandin concentrations observed during the course of labor[101-105] have been considered invalid because fluid for these studies was retrieved transvaginally and may have yielded spurious results.[106] Indeed, contamination of the sample with vaginal secretions which has a high prostaglandin content may provide an inaccurate estimation of the physiologic changes in amniotic fluid prostaglandin levels.[100,107] Moreover, amniotic fluid prostaglandin concentrations obtained transvaginally from the forebag may not be representative of the events that occur in the entire amniotic cavity and membranes.[107] Indeed, prostaglandin levels in fluid obtained transvaginally are higher than those obtained transabdominally from the same women.[107] This difference can be attributed to the effect of the vaginal or cervical microorganisms and cytokines on prostanoid biosynthesis by the chorioamniotic membranes of the forebag.[101,105] However, a recent study has demonstrated that an early and significant increase in amniotic fluid prostaglandin concentrations occurs in fluid retrieved transabdominally in patients in early spontaneous labor at term.[108] These observations are consistent with those found in premature rupture of membranes at term;[109] an increase in amniotic fluid concentrations of prostanoids was observed in early labor. Similar findings have been reported in longitudinal studies performed in nonhuman primates.[110] More importantly, a recent study in which women underwent serial amniocenteses prior to the onset of labor demonstrated that amniotic fluid prostaglandin concentrations increase before the onset of spontaneous labor.[111] Therefore, most of the available evidence in humans, as well as in animals, suggests that prostaglandin concentrations increase prior to the onset of labor or during early labor.[101-105,108-111] Although these data do not prove that prostaglandins are the only mediators for the onset of labor, they provide support for the concept that the correct temporal relationship exists between an increase in prostaglandins and the subsequent onset of labor.

## *What Are the Regulatory Mechanisms Responsible for the Increase Bioavailability of Prostaglandins?*

Prostaglandins are produced by intrauterine tissues including amnion, chorion, decidua, myometrium and placenta.[112-118] Although there are many substances which can increase prostaglandin biosynthesis, the precise signals responsible for their increase during the course of labor have not been determined. Candidates include cytokines,[116-118] growth factors (*i.e.*, epidermal growth factor),[119] cortisol[120] and others. Regardless of the specific factor, a role for the fetus in the control of the timing of parturition has been suggested by the classical studies of Liggins *et al.*[121,122]

Recent studies indicate that destruction of the paraventricular nucleus of the fetal hypothalamus results in prolongation of pregnancy in sheep.[123] The human counterpart to this animal experiment is anencephaly where there is also a tendency to have a prolonged pregnancy[124] (if patients with polyhydramnios are excluded). However, the situation in human anencephaly is considerably more complicated than that described in animal experiments. The discrepancy can be explained by the wide range of CNS and pituitary lesions found in human anencephaly.

It can be surmised that the fetus must have a means of knowing how old or how mature he/she is. Once maturity has been reached, the fetal brain and specifically the hypothalamus increases CRH secretion, which in turn stimulates ACTH production and cortisol production by the fetal adrenals.[125,126] This increase in cortisol in sheep and DHEA-S in primates eventually leads to activation of the common terminal pathway of parturition.[127,128]

### The Premature Labor Syndrome

Although term and preterm labor share a common terminal pathway, we propose that while term labor is the result of physiologic activation of this terminal pathway, preterm labor is the consequence of pathologic activation. We view preterm labor as a pathologic event; labor may be considered as the response of the fetomaternal pair to a variety of insults (infection, ischemia, etc.). If these insults cannot be effectively handled in the context of a continuing pregnancy, then labor and delivery may occur.

A considerable body of clinical evidence supports the existence of a relationship between complications of pregnancy and spontaneous preterm labor/delivery. For example, the prevalence of intrauterine infection, fetal growth retardation, congenital anomalies and abruptio placenta is higher in patients delivering preterm neonates than in those delivering at term.[17,129-135] Although it could be argued that many of these complications could be the consequence rather than the cause of premature labor, this view is difficult to accept for conditions which are chronic in nature, and therefore, must have occurred prior to preterm labor/delivery (*i.e.*, growth retardation and congenital anomalies).

Much effort has been invested in the study of the role of infection as an etiologic agent for premature labor. Four lines of evidence support a role for infection: 1) systemic or intrauterine infection of pregnant animals can result in preterm labor and delivery;[86,136-145] 2) antibiotic treatment of ascending intrauterine infections can prevent prematurity in experimental models of chorioamnionitis;[136] 3) systemic maternal infection such as pyelonephritis and pneumonia are frequently associated with the onset of premature labor in humans[146-158] and 4) subclinical intrauterine infections are associated with preterm birth.[11,159-161] We have critically reviewed this evidence elsewhere.[129]

Infection is, however, only one of the insults that may compromise the fetomaternal survival and lead to preterm labor. Placental histopathologic studies would suggest that inflammation may account for probably no more than 30–40% of cases of preterm delivery.[162] This estimate correlates well with our studies of amniotic fluid microbiology.[159] Therefore, other pathologic processes must be responsible for the initiation of preterm labor in the remainder of cases. We recently presented biochemical, cytologic, immunologic, microbiologic, and clinical evidence that preterm labor is a heterogenous condition.[163] Using cluster analysis, we established that there are two main subgroups of patients presenting with preterm labor and intact membranes delivering preterm: Those with acute inflammatory lesions of the placenta, and those without these lesions.[163] The second group is also heterogenous and includes patients with vascular lesions in

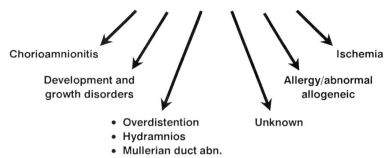

**FIGURE 1.** The preterm labor syndrome.

the placental bed, chronic villitis, extensive fibrinoid necrosis, etc.[163] By far, the most common noninflammatory lesion of the placenta in the setting of preterm delivery, is vascular pathology (decidual thrombosis, acute atherosis, failure of physiologic transformation of the spiral arteries, etc.).[164] We propose that these vascular lesions may lead to uteroplacental ischemia and to the initiation of preterm labor and delivery. Clinical and experimental observations supporting this include (a) that there is an excess of intrauterine growth retardation and abruptio placenta in the setting of premature birth[165] and (b) that experimental uterine ischemia in monkeys often results in the initiation of labor.

Another distinct clinical group of patients with a potentially different mechanism for preterm labor and delivery is composed of women with congenital anomalies[166] and polyhydramnios.[167,168] Uterine overdistension may activate a uterine pressor sensitive system capable of initiating uterine contractility and labor.[169,170] This mechanism can be invoked to also explain the excees rate of preterm labor observed in multiple gestations.[171,172]

Yet another potential mechanism for preterm labor and delivery is an immunologically mediated phenomenon induced by an allergic mechanism. Indeed, the uterus contains a large number of mast cells, and the trophoblast may constitute the antigen required for eliciting an allergic reaction. Garfield *et al.* recently reported that products of mast cell degranulation are capable of inducing myometrial contractions.[173] We have also identified a group of patients in preterm labor with clinical and laboratory findings consistent with an allergy-mediated event.[174]

The emerging picture is that preterm labor and delivery is a syndrome (FIG. 1). Multiple pathological processes may lead to myometrial and membrane/decidual activation and cervical ripening. The clinical presentation (*i.e.*, uterine contractility, preterm cervical ripening without significant clinical contractility or PROM) will depend upon the differential effect of the insults on the various components on the common terminal pathway (FIG. 2). This view of preterm labor has considerable implications for the diagnosis, treatment, and understanding of the cellular and biochemical mechanisms responsible for the initiation of parturition. Since preterm labor is a heterogenous condition, it is unlikely that it will have a single treatment (*i.e.*, tocolysis). Moreover, if preterm labor is the result of a chronic insult, it is extremely unlikely that tocolysis will be successful in preventing preterm birth. We consider tocolysis as a treatment for only one of the manifestations of activation

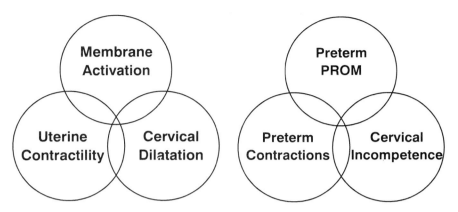

**FIGURE 2.** Components of the common terminal pathway of human parturition (*left*) and the clinical manifestations of their premature activation (*right*).

of the common terminal pathway, (*i.e.*, uterine contractility) but not for the underlying pathologic process responsible for this activation.

## REFERENCES

1. VAN DEN BERG, B. J. & F. W. OESHSLI. 1984. Prematurity. *In* Perinatal Epidemiology. M. B. Bracken, Ed. 69. Oxford University Press. London.
2. RUSH, R. W., M. J. N. C. KEIRSE, P. HOWAT *et al.* 1976. Contribution of preterm delivery to perinatal mortality. Br. Med. J. **2**: 965.
3. MAIN, D. M. & E. K. MAIN. 1986. Management of preterm labor and delivery. *In* Obstetrics: Normal and Problem Pregnancies. S. G. Gabbe, J. Niebyl & J. L. Simpson, Eds. 689. Churchill Livingstone. New York.
4. KESSEL, S. S., J. VILLAR, H. W. BERENDES *et al.* 1984. The changing pattern of low birth weight in the United States (1970 to 1980). J. Am. Med. Assoc. **251**: 1978.
5. BROWN, E. 1993. Long term sequelae of preterm birth. *In* Preterm Birth: Causes, Prevention and Management. Second Edit. A. R. Fuchs, F. Fuchs & P. Stubblefield, Eds. 477. McGraw-Hill, Inc. New York.
6. AVERY, M. E., W. T. TOOLEY, J. B. KELLER *et al.* 1987. Is chronic lung disease in low birth weight infants preventable? A survey of eight centers. Pediatrics **79**: 26.
7. EDWARDS, D. K., M. D. WAYNE & W. H. NORTHWAY. 1977. Twelve years' experience with bronchopulmonary dysplasia. Pediatrics **59**: 839.
8. HOLDE, K. R., D. MELLITS & J. M. FREEMAN. 1982. Neonatal seizures, I: correlation of prenatal and perinatal events with outcomes. Pediatrics **70**: 165.
9. MELLITS, D., K. R. HOLDEN & J. M. FREEMAN. 1982. Neonatal seizures II: a multivariate analysis of factor associated with outcome. Pediatrics **70**: 177.
10. AMON, E., 1992. Premature labor. *In* Medicine of the Fetus & Mother. A. E. Reece, J. C. Hobbins, M. J. Mahoney & R. H. Petrie, Eds. 1398. JB Lippincott Company. Philadelphia.
11. ROMERO, R., C. AVILA, C. A. BREKUS & M. MAZOR. 1990. The role of systematic and intrauterine infection in preterm parturition. *In* Uterine Contractility. R. E. Garfield, Ed. 319. Serono Symposia. Norwell, MA.
12. NATHANIELSZ, P. W. N. & M. B. O. M. HONNEBIER. 1992. Myometrial function. *In* Prostaglandins and the Uterus. J. O. Drife & A. A. Calder, Eds. 161. Springer-Verlag. London, Berlin, Heidelberg, New York, Paris, Tokyo, Hong Kong, Barcelona, Budapest.
13. HSU, H. W., J. P. FIGUEROA, M. B. O. M. HONNEBIER, R. WENTWORTH & P. W. NATHANIELSZ. 1989. Power spectrum analysis of myometrial electromyogram and

intrauterine pressure changes in the pregnant monkey in late gestation. Am. J. Obstet. Gynecol. **161:** 467.
14. TAYLOR, N. F., M. C. MARTIN, P. W. NATHANIELSZ & M. SERON-FERRE. 1983. The fetus determines circadian oscillation of myometrial electromyographic activity in the pregnant rhesus monkey. Am. J. Obstet. Gynecol. **146:** 557.
15. BINIENDA, Z., E. D. ROSEN, A. KELLEMAN, D. W. SADOWSKY, M. D. MITCHELL & P. W. NATHANIELSZ. 1990. Maintaining fetal normoglycemia prevents the increase in myometrial activity and uterine 13,14-dihydro-15-keto-prostaglandin $F_{2a}$ production during food withdrawal in late pregnancy in the ewe. Endocrinology **127:** 307.
16. NATHANIELSZ, P. W., E. R. POORE, A. BRODIE, N. F. TAYLOR, G. PIMENTEL, J. P. FIGUEROA & D. FRANK. 1987. Update on molecular events of myometrial activity during pregnancy. In Research in Perinatal Medicine. P. W. Nathanielsz & J. T. Parer, Eds. 111. Perinatology Press. Ithaca, N.Y.
17. ROMERO, R., C. AVILA & W. SEPULVEDA. 1993. The role of systemic and intrauterine infection in preterm labor. In Preterm Birth: Causes, Prevention, and Management. 2nd edit. A. R. Fuchs, F. Fuchs & P. G. Stubblefield, Eds. 97. McGraw-Hill, Inc. New York.
18. HONNEBIER, M. B. O. M., S. L. JENKINS, R. A. WENTWORTH, J. P. FIGUEROA & P. W. NATHANIELSZ. 1991. Temporal structuring of delivery in the absence of a photoperiod: preparturient myometrial activity of the rhesus monkey is related to maternal body temperature and depends on the maternal circadian system. Biol. Reprod. **45:** 617.
19. KATZ, M., R. NEWMAN & P. GILL. 1986. Assessment of uterine activity in ambulatory patients at high risk of preterm labor and delivery. Am. J. Obstet. Gynecol. **154:** 44.
20. OWINY, J. R., L. C. CHAVIN, M. D. MITCHELL & P. W. NATHANIELSZ. 1991. Effect of 48 hour infusion of oxytocin antagonist (OTA) on myometrial activity of pregnant sheep at 139 days' gestational age (dGA). Presented at the 38th Annual Meeting of the Society for Gynecologic Investigation, March 20–23, 1991, San Antonio, Texas, Abstract #101.
21. WILSON, L., JR., M. T. PARSONS & G. FLOURET. 1990. Inhibition of spontaneous uterine contractions during the last trimester in pregnant baboons by an oxytocin antagonist. Am. J. Obstet. Gynecol. **163:** 1875.
22. HONNEBIER, M. B. O. M., J. P. FIGUEROA, J. RIVIER, W. VALE & P. W. NATHANIELSZ. 1989. Studies on the role of oxytocin in late pregnancy in the pregnant rhesus monkey (I): plasma concentration of oxytocin in the maternal circulation throughout the 24 h day and the effect of the synthetic oxytocin antagonist [1-$\beta$-Mpa($\beta$-(CH2)5)1,)Me)Tyr2,Orn8]OT on spontaneous nocturnal myometrial contractions. J. Dev. Physiol. **12:** 225.
23. FOWDEN, A. L., R. HADING, M. M. RALPH & G. D. THORBURN. 1987. The nutritional regulation of plasma prostaglandin E concentrations in the fetus and pregnant ewe during late gestation. J. Physiol. **394:** 1.
24. BINIENDA, Z., A. MASSMANN, M. D. MITCHELL, R. D. GLEED, J. P. FIGUEROA & P. W. NATHANIELSZ. 1988. The effect of food withdrawal on arterial blood glucose and plasma 13,14-dihydro-15-keto-prostaglandin $F_{2a}$ (PGFM) concentrations and nocturnal myometrial electromyograph activity in the pregnant rhesus monkey in the last third of gestation: a model for preterm labor? Am. J. Obstet. Gynecol. **160:** 746.
25. FOWDEN, A. L. & M. SILVER. 1983. The effect of the nutritional state on the uterine prostaglandin F metabolite concentrations in the pregnant ewe during late gestation. J. Exp. Physiol. **68:** 337.
26. KAPLAN, M., A. I. EIDELMAN & Y. ABOULAFIA. 1983. Fasting and the precipitation of labor. The Yom Kippur effect. JAMA **250:** 1317.
27. GARFIELD, R., T. TABB & G. THILANDER. 1990. Intercellular coupling and modulation of uterine contractility. In Uterine Contractility. R. E. Garfield, Ed. 21. Serono Symposia. Norwell, MA.
28. GARFIELD, R. E., S. SIMS & E. E. DANIEL. 1977. Gap junctions: their presence and necessity in myometrium during gestation. Science **198:** 958.

29. GARFIELD, R. E., S. SIMS, M. S. KANNAN & E. E. DANIEL. 1978. Possible role of gap junctions in activation of myometrium during parturition. Am. J. Physiol. **235**: C168.
30. GARFIELD, R. E. & R. H. HAYASHI. 1981. Appearance of gap junctions in the myometrium of women during labor. Am. J. Obstet. Gynecol. **140**: 254.
31. GARFIELD, R. E., C. P. PURI & A. I. CSAPO. 1982. Endocrine, structural and functional changes in the uterus during premature labor. Am. J. Obstet. Gynecol. **142**: 21.
32. COLE, W. C., R. E. GARFIELD & J. S. KIRKALDY. 1985. Gap junctions and direct intercellular communication between rat uterine smooth muscle cells. Am. J. Physiol. **249**: C20.
33. BALDUCCI, J., B. RISEK, N. B. GILULA, A. HAND, J. F. X. EGAN & A. M. VINTZILEOS. 1993. Gap junction in human myometrium: a key to preterm labor? Am. J. Obstet. Gynecol. **168**: 1609.
34. SCHWAHN, H. & V. DUBRAUSKY. 1966. The structure of the musculature of the human uterus-muscles and connective tissue. Am. J. Obstet. Gynecol. **94**: 391.
35. DANFORTH, D. & I. EVANSTON. 1954. The distribution and functional activity of the cervical musculature. Am. J. Obstet. Gynecol. **68**: 1261.
36. ULDBJERG, N., A. FORMAN, L. PETERSEN, *et al.* 1992. Biomechanical and biochemical changes of the uterus and cervix during pregnancy. *In* Medicine of the Fetus and Mother. E. A. Reece, J. C. Hobbins, M. J. Mahoney & R. H. Petrie, Eds. 849. JB Lippincott Co.
37. ULDBJERG, N., G. EKMAN, A. MALMSTROM *et al.* 1982. Ripening of the human uterine cervix related to changes in collagen, glycosaminoglycans and collagenolytic activity. Am. J. Obstet. Gynecol. **147**: 662.
38. LIGGINS, G. C. 1981. Cervical ripening as an inflammatory reaction. *In* The Cervix in Pregnancy and Labour: Clinical and Biochemical Investigations. D. A. Ellwood & A. B. M. Anderson, Eds. 1. Churchill Livingstone. Edinburgh.
39. ITO, A., D. HIRO, Y. OJIMA & Y. MORI. 1988. Spontaneous production of interleukin-1-like factors from pregnant rabbit uterine cervix. Am. J. Obstet. Gynecol. **159**: 261.
40. ITO, A., P. LEPPERT & Y. MORI. 1990. Human recombinant interleukin-1 increases elastase-like enzyme in human uterine cervical fibroblasts. Gynecol. Obstet. Invest. **30**: 239.
41. ITO, A., D. HIRO, K. SAKYO & Y. MORI. 1987. The role of leukocyte factors on uterine cervical ripening and dilation. Biol. Reprod. **37**: 511.
42. PINTO, R. M., W. RABOW & R. A. VOTTA. 1965. Uterine cervix ripening in term pregnancy due to the action of estradiol-17β. Am. J. Obstet. Gynecol. **92**: 319.
43. RAJABI, M. R., G. R. DODGE, S. SOLOMON & P. ROBIN. 1991. Immunochemical and immunohistochemical evidence of estrogen-mediated collagenolysis as a mechanism of cervical dilation in the Guinea pig at parturition. Endocrinology **128**: 371.
44. CHWALISZ, K., O. SHI SHAO, G. NEFF & J. V. ELGER. 1987. The effect of antigestagen ZK 98, 199 on the uterine cervix. Acta Endocrinol. **283**: 113.
45. BISHOP, E. H. 1964. Pelvic scoring for elective induction. Obstet. Gynecol. **24**: 266.
46. WOOD, C., R. BANNERMAN, R. BOOTH & J. PINKERTON. 1965. The prediction of premature labor by observation of the cervix and external tocography. Am. J. Obstet. Gynecol. **91**: 396.
47. PAPIERNIK, E., J. BOUYER & D. COLLIN. 1986. Precocious cervical ripening and preterm labor. Obstet. Gynecol. **67**: 238.
48. BOUYER, J., E. PAPIERNIK, J. DREYFUS *et al.* 1986. Maturation signs of the cervix and prediction of preterm birth. Obstet. Gynecol. **68**: 209.
49. ANDERSON, A. & A. TURNBULL. 1969. Relationship between length of gestation and cervical dilatation, uterine contractility, and other factors during pregnancy. Am. J. Obstet. Gynecol. **105**: 1207.
50. STUBBS, T. M., P. VAN DORSTEN & M. MILLER III. 1986. The preterm cervix and preterm labor: relative risks, predictive values, and change over time. Am. J. Obstet. Gynecol. **155**: 829.
51. LEVENO, K. J., K. COX & M. ROARK. 1986. Cervical dilatation and prematurity revisited. Obstet. Gynecol. **68**: 434.

52. HOLBROOK, R. H., J. FALCON, M. HERRON et al. 1987. Evaluation of the weekly cervical examination in a preterm birth prevention program. Am. J. Perinatol. **4:** 240.
53. CATALANO, P. M., T. ASHIKAGA & L. I. MANN. 1989. Cervical change and uterine activity as predictors of preterm delivery. Am. J. Perinatol. **6:** 185.
54. STYS, S. J., W. H. CLEWELL & G. MESCHIA. 1978. Changes in cervical compliance at parturition independent of uterine activity. Am. J. Obstet. Gynecol. **130:** 414.
55. LOCKWOOD, C. J., A. E. SENYEI, M. R. DISCHE et al. 1991. Fetal fibronectin in cervical and vaginal secretions as a predictor of preterm delivery. N. Engl. J. Med. **325:** 669.
56. NAGEOTTE, M. P., K. A. HOLLENBACH, B. A. VANDERWAHL & K. M. HUTCH. 1992. Oncofetal fibronectin in patients at increased risk for preterm delivery (abstract). Am. J. Obstet. Gynecol. **166:** 274.
57. LOCKWOOD, C. J., R. WEIN, M. ALVAREZ & R. BERKOWITZ. 1993. Fetal fibronectin predicts preterm delivery in asymptomatic patients (abstract). Am. J. Obstet. Gynecol. **168:** 311.
58. BENNETT, P. R., M. G. ELDER & L. MYATT. 1987. The effects of lipoxygenase metabolites of arachidonic acid on human myometrial contractility. Prostaglandins **33:** 837.
59. CARRAHER, R., D. W. HAHN, D. M. RITCHIE et al. 1983. Involvement of lipoxygenase products in myometrial contractions. Prostaglandins **26:** 23.
60. RITCHIE, D. M., D. W. HAHN & J. L. MCGUIRE. 1984. Smooth muscle contraction as a model to study the mediator role of endogenous lipoxygenase products of arachidonic acid. Life Sci. **34:** 509.
61. WIQVIST, N., B. LINDBLOM, M. WIKLAND & L. WILHELMSSON. 1983. Prostaglandins and uterine contractility. Acta Obstet. Gynecol. Scand. **113:** 23.
62. GREER, I. A. 1992. Cervical ripening. In: Prostaglandins and the Uterus. J. O. Drife & A. A. Calder, Eds. 191. Springer-Verlag. London, Berlin, Heidelberg, New York, Paris, Tokyo, Hong Kong, Barcelona, Budapest.
63. RAJABI, M. R., S. SOLOMON & A. R. POOLE. 1991. Hormonal regulation of interstitial collagenase in the uterine cervix of the guinea pig. Endocrinology **128:** 863.
64. ELLWOOD, D. A., M. D. MITCHELL & A. B. M. ANDERSON. 1980. The in vitro production of prostanoids by the human cervix during pregnancy: preliminary observations. Br. J. Obstet. Gynaecol. **87:** 210.
65. CALDER, A. A. 1980. Pharmacological management of the unripe cervix in the human. In Dilatation of the Uterine Cervix. F. Naftolin & P. G. Stubblefield, Eds. 317. Raven Press. New York.
66. CALDER, A. A. & I. A. GREER. 1991. Pharmacological modulation of cervical compliance in the first and second trimesters of pregnancy. Semin. Perinatol. **15:** 162.
67. NOVY, M. J. & G. C. LIGGINS. 1980. Role of prostaglandins, prostacyclin, and thromboxanes in the physiological control of the uterus and in parturition. Semin. Perinatol. **4:** 45.
68. MITCHELL, M. D. 1984. The mechanism(s) of human parturition. J. Dev. Physiol. **6:** 107.
69. MACDONALD, P. C., F. M. SCHULTZ, J. H. DUENHOELTER, N. F. GANT, J. M. JIMENEZ, J. A. PRITCHARD, J. C. PORTER & J. M. JOHNSTON. 1974. Initiation of human parturition. Obstet. Gynecol. **44:** 629.
70. CHALLIS, J. R. G. & D. M. OLSON. 1988. Parturition. In The Physiology of Reproduction. E. Knobil & J. Neill, Eds. 2177. Raven Press. New York.
71. BLEASDALE, J. E. & J. M. JOHNSTON. 1985. Prostaglandins and human parturition: regulation of arachidonic acid mobilization. Rev. Perinatal. Med. **5:** 151.
72. THRONBURN, G. D. & J. R. G. CHALLIS. 1979. Endocrine control of parturition. Physiol. Rev. **59:** 863.
73. CHALLIS, J. R. G. 1979. Endocrine control of parturition. Physiol. Rev. **59:** 863.
74. MACKENZIE, I. Z. 1992. Prostaglandins and midtrimester abortion. In Prostaglandins and the Uterus. J. O. Drife & A. A. Calder, Eds. 119. Springer-Verlag. London, Berlin, Heidelberg, New York, Paris, Tokyo, Hong Kong, Barcelona, Budapest.
75. KARIM, S. M. M. & G. M. FILSHIE. 1970. Therapeutic abortion using prostaglandin $F_{2a}$. Lancet **i:** 157.

76. EMBREY, M. P. 1970. Induction of abortion by prostaglandin $E_1$ and $E_2$. Br. Med. J. **2:** 258.
77. World Health Organisation Task Force. 1976. Comparison of intra-amniotic prostaglandin $F_{2a}$ and hypertonic saline for second trimester abortion. Br. Med. J. **i:** 1373–1376.
78. World Health Organisation Task Force. 1982. Termination of second trimester pregnancy by intra-muscular injection of 16-phenoxy-$w$-17,18,19,20-tetranor $PGE_2$ methyl sulfanilamide. Int. J. Gynaecol. Obstet. **20:** 383.
79. World Health Organisation Task Force. 1977. Repeated vaginal administration of 15-methyl $PGF_{2a}$ for termination of pregnancy in the 13th to 20th week of gestation. Contraception **16:** 175.
80. HUSSLEIN, P. 1992. Prostaglandins for induction of labour. In Prostaglandins and the Uterus. J. O. Drife & A. A. Calder, Eds. 181. Springer-Verlag. London, Berlin, Heidelberg, New York, Paris, Tokyo, Hong Kong, Barcelona, Budapest.
81. HUSSLEIN, P. 1991. Use of prostaglandins for induction of labor. Semin. Perinatol. **15:** 173.
82. MACER, J., M. BUCHANAN & L. YONEKURA. 1984. Induction of labor with prostaglandin $E_2$ vaginal suppositories. Obstet. Gynecol. **63:** 664.
83. GORDON-WRIGHT, A. P. & M. ELDER. 1979. Prostaglandin $E_2$ tablets used intravaginally for induction of labor. Br. J. Obstet. Gynaecol. **86:** 32.
84. EKMAN, G. A., K. FORMAN, U. MARSAL et al. 1983. Intravaginal versus intracervical applications of prostaglandin $E_2$ in viscous gel of cervical priming and induction of labor at term in patients with unfavorable cervical state. Am. J. Obstet. Gynecol. **147:** 657.
85. KEIRSE, M. J. N. C. 1990. Eicosanoids in human pregnancy and parturition. In M. Mitchell, Ed. Eicosanoids in Reproduction. 199. CRC Press. Boca Raton, FL.
86. SKARNES, R. C. & M. J. K. HARPER. 1972. Relationship between endotoxin-induced abortion and the synthesis of prostaglandin F. Prostaglandins **1:** 191.
87. HARPER, M. J. K. & R. C. SKARNES. 1972. Inhibition of abortion and fetal death produced by endotoxin or prostaglandin $F_{2a}$. Prostaglandins **2:** 295.
88. GIRI, S. N., G. H. STABENFELD, T. A. MOSELEY, T. W. GRAHAM, M. L. BRUSS, R. H. BONDURANT, J. S. CULLOR & B. I. OSBURN. 1991. Role of eicosanoids in abortion and its prevention by treatment with flunixin meglumine in cows during the first trimester of pregnancy. J. Vet. Med. **A38:** 445.
89. KEIRSE, M. J. N. C. 1979. Endogenous prostaglandins in human parturition. In Human Parturition. M. Keirse, A. Anderson & J. Gravenhorst, Eds. 101. Martinus Nijhoff Publishers. The Hague.
90. SELLERS, S. M., M. D. MITCHELL, A. B. ANDERSON & A. C. TURNBULL. 1981. The relationship between the release of prostaglandins at amniotomy and the subsequent onset of labour. Br. J. Obstet. Gynaecol. **88:** 1211.
91. ROMERO, R., M. EMAMIAN, M. WAN, C. GRZBOSKI, J. C. HOBBINS & M. D. MITCHELL. 1987. Increased concentrations of arachidonic acid lipoxygenase metabolites in amniotic fluid during parturition. Obstet. Gynecol. **70:** 849.
92. ROMERO, R., Y. K. WU, M. MAZOR, J. C. HOBBINS & M. D. MITCHELL. 1988. Increased amniotic fluid leukotriene C4 concentration in term human parturition. Am. J. Obstet. Gynecol. **159:** 655.
93. ROMERO, R., Y. K. WU, M. MAZOR, J. C. HOBBINS & M. D. MITCHELL. 1989. Amniotic fluid concentration of 5-hydroxyeicosatetraenoic acid is increased in human parturition at term. Prostaglandins Leukotrienes Essent. Fatty Acids **35:** 81.
94. ROMERO, R., M. EMAMIAN, R. QUINTERO, M. WAN, J. C. HOBBINS & M. D. MITCHELL. 1986. Amniotic fluid prostaglandin levels and intra-amniotic infection. Lancet **1:** 1380.
95. ROMERO, R., Y. K. WU, M. MAZOR, J. C. HOBBINS & M. D. MITCHELL. 1988. Amniotic fluid prostaglandin $E_2$ in preterm labor. Prostaglandins Leukotrienes Essent. Fatty Acids **34:** 141.
96. ROMERO, R., M. EMAMIAN, M. WAN, R. QUINTERO, J. C. HOBBINS & M. D. MITCHELL. 1987. Prostaglandin concentrations in amniotic fluid of women with intra-amniotic infection and preterm labor. Am. J. Obstet. Gynecol. **157:** 1461.

97. ROMERO, R., Y. K. WU, M. SITORI, E. OYARZUN, M. MAZOR, J. C. HOBBINS & M. D. MITCHELL. 1989. Amniotic fluid concentrations of prostaglandin $F_{2a}$, 13,14-dihydro-15-keto-prostaglandin $F_{2a}$ (PGFM) and 11-deoxy-13,14-dihydro 15-keto-11, 16-cyclo-prostaglandin E2 (PGEM-II) in preterm labor. Prostaglandins **37:** 149.
98. MACDONALD, P. C., F. M. SCHULTZ, J. H. DUENHOELTER et al. 1974. Initiation of human parturition. Obstet. Gynecol. **44:** 629.
99. CUNNINGHAM, F. G., P. D. MACDONALD, N. F. GANT, K. J. LEVENO & L. C. GILSTRAP. 1993. Williams Obstetrics, 19th Edition. Section IV. Normal labor and delivery and the puerperium. Chapter 12. Parturition: Biomolecular and physiologic processes. 297. Appleton and Lange. Norwalk, CT.
100. MACDONALD, P. C. & M. L. CASEY. 1993. The accumulation of prostaglandins (PG) in amniotic fluid is an aftereffect of labor and not indicative of a role for $PGE_2$ or $PGF_{2a}$ in the initiation of human parturition. J. Clin. Endocrinol. Metab. **76:** 1332.
101. KEIRSE, M. J. N. C. & A. C. TURNBULL. 1973. F prostaglandins in amniotic fluid during pregnancy and labour. J. Obstet. Gynaecol. Br. Commonw. **80:** 970.
102. SALMON, J. A. & J. J. AMY. 1973. Levels of prostaglandin $F_{2a}$ in amniotic fluid during pregnancy and labour. Prostaglandins **4:** 523.
103. KEIRSE, M. J. N. C., A. F. P. FLINT & A. C. TURNBULL. 1974. F prostaglandins in amniotic fluid during pregnancy and labor. J. Obstet. Gynaecol. Br. Commonw. **81:** 131.
104. DRAY, F. & R. FRYDMAN. 1976. Primary prostaglandin in amniotic fluid in pregnancy and spontaneous labor. Am. J. Obstet. Gynecol. **126:** 13.
105. KEIRSE, M. J. N. C., M. D. MITCHELL & A. A. TURNBULL. 1977. Changes in prostaglandin F and 13,14-dihydro-15-keto-prostaglandin F concentrations in amniotic fluid at the onset of labour. Br. J. Obstet. Gynaecol. **84:** 743.
106. MCDONALD, P. C., S. KOGA & M. L. CASEY. 1991. Decidual activation in parturition: examination of amniotic fluid for mediators of the inflammatory response. Ann. N.Y. Acad. Sci. **622:** 315.
107. ROMERO, R., R. GONZALEZ, P. BAUMANN, E. BEHNKE, L. RITTENHOUSE, D. BARBERIO, D. B. COTTON & M. D. MITCHELL. 1994. Topographic differences in amniotic fluid concentrations of prostanoids in women in spontaneous labor at term. Prostaglandins Leukotrienes Essent. Fatty Acids **50:** 97.
108. ROMERO, R., P. BAUMANN, R. GONZALEZ, R. GOMEZ, L. RITTENHOUSE, D. BARBERIO, E. BEHNKE, D. B. COTTON & M. MITCHELL. Amniotic fluid prostanoid concentrations increase early during the course of spontaneous labor at term. Am. J. Obstet. Gynecol. Submitted.
109. ROMERO, R., P. BAUMANN, R. GOMEZ, C. SALAFIA, L. RITTENHOUSE, D. BARBERIO, E. BEHNKE, D. B. COTTON & M. D. MITCHELL. 1993. The relationship between spontaneous rupture of membranes, labor and microbial invasion of the amniotic cavity and amniotic fluid concentrations of prostaglandins and thromboxane $B_2$ in term pregnancy. Am. J. Obstet. Gynecol. **168:** 1654.
110. HALUSKA, G. J., F. Z. STANCZYK, M. J. COOK & M. J. NOVY. 1987. Temporal changes in uterine activity and prostaglandin response to RU486 in rhesus macaques in late gestation. Am. J. Obstet. Gynecol. **157:** 1487.
111. ROMERO, R., H. MUNOZ, R. GOMEZ et al. An increase in prostaglandin bioavailability precedes the onset of spontaneous parturitions in humans. Am. J. Obstet. Gynecol. Submitted.
112. OLSON, D. M., T. ZAKAR, Z. SMIEJA, E. A. MACLEOD & S. L. BROWN. 1992. A pathway for the regulation of prostaglandins and parturition. *In* Prostaglandins and the Uterus. J. O. Drife & A. A. Calder, Eds. 149. Springer-Verlag. London, Berlin, Heidelberg, New York, Paris, Tokyo, Hong Kong, Barcelona, Budapest.
113. OKAZAKI, T., M. L. CASEY, J. R. OKITA, P. C. MACDONALD & J. M. JOHNSTON. 1981. Initiation of human parturition. XII. Biosynthesis and metabolism of prostaglandins in human fetal membranes and uterine decidua. Am. J. Obstet. Gynecol. **139:** 373.
114. OLSON, D. M., T. ZAKAR, F. A. POTESTIO & Z. SMIEJA. 1990. Control of prostaglandin production in human amnion. News Physiol. Sci. **5:** 259.

115. DUCHESNE, M. J., H. THALER-DAO & A. CRASTES DE PAULET. 1978. Prostaglandin synthesis in human placenta and fetal membranes. Prostaglandins **15:** 19.
116. ROMERO, R., S. DURUM, C. DINARELLO, E. OYARZUN, J. C. HOBBINS & M. D. MITCHELL. 1989. Interleukin-1 stimulates prostaglandin biosynthesis by human amnion. Prostaglandins **37:** 13.
117. ROMERO, R., K. MANOGUE, E. OYARZUN, Y. K. WU & A. CERAMI. 1991. Human decidua: a source of tumor necrosis factor. Eur. J. Obstet. Gynecol. Reprod. Biol. **41:** 123.
118. ROMERO, R., K. R. MANOGUE, M. D. MITCHELL, Y. K. WU, J. C. HOBBINS & A. CERAMI. 1989. Cachectin-tumor necrosis factor in the amniotic fluid of women with intraamniotic infection and preterm labor. Am. J. Obstet. Gynecol. **161:** 336.
119. ROMERO, R., Y. K. WU, E. OYARZUN, J. HOBBINS & M. MITCHELL. 1989. A potential role for epidermal growth factor/alpha-transforming growth factor in human parturition. Eur. J. Obstet. Gynaecol. Rep. Biol. **33:** 55.
120. NOVY, M. J. & S. W. WALSH. 1983. Dexamethasone and estradiol treatment in pregnant rhesus macaques: effects on gestational length, maternal plasma hormones, and fetal growth. Am. J. Obstet. Gynecol. **145:** 920.
121. LIGGINS, G. C., R. J. FAIRCLOUGH, S. A. GRIEVES, C. S. FORSTER & B. S. KNOX. 1977. Parturition in the sheep. *In* The Fetus and Birth. Ciba Foundations Symposium. J. Knight & M. O'Connor, Eds. 5. Elsevier. Amsterdam.
122. LIGGINS, G. C., R. J. FAIRCLOUGH, S. A. GRIEVES, J. Z. KENDALL & B. S. KNOX. 1973. The mechanism of initiation of parturition in the ewe. Recent Prog. Horm. Res. **29:** 111.
123. MCDONALD, T. J. & P. W. NATHANIELSZ. 1991. Bilateral destruction of the fetal paraventricular nuclei prolongs gestation in sheep. Am. J. Obstet. Gynecol. **165:** 764.
124. HONNEBIER, W. J. & D. F. SWAAB. 1973. The influence of anencephaly upon intrauterine growth of foetus and placenta and upon gestation length. Br. J. Obstet. Gynaecol. **80:** 577.
125. LIGGINS, G. C., L. W. HOLM & P. C. KENNEDY. 1966. Prolonged pregnancy following surgical lesions of the foetal lamb pituitary. J. Reprod. Fertil. **12:** 419.
126. KENDALL, J. Z., J. R. G. CHALLIS, I. C. HART *et al.* 1977. Steroid and prostaglandin concentrations in the plasma of pregnant ewes during infusion of adrenocorticotrophin or dexamethasone to intact or hypophysectomized foetuses. J. Endocrinol. **75:** 59.
127. LIGGINS, G. C. 1968. Premature parturition after infusion of corticotrophin or cortisol into foetal lambs. J. Endocrinol. **42:** 323.
128. REES, L. H., P. M. B. JACK, A. L. THOMAS & P. W. NATHANIELSZ. 1975. Role of foetal adrenocorticotrophin during parturition in sheep. Nature **253:** 274.
129. ROMERO, R. & M. MAZOR. 1988. Infection and preterm labor. Clin. Obstet. Gynecol. **31:** 553.
130. TAMURA, R. K., R. E. SABBAGHA, R. DEPP, N. VAISRUB, S. L. DOOLEY & M. L. SOCOL. 1984. Diminished growth in fetuses born preterm in spontaneous labor or rupture of membranes. Am. J. Obstet. Gynecol. **148:** 1105.
131. WEINER, C. R., R. E. SABBAGHA, N. VAISRUB & R. DEPP. 1985. A hypothetical model suggesting suboptimal intrauterine growth in infants delivered preterm. Obstet. Gynecol. **65:** 323.
132. MACGREGOR, S. N., R. E. SABBAGHA, R. K. TAMURA, B. W. PIELET & S. L. FEIGENBAUM. 1988. Differing fetal growth patterns in pregnancies complicated by preterm labor. Obstet. Gynecol. **72:** 834.
133. RODECK, C. H. 1985. Fetal abnormality and preterm labor. *In* Preterm Labour and Its Consequences. R. W. Beard & F. Sharp, Eds. 163. Royal College of Obstetricians and Gynecologists. London.
134. STUBBLEFIELD, P. G. 1984. Causes and prevention of preterm birth: an overview. *In* Preterm Birth: Causes, Prevention and Management. F. Fuchs & P. G. Stubblefield, Eds. 3. MacMillian Publishing Company. New York.
135. PAPIERNICK, E. & M. KAMINSKI. 1978. Multifactored study of the risks of prematurity at 32 weeks' gestation. J. Perinatol. Med. **2:** 30.

136. ROMERO, R., H. MUNOZ, M. RAMIREZ *et al.* 1994. Antibiotic therapy reduces the rate of infection-induced preterm delivery and perinatal mortality. 14th Annual Meeting of the Society of Perinatal Obstetricians, January 24–29, 1994, Las Vegas, Nevada (Abstract #418).
137. FIDEL, P., R. ROMERO, N. WOLF *et al.* Systemic and local cytokine profiles in endotoxin-induced preterm parturition in mice. Am. J. Obstet. Gynecol. In press.
138. MCDUFFIE, R. S., M. P. SHERMAN & R. S. GIBBS. 1992. Amniotic fluid tumor necrosis factor and interleukin-1 in a rabbit model of bacterially induced preterm pregnancy loss. Am. J. Obstet. Gynecol. **167:** 1583.
139. BANG, B. 1987. The etiology of epizootic abortion. J. Comp. Anthol. Ther. **10:** 125–150.
140. ZAHL, P. A. & C. BJERKNES. 1943. Induction of decidua-placental hemorrhage in mice by the endotoxins of certain gram-negative bacteria. Proc. Soc. Exp. Biol. Med. **54:** 329.
141. TADEKA, Y. & I. TSUCHIYA. 1953. Studies on the pathological changes caused by the injection of the Shwartzman filtrate and the endotoxin into pregnant rabbits. Jpn. J. Exp. Med. **21:** 9.
142. TADEKA, Y. & I. TSUCHIYA. 1953. Studies on the pathological changes caused by the injection of the Shwartzman filtrate and the endotoxin into pregnant animals, II. On the relationship of the constituents of the endotoxin and the abortion-producing factor. Jpn. J. Exp. Med. **23:** 105.
143. RIEDER, R. F. & L. THOMAS. 1960. Studies on the mechanisms involved in the production of abortion by endotoxin. J. Immunol. **84:** 189.
144. MCKAY, D. G. & T.-C. WONG. 1963. The effect of bacterial endotoxin on the placenta of the rat. Am. J. Pathol. **42:** 357.
145. KULLANDER, S. 1977. Fever and parturition: an experimental study in rabbits. Acta Obstet. Gynecol. Scand. **66:** 77.
146. FINLAND, M. & T. D. DUBLIN. 1939. Pneumococcic pneumonias complicating pregnancy and the puerperium. JAMA **112:** 1027.
147. OXHORN, H. 1955. The changing aspects of pneumonia complicating pregnancy. Am. J. Obstet. Gynecol. **70:** 1057.
148. BENEDETTI, T. J., R. VALLE & W. J. LEDGER. 1976. Antepartum pneumonia in pregnancy. Am. J. Obstet. Gynecol. **144:** 413.
149. MADINGER, N. E., J. S. GREENSPOON & A. G. ELLRODT. 1989. Pneumonia in pregnancy: has modern technology improved maternal and fetal outcome? Am. J. Obstet. Gynecol. **161:** 657.
150. MCLANE, C. M. 1939. Pyelitis of pregnancy: a five year study. Am. J. Obstet. Gynecol. **38:** 117.
151. KASS, E. 1962. Maternal urinary tract infection. N.Y. State J. Med. **1:** 2822.
152. HIBBARD, L., L. THRUPP, S. SUMMERIL, M. SMALE & R. ADAMS. 1967. Treatment of pyelonephritis in pregnancy. Am. J. Obstet. Gynecol. **98:** 609.
153. CUNNINGHAM, F. G., G. B. MORRIS & A. MIKAL. 1973. Acute pyelonephritis of pregnancy: a clinical review. Obstet. Gynecol. **42:** 112.
154. FAN, Y.-D., J. G. PASTOREK, J. M. MILLER & J. MULVEY. 1987. Acute pyelonephritis in pregnancy. Am. J. Perinatol. **4:** 324.
155. WING, E. S. & D. V. TROPPOLI. 1930. The intrauterine transmission of typhoid. JAMA **95:** 405.
155a. DIDDLE, A. W. & R. L. STEPHENS. 1938. Typhoid fever in pregnancy: probable intrauterine transmission of the disease. Am. J. Obstet. Gynecol. **38:** 300.
156. STEVENSON, C. S., A. J. GLASKO, & E. C. GILLESPIE. 1951. Treatment of typhoid in pregnancy with chloramphenicol (chloromycetin). JAMA **146:** 1190.
157. HERD, N. & T. JORDAN. 1981. An investigation of malaria during pregnancy in Zimbabwe. A. Afr. J. Med. **27:** 62.
158. GILLES, H. M., J. B. LAWSON, M. SIBELAS, A. VOLLER & N. ALLAN. 1969. Malaria, anaemia and pregnancy. Ann. Trop. Med. Pharmacol. **63:** 245.
159. ROMERO, R., M. SIRTORI, E. OYARZUN *et al.* 1989. Infection and labor, V. Prevalence, microbiology, and clinical significance of intraamniotic infection in women with preterm labor and intact membranes. Am. J. Obstet. Gynecol. **161:** 817.

160. ROMERO, R., F. SHAMMA, C. AVILA *et al.* 1990. Infection and labor. VI. Prevalence, microbiology, and clinical significance of intraamniotic infection in twin gestations with preterm labor. Am. J. Obstet. Gynecol. **163:** 757.
161. ROMERO, R., C. AVILA, C. A. BREKUS & R. MOROTTI. 1991. The role of systemic and intrauterine infection in preterm parturition. *In:* The Primate Endometrium. C. Bulletti & E. Gurpide, Eds. Ann. N.Y. Acad. Sci. **622:** 355.
162. ROMERO, R., C. M. SALAFIA, A. P. ATHANASSIADIS *et al.* 1992. The relationship between acute inflammatory lesions of the placenta and amniotic fluid microbiology. Am. J. Obstet. Gynecol. **166:** 1382.
163. ROMERO, R. 1993. The preterm labor syndrome: biochemical, cytologic, immunologic, pathologic, microbiologic, and clinical evidence that preterm labor is a heterogeneous disease. Am. J. Obstet. Gynecol. **168:** 288.
164. ARIAS, F. 1990. Placental insufficiency: an important cause of preterm labor and preterm premature ruptured membranes. Presented at the 10th Annual Meeting of the Society of Perinatal Obstetricians, January 23–27, 1990, Houston, Texas.
165. CHELLAM, V. G. & D. I. RUSHTON. 1985. Chorioamnionitis and funiculitis in the placentas of 200 births weighing less than 2.5 kg. Br. J. Obstet. Gynaecol. **92:** 808.
166. LUDMIR, J., P. SAMUELS, S. BROOKS & M. T. MENNUTI. 1990. Pregnancy outcome of patients with uncorrected uterine anomalies managed in a high-risk obstetric setting. Obstet. Gynecol. **75:** 906.
167. HILL, L., R. BRECKEL, M. L. THOMAS & J. K. FRIES. 1987. Polyhydramnios: ultrasonically detected prevalence and neonatal outcome. Obstet. Gynecol. **69:** 21.
168. PHELAN, J. P., Y. W. PARK, M. O. AHN & S. E. RUTHERFORD. 1990. Polyhydramnios and perinatal outcome. J. Perinatol. **4:** 347.
169. CSAPO, A., H. TAKEDA & C. WOOD. 1963. Volume and activity of the parturient rabbit uterus. Am. J. Obstet. Gynecol. **85:** 813.
170. FUCHS, A.-R., S. PERIYASAMI, M. ALEXANDROVA & M. S. SOLOFF. 1983. Correlation between oxytocin receptor concentration and responsiveness to oxytocin in pregnant rat myometrium: effect of ovarian steroids. Endocrinology **113:** 742.
171. CASPI, E., J. RONEN & P. SCHREYER. 1976. The outcome of pregnancy after gonadotrophin therapy. Br. J. Obstet. Gynaecol. **83:** 967.
172. MCCARTHY, B., B. SACHS, P. LAYDE *et al.* 1981. The epidemiology of neonatal death in twins. Am. J. Obstet. Gynecol. **141:** 242.
173. GARFIELD, R. E. 1989. Uterine mast cells: immunogenic control of myometrial contractility. Presented at the 36th Annual Meeting of the Society of Gynecologic Investigation, San Diego, CA, March 15–16, 1989.
174. ROMERO, R., M. MAZOR, C. AVILA, R. QUINTERO & H. MUNOZ. 1991. Uterine "allergy": a novel mechanism for preterm labor. Am. J. Obstet. Gynecol. **164:** 375.

# Morphometric Characteristics of the Decidua, Cytotrophoblast, and Connective Tissue of the Prelabor Ruptured Fetal Membranes[a]

T. M. MALAK, G. MULHOLLAND, AND S. C. BELL

*Department of Obstetrics and Gynaecology
Clinical Sciences Building
Leicester Royal Infirmary
P.O. Box 65
Leicester LE2 7LX, United Kingdom*

Preterm birth (PTB) is the most challenging problem in modern obstetrics. It may be medically or obstetrically indicated, preceded by prelabor rupture of the fetal membranes (PROM) or preceded by spontaneous preterm labor. PROM precedes 40% of PTB cases. The pathophysiology of PROM and preterm birth is not fully established. However, infection is a known association with PROM and PTB[1] and it causes marked dissociation of the connective tissue of the fetal membranes.[2] The morphometric features of the connective and cellular (decidua and cytotrophoblast) tissues of the fetal membranes in noninfected cases of preterm PROM are not fully characterized. We have reported their morphometric characteristics following term birth[3,4] by determining the thickness of the connective and cellular tissues in different regions of the fetal membranes at the light microscopic level. We also reported the ultrastructural features associated with these light microscopic findings.[3,4] In this study we report the morphometric characteristics of the decidua and amniochorion of the noninfected cases of preterm PROM in comparison to other cases of preterm birth.

## MATERIAL AND METHODS

The study included 13 cases preceded by PROM (cases with PROM), 14 cases of spontaneous preterm birth not preceded by PROM (cases without PROM) and 14 underwent emergency caesarean sections (CS) for placental abruption or fetal distress and were not in labor. Immediately after delivery, multiple samples were obtained from decidua and amniochorion halfway between the rupture site (or that over the cervix) and the placental edge. We termed this region the mid-zone. Hematoxylin- and eosin-stained cryostat sections were used to assess the thickness of the connective and cellular tissues using an image analysis system.

## RESULTS

Cases associated with chorioamnionitis, diagnosed histologically[5] were not included in the analysis. The incidence of chorioamnionitis was 0% (CS cases),

---

[a] This work was supported by WellBeing, UK.

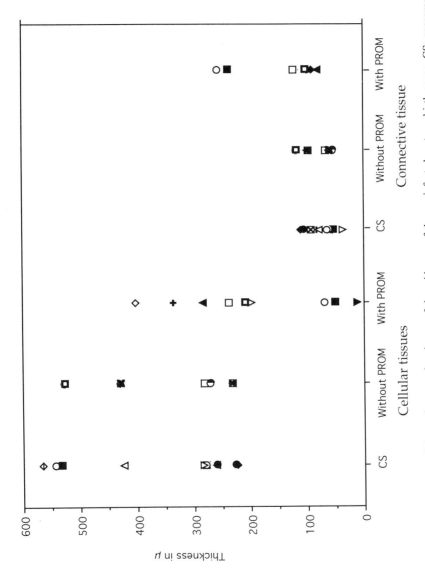

**FIGURE 1.** The thickness of the cellular and connective tissues of the mid-zone of the noninfected preterm birth cases. CS: caesarean section group; PROM: prelabor rupture of fetal membranes group.

TABLE 1. The Mean Thickness in $\mu$ (Standard Error) of the Cellular and Connective Tissue of the Mid-Zone of the Fetal Membranes in Noninfected Cases of Preterm Birth[a]

|  | CS | Without PROM | With PROM |
|---|---|---|---|
| Cellular tissue | 341.6 (8.3) | 349.7 (7.2) | 212.6 (7.4) |
| Connective tissue | 73.1 (1.3) | 67 (1.6) | 135.7 (5.5) |

[a] CS: caesarean section group; PROM: prelabor rupture of fetal membranes group.

28.5% (cases without PROM) and 30.7% (cases with PROM). The mean gestational age of all patients was 31.9 weeks (no statistical difference was found between the subroups). Using one factor analysis of variance and Scheffe's test, a statistically significant increase in the thickness of the connective tissue and a decrease in that of cellular tissues ($p < 0.0001$) were found in cases with PROM in comparison to cases without PROM and the CS group (FIG. 1 & TABLE 1). No significant difference was found between the last two groups.

## DISCUSSION

Infection is a well established association with PROM and PTB and our results are in agreement with this finding. In this study morphometric alteration, characterized by decrease of thickness of cellular tissues of the chorio-decidual interface and increase in thickness of the connective tissue of the amniochorion in the mid-zone, was found to be marked in PROM cases in comparison to other cases of PTB. We previously found that the decreased thickness of the cellular layers was associated with a decrease in the total cell mass and cellular degenerative changes diagnosed ultrastructurally.[3,4] We have also found that the increased thickness of the connective tissue of the amniochorion reflected its disruption and degradation that were diagnosed ultrastructurally.[3,4] This marked morphometric alteration associated with PROM cases may, therefore, indicate a membrane disruption that may predispose the membrane to rupture. Whether the cellular changes (loss of cell mass and cellular degeneration) are the cause of the connective tissue disruption remains to be studied. Further characterization of these changes may help to understand the mechanisms associated with preterm PROM.

## REFERENCES

1. GIBBS, R., R. ROMERO, S. HILLIER et al. 1992. Am. J. Obstet. Gynecol. **166:** 1515–1528.
2. MCGREGOR, J., J. FRENCH, D. LAWELLIN et al. 1987. Obstet. Gynecol. **69:** 167–174.
3. ABDEL-MALAK, T., S. BELL, S. CROSIER et al. 1993. Br. J. Obstet. Gynaecol. **100:** 289.
4. MALAK, T. & S. BELL. 1993. Contemp. Rev. Obstet. Gynaecol. **5:** 117–123.
5. SALAFIA, C., C. WEIGL & L. SILBERMAN. 1989. Obstet. Gynecol. **73:** 383–389.

# Operative Laparoscopy

## Videolaparoscopy and Videolaseroscopy

CAMRAN NEZHAT,[a,b,c] FARR NEZHAT,[a,b]
AND CEANA NEZHAT[a,b]

[a]Department of Obstetrics and Gynecology
Mercer University School of Medicine
Macon, Georgia

[b]Department of Obstetrics and Gynecology
Stanford University
Palo Alto, California

## INTRODUCTION

Since the first attempt at endoscopy by Philip Bozzini of Italy in 1805, the instrumentation for laparoscopy has developed at an acceptable rate although the applications have lagged. Laparoscopy was moderately successful in Europe during the first half of the twentieth century.[1] The technique was applied to diagnostic and simple sterilization procedures and while the results were promising, the procedure was not accepted in the United States. The advantages of the laparoscope were diminished by several drawbacks. The surgoen had to work crouched over the patient, peering with one eye through the scope; visibility was limited, the position was uncomfortable, and the surgeon became easily fatigued. The surgical team was unable to view the procedure. Auxiliary instruments were not available to perform complicated procedures.

In the 1970s Victor Gomel[1] reported successful salpingo-ovariolysis, salpingo-oophorectomy, fimbrioplasty and management of ectopic pregnancy. At the same time, Kurt Semm headed the German-based Kiel School's development of instruments for operative laparoscopy.[2] Gomel,[3] Bruhat,[4] Semm and others[5] contributed to this technique, but it was not integrated into the operating room.

In 1965, as laparoscopy stagnated, the $CO_2$ laser was used in experimental surgery. The high-tech concept of the laser gained public attention. Through lay publications, attention was focused on this new surgical tool and it was used with the laparoscope. Bruhat[6] and Tadir[7] were among the first to report laser laparoscopy, using the second puncture and a joystick arrangement, respectively. Fiber lasers[8-11] were used with the laparoscope to treat various pelvic disorders with acceptable results. However, gynecologists continued primarily to use the $CO_2$ laser. These combinations were subject to the mentioned limitations and not frequently used.

Experiments were conducted in human and animal laboratories with a video camera attached to the eyepiece of the scope.[12] The camera magnified the image and projected it onto monitors in the operating room, eliminating the major disadvantages of the laparoscope. The early cameras were cumbersome and the first

---

[c] Corresponding author: Camran Nezhat, M.D., 5555 Peachtree Dunwoody Road, N.E., Suite 276, Atlanta, Georgia 30342.

videolaparoscopic surgeries on humans were difficult due to the cameras' weight, inadequate light source, and poor resolution. Its use was criticized. However, the senior author persisted in developing his concept of videolaparoscopy. In the early 1980s, equipment companies recognized the market for a miniature video camera. Lighter versions with higher resolution and better light sources were produced. The elements were in place for a revolution in abdominal and pelvic surgery.[13]

At the combined annual meetings of the American Fertility Society and Canadian Fertility and Andrology Society in November, 1986, the senior author presented the benefits and results of videolaparoscopy in over 600 endometriosis surgeries.[13] Using more refined cameras and the combined $CO_2$ laser and laparoscope, we successfully performed laparoscopic procedures on over 1,000 patients including those with extensive endometriosis.[14] Through the publication and presentation of case reports and detailed studies, we have promulgated the use of videolaparoscopy and videolaseroscopy in gynecology (benign and malignant pathology),[15-20] lower gastroenterology[21,22] and urology.[23] The demand for the technique was finally created when patients recommended the procedure to acquaintances. Public interest articles focused on patients who had benefited from videolaseroscopy.[24-26] Media attention and word-of-mouth made operative laparoscopy one of the first truly consumer-driven medical advances.

The applications of operative laparoscopy and the number of surgeons learning the technique are increasing. Operative videolaparoscopy offers several benefits over an open procedure. First, pelvic and abdominal anatomy are magnified by the video camera and scope, allowing the surgeon to perform microsurgical procedures. Second, pneumoperitoneum decreases bleeding and provides a cleaner operating field. Third, areas like the upper abdomen, posterior cul-de-sac and posterior aspect of the broad ligaments may be more thoroughly evaluated, and with technological advances such as the development of the $CO_2$ laser, disease may be treated more precisely and possibly with a greater margin of safety. Fourth, operative laparoscopy produces fewer de novo adhesions[27,28] and requires a shorter recovery period. Finally, when performed by a trained and experienced surgeon, intraoperative and postoperative complications, and morbidity, such as small bowel ileus, infection, etc. are decreased compared to laparotomy. An added benefit of the addition of video is the permanent record created by taping the procedure which may be used for future reference. This tape can be used to demonstrate techniques to other physicians, explain a procedure to a patient, review a patient's condition should further treatment become necessary, or provide information for research.

For several years, we have avoided over 98% of all laparotomies which would have been performed to treat benign, and in some cases, malignant gynecologic disease. It is our belief that this same percentage of all pelvic and abdominal surgeries will be performed via laparoscopy by the 21st century. The following is our experience with various applications of this technique.

## *Appendectomy*

During laparoscopic treatment of diverse pelvic pathologies, incidental appendectomy is often performed.[16] Ancillary instruments are introduced through 5 mm accessory trocars, and include grasping forceps, endoloop suture applicators, a suction-irrigator probe (American Hydro-Surgical Instruments, Delray Beach, FL) and bipolar forceps. Appendectomy may be concomitant with surgeries for pelvic endometriosis and/or adhesions.

In a series of 254 appendectomies, no major intraoperative complications were noted. Postoperatively, one woman had a small pelvic abscess which required surgical intervention. All patients were discharged from the hospital within 24 hours of surgery.[16]

### Bladder Resection for Severe Endometriosis

The $CO_2$ laser, hydrodissection and bipolar electrocoagulation are used to excise the endometriosis nodule, including the mucosal layer.[29] After the lesion is removed and the bladder closed,[30] cystoscopic evaluation is performed to determine if the closure is watertight.

We have performed 3 partial cystectomies for severe bladder endometriosis. All patients are doing well, with postoperative follow-up ranging from 12 to 48 months.[31]

### Ectopic Pregnancy Management

The chance of managing unruptured ectopic pregnancy laparoscopically has increased with rapid serum human chorionic gonadotropic (HCG) assays and high-resolution vaginal ultrasounds.[32-34] New medical management techniques utilizing ultrasonically guided injection of methotrexate, potassium or prostaglandin $F_2$ alpha, may some day replace primary laparoscopic management of ectopic pregnancy.

When an unruptured tubal pregnancy is confirmed laparoscopically, surgical management should be instituted at that procedure. The surgeon should talk to the patient preoperatively to ascertain her desire for fertility preservation and to determine whether or not she has had previous ectopic pregnancies. The patient must understand that salpingectomy or laparotomy may become necessary. However, an experienced endoscopic surgeon can laparoscopically manage ectopic pregnancies, regardless of size and independent of location.[34] Finally, the need for careful follow-up with conservative management must be explained to the patient.

In patients who prefer permanent sterilization, coagulation using bipolar Kleppinger forceps over a small ectopic pregnancy will destroy the tubal pregnancy and sterilize the patient. For larger ectopics (greater than 6 cm), cases of spontaneous tubal rupture or more than one recurrent ipsilateral ectopic pregnancy, salpingectomy may be indicated.[18] An alternative to salpingectomy involves using an automatic stapling device[29] which is placed along the mesosalpinx, parallel to the fallopian tube and triggered, simultaneously clamping and cutting the pedicle. This technique, which is expensive, has been associated with postoperative hematoma and other injuries.

Salpingotomy has been shown to produce higher subsequent pregnancy rates and lower recurrence rates of ectopic pegnancy than salpingectomy.[32] Linear salpingotomy should be performed in patients who want to preserve the affected tube and are hemodynamically stable.

Weekly hCG levels must be followed until they decrease to nonpregnant levels. Consistent or rising levels require further medical or surgical management.

Segmental resection of the tube has a better prognosis in the narrow isthmus portion of the tube, possibly because pregnancies in this site tend to infiltrate deeper into tubal tissue layers and are smaller, and therefore less well-defined for surgical manipulation.[32] Segmental resection may also be utilized in cases of spontaneous rupture without active bleeding, and persistent tubal pregnancies. As much fallopian tube as possible should be preserved so that microsurgical reanastomosis can be attempted at a later date.

### Hysterectomy

Laparoscopic hysterectomy (LH) may be defined as the complete endoscopic excision of the uterus from its attachments. In a total hysterectomy, the vaginal cuff is repaired laparoscopically. In a laparoscopic supracervical hysterectomy (LSH), the cervical stump is closed laparoscopically. All other combinations are variations of laparoscopically-assisted hysterectomy.[35]

Gynecologists recognize that vaginal hysterectomy patients experience less postoperative morbidity and pain, and require a shorter period of recuperation when compared to abdominal hysterectomies. However, approximately 70 percent of hysterectomies are still done by laparotomy. Laparoscopic and laparoscopically-assisted vaginal hysterectomy have been introduced to provide an alternative to abdominal hysterectomy. Preliminary results confirm less intraoperative blood loss and shorter recuperation, without increased complications.[19]

We have been favorably impressed with the postoperative recovery of and low morbidity in these patients, particularly those with significant pelvic pathology.

In a series of 361 laparoscopic and laparoscopically-assisted hysterectomies for a variety of indications, all women are doing well.[36]

We do not advocate converting vaginal hysterectomies to laparoscopic or laparoscopically-assisted hysterectomies. Rather, the laparoscopic approach is an appropriate alternative to those procedures which would otherwise require laparotomy.[36]

### Radical Hysterectomy

We have developed a technique to perform radical hysterectomy and lymphadenectomy laparoscopically.[12,22] During the laparoscopic portion of the procedure, all pedicles are coagulated with bipolar electrocoagulator and incised with $CO_2$ laser, scissors or unipolar electrocoagulator.[17] Sutures are not necessary, and peritoneal incisions may be left to heal secondarily.

The role of operative laparoscopy in gynecologic oncology remains controversial, and it has not yet been determined which cases are best served by this technique. Laparoscopy has been used successfully to treat cervical cancer,[12,20,38] endometrial cancer,[20,39] and early ovarian cancer.[40] We began reporting our experience with paraaortic node dissection in 1989.[20,41]

### Marshall-Marchetti-Krantz and Burch Procedure

Preoperative evaluation includes history, physical, pelvic exam, imaging techniques, and urodynamic testing (basic; or complex with or without urologic consult).

In a series of 21 patients, operative time for the Marshall-Marchetti-Krantz and Burch procedure ranged from 25 to 45 minutes and blood loss was from 10 to 60 mL.

No intraoperative or postoperative complications were noted, except for one woman who was unable to void. She required self-catheterization for 10 days. All other women voided following removal of the Foley catheter. To date, all patients have reported subjective and objective success.

The preliminary results from our 2 to 24 month follow-up are encouraging, and our work in this area is ongoing.[42]

## Myomectomy

Patients with indications for myomectomy are managed with GnRH analogs (Lupron, Tapp Pharmaceuticals, North Chicago, IL or Synarel, Syntex, Palo Alto, CA) for up to 3 months preoperatively. Three months of amenorrhea does improve preoperative hematocrits; patients are also given the option of autologous blood donation.[43]

We have developed a combined laparoscopic and minilaparotomy approach to myomectomy (LAM) with excellent results.[44]

Fifty-seven LAMs were reviewed. Each woman had one or multiple leiomyomas weighing between 28 and 998 g. The average blood loss was 267 mL; in 36 patients, the blood loss was less than 200 mL. The average operative time was 127 minutes.

The patients were usually discharged from the hospital the day of surgery or the morning of postoperative day one. The mean time of 1.28 days is skewed because the first patients were hospitalized for observation. Forty-one patients were discharged on or before postoperative day one, 12 women were discharged on postoperative day 2, and 4 were in the hospital over 72 hours.

The patients have been observed postoperatively for 3 to 24 months (mean, 11.35 months; median, 9 months). All women with menometrorrhagia reported improvement of their symptoms. Four women who were infertile and whose preoperative infertility workup was otherwise negative, conceived between 6 and 9 months postoperatively. Three patients underwent second look laparoscopy. One had minor filmy adhesions between the uterus and omentum; another had moderately thick, avascular adhesions of omentum to uterine fundus. One had avascular adhesions involving the uterine fundus, adnexa and pelvic sidewall. These women were all found to have adhesions at the initial laparoscopy.

## Oophorectomy and Adnexal Mass Management

Doubts remain about the laparoscopist's ability to diagnose and properly manage early ovarian cancer if the adnexal mass in question is found to be malignant.[45] One concern is that the spillage of a cancer confined to the ovary may worsen prognosis. However, when a competent surgeon follows proper protocol adnexal masses may be safely evaluated and most treated laparoscopically.

Patients are evaluated clinically with a pelvic exam and vaginal ultrasound, along with a review of previous intraoperative records. Simple (unilocular) cysts in premenopausal women are initially managed with hormonal suppressive therapy using oral contraceptive pills containing 50 micrograms of estrogen, Depo-Provera or danazol. A serum CA 125 level or other tumor marker, if indicated, should also be obtained for postmenopausal patients. Cystic, complex or solid masses up to 25 cm have been laparoscopically managed by the authors, including endometriomas, benign cystic teratomas and intraligamentous myomata.[40]

Informed consent should include a statement to the patient that laparoscopic diagnosis and treatment of adnexal mass are not standard medical practice at this time (1993). Patients are further informed that if a cancer is found, intraoperative cancer cell spillage could influence survival. In addition, patients must understand that a second surgery, specifically a laparotomy, might be required if the findings at laparoscopy cannot be properly managed laparoscopically.

Intraoperative management of all patients with masses is carefully standardized, and includes inspecting the pelvis, ovaries, upper abdomen and diaphragmatic surfaces for any vegetation or other sign of malignancy. Peritoneal washings are obtained for cytology. If a strong suspicion of malignancy based on intraoperative findings exists, an attempt is made to obtain frozen section biopsies without rupturing the cyst. If that is not possible, the laparoscopic procedure is terminated, and the patient will undergo a laparotomy.

The management of the cystic mass itself includes aspirating the fluid and sending it for cytology, followed by opening the cyst and inspecting the wall for excrescences or irregular thickening. Frozen section biopsies are obtained if the surgeon feels any surfaces appear suspicious. Finally, depending on the patient's age and pertinent clinical history, an ovarian cystectomy or oophorectomy may be performed.[17]

No substitute exists for sound clinical judgement. A surgeon should perform the techniques he/she is comfortable with, and should conduct careful preoperative patient screenings.[40]

*Endometriomas*

Superficial ovarian endometriosis can be vaporized, and those <2 cm which may be difficult to remove can be biopsied and then vaporized. Larger endometriomas, however, must be removed to reduce the risk of recurrence.[46,47]

Endometriomas must be approached as are all other adnexal masses; endometrioid carcinoma can coexist with endometriosis, and is indistinguishable at surgery until histology is reported. We have encountered an endometriosis, and is indistinguishable at surgery until histology is reported. We have encountered an endometrioid adenocarcinoma while managing bilateral endometriomas. Histologic examination of the cyst wall is mandatory in even the most typical appearing case.[40]

In a prospective study of 216 hemorrhagic, or "chocolate," ovarian cysts, three types of endometriomas were identified, both clinically and pathologically.[48] They were classified based on gross appearance, size, content, ease of removal of the capsule and pathological findings. We have postulated that large ovarian endometriomas represent secondary involvement of functional cysts with superficial endometriosis.

### Ovarian Remnant Management

Ovarian remnant syndrome can be treated laparoscopically. Intraabdominal adhesions are lysed and ovarian remnants dissected using hydrodissection[49] and videolaseroscopy.[29] Excellent results with few complications have been reported following this procedure.[50]

## Peritoneal Endometriosis

As the $CO_2$ laser does not penetrate water, a fluid backstop (hydrodissection) allows the surgeon to work on selected tissue with a more comfortable margin than would otherwise be available.[49]

To treat endometriosis of the bladder, for example, an aspiration needle is used to inject 20 to 30 mL of lactated Ringer's (Baxter) subperitoneally in an avascular area approximately 2 cm from the endometrial lesion. This elevates the peritoneum and backs it with a fluid bed. A 0.5-cm incision is made with the laser on this elevation, through which 100 to 200 mL of lactated Ringer's are injected subperitoneally. The lesion may then be vaporized or excised using the $CO_2$ laser in the ultrapulse mode. The manipulation of and trauma to the pelvic organs should be kept to a minimum. Any excessive resection, vaporization, coagulation or manipulation in this area may predispose the patient to adhesion formation.

Rock has reported good results using electrocoagulation to treat endometriosis.[51]

## Presacral Neurectomy

Presacral neurectomy offers a surgical alternative for the amelioration of intractable dysmenorrhea.[52] This procedure utilizes a single umbilical laser laparoscope and two or three suprapubic accessory trocars.[29] We have performed presacral neurectomy in over 150 patients with severe dysmenorrhea and central pain associated with different stages of endometriosis without intraoperative or postoperative complications, except for one case of active bleeding. The source was a branch of the inferior mesenteric artery, and the bleeding was controlled laparoscopically. Blood loss was minimal and no patient required a laparotomy. All patients left the hospital within 24 hours of surgery.[52]

## Bowel Endometriosis and Bowel Resection

Patients with severe endometriosis frequently have uterosacral ligament, rectovaginal septum and deep rectosigmoid involvement with partial or complete obliteration of the posterior cul-de-sac. This disease can be excised or vaporized, and requires maximal cooperation between the assistant and surgeon.

Small perforations can be repaired laparoscopically with 3 to 4 interrupted 3-0 silk or 4-0 polydioxanone sutures (Ethicon).[29] Patients may be discharged within 24 hours, except those who had bowel perforations or resection.[53]

### Bowel Resection

The laparoscopic bowel resection is identical to a laparotomy except that biopolar electrocoagulator and laser replace sutures and scissors. We have developed a technique for partial colon resection and reported the results from a series of several women. They were evaluated preoperatively and intraoperatively, including barium enema and sigmoidoscopy. In addition, a rectovaginal examination confirmed severe lower colon endometriosis in all patients. All had previous surgical intervention during which bowel endometriosis was diagnosed. All patients had preoperative mechanical and antiobiotic bowel preparation as previously described.[21,23]

In a series of 356 women who underwent laparoscopic treatment of bowel endometriosis using different techniques, two patients required intraoperative laparotomy early in our experience. The first patient underwent laparotomy for repair of culdotomy after treatment of infiltrative rectal endometriosis. The other patient required laparotomy for anastomosis due to an unsuccessful attempt to place a purse-string suture around the patulous rectal ampulla. Significant postoperative complications occurred in 1.7% of patients. Two women developed leaks and pelvic infections. One required a laparoscopic temporary colostomy with subsequent takedown and repair by laparotomy, and one was managed by prolonged drainage under CT scan guidance. One woman had bowel stricture requiring resection and reanastomosis by laparotomy. One developed a pelvic abscess which after failed drainage required subsequent laparoscopic right salpingo-oophorectomy. One patient who had anterior wedge resection of the rectum experienced immediate rectal prolapse which was reduced without surgical management. Her original bowel symptoms persisted, and she finally had a colectomy. Minor complications included skin ecchymosis, temporary urinary retention, temporary diarrhea or constipation, and dyschezia.

### *Tubal Adhesiolysis & Hydrosalpinges*

Using videolaseroscopy to lyse and remove peritubal adhesions has proved effective in preserving fertility, providing the anatomy of the lumen, including major and minor folds of the mucosa and cilia, has not been destroyed by disease.[29] Fimbrioscopy[54] can be used to further evaluate the tubes intraoperatively. When compared to reported pregnancy rates following laparotomy, the results by laparoscopy are more encouraging.

### *Sacral Colpopexy*

To date, we have performed 6 sacral colpopexy procedures.[29] With the exception of one case, all procedures were completed laparoscopically. During application of the staples, one patient (77 years old and obese) had significant bleeding and eventually underwent laparotomy. All patients have been followed for 6 months to 2 years and all had complete relief of their symptoms with excellent vaginal vault support.

### *Ureteroureterostomy*

In patients with partial or complete ureteral obstruction which is unresponsive to medical therapy, ureteroureterostomy is necessary.[23] We have had excellent results with this technique, which may also be used to repair ureter injury.[54,55] The ureter is dissected from surrounding tissues. The proximal ureter is transected, and a 7F ureteral catheter is introduced cystoscopically into the distal ureter. The distal ureter is transected over the stent and the obstructed portion removed. The ureteral stent is introduced into the proximal ureter and advanced into the renal pelvis. Four interrupted 4-0 polydioxanone sutures are placed to approximate ureteral edges.

TABLE 1. Summary of Complications and Method of Treatment

| Complication: | Vascular | | Gastrointestinal | | Genitourinary | | Other[a] |
|---|---|---|---|---|---|---|---|
| | Abdominal Wall | Intra-abdominal | Small Bowel | Large Bowel | Bladder | Ureter | |
| Intraoperative | 117 | 6 | 22 | 9 | 8 | 3 | 3 |
|   Laparoscopy | 116 | 2 | 15 | 8 | 5 | 2 | 0 |
|   Minilaparotomy | 1 | 4 | 3 | 1 | 0 | 0 | 0 |
|   Laparotomy | 0 | 0 | 4 | 0 | 2 | 0 | 0 |
|   Medical treatment | 0 | 0 | 0 | 0 | 1 | 1 | 3 |
| Postoperative | 12 | 5 | 6 | 5[b] | 3 | 1 | 17 |
|   Laparoscopy | 6 | 2 | 1 | 1 | 1 | 1 | 3 |
|   Laparotomy | 1 | 2 | 1 | 3 | 0 | 0 | 3 |
|   Medical treatment | 5 | 1 | 4 | 1 | 2 | 0 | 12 |

[a] Other includes pelvic infection, subcutaneous emphysema, pulmonary edema, incisional hernia, deep vein thrombosis, pleural effusion, vaginal cuff dehiscence and severe dehydration.
[b] Some patients had a combination of laparoscopy and laparotomy or laparoscopy and medical treatment.

## Complications

TABLE 1 summarizes our experience with complications. From July 1982 until the end of December 1993, we performed 6949 cases with an overall complication rate of 3.08%. Many of the surgeries involved patients with severe endometriosis and adhesions. As we became more experienced, we incorporated more procedures from different disciplines.

### REFERENCES

1. GOMEL, V. 1989. Operative laparoscopy: time for acceptance. Fertil. Steril. **52:** 1–11.
2. METTLER, L., H. GIESEL & K. SEMM. 1979. Treatment of female infertility due to tubal obstruction by operative laparoscopy. Fertil. Steril. **32:** 384–388.
3. GOMEL, V. 1977. Salpingostomy by laparoscopy. J. Reprod. Med. **18:** 265.
4. BRUHAT, M. A., G. MAGE, H. MANHES & J. L. POULY. 1980. Treatment of ectopic pregnancy by means of laparoscopy. Fertil. Steril. **33:** 411–418.
5. LEVENTHAL, J. M., L. R. SIMON & S. S. SHAPIRO. 1971. Laparoscopic removal of intrauterine contraceptive devices following perforation. Am. J. Obstet. Gynecol. **111:** 102.
6. BRUHAT, M., G. MAGE & M. MANHES. 1979. Use of the $CO_2$ laser via laparoscopy. In Laser Surgery III. Proceedings of the 3rd International Society for Laser Surgery. I. Kaplan, Ed. 175–176. International Society for Laser Surgery. Tel Aviv.
7. TADIR, Y., I. KAPLAN, Z. ZUCKERMAN, T. EDELSTEIN & J. OVADIA. 1984. New instrumentation and technique for laparoscopic carbon dioxide laser operations: a preliminary report. Obstet. Gynecol. **63**(4): 582–585.
8. LOMANO, J. M. 1983. Laparoscopic ablation of endometriosis with the YAG laser. Lasers Surg. Med. **3:** 179.
9. NEZHAT, C., W. K. WINER & F. NEZHAT. 1988. A comparison of the $CO_2$, Argon, and KTP/532 lasers in the videolaseroscopic treatment of endometriosis. Colposc. Gynecol. Laser Surg. **4:** 41.
10. KEYE, W. R., JR., L. W. HANSEN, M. ASTIN & A. M. POULSON, JR. 1987. Argon laser therapy of endometriosis: a review of 92 consecutive patients. Fertil. Steril. **47:** 208.
11. DANIELL, J. R., W. MILLER & R. TOSH. 1986. Initial evaluation of the use of the potassium-titanyl-phosphate (KTP-532) laser in gynecologic laparoscopy. Fertil. Steril. **46:** 373.
12. NEZHAT, C. 1986. Videolaseroscopy: a new modality for the treatment of endometriosis and other diseases of the reproductive organs. Colposc. Gynecol. Laser Surg. **2:** 221–224.
13. NEZHAT, C. and staff writer. 1986. Videolaseroscopy for endometriosis care. Obstet. Gynecol. News (November 15–30): 41–42.
14. NEZHAT, C., S. R. CROWGEY & C. P. GARRISON. 1986. Surgical treatment of endometriosis via laser laparoscopy. Fertil. Steril. **45:** 778–783.
15. NEZHAT, C., S. CROWGEY & F. NEZHAT. 1989. Videolaseroscopy for the treatment of endometriosis associated with infertility. Fertil. Steril. **51:** 237–240.
16. NEZHAT, C. & F. NEZHAT. 1991. Incidental appendectomy during videolaseroscopy. Am. J. Obstet. Gynecol. **165;** 559–564.
17. NEZHAT, F., C. NEZHAT & S. L. SILFEN. 1991. Videolaseroscopy for oophorectomy. Am. J. Obstet. Gynecol. **165:** 1323–1330.
18. NEZHAT, C., F. NEZHAT & W. WINER. 1991. Salpingectomy via laparoscopy: a new surgical approach. J. Laparosc. Surg. **1:** 91–95.8.
19. NEZHAT, C., F. NEZHAT, S. GORDON & E. WILKINS. 1992. Laparoscopic versus abdominal hysterectomy. J. Reprod. Med. **37:** 247–250.
20. NEZHAT, C., M. O. BURRELL, F. R. NEZHAT, B. B. BENIGNO & C. E. WELANDER. 1992. Laparoscopic radical hysterectomy with para-aortic and pelvic node dissection. Am. J. Obstet. Gynecol. **166:** 864–865.

21. NEZHAT, F., C. NEZHAT & E. PENNINGTON. 1992. Laparoscopic proctectomy for infiltrating endometriosis of the rectum. Fertil. Steril. **57:** 1129–1132.
22. NEZHAT, C., F. NEZHAT, E. PENNINGTON & C. H. NEZHAT. 1994. Laparoscopic partial colon resection and reanastomosis for deeply infiltrative endometriosis. Surg. Endosc. **8:** 682–685.
23. NEZHAT, C., F. NEZHAT & B. GREEN. 1992. Laparoscopic treatment of obstructed ureter due to endometriosis by resection and ureteroureterostomy. A case report. J. Urol. **148:** 865–868.
24. WALLIS, C. 1986. The career woman's disease? Time April **28:** 62.
25. CLARK, M. & G. CARROLL. 1986. Conquering endometriosis. Newsweek October **13:** 95.
26. COWLEY, G. 1990. Hanging up the knife. Newsweek February **12:** 58–59.
27. NEZHAT, C., F. NEZHAT, D. A. METZGER & A. A. LUCIANO. 1990. Adhesion reformation after reproductive surgery by videolaseroscopy. Fertil. Steril. **53**(6): 1008–1011.
28. Operative Laparoscopy Study Group. 1991. Postoperative adhesion development after operative laparoscopy: evaluation at early second-look procedures. Fertil. Steril. **55:** 700–704.
29. NEZHAT, C., F. NEZHAT & C. NEZHAT. 1992. Operative laparoscopy (minimally invasive surgery): state of the art. J. Gynecol. Surg. **8:** 111–141.
30. SMITH, M. S. 1991. Cystostomy and vesicostomy. *In* Urologic Surgery. 4th edit. J. F. Glenn, Ed. Lippincott. Philadelphia.
31. NEZHAT, F. & C. NEZHAT. 1993. Laparoscopic segmental bladder resection for endometriosis: a report of two cases. Obstet. Gynecol. **81:** 882–884.
32. DECHERNEY, A. & M. P. DIAMOND. 1987. Laparoscopic salpingostomy for ectopic pregnancy. Obstet. Gynecol. **70:** 948–950.
33. STANGEL, J. J. & V. GOMEL. Techniques in conservative surgery for tubal gestation. Clin. Obstet. Gynecol. **23:** 1221–1228.
34. NEZHAT, C. & F. NEZHAT. 1990. Conservative management of ectopic gestation, letter-to the editor. Fertil. Steril. **53:** 382–383.
35. NEZHAT, C., F. NEZHAT & M. BURRELL. 1992. Laparoscopically assisted hysterectomy for the management of a borderline ovarian tumor: a case report. J. Laparoendosc. Surg. **2:** 167–169.
36. NEZHAT, F., C. H. NEZHAT, D. ADMON, S. GORDON *et al.* 1994. Complications and results of 361 hysterectomies performed at laparoscopy. J. Am. Coll. Surg. Accepted for publication.
37. SUMMIT, R. L., T. G. STOVALL, F. W. LING & G. H. LIPSCOMB. 1992. Laparoscopic-assisted vaginal hysterectomy using endoscopic staples. American College of Obstetricians and Gynecologists, 40th Annual Clinical Meeting, April 25–30, 1992, Las Vegas, Nevada.
38. CANIS, M., G. MAGE, A. WATTIEZ, J. L. POULY, C. CHAPRON & M. A. BRUHAT. 1992. Vaginally assisted laparoscopic radical hysterectomy. J. Gynecol. Surg. **8:** 103–105.
39. CHILDERS, J., P. BRZECHFFA, K. HATCH & E. SURWIT. 1993. Laparoscopically assisted surgical staging (LASS) of endometrial cancer. Gynecol. Oncol. **51:** 33–38.
40. NEZHAT, C., F. NEZHAT, C. E. WELANDER & B. BENIGNO. 1992. Four ovarian cancers diagnosed during laparoscopic management of 1,011 adnexal masses. Am. J. Obstet. Gynecol. **167:** 790–796.
41. NEZHAT, C. 1989. Tenth Annual Baltimore-Washington Seminar & Tutorial, December 13–15, 1989.
42. NEZHAT, C. H., F. NEZHAT, C. NEZHAT & H. ROTTENBERG. 1994. Laparoscopic retropubic cystourethropexy: a preliminary study. Obstet. Gynecol. In press.
43. NEZHAT, C., F. NEZHAT, S. L. SILFEN, N. SCHAFFER & D. EVANS. 1991. Laparoscopic myomectomy. Int. J. Fertil. **36:** 275–280.
44. NEZHAT, C., F. NEZHAT, O. BESS & C. H. NEZHAT. 1993. Laparoscopically assisted myomectomy: a report of a new technique in 57 cases. Int. J. Fertil. Accepted for publication.
45. MAIMON, M., V. SELTZER & J. BOYCE. 1991. Laparoscopic excision of ovarian neoplasms subsequently found to be malignant. Obstet. Gynecol. **77:** 536–565.

46. NEZHAT, C., W. K. WINER & F. NEZHAT. 1988. Is endoscopic treatment of endometriosis and endometrioma associated with better results than laparotomy? Am. J. Gynecol. Health. **2**(3): 10–16.
47. HASSON, H. M. 1990. Laparoscopic management of ovarian cysts. J. Reprod. Med. **25**: 863–867.
48. NEZHAT, F., C. NEZHAT, C. ALLAN, D. METZGER *et al.* 1992. Clinical and histologic classification of endometriomas. J. Reprod. Med. **37**: 771–776.
49. NEZHAT, C. & F. NEZHAT. 1989. Safe laser excision or vaporization of peritoneal endometriosis. Fertil. Steril. **52**(1): 149–151.
50. NEZHAT, C. & F. NEZHAT. 1992. Operative laparoscopy for the management of ovarian remnant syndrome. Fertil. Steril. **57**: 1003–1007.
51. ROCK, J. A. 1991. Laparoscopic cautery in the treatment of endometriosis-related infertility. Fertil. Steril. **55**: 246–251.
52. NEZHAT, C. & F. NEZHAT. 1992. A simplified method of laparoscopic presacral neurectomy for the treatment of central pelvic pain due to endometriosis. Br. J. Obstet. Gynecol. **99**: 659–663.
53. NEZHAT, C., F. NEZHAT & E. PENNINGTON. 1992. Laparoscopic treatment of lower colorectal and infiltrative rectovaginal septum endometriosis by the technique of videolaseroscopy. Br. J. Obstet. Gynaecol. **99**: 664–667.
54. NEZHAT, F., W. K. WINER & C. NEZHAT. 1990. Fimbrioscopy and salpingoscopy in patients with minimal to moderate pelvic endometriosis. Obstet. Gynecol. **75**: 15–17.
55. GOMEL, V. & C. JAMES. 1991. Intraoperative management of ureteral injury during operative laparoscopy. Fertil. Steril. **55**: 416–419.
56. NEZHAT, C. & F. NEZHAT. 1992. Laparoscopic repair of resected ureter during operative laparoscopy to treat endometriosis. A case report. Obstet. Gynecol. **80**: 543–544.

# The Rationale for Use of Medical Suppressive Therapy Prior to Endoscopic Surgery

VEASY C. BUTTRAM, JR.[a]

*Baylor University College of Medicine*
*Houston, Texas*

Three modes of therapy are now available for the conservative management of endometriosis. They are surgery, medical suppression and a combination of surgery and medical suppression. The mode chosen will generally depend upon the severity of the disease and the magnitude of the symptoms (*i.e.*, infertility, dysmenorrhea, dyspareunia, etc.).

### *Surgery*

Until recently the usual treatment of endometriosis had been surgery through restoration of normal anatomy by excision, laser, or cautery of implants or endometriomas and often lysis of adhesions. During the past two decades the surgical route has been modified by using laparoscopic techniques, which allows much of the surgery to be performed by endoscopy.

There are several reasons why surgery alone may not be the best method of treatment. These include:

1. Postoperative adhesions which can cause infertility.
2. Endometriosis not removed because of fear of injury to a vital organ.
3. Non-visualized endometriosis. (It is speculated that microscopic disease is often left unattended.)
4. Health risks and pain.
5. Expense.

### *Medical Suppression*

Many different drugs have been used in the treatment of endometriosis. They include androgens, progestins, estrogen-progestin combinations, danazol, gestrinone, and more recently GnRH agonists. (The author has no experience with gestrinone and will confine his comments to the use of danazol and GnRH agonists.)

---

[a] Correspondence: Obstetrical & Gynecological Associates, P.A., 7550 Fannin, Houston, TX 77054-1989.

There are several reasons why medical therapy alone may not be as effective as desired including:

1. The temporizing nature of drug therapy. Endometrial implants and endometriomas tend to recur shortly after medical therapy has been discontinued.
2. Improvement of fertility is questionable.
3. The inability of medical therapy to affect dense adhesions (a part of the pathology of endometriosis).
4. Response variability (*i.e.*, not all patients respond *the same*).
5. Occasionally intolerable or possibly harmful side effect to the drug.
6. Expense.

## *Combined Medical Suppression and Surgery*

Pre- and postoperative medical suppression have been used for many years in the treatment of endometriosis. Some studies have indicated that this form of therapy in the infertile female results in a higher pregnancy rate than surgery or medical suppression alone.[1,2]

There are several reasons why combined therapy may not be as effective as desired including:

1. The same reasons that surgery alone may not be as effective as desired.
2. The same reasons that medical suppression alone may not be as effective as desired.
3. A combination mode of treatment generally requires two surgical procedures (*i.e.*, diagnostic laparoscopy followed by laparoscopic surgery or laparotomy after completion of medical suppression for 3–6 months).

Because a combination mode of therapy requires two surgical procedures, this form of treatment must be justified. It should be pointed out that:

1. To date no study has documented that medical suppression alone enhances the pregnancy rates regardless of the stage of the disease.
2. In several studies, surgery (both laparoscopic and laparotomy) has been shown to be effective in enhancing conception rates and the degree of surgical success is dependent upon the stage of the disease.[2-4]
3. When surgery has been unsuccessful it has been the author's observation that:
   a. Repeat laparoscopy often reveals persistent or new endometriosis. There is no way to prevent the development of new endometriosis, but more meticulous surgery will reduce persistent disease.
   b. Repeat laparoscopy often reveals severe adnexal adhesions, most likely a result of the surgery. One could conclude that the main reason surgery for endometriosis is less effective than desired is the development of postoperative adhesions. One major potential way to reduce the risk of postoperative adhesions is to treat the patient with medical suppression prior to surgery. (This is particularly true for patients with moderate or severe disease.) To provide the rationale for its use, a review of the pathophysiology of adhesions formation is needed.

## Pathophysiology of Adhesion Formation

The peritoneum is composed of two layers including a superficial layer of polygonal mesothelial cells and the submesothelial-stromal layer composed of connective tissue, collagen, reticular and elastic fibers which contains abundant vasculature and lymphatic structures.[5] Pelvic adhesions can be caused by anything that causes peritoneal tissue to be injured or inflamed. Thus, surgical trauma, infection, or noninfectious conditions such as endometriosis can cause adhesions to form. It has been postulated that such injuries to the peritoneal surface cause a disruption of stromal mast cells resulting in the release of histamine and vasoactive kinins.[5] These substances cause an increase in capillary permeability which leads to the formation of a serosanguinous exudate, which in turn results in deposition of fibrin. Under normal conditions, plasminogen activator is released which causes a release of plasmin resulting in fibrinolysis. Normal healing then occurs without adhesion formation.

In a hypoxic state the release of plasminogen activator is reduced.[5] With less plasminogen activator and plasmin, fibrinolysis is decreased. A fibrin matrix develops, with fibroblasts and capillary proliferating within the matrix in the usual manner of tissue healing leading to scar formation. This adhesion becomes permanent. More injury or inflammation results in an increased amount of fibrin deposition. A greater hypoxic state results in less fibrinolysis. The severity of the inflammation or injury determines the amount and density of the adhesions.

This model for pelvic adhesion formation may thus provide some insight into the etiology of pelvic adhesions associated with endometriosis. Theoretically the inflammation associated with endometriosis could initiate the exudative process leaving the formation of fibrin deposition. It is possible that the fibrin deposition is greater in patients with inflammation secondary to endometriosis because the normal fibrinolytic mechanisms are overwhelmed resulting in peritoneal adhesions. Although plausible, this possibility has not been examined.

## Preoperative Use of Medical Suppression Therapy

In a study conducted nearly 20 years ago a preoperative pseudopregnancy regimen was combined with surgery in an attempt to increase the pregnancy rates of patients with infertility attributed to endometriosis.[6] The rates were reduced. Although the exact reasons for the results remain unknown, the pseudopregnancy regimen may have created a pelvic environment wherein the surgery would more likely result in the development of postoperative adhesions. This pseudopregnancy state may result in increased capillary proliferation or vasodilation, both conditions conducive to trauma and increased fibrin deposition.

In 1982 we published a report on the efficacy of danazol in the treatment of endometriosis.[4] We noted that after six months of therapy, peritoneal disease tended to regress by about two thirds. Some patients (41%) had total resolution of the disease, whereas others (7%) experienced no effect of treatment. Ovarian disease regressed but to a lesser extent than did peritoneal disease. Large endometriomas were reduced minimally, but those <1 cm in diameter were, like peritoneal disease, decreased in size by approximately two thirds.

One finding from this study is clear. Six months of preoperative danazol treatment creates a pelvic environment much different from that of a pseudopregnant or normal ovulatory state. There is much less hyperemia in a hypoestrogenic state. Capillaries are less abundant and less dilatated. Inflammatory reaction is reduced making the identification of endometrial implants and/or endometriomas easier. (The author does not agree with the proposal that preoperative suppression therapy reduces endometrial implants to the extent that they or their remnants cannot be visualized. At initial laparoscopy, the endometriosis should be documented preferably by schematic pictures and photographs.) Following danazol treatment peritoneal fluids are not only diminished in quantity but appear clear suggesting less fibrin content. The ovaries are inactive. Easily traumatized functional cysts are absent. Endometriomas of the ovaries are easier to remove and can often be enucleated causing less trauma to the ovary than an excisive procedure. Adhesions also seem easier to lyse without trauma to adjacent tissue.

One can conclude that preoperative danazol creates a hypoestrogenic pelvic environment that significantly reduces the risk of postoperative adhesions. Although randomized control trials have not been performed to establish this contention, we are confident that it is the case. In addition, as Dmowski observed we found that filmy adhesions often disappear in patients taking danazol for six months. We postulated that danazol reduces the inflammatory process and that the motion of pelvic viscera lyses filmy adhesions.

In 1985 we reported that six months of preoperative danazol therapy resulted in a 12% improvement in pregnancy rates of patients with mild, moderate, and severe endometriosis.[2] This increase in pregnancy rates was attributed primarily to the improved pelvic environment and a reduction in postoperative adhesion formation. Other factors possibly contributing to the increased rates were the improvement in surgical skills or surgical adjuvants.

GnRH agonists produce a hypoestrogenic state (probably more than does danazol). Our observation has been that agonists have the same effect on the pelvic environment as does danazol. They also have a similar effect on endometriosis (implants, endometriomas, and adhesions). Currently, data substantiating higher pregnancy rates with the use of preoperative GnRH agonists over surgery alone are not available. However, we anticipate studies on this subject in the near future.

## *Length of Medical Treatment*

How long should danazol or GnRH agonist be used to create a pelvic environment which reduces the risk of postoperative adhesions? Is a three-month regimen sufficient? We have been studying this question for several years, and although a clear conclusion has not been reached, we believe that an improved pelvic environment is created after three months of therapy. However, there is less resolution of disease in 3 months after treatment compared to 6 months.

## *The Use of Postoperative Medical Suppression Therapy*

Some practitioners believe that medical suppressive therapy should be used postoperatively. In 1981 Wheeler and Malinak retrospectively analyzed surgical treatment of endometriosis with and without three to six months of danazol used postoperatively.[1] The patients who received danazol had a higher cumulative pregnancy rate than those who did not receive the drug. They concluded that postoperative danazol suppressed disease not completely removed at the time of surgery. This is logical. However, we know that medical therapy does not eradicate the disease and that temporary suppressive therapy will result in recurrence of the disease. The use of medical therapy preoperatively seems more logical since it creates a pelvis more amenable to surgical correction of endometriosis without as much risk of postoperative adhesions. In addition, it has its suppressive effect upon endometriosis as does postoperative therapy.

## CONCLUSION

In all cases of minimal and most cases of mild endometriosis the disease can be eradicated through the laparoscope with laser or cautery. The risk of postoperative adhesions is probably not sufficient to warrant medical suppressive therapy and a second surgical procedure. However, in some infertile patients with mild disease and *almost* all with moderate or severe disease, medical suppressive treatment followed by a second operation will result in an improved pregnancy rate.

## REFERENCES

1. WHEELER, J. & L. R. MALINAK. 1981. Postoperative danazol therapy in infertility patients with severe endometriosis. Fertil. Steril. **36:** 460.
2. BUTTRAM, V. C., R. C. REITER, S. M. WARD & R. N. WARD. 1985. Treatment of endometriosis with danazol: Report of a six-year prospective study. Fertil. Steril. **43:** 353.
3. BUTTRAM, V. C. 1979. Conservative surgery for endometriosis in the infertile female: a study of 206 patients with implications for both medical and surgical therapy. Fertil. Steril. **31:** 117.
4. BUTTRAM, V. C., J. B. BELUE & R. C. REITER. 1982. Interim report of a study of danazol for the treatment of endometriosis. Fertil. Steril. **37:** 478.
5. BUTTRAM, V. C. & R. C. REITER. 1985. Surgical Treatment of the Infertile Female. 69–72. Williams & Wilkens, Publishers.
6. ANDREWS, W. C. & G. D. LARSON. 1974. Endometriosis treatment with hormonal pseudopregnancy and/or operation. Am. J. Obstet. Gynecol. **118:** 643.

# Laparoscopic Myomectomy
## Operative Procedure and Results

JEAN-BERNARD DUBUISSON AND CHARLES CHAPRON[a]

*Service de Chirurgie Gynécologique du Professeur Dubuisson*
*Clinique Universitaire Baudelocque*
*C.H.U. Cochin Port-Royal*
*123, Boulevard Port-Royal*
*75014 Paris, France*

## INTRODUCTION

The indications for laparoscopic surgery have increased considerably over the past few years, thanks essentially to surgeons' growing expertise and technological improvements.[1-3] The many improvements to the equipment have permitted new techniques to be developed. Alongside the high quality videolaparoscopes and $CO_2$ lasers available, the importance of high frequency generators, irrigation/aspiration devices and certain disposable instruments should also be stressed. Myomectomy has recently become an indication for laparoscopic surgery.[3-5]

## OPERATIVE TECHNIQUE

### Surgical Equipment

In addition to the standard equipment required for any laparoscopic surgical procedure (automatically controlled insufflator, axial panoramic optics system, video system, irrigation and aspiration device) we find several other instruments are necessary when carrying out myomectomy. The monopolar hook provides coagulation and uterine section, with either a purely cutting action or accompanied by coagulation depending on the uterine vascularization. A bipolar coagulating wide-jawed forceps is essential to obtain perfect hemostasis. Two grasping forceps are often used to help when dissecting the myoma. A laparoscopic forceps with 10-mm jaws is used to provide traction on the myoma during enucleation. Laparoscopic suture equipment required for uterine closure comprises a laparoscopic needleholder, atraumatic grasping forceps without claws, and suture material. We use 10 cm of 3/0 vicryl with a straight needle 20 mm long, or on occasion 10 cm of 3/0 or 4/0 PDS with a 3/8 circle needle which can be introduced via a 10-mm trocar (Ethicon, Ethnor, France).

### Patient Setup

This should include the installation of a urinary catheter to be left in place until the end of the operation, together with a rigid cannula of the vacurette 8

---

[a] Reprint request and correspondence: Doctor Charles Chapron.

type placed in the uterine cavity. This enables optimum exposure of the uterus. For example, when dealing with a posterior fibroma, the uterus is anteverted using the cannula. After installing the laparoscope at the umbilicus, three supra pubic routes must be ensured: two lateral 5-mm trocars located outside the epigastric vessels, and a 10-mm trocar on the midline. The latter will serve to introduce the 10-mm grasping forceps and the curved needles. Where these three suprapubic torcars should be placed relative to the pubis depends on the volume of the uterus: the bigger the uterus the higher the trocars need to be. Finally, when the patient is of childbearing age, we carry out a methylene blue test. This enables the endometrium to be stained (except in women under LHRH treatment), thus facilitating submucosal dissection of intramural myomas without opening the cavity, and suture of the myometrium when the cavity is opened.

## *Myomectomy*

Proper exposure of the myomas is crucial and is facilitated by the uterine cannulation. When looking for intramural myomas, it is important to identify the slightest hump and investigate any asymmetry relative to the round ligaments. In the case of a myoma on the broad ligament or posterior to the isthmus, it is important to locate the ureter. The technique is relatively simple for a pedunculated myoma, consisting simply of coagulating and sectioning the pedicle. Once complete hemostasis has been achieved, no suture is generally needed.

Intramural myomas or pedunculated myomas with a broad base require hysterotomy level with the myoma. The incision is usually vertical, although it may be horizontal. We use the monopolar hook, and the bipolar forceps for additional hemostasis of the myometrium vessels. We do not use any vasoconstrictor agents. Once the myoma has been located, it is grasped using the grasping forceps, then traction on the myoma exposes the cleavage plane. The hook is used for dissection. In the case of a myoma located on the broad ligament, it can be an advantage to start dissection anteriorly by sectioning the round ligament.

## *Closing the Uterus*

After first ensuring perfect hemostasis, we close the uterus by suturing along a seromuscular plane (most often with straight needles swaged to 10-cm suture material). This is usually achieved using separate intraperitoneal knots. It is easier to take the suture material through with a straight needle, and intraperitoneal knots reduce the risk of tearing the myometrium when the knot is tied. Under certain circumstances, however, curved needles and extra corporeal knots are used.

## *Extracting the Myoma*

Two different techniques can be used for this. The suprapubic route is suitable for small or medium sized myomas only (<3 cm). The midline trocar is removed and a tenaculum forceps introduced under laparoscopic control. The myoma is grasped and brought up to the opening in order to avoid $CO_2$ leakage. Then, depending on the size, the myoma is fragmented using a cold knife, small retractors and another tenaculum forceps. Once all the fragments of myoma have been removed, the incision is closed along two planes.

For obvious aesthetic reasons, this technique is destined for myomas of moderate size. For large myomas (>3 cm) a posterior colpotomy is preferable. The myoma is taken down into the Pouch of Douglas; the latter is made to bulge using a laparoscopic forceps thus making it easier to open. Next the myoma is grasped using a tenaculum forceps after which it may be necessary to reduce it to fragments. The vagina is then closed using the standard technique. The colpotomy can also be carried out via laparoscopy using the monopolar hook: a vaginal compress placed in the posterior cul de sac makes the incision easier to achieve.

Finally, when the suprapubic incision or colpotomy is closed, the use of laparoscopy enables a careful peritoneal cleansing to be carried out together with a check that there is no bleeding. No suction drains are left in place.

## DISCUSSION

Endoscopic surgery and preoperative treatment using LHRH agonists have resulted in changes in the operative techniques for myomectomy. When fibromas give rise to symptoms indicating surgery, it is important to know how many there are, where they are and how big they are when endoscopic surgery is planned, in order to keep the risk of recurrence to a minimum.[6] Pelvic ultrasonography can provide this essential information. Diagnostic hysteroscopy completes the workup for women suffering from menometrorrhagia, when there are multiple myomas, in cases of sterility or endouterine abnormalities revealed during ultrasonography and hysterography.

Laparoscopic surgery can be envisaged for subserosal or intramural myomas.[4]

A number of publications have confirmed the advantages of using LHRH agonists to reduce the volume of myomas. They make conservative surgery easier when surgery is indicated. This is because the LHRH agonists reduce uterine vascularization by hypoestrogenia and consequently also reduce preoperative bleeding.[11] It takes about 8 to 12 weeks for the effects of agonist treatment to become obvious.[8] Preoperative treatment with agonists is indicated essentially for large fibromas which Doppler ultrasonography has shown to be highly vascularized.

Our experience demonstrates that laparoscopic myomectomy can be carried out perfectly safely, provided certain conditions are respected which basically concern the volume and number of myomas. Laparoscopic myomectomy can be carried out without risk when the number of myomas is, for myomas of at least 4 cm, less than 4. In excess of this, the bleeding and duration of the operation go against laparoscopy. It has now been amply proved that laparoscopic myomectomy is feasible.[3-5] In most cases it is not difficult to enucleate the myoma. However, we did come across two problems in obtaining cleavage (2%) and had to have recourse to laparotomy. One of these cases was an adenomyoma.

One of the special points in this technique is the use of intraperitoneal sutures for closing the uterus. This should be considered when dealing with a deep intramural myoma. Suturing gives extra hemostasis action and helps prevent the uterus from becoming fragile. On the other hand, when dealing with a superficial subserous myoma, there is no need to suture if hemostasis has been achieved by electrocoagulation. If it is decided to proceed with a uterine suture, it must be carried out with great care especially if the patient desires pregnancy later. We have observed no ruptures of the uterus in our series. Nevertheless, a case of uterine rupture at the end of pregnancy was reported recently.[12] We feel the risk of uterine rupture following laparoscopic myomectomy is slight but needs to be assessed by larger studies.

Pelvic adhesions after myomectomy are a problem which needs to be looked at, especially in women of childbearing age, and all the more so in that a certain proportion of women with myomas suffer from infertility which can be explained by no other cause.[13] The risk of postmyomectomy adhesions after laparoscopic surgery is low for our series (2/17). These preliminary results again need confirming by larger studies.

In conclusion we can state that laparoscopic myomectomy as a technique presents distinct advantages, with no risk if the patients are rigorously selected. Larger studies should ensure a more precise assessment of the indications and clarify the technique even further.

## SUMMARY

Myomectomy was performed by laparoscopy in 102 patients, according to a precise technique using the monopolar hook for the uterine incision and intraperitoneal sutures.

Myomas were mostly removed through the suprapubic puncture site after fragmentation or by colpotomy. Conversion to laparotomy during the laparoscopic procedure was necessary in 2 cases. No complications were observed. A second-look laparoscopy was performed in 17 cases. Postoperative adhesions were noted in 2 cases. In our experience, operative laparoscopy has several advantages over laparotomy and the risk of complications is low in selected cases.

## REFERENCES

1. BRUHAT, M. A., H. MANHES, J. CHOUKROUN & F. SUZANNE. Essai de traitement per coelioscopique de la grossesse extra-utérine. A propos de 26 observations. Rev. Fr. Gynécol. Obstét. **72:** 667–672.
2. MURPHY, A. A. 1987. Operative laparoscopy. Fertil. Steril. **47:** 1–18.
3. SEMM, K. & L. METTLER. 1980. New techniques in advanced laparoscopic surgery. Ballière's Clin. Obstet. Gynecol. C. J. C. Sutton, Ed. **138:** 121–127.
4. DUBUISSON, J. B., F. LECURU, H. FOULOT, L. MANDELBROT, F. X. AUBRIOT & M. MOULY. 1992. Myomectomy by laparoscopy: a preliminary report of 43 cases. Fertil. Steril. **56:** 827–830.
5. NEZHAT, C., F. NEZHAT, S. SILFEN, N. SCHEFFER & D. EVANS. 1991. Laparoscopic myomectomy. Int. Fertil. **36:** 275–280.
6. FEDELE, L., P. VERCELLIN, S. BIANCHI, D. BRIOSCHI & M. DORTA. 1990. Treatment with GnRH agonists before myomectomy and the risk of short-term myoma recurrence. Br. J. Obstet. Gynaecol. **97:** 393–396.
7. LUMSDEN, M. A., C. P. WEST & D. T. BAIRD. 1987. Goserelin therapy before surgery for uterine fibroids. Lancet **1:** 36.
8. FRIEDMAN, A. J., D. HARRISON-ATLAS, R. L. BARBIERI et al. 1989. A randomized, placebo-controlled, double-blind study evaluating the efficacy of leuprolide acetate depot in the treatment of uterine leiomyomata. Fertil. Steril. **51:** 251–256.
9. FRIEDMAN, A. J., M. S. REIN, D. HARRISON-ATLAS, J. M. GARFIELD & P. M. DOUBILET. 1989. A randomized placebo-controlled, double-blind study evaluating leuprolide acetate depot treatment before myomectomy. Fertil. Steril. **52:** 728–733.

10. SHAW, R. W. 1989. Mechanism of LHRH analogue action in uterine fibroids. Horm. Res. **32:** 150–153.
11. MATTA, W. H. M., I. STABILE, R. W. SHAW & S. CAMPBELL. 1988. Doppler assessment of uterine blood flow changes in patients with fibroids receiving the gonadotropin-releasing hormone agonist Buserelin. Fertil. Steril. **49:** 1083–1085.
12. HARRIS, W. H. 1992. Uterine dehiscence following laparoscopic myomectomy. Obstet. Gynecol. **80:** 545–546.
13. COHEN, J., J. B. COCHINI & V. LOFFREDO. 1981. Cent sept myomectomies: relations avec la fertilité. Gynécologie **32:** 43.

# Endoscopic Treatment of Dermoid Cyst

MAURIZIO ROSATI

*Clinique et Maternité Sainte-Elisabeth*
*Service de Gynécologie*
*(Chef de Service P. Degeest)*
*Place Louise Godin, 15*
*5000 Namur, Belgium*

## INTRODUCTION

Benign cystic teratoma (dermoid cyst) accounts for 10–20% of ovarian neoplasms,[1] with one estimate up to 44%, according to a 10-year retrospective review of 861 women treated for ovarian neoplasm.[2]

It is also the most common teratoma, with highest prevalence in ovulating women.[3] Both ovaries are involved in 10–15% of cases.[4]

Ovarian torsion, infection and rupture have been reported as the most frequent complications of dermoid cyst.[1,5,6]

Malignant degeneration is possible in 1–2% of cases,[1,4,5,7] or in 0.3% of cases according to a recent review of 286 teratomas[5] (TABLE 1).

Laparotomic cystectomy or oophorectomy has been the traditional management of dermoid cyst. Laparoscopic oophorectomy with culdotomy extraction has been described as an option when a woman does not desire future fertility and has a normal controlateral ovary; in these cases spillage has been directed through the culdotomy incision.[8,9]

More recently, Reich and colleagues described techniques to excise large cysts without spillage while preserving the ovary, including the use of an impermeable bag to enclose the cyst or ovary prior to withdrawal.[10]

This report assesses the efficacy of laparoscopic cystectomy or oophorectomy and confirms the safety of an impermeable bag to enclose the teratoma prior to decompression and removal.

## MATERIALS AND METHODS

For 10 months, from September 1992 to June 1993, 66 women were treated for adnexal cyst, most of whom were diagnosed by vaginal ultrasound at "Clinique et Maternité Sainte-Elisabeth" of Namur in Belgium. Thirteen of the 66 had laparotomic treatment; 2 of them for benign cystic teratoma (the first for unilateral teratoma 15 cm in diameter, the second for bilateral teratoma, the larger measuring 12 cm in diameter; both cases had an associated uterine myoma).

Fifty-three of the 66 cases underwent laparoscopic management. For 7 of them the diagnosis was dermoid cyst and in these cases, after excision, an impermeable bag was used in order to avoid spillage during evacuation (TABLE 2).

The average age of the 7 women laparoscopically managed was 33 (range, 20–45).

TABLE 1. Dermoid Cysts: Epidemiological Data

| | | |
|---|---|---|
| | Frequence | 10–44% |
| | Bilaterality | 10–15% |
| | Complications | |
| | Torsion | 7–10% |
| | Infection | 2.5% |
| | Rupture | 3.8% |
| | Malignancy | 0.3–2% |

Prior to surgery, 4 patients had appreciable pelvic mass confirmed by vaginal ultrasound; in 2 cases a dermoid cyst was incidentally discovered by vaginal ultrasound at the time of a routine check-up; in 1 case of infertility, the teratoma was detected by hysterosalpingography and a pelvic mass was confirmed by vaginal ultrasound. CA 125s were obtained in 5 cases; all were negative.

Of 4 women with appreciable pelvic mass, one a 45 year old with a mass about 8 cm in diameter, required CT scan and CA 125, as the findings of ultrasound were doubtful. Neither calcifications nor adipose tissue were found in the lesion at the CT scan and the CA 125 was normal. In this case a unilateral adnexectomy was performed. A "struma ovarii" formed by multiple colloid cysts was found on microscopic examination.

In all seven cases the teratoma was unilateral.

## SURGICAL TECHNIQUES

Laparoscopy under general anesthesia was performed in all cases, the pelvis and abdomen were carefully inspected and the ovaries were evaluated for visual evidence of malignancy.

Cystectomy without spillage was accomplished by using the $CO_2$ laser at 20 watts in continuous mode to vaporize a superficial incision through the ovarian cortex, avoiding rupture of the underlying cyst wall.

Spillage occurred in 1 case, when electrosurgical electrodes were used to perform the incision, consistent with the findings of Reich and colleagues.[10]

After locating the cleavage plane between the cyst wall and the ovarian cortex, aquadissection and forceps traction were used to separate the dermoid cyst from surrounding ovarian tissue. Laser was used to vaporize fibrous adherences and vessels near the hilum.

TABLE 2. Adnexal Cysts Treated between September 1992 and June 1993

| | No. Patients | No. Cysts | No. Dermoid Cysts |
|---|---|---|---|
| Vaginal ultrasound diagnosis | 66 | 75 | 10[a] |
| Laparotomic treatment | 13 | 15 | 3[b] |
| Laparoscopic-minilaparotomic treatment | 10 | 12 | 1 |
| Laparoscopic treatment | 43 | 48 | 6 |

[a] 9 patients, 13.3%.
[b] 2 patients.

TABLE 3. Technical Modalities of Laparoscopic Surgery for 7 Dermoid Cysts between 5 and 9 cm in Diameter

|  | No. Cases | No. Unruptured Cysts | No. Ruptured Cysts |
|---|---|---|---|
| Excision |  |  |  |
| Annexectomy | 1 | 1 | — |
| Cystectomy | 6 | 5 | 1 |
| Extraction |  |  |  |
| Within the bag | 6 |  |  |
| Without bag | 1 |  |  |
| By minilaparotomy | 1 |  |  |
| By culdotomy | 6 |  |  |

In one case, following excision of the intact cyst from inside the ovary, electrosurgical fulguration was necessary to obtain complete hemostasis inside the ovary.

The edges were reapproximated, so that suturing was not required.

In these 6 cases (5 cyst excision, 1 adnexectomy) an impermeable bag, 10 cm in diameter, was pushed into the peritoneal cavity through the 12-mm umbilical trocar of the laparoscope. The free, intact specimen was placed in the bag, which was closed by pulling the drawstring. Then a culdotomy incision 1 cm in diameter was performed. The drawstring and the edge of the bag were withdrawn through the incision in the posterior vagina; the tip of a finger was inserted into the opened edges of the bag through the vaginal incision in order to touch the surface of the cyst; then, under finger control the smooth tip of a Menghini needle was pushed onto the cyst surface and its sharp tip pierced the cyst wall.

Cyst decompression and removal was obtained in 3 cases by aspirating through the Menghini needle in a syringe about 100 cc of fluid (colloid tissue in one case); in the remainder of cases the cyst contents were drained by introducing small atraumatic forceps to fragment the cyst.

The culdotomy incision was then closed vaginally with a single cross suture by using 0 dexon II (Davis Geck, Cyanamid, Leuven, Belgium) on a curved needle.

In the one case where the spillage occurred, a minilaparotomy and direct aspiration of fatty and epithelial element by a large suction cannula was quickly performed; the cyst was pulled out of the abdominal wall and the ovary repaired using microsurgical techniques. At the end of the procedure the minilaparotomy was sutured and the abdominal cavity was inspected laparoscopically, removing the remaining fatty tissue in order to prevent chronic granulomatous reaction, as recommended by Audebert and colleagues.[11]

## RESULTS

A summary of results of surgery is shown in TABLE 3.

Operating time averaged 123 minutes (range, 90–180). No postoperative complications occurred. Six patients were ready to be discharged on day 1. One patient was discharged on day 2 after surgery, because of the minilaparotomy.

## DISCUSSION

A variety of techniques can be employed to manage ovarian dermoid cyst, depending on the patient's desire for future fertility and the surgeon's skill and confidence.[10]

Laparoscopy is a surgical method which has been successfully used for the excision of ovarian teratomas; but the most delicate stage in the operation is extraction of the cyst, especially when it is large and has an important solid component. Spillage from dermoid cyst should be avoided not only to reduce the risk of a granulomatous reaction, but also in recognition of the possibility of malignant elements occurring within the teratoma.[12]

## CONCLUSION

This series demonstrates that endoscopic treatment of dermoid cyst by using a bag during the culdotomy evacuation is an effective and safe method with good surgical outcome in all cases, even when voluminous cysts were removed.

## SUMMARY

Seven cases of benign cystic teratoma (dermoid cyst) were managed laparoscopically (six cyst excisions and one adnexectomy) using a surgical procedure to avoid spillage.

Outcome was good in all cases without any complications.

## ACKNOWLEDGMENTS

Thanks are due to Dr. P. Degeest, Dr. J.-P. Delforge, Dr. A. Godart, Dr. Ph. Goffin, and Dr. N. Royer for their contributions.

## REFERENCES

1. PETERSON, W. F., E. C. PREVOST, T. T. EDMUNDS, J. M. HANDLEY & F. K. MORRIS. 1955. Benign cystic teratomas of the ovary: a clinico-statistical study of 100 cases with a review of the literature. Am. J. Obstet. Gynaecol. **70:** 368.
2. KOONINGS, P. P., K. CAMPBELL, D. R. MISHELL & D. A. GRIMES. 1989. Relative frequency of primary ovarian neoplasm. A 10-year review. Obstet. Gynaecol. **74:** 291.
3. GERALD, P. S. 1975. Origin of teratomas. N. Engl. J. Med. **292:** 103.
4. MATZ, M. H. 1961. Benign cystic teratoma of the ovary. A review. Obstet. Gynaecol. Surv. **16:** 591.
5. AYHAN, A., T. AKSU, O. DEVEGLIOGLU, S. TUNCER & A. AYHANA. 1991. Complications and bilaterality of mature ovarian teratomas (clinicopathological evaluation of 286 cases). Aust. N.Z. Obstet. Gynaecol. **31:** 33.
6. HOLDSTWORTH, K. J., A. A. MCCULLOCH & I. D. DUNCAN. 1990. Mucinous ascite associated with rupture of benign ovarian teratoma. Case report. Br. J. Obstet. Gynaecol. **97:** 952.
7. CRISTOPHERSON, W. A. & R. B. COUNCEL. 1989. Malignant degeneration of a mature ovarian teratoma. Int. J. Gynaecol. Obstet. **30:** 379.

8. REICH, H. 1987. Laparoscopic oophorectomy and salpingo-oophorectomy in the treatment of benign tubo ovarian disease. Int. J. Fertil. **32:** 233.
9. LEVINE, R. L. 1990. Pelviscopic surgery in women over 40. J. Reprod. Med. **35:** 597.
10. REICH, H., F. MCGLYNN, L. SEKEL & P. TAYLOR. 1992. Laparoscopic management of ovarian dermoid cyst. J. Reprod. Med. **37:** 640.
11. AUDEBERT, A. J. M., K. GAAFAR & CL. EMPERAIRE. 1993. Traitement par coeliochirurgie des kystes dermoides. A propos d'une serie de 33 kystes. J. Gynécol. Obstet. Biol. Reprod. **22:** 27.
12. SHIRLEY, R. L., A. J. PIRO & D. W. CROCKER. 1971. Malignant neural elements in a benign cystic teratoma. Obstet. Gynaecol. **37:** 402.

# Therapeutic Strategy in Tubal Infertility

FRANÇOIS AUDIBERT

*Service de Gynécologie Obstérique*
*Hopital Arnaud de Villeneuve*
*555 route de Ganges*
*34059 Cedex Montpellier, France*

*and*

*24 rue Thiers*
*13100 Aix en Provence, France*

## INTRODUCTION

During the last fifteen years, many changes have occurred in the treatment of the tubal lesions which are responsible for tubal infertility.

Developed by several physicians during the sixties, particularly by Doctors Palmer,[1] Winston,[2] and Gomel,[3] conventional surgery was later improved by the use of the microscope, which produced more accuracy and less trauma. But, whatever the type of surgery, results were strongly correlated with tubal mucosal potential, and only an average of 30% of all patients were able to obtain a child by these methods.

New therapeutic possibilities have been introduced with *in vitro* fertilization (IVF). Initially IVF was applied only to patients in whom microsurgery had failed. However, with improving pregnancy rates, IVF has become a possible first therapeutic choice.

Since 1987, endoscopic surgery has also been increasingly promoted as an effective treatment for tubal lesions.

In this article we give an overview of all the treatment procedures available in tubal pathology, and try to define the most effective current strategy.

## METHODS

### Microsurgery

Conventional surgery and then microsurgery became widespread during the eighties. Different prognoses[4] were established depending on the type of tubal lesions and the location of the lesion in the tube.

### Restoration of Ligated Tubes

The most successful results in a large number of patients were obtained in the restoration of ligated tubes. An average of 50 to 80% intrauterine pregnancy rates was obtained after 2 years of attempts with a 2 to 4% rate of ectopic pregnancies. These rates reflect that the surgery is performed on a normal tube simply blocked by clips or knotted with a functional mucosa. In addition, this surgery is usually performed on isthme with the least removal of isthmic tissue, pregnancy rates being directly proportional to isthmic tubal length.

## Proximal Tubal Pathology

Results were different when surgery was performed for tubal proximal pathology. The pregnancy rates expected with microsurgery were about 30 to 50% intrauterine pregnancies and 6% ectopic pregnancies. The results[5] were the same whether surgery was interstitiel, cornual or very proximal isthmic.

With microsurgery on proximal lesion, we can expect half the number of intrauterine pregnancies and twice as many ectopic pregnancies.

Suture technique, permeability obtained and the state of proximal and distal mucosae all explain results which, while varying, are still very acceptable.

## Distal Tubal Pathology

When we consider distal pathology, results depend on the severity of the distal tube pathology.[6] Effectively, for fimbrioplasty, intrauterine pregnancy rates are 50%, and ectopic pregnancy 12%. However, when the tube is closed and a salpingoplasty must be performed, intrauterine pregnancies decrease to 35 to 40%, and ectopic pregnancies remain at 12%.

This means that when the patient becomes pregnant after distal surgery, there is a 25% chance that the pregnancy will be ectopic.

Results are directly correlated with tubal mucosa and ciliary epithelium.

When the lesion is a phimosis, the mucosa is still present and efficient by tubal serosae progressively surrounds the fimbria.

When the lesion is a hydrosalpinx, the mucosa disappears progressively, replaced by thick inefficient serosa. In this case, the ectopic pregnancy rate is not higher because the reopened tube is totally inefficient.

## Proximal and Distal Tubal Pathology

Some times proximal and distal surgery were performed on the same tube, with 10% intrauterine and 10% extrauterine pregnancy rates. The low rate of intrauterine pregnancies explains why this technique is no longer used.

Reestablishment of tubal patency does not necessarily indicate the possibility of pregnancy if the lesions are very deep. In another sense, the lack of function protects against ectopic pregnancy.

## Iterative Tubal Surgery

When surgery was repeated on the same tube, the average rate of intrauterine pregnancy was 20% and ectopic pregnancy 10%. The excessive rate of ectopic pregnancy explains why this type of surgery is no longer used.

## Conclusion

The large quantity of statistics available has allowed physicians to define a strategy for the microsurgical treatment of tubal lesions and has indicated that the proper indications for this surgery are ligated tubes or tubes with proximal lesions. This procedure is no longer indicated in distal pathology.

## Endoscopy

Endoscopy has brought simplifications to surgical techniques, permitting tubal evaluation and treatment during the same procedure, short hospitalization and minimal physical trauma. But the challenge of the last eighteen years has been to demonstrate that this technique results in similar chances of pregnancy, as compared with microsurgery.

Different endoscopic techniques have been proposed, depending on the location of tubal pathology. For proximal pathologies, several authors have tested the efficacy of classic intraabdominal laparoscopy. One of them, Madalenat, in 1989 performed the technique on 6 previously ligated patients. After removal of the obstacle and reopening of the tube, a plastic guide was passed through the tube. Correction was performed by glue, and the guide was removed several days later. No pregnancy occurred, but in 3 cases tubes were patent on hysterography after 6 months. Much more interesting was the utilization of catheterization using hysteroscopy.

For distal surgery, results were very successful and progressively eliminated the use of microsurgery for this indication. Tuboscopy, widely used by some physicians, allows screening of the ampulla.

### Catheterization under Hysteroscopic Control

Over the last several years, one of the more exciting endoscopic techniques for proximal pathology has been developed: catheterization under hysteroscopic control.

The removal of an obstruction in the tube was previously done by tubal insufflation with gas under high pressure, and later by selective salpingography with direct introduction of liquid and placement of a catheter into the tube. Progressively, technological evolution permitted the physician to pass this catheter under hysteroscopic control.

*Technique.* Some aspects of the technique should be emphasized:

The patient must be under general anesthesia.

Hysteroscopy may be performed with different media: $CO_2$, glycocol or physiological serum under pressure control (<180 mmHg).

The preferred transfer set is the Jansen-Anderson catheter from Cook Laboratories. It consists of a catheter guide with a mouth and a round top, which allows an atraumatic tubal ostium catheterization; a metallic guide which is introduced into the catheter guide for more rigidity; and the catheter with an external diameter of 1.05 mm and an internal diameter of 0.74 mm. Introduced, its top extends 2.5 cm above the catheter guide.

The catheter is introduced close to the hysteroscope after global endometrial and tubal sphincter evaluation. Several steps must be followed:

a) the catheter guide is brought close to the ostium;
b) then, the metallic guide is eased a little to give a smooth and normal curve to the catheter guide, which is introduced with its round top into the ostium;

c) the metallic guide is removed completely and the smooth catheter is replaced through the proximal lesions;
d) after filling it with a syringe of water to give rigidity, the catheter is pushed into the tube.

*Results.*[7] The failure of rate is about 10%, due to fibrosis, polyps or synechis of the ostium.

When catherization is "apparently" successful, about 80% of tubes are effectively reopened.

After 6 months, about 30% of successfully catheterized tubes again become blocked.

The pregnancy rate is about 25%, mostly in the first 6 months of exposure.

The ectopic pregnancy rate is low, about 3%.

Compared with microsurgery, results seem to be poorer. But we must remember that catheterization is a very recent technique with limited statistics, and control of the distal tube is not always known and depends on laparoscopy.

*Complications, Failure, Contraindications.* The main complication of this technique is an 8% rate of proximal tubal perforation. The prognosis seems to be good, because a pregnancy was described after perforation. However, when perforation occurs, the physician usually stops the catherization and the tube remains closed.

Some parameters explain the failure of the technique such as previous microsurgery, which tends to result in low tubal patency and a high rate of ectopic pregnancy, previous ectopic pregnancy and previous pelvic infection, with a higher risk of reobstruction (60%).

There are three contraindications to this technique: proximal and distal pathology on the same tube; a proximal nodule, which causes high risk of tubal perforation and of re-occlusion, and distal isthmic pathology.

Finally, the indications for catheterization depend on occlusion histology: a) tubal obstruction may be due to mud or mucosae agglutination (40%) in which case, catheterization will be very successful; b) on the contrary, failure seems to be mostly due to severe tubal lesions (60%) with a high risk of reobstruction.

However, most of the time there is no way of knowing in advance which type of histology we are dealing with. But, because there is a more than 50% chance of opening the tube, even in the presence of severe pathology, this technique appears to us to be important for the first attempt. This is a simple technique which does not preclude classic microsurgery in case of failure.

## Laparoscopy for Distal Pathology

More widespread at present is the use of endoscopy in distal pathology. Both techniques, microsurgery and endoscopy, have shown that the prognosis after surgery depends on tubal status. The technique is variable, and depends on the severity of distal occlusion.

*Technique.* In case of phimosis, the forceps is introduced into the luminal tube and removed, opened slightly, to allow section of the peritoneal serosa. When the lumen is closed, the tube is filled with blue liquid and the ostium located. A new fimbria is formed with sections from the ostium and eversion is fixed by low coagulation, either by electricity or laser, at 1 cm from the fimbria. The quality of the mucosa is critical to the ease of eversion.

**TABLE 1.**


*Classification.* Because of the importance of tubal status, some authors have proposed various classifications. We use the French system (TABLE 1), with criteria of fimbrial permeability, mucosal quality, and thickness of the tubal wall. Four stages are proposed function of scores.

*Results.* Many authors have published rather similar results of distal endoscopy. TABLE 2 gives the results of Professeur Bruhat[8] from Clermont Ferrand published in 1990. Some differences in pregnancy rates between microsurgery and endoscopy in stages I and II disappeared when the number of subjects increased and after normal fertility exposure.

The rate of ectopic pregnancies was almost the same with both techniques, and in stages III and IV, results are very poor.

Since endoscopy can be performed during the initial laparoscopic evaluation, there is no longer a place for microsurgery in distal tubal infertility.

## Transfimbria Tuboscopy

Salpingoscopy, or transfimbria tuboscopy, promoted by Doctors Cornier,[9] Henri Suchet[10] and Brossens, is not often used by endoscopists, probably due to the longer duration of this technique, the cost of material and the belief by many physicians that hysterography is sufficient for evaluating the state of tubal mucosa.

However, tuboscopy is the only means of evaluating the state of tubal mucosa and intraampullary lesions. Tuboscopy allows the section of adhesions, the freeing of syncheses of ampullar folds, biopsies, and the removal of polyps.

In a study done by Cornier on a group of 171 patients with unexplained infertility, about 37% of the patients had intraluminal pathology with no proof on hysterography. A pregnancy rate of 72% was obtained after treatment of intraampullary adhesions.

## Transcervical Tuboscopy

Recently developed, and still to be evaluated, is transcervical tuboscopy. The essential part of this technique is due to the development of optic fibers, thin enough to pass through the length of proximal tube and allowing, with a water flash system and video, an ampullary exploration. The cost of optic fiber remains a problem.

**TABLE 2.**

TABLE 3.

### Recanalization under Fluoroscopic Evaluation

After microsurgery and endoscopy, tubal recanalization under fluoroscopic evaluation is a well-known technique, with studies of more than 200 patients published. The first attempt was performed in 1977 with a bronchial catheter.[11]

*Technique.* This technique is similar to hysteroscopic catheterization, but with some particularities: no anesthesia is necessary; recanalization is performed at the same time as hysterography; the method can easily be repeated; and ultrasonographic control of catheterization can be used.

*Results.* An evaluation of different types of obstruction is possible:
In 70% of cases, a simple injection of contrast medium allows tubal opacification and permeability. We can assume that the abnormality of the tubes consists of amorphous debris or light adhesions.
In 30% of cases, proximal obstruction persists. Guide and catheter are advanced into the tube and an attempt is made to remove the obstruction with short back-and-forth movements of the guide wire. The abnormalities of the tubes in these cases are mostly due to endometriosis or salpingitis. Some practitioners add to this technique a transcervical balloon tuboplasty, but the tubes can be perforated or otherwise damaged.

### In Vitro *Fertilization*

Another method is *in vitro* fertilization, which has changed completely the prognosis of tubal infertility, particularly when the tube is in poor condition.

*Prognosis.* Compared with other infertility groups,[12] tubal infertility (TABLE 3) is characterized by about the same mean number of pregnancies per harvest (18%) and transfer (22%).
If we consider the pregnancy rate per embryo transferred, we are surprised to find a significantly lower pregnancy rate for 2, 3, 4 and more embryos transferred in tubal infertility than in unexplained infertility.

*Role of the Tube on Prognosis.* With the idea that tubal pathology could decrease the embryo implantation, we did a retrospective study (results not published) of patients involved in IVF in our center over a period of 2 years. Criteria for inclusion in the study were tubal infertility with tubes closed (proximal and/or distal) bilateral or unique, the patient less than 40 years old and less than 3 IVF attempts. In some cases, both tubes had previously been removed. One hundred and fifty-six IVF attempts were retained for the study.
Results were interesting with a pregnancy rate per transfer, and per embryo transferred somewhat low in distal pathology (22% and 8.4%). Proximal pathology

(35% and 14%) plays the same role as salpingectomy (34% and 13.8%), with high incidence of embryo implantation.

This study does not constitute a proof of interaction between tube and endometrium, particularly when there is tubal pathology such as distal occlusion. The best results were obtained in the presence of a proximal lesion or after salpingectomy. These findings represent an area for further research. The correlation of salpingectomy to IVF results has still to be demonstrated.

In our team, the idea of clipping or removing the tube when pathology is important is discussed after 3 IVF attempts have been performed without results.

## *GnRH Agonist*

Proximal tubal obstruction associated with salpingitis isthmica nodosa is a known complication of endometriosis. In contrast to surgical approaches, some authors are trying to evaluate a medical approach using ovarian suppression with a long-acting agonist of GnRH.

*Materials and Methods.* In a recent study performed by de Ziegler,[13] 6 women suffering from endometriosis documented by laparoscopy with bilateral proximal tubal obstruction received 3 months of therapy with GnRH agonist and underwent a new evaluation of their status. No distal pathology was found in this group.

*Results.* Hysterographic control showed that all patients had at least one tube reopened.

Fourteen hyperstimulation cycles were performed after the GnRH therapy, with a 29% pregnancy rate per cycle and 67% per patient.

Because of the limited number of patients no conclusion can be drawn, but GnRH agonist could represent a good alternative for proximal lesions in endometriosis.

The successful use of Danatrol in proximal pathology as a treatment of choice before microsurgery was described by Professor Tran in 1980.

## SUMMARY

The foregoing description of various methodologies reveals how rich and evolutive the possibilities are for treating tubal disease with a rational approach. Different solutions are possible.

### *Proximal Pathology without Distal Pathology*

The isthmic lumen can be obstructed or permeable with pathology.

If obstructed, the first approach is catheterization, hysteroscopic or fluoroscopic.

If permeable with diverticula, polyp or irregularity, indications can be GnRH agonist, catheterization, or microsurgery as a last resort.

When patency is obtained, a pregnancy is a normal consequence, but after a one-year trial with no pregnancy, IVF should be proposed. If no patency is obtained, IVF is the only possibility.

### Proximal Pathology Associated with Distal Pathology

The indication depends on distal pathology. If stage I, or phimotic with normal mucosa, proximal treatment with distal laparoscopy can be performed. If no pregnancy occurs, IVF should be proposed. In other situations, IVF represents the only possibility. Salpingectomy for widespread lesions can be performed to improve the results of IVF.

### Distal Pathology without Proximal Pathology

Treatment depends on the regenerative possibility of the mucosa and in this situation, tuboscopy can assist the decision. If the quality of the tube is stage I and II, distal laparoscopy is the best possibility. For other stages the best method is IVF. In every case, a one-year attempt at pregnancy seems to be enough to prove infertility.

### Adhesions

If adhesions are light or vascular, laparoscopy can be performed to liberate tubes and ovaries as much as possible. This procedure does not change the results of distal surgery.

When adhesions are very sclerotic, laparoscopy should be avoided in favor of IVF. Experience has shown that adhesions recur very quickly.

## CONCLUSION

The treatment of tubal infertility today is dominated by endoscopic techniques, which are becoming more and more effective as a result of technological improvements. But when these methods fail, or are contraindicated, IVF provides a useful alternative.

## REFERENCES

1. PALMER, R. 1979. Remarques d'un chirurgien conventionnel, mais respectueux de la fragilité tubaire. *In* Oviducte et Fertilité. 337–340. Masson.
2. WINSTON, R. M. L. 1980. Microsurgery of the fallopian tube: from fantasy to reality. Fertil. Steril. **34**(6): 521–530.
3. GOMEL, V. 1978. Salpingostomy by microsurgery. Fertil. Steril. **29**: 380–387.
4. AUDEBERT, A. J. M. 1979. Résultats d'ensemble des salpingoplasties a travers la chirurgie traditionnelle et la microchirugie. *In* Oviducte et Fertilité. 337–340. Masson.
5. DUBUISSON, J. B., F. X. AUBRIOT, C. RANOUX & R. HENRION. 1985. Places actuelles de la microchirurgie et de la fécondation in vitro dans les traitements des stérilités tubaires. Rev. Fr. Gynécol. Obstét. **80**: 607–612.
6. HEDON, B., R. DENJEAN, J. P. DAURES, P. MARES, B. VALENTIN, J. L. VIALA & G. DURAND. 1984. Stérilités tubaires: fécondation in vitro ou microchirurgie. Presse méd. **13**: 33–37.
7. NAGY, P. 1992. Traitement des obstructions tubaires proximales par cathétérisme selectif de l'ostium sous hysteroscope. These d'état. Montpellier.

8. BRUHAT, M. A., G. MAGE, J. L. POULY, H. MANHES, M. CANIS & A. WATTIEZ. 1989. Néostomies. *In* Cœlioscopie opératoire, 95–108. Medsi/McGraw-Hill. Paris.
9. CORNIER, E. 1985. L'ampulloscopie per-cœlioscopique. J. Gynécol. Obstét. Biol. Reprod. **14:** 459–466.
10. HENRI-SUCHET, J., L. TESQUIER, J. P. PEZ & V. LOFREDO. 1985. Tuboscopie. Rev. Fr. Gynécol. Obstét. **80**(11): 841–842.
11. ROUANET, J. P., P. MARES, A. MAUBON & H. SAUCEROTTE. 1993. Selective Salpingogrpahy. Ref. Gynécol. Obstét. **1:** 7–14.
12. GEFF. 1993. Compte rendu annuel. Serono.
13. DE ZIEGLER, D., J. THURRE DI BERNARDO, CHIN LHINH & J. SANCHES. 1993. Endometriose et blocage tubaire proximal: une indication à l'utilisation des agonistes de la gonadolibérine (GnRH-a). Ref. Gynécol. Obstét. **1:** 58–62.

# Operative Hysteroscopy

## Ten Years' Experience

A. PERINO,[a] P. CRISTOFORONI,[b] AND N. CHIANCHIANO

*Chair of Physiopathology of Human Reproduction*
*Department of Obstetrics and Gynecology*
*University of Palermo*
*Palermo, Italy*

*and*

[b]*Department of Obstetrics and Gynecology*
*University of Genoa*
*Genoa, Italy*

## INTRODUCTION

The use of hysteroscopic surgery for the treatment of endouterine pathologies such as synechias, septa, myomas, and abnormal uterine bleeding (AUB) is rapidly spreading all over the world. Many reports stress the advantages of this technique as compared with traditional surgery in terms of saving of the hospital stay, the postoperative recovery and the early return to work, the fewer complications and a better reproductive outcome.[1-5]

Our group started performing operative hysteroscopy in the early 1980s, when the first synechias were excised with endosurgical scissors, considering it as the natural consequence of the introduction of diagnostic hysteroscopy.[6] Since then, improved operators' skill together with advances in technology have allowed the treatment of more difficult cases and increased the indications.

In this study the criteria used for selecting patients to undergo operative hysteroscopy are reviewed, and data regarding the three most significant hysteroscopic procedures (metroplasty for uterine septa, resection of submucous myomas and endometrial ablation for AUB) are reported. Finally, some of the guidelines used by our group in selecting patients and in performing the procedures, in order to best minimize the chances of complications are expounded.

## MATERIALS AND METHODS

We report our experience regarding 376 patients who underwent endoscopic uterine surgery at the Department of Obstetrics and Gynecology, University of Palermo, between January 1984 and June 1992. We used data from 308 patients who fulfilled our study criteria and had a follow-up period of at least one year. The patients were divided into three groups according to clinical criteria.

---

[a] Reprint request: Prof. A. Perino, Cattedra di Fisiopatologia della Riproduzione Umana, Istituto Materno Infantile, Via Cardinale Rampolla, 1, 90133 Palmero, Italy.

One hundred and sixty-five women (group A) had a diagnosis of uterine septum: 120 of them had suffered two or more miscarriages or preterm deliveries due to the septum; the other 45 were nulliparous. Their mean age was 27.9 years (range, 21 to 38). Group B included 75 women with submucous fibroids diagnosed during investigation because of infertility or menstrual disorders. Their uterine size varied from normal to that of a 16-week pregnancy, with a median size of 8 weeks. Submucous myomas ranged in size from 1 to 7 cm. The mean age was 36.4 years (range, 27 to 44). The third group of patients (group C) included 76 women with dysfunctional uterine bleeding (DUB), with uterine cavity smaller than 14 cm and without any endometrial malignancy or precursor. Their mean age was 43.9 years (range, 32 to 48).

The equipment utilized consisted of an operative hysteroscope with rigid scissors (Operating Micro-Hysteroscope Hamou 2, with an outer diameter of 7 mm; Karl Storz GmbH, Tuttlingen, Germany) for 66 cases of uterine septa, while a 26 French resectoscope with a conventional telescope having a 30° field of vision and a working element with a passive cutting action (Karl Storz GmbH) for all other procedures. It included a high frequency electrosurgical unit with automatic cut and coagulation control (Autocon, Karl Storz GmbH). The uterine cavity was distended with $CO_2$ when the operative Hamou 2 hysteroscope was used (MicroHysteroflator, Karl Storz GmbH) and with a urologic liquid medium with the resectoscope. The latter medium was introduced by a new irrigating system that allows an electronic control of flow and intrauterine pressure (Hamou Hysteromat, Karl Storz GmbH).

Several parameters were used to assess the outcome of surgery: operating time, intraoperative bleeding, failure rate, need of subsequent operations and, for the metroplasty, reproductive results. Intraoperative bleeding was graded on a three-point scale: severe (which was never found in our study) would have necessitated immediate suspension of the hysteroscopic procedure in favor of laparotomy; moderate, requiring coagulation of bleeding vessels; and mild, insufficient to interfere with the operation.

The first control was made one to two months after surgery in group A, and failure was defined as persistence of a uterine septum larger than 1 cm as diagnosed by hysteroscopy and/or hysterosalpyngography (HSG). In group B, the procedure was considered to have failed when the myoma had not been completely removed at the first hysteroscopic control done two months after surgery, or if the menstrual cycle still showed abnormalities at the end of the one-year follow-up. In group C, the patients were controlled 3, 6, 9 and 12 months postoperatively, and the therapeutic failure was defined as persistence or relapse into AUB when assessed after one year.

## RESULTS

The parameters used to evaluate surgical results of 165 resections of uterine septa are given in TABLE 1. The operating time refers to the time (minutes ± SD) actually employed in the resection: the exploration and dilatation time is not included in the calculation (FIG. 1). No case of severe bleeding, requiring the interruption of the procedure and the execution of the laparotomy was recorded. In this group two uterine perforations, both of them on nulliparous women with small size uterus, were recorded: neither of them became pregnant during the follow-up. Ten patients (eight of them incised with rigid scissors) had an incom-

TABLE 1. Hysteroscopic Metroplasty: Surgical Results in 165 Patients

| Parameter | |
|---|---|
| No. of patients | 165 |
| Operating time (min) | 11.3 ± 2.2 |
| No. of cases of intraoperative bleeding | |
|   Severe | 0 |
|   Moderate | 10 (6.1%) |
|   Mild | 155 (93.9%) |
| No. of uterine perforations | 2 (1.2%) |
| No. of failures (septa not completely removed) | 10 (6.1%) |
| No. of subsequent obstetric uterine ruptures | 0 |

pletely removed septum and required a subsequent hysteroscopic procedure. No case of long-term complication (*i.e.*, obstetric uterine rupture) was recorded. The results regarding the obstetric outcome of this group of patients are reported in TABLE 2. Sixty-five patients experienced a vaginal delivery after the hysteroscopic metroplasty (one had a twin-pregnancy). Ten patients underwent a caesarean section. No case of abnormal delivery of the placenta was recorded.

The results of the 75 performed hysteroscopic myomectomies having at least one year follow-up are reported in TABLE 3. Ten patients had moderate bleeding during surgery requiring only vessels coagulation. No uterine perforation was recorded in this group (FIG. 2). The failure rate (incompletely removed fibroids or persistent AUB) was 16% (12 cases). In TABLE 4 surgical results are compared to the size of the fibroids. Four (25%) of the 16 patients with fibroids larger than 4 cm later required abdominal myomectomy or vaginal or abdominal hysterectomy.

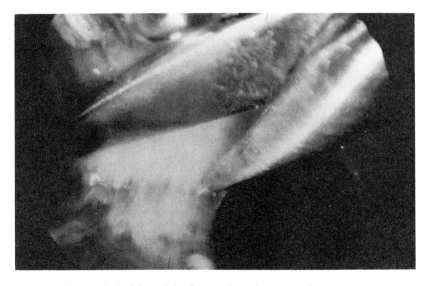

**FIGURE 1.** Incision of the fibrous tissue in a case of septate uterus.

**TABLE 2.** Obstetric Outcome of 165 Hysteroscopic Metroplasties (Follow-Up >1 year)

| Parameter | Previous Fertile Patients | Infertile Patients | Total |
|---|---|---|---|
| Vaginal delivery | 55[a] (52.8%) | 10 (38.4%) | 65 |
| Cesarean section | 31 (29.8%) | 9 (34.6%) | 40 |
| Ongoing pregnancies | 8 (7.7%) | 2 (7.6%) | 10 |
| Miscarriages | 9 (8.6%) | 4 (15.3%) | 13 |
| Ectopic pregnancies | 1 (1.0%) | 1 (3.8%) | 2 |
| Total pregnancies | 104 (86.6%) | 26 (57.7%) | 130 |
| Total patients | 120 | 45 | 165 |

[a] There was one twin pregnancy.

Two (3.4%) of the women with fibroids smaller than 4 cm required a second hysteroscopic myomectomy because of an unresolved first procedure.

In TABLE 5 the surgical results of the 76 analyzed endometrial ablations performed on patients with DUB resistant to medical therapy are shown (FIG. 3). Eight patients (10.5%) had moderate intraoperative bleeding. The outcome of the procedure was unsatisfactory in 13 (17.1%) patients: therefore, 63 patients of this group could avoid an otherwise necessary major uterine surgery.

## DISCUSSION

Hysteroscopic operative procedures are not as easy as they might first appear. The operator must become skilled in mastering the technique as well as understand the capabilities and limitations of the instruments used for each indication. In this regard, recent reports stress that particular attention must be paid by the operator to the careful selection of each case, evaluating specific indications and contraindications. Failure to do so, because of carelessness or presumption, might lead to possible complications.[7-9] The indications for resection of uterine septa have been discussed in many reports: there is presently general agreement that hysteroscopic metroplasty is the first choice treatment for this mullerian malformation.[2,8,10-11]

**TABLE 3.** Intraoperative and Long-Term Results of 75 Hysteroscopic Resections of Myomas

| Parameter | |
|---|---|
| No. of patients | 75 |
| Operating time (min) | 34.9 ± 9.5 |
| No. of cases of intraoperative bleeding | |
|   Severe | 0 |
|   Moderate | 10 (13.3%) |
|   Mild | 65 (86.7%) |
| No. of uterine perforations | 0 |
| No. of failures (myomas not completely removed and/or persistence of AUB) | 12 (16.0%) |

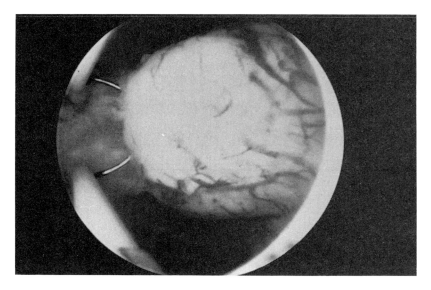

**FIGURE 2.** Electroresection of a submucous myoma.

Our operative results further prove that hysteroscopic resection is a safe and effective alternative to transabdominal metroplasty.

Major attention must be paid to the prevention of long-term complications following uterine septa resection. Two very recent case reports (12, 13) describe spontaneous uterine rupture during the second and third trimester of pregnancy following uterine perforation during hysteroscopic metroplasty performed under laparoscopic control. To the best of our knowledge, at least three other unpublished cases have occurred at other institutions in the past.[14] As a matter of fact, we think that uterine perforation is not the *conditio sine qua non* to cause a successive obstetric uterine rupture. The weakness resulting from an exaggerated incision of the uterine fundus might lead to the same risk. We and other groups[15] are presently performing operative hysteroscopy under real-time abdominal ultrasonic control; this technique is, in our experience, more effective than laparoscopy in preventing uterine perforation. Moreover, sonography permits real-time control of the residual thickness of the uterine wall: a "safety area" at least 10 mm thick (more often 12–13 mm) between cavity and uterine serosa is usually left (FIG. 4). Our short- and long-term results seem to support our technique: since the introduction of

**TABLE 4.** Hysteroscopic Myomectomy: Relationship between Fibroid Size and Results

| Size of Myoma | No. of Patients | Failures | No. of Hysteroscopic Reoperations | No. of Hysterectomies |
|---|---|---|---|---|
| <4 cm | 59 | 5 (8.5%) | 2 (3.4%) | 1 (1.7%) |
| >4 cm | 16 | 7 (43.4%) | 1 (6.2%) | 4 (25.0%) |

TABLE 5. Endometrial Ablation: Results of 76 Patients with Follow-Up >1 Year

| Parameter | |
|---|---|
| No. of patients | 76 |
| Operating time (min) | 23.2 ± 4.9 |
| No. of cases of intraoperative bleeding | |
| Severe | 0 |
| Moderate | 8 (10.5%) |
| Mild | 68 (89.5%) |
| No. of uterine perforations | 0 |
| No. of failures | 13 (17.1%) |

ultrasonic control, we have not recorded any perforation or subsequent uterine rupture (data from 84 patients).

In the past few years increasing attention has been devoted to hysteroscopic treatment of submucous myomas.[16,17] Derman et al.,[17] referring to 108 hysteroscopic myomectomies, reported a 2.1% incidence of serious complications during the procedure, necessitating a laparotomy, and a 24.5% failure rate at follow-up. Corson and Brooks,[18] presenting their operative cases series of 92 myomas, reported that 16 patients needed further surgical procedures, i.e., 11 had a second operative hysteroscopy, and 5 underwent abdominal myomectomy or hysterectomy. The analysis of our results shows an overall failure rate of 16.0%. Our data strongly indicate that a higher incidence of failures is found in the group of patients with myomas larger than 4 cm in diameter. Thus, based on our experience, we presently consider patients with: (1) fibroids larger than 4 cm in diameter or with

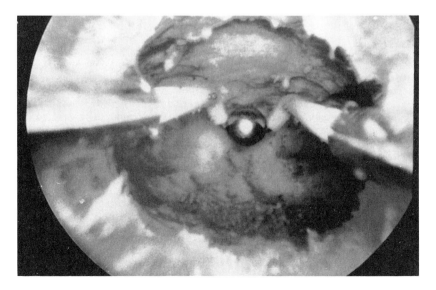

FIGURE 3. Endometrial ablation: the rollerball is particularly useful for coagulating endometrial mucosa in the horn.

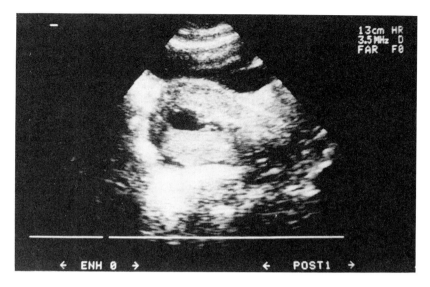

**FIGURE 4.** Incision of uterine septum under ultrasonic control.

an intramural portion greater than one third of their volume, (2) presence of other intramural myomas, and (3) global uterine size greater than that of a twelve-week pregnancy, as at risk of additional surgery.

Ultrasounds have been utilized in selecting patients for hysteroscopic treatment; however, they do not seem to have a very high specificity in differentiating between submucous and intramural myomas.[19] We are presently performing transvaginal hysterosonography in all patients scheduled to undergo hysteroscopic myomectomy: the initial impression is that this new method is very sensitive in differentiating submucous and intramural fibroids.

Endometrial ablation is certainly the most promising form of conservative intervention in women with menorrhagia.[20,21] The precise criteria for patients selection are yet to be defined. At present, we believe that it should only be carried out in women with a diagnosis of DUB not responding to medical therapies and who have no further desire for pregnancy. The preoperative work-out must include careful exclusion of malignant or premalignant endometrial lesions by hysteroscopy and direct biopsy. Piper et al.[22] reported 80 endometrial ablations with a follow-up of at least one year. They presented a success rate of 72.0%, and some complications, including 3 uterine perforations and 4 women requiring successive hysterectomy. Magos et al., in a large series of cases, reported a higher success rate, up to 90.0%.[23] Our results do not significantly differ as regards success rate (84.2%); no major intraoperative complications occurred in our experience. Thus, endometrial ablation appears to be a procedure capable of avoiding hysterectomy in a potentially large group of patients.

Recent reports showed that pretreatment therapy with GnRH analogue agonists before hysteroscopic surgery is effective in making easier endometrial ablation and resection of submucous myomas.[24,25]

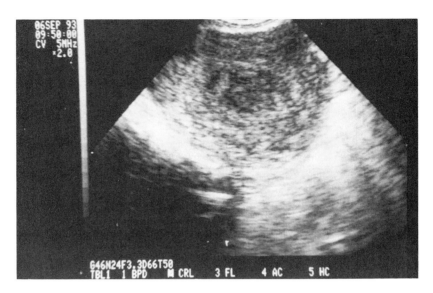

**FIGURE 5.** Transvaginal sonography (longitudinal scan) in a case of submucous myoma: the localizaiton of the lesion is not completely clear.

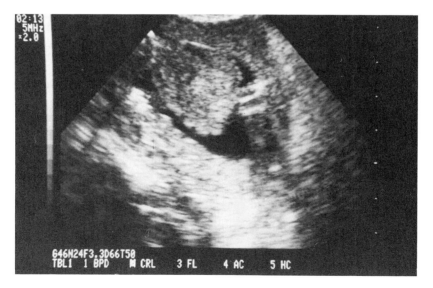

**FIGURE 6.** Transvaginal hysterosonography (longitudinal scan) of the same case as FIGURE 5: once saline solution is injected through a catheter into the uterine cavity, the lesion is well clarified.

However, long-term follow-up data must be collected in order to better define the actual risk and benefits of hysteroscopic endometrial ablation.

## REFERENCES

1. Fayez, J. A. 1986. Comparison between abdominal and hysteroscopic metroplasty. Obstet. Gynecol. **68:** 399–403.
2. Perino, A., L. Mencaglia, J. Hamou & E. Cittadini. 1987. Hysteroscopy for metroplasty of uterine septa. Fertil. Steril. **48:** 321–323.
3. Loffer, F. D. 1987. Hysteroscopic endometrial ablation with the Nd:Yag laser using a nontouch technique. Obstet. Gynecol. **69:** 679–682.
4. Baggish, M. S., J. Barbot & R. F. Valle. 1989. Operative hysteroscopy I. *In* Diagnostic and Operative Hysteroscopy: a Text and Atlas. M. S. Baggish, J. Barbot & R. F. Valle, Eds. 163–178. Year Book Medical Publisher, Inc. Chicago.
5. DeCherney, A. H., M. P. Diamond, G. Lavy & M. L. Polan. 1987. Endometrial ablation for intractable uterine bleeding: hysteroscopic resection. Obstet. Gynecol. **70:** 668–670.
6. Perino, A., J. Hamou & E. Cittadini. 1983. Diagnosis and management of intrauterine adhesions by mycrohysteroscopy. Acta Eur. Fertil. **14:** 117–121.
7. Hamou, J. 1991. Hysteroscopy and Mycrohysteroscopy. A Text and Atlas. Appleton and Lange. San Mateo, CA.
8. Perino, A., J. Hamou, L. Carlino, M. Petronio & F. Ubaldi. 1993. L'isteroscopia operatoria. Cofese Ed. Palermo.
9. Blanc, B. & L. Boubli. 1991. Manuel d'hystéroscopie opératoire. Edt. Vigot. Paris.
10. Israel, R. & C. M. March. 1984. Hysteroscopic incision of the septate uterus. Am. J. Obstet. Gynecol. **149:** 66–73.
11. Valle, R. F. & J. J. Sciarra. 1986. Hysteroscopic treatment of the septate uterus. Obstet. Gynecol. **67:** 253–257.
12. Halvorson, L. M., R. D. Aserkoff & S. P. Oskowitz. 1993. Spontaneous uterine rupture after hysteroscopic metroplasty with uterine perforation. A case report. J. Reprod. Med. **38:** 236–238.
13. Howe, R. S. 1993. Third-trimester uterine rupture following hysteroscopic uterine perforation. Obstet. Gynecol. **81:** 827–829.
14. Hamou, J. Personal communication.
15. Perino, A., E. Catinella, G. Comparetto, R. Venezia, P. Candela, C. Cimino *et al.* 1987. Hysteroscopic metroplasty: the role of ultrasound in the diagnosis and monitoring of patients with uterine septa. Acta Eur. Fertil. **18:** 349–352.
16. Donnez, J., B. Schrurs, S. Gillerot, J. Sandow & F. Clerckx. 1989. Treatment of uterine fibroids with implants of gonadotropin-releasing hormone agonist: assessment by hysterography. Fertil. Steril. **51:** 947–950.
17. Derman, S. G., J. Rehnstrom & R. S. Neuwirth. 1991. The long-term effectiveness of hysteroscopic treatment of menorrhagia and leyomiomas. Obstet. Gynecol. **77:** 591–594.
18. Corson, S. L. & P. G. Brooks. 1991. Resectoscopic myomectomy. Fertil. Steril. **55:** 1041–1046.
19. Fukuda, M., T. Shimizu, K. Fukuda, W. Yomura & S. Shimizu. 1993. Transvaginal hysterosonography for differential diagnosis between submucous and intramural myoma. Gynecol. Obstet. Invest. **35:** 236–239.
20. Goldrath, M. H., T. A. Fuller & S. Segal. 1981. Laser vaporization of the endometrium for the treatment of menorrhagia. Am. J. Obstet. Gynecol. **140:** 14–19.
21. Garry, R., J. Erian & S. A. Grochmal. 1991. A multi-centre collaborative study into the treatment of menorrhagia by Nd:Yag laser ablation of the endometrium. Br. J. Obstet. Gynaecol. **98:** 357–362.
22. Pyper, R. J. D. & A. D. Haeri. 1991. A review of 80 endometrial resections for menorrhagia. Br. J. Obstet. Gynaecol. **98:** 1049–1054.

23. MAGOS, A. L., R. BAUMANN, G. M. LOCKWOOD & A. C. TURNBULL. 1991. Experience with the first 250 endometrial resections for menorrhagia. Lancet **337:** 1074–1078.
24. BROOKS, P. G., S. P. SERDEN & I. DAVOS. 1991. Hormonal inhibition of the endometrium for resectoscopic endometrial ablation. Am. J. Obstet. Gynecol. **164:** 1601–1606.
25. PERINO, A., N. CHIANCHIANO, M. PETRONIO & E. CITTADINI. 1993. Role of leuprolide acetate depot in hysteroscopic surgery: a controlled study. Fertil. Steril. **59:** 507–510.

# Ultrasound, Hysteroscopy, and Histological Assessment of the Endometrium in Postmenopausal Women

G. POSSATI, V. M. JASONNI, S. NALDI, S. MAZZONE,
S. GABRIELLI,[a] M. BEVINI,[a] G. MUSERRA,
A. PARESCHI, AND C. FLAMIGNI

*Department of Obstetrics and Gynecology*
*Reproductive Medicine Unit*
*[a]Section of Prenatal Pathophysiology*
*University of Bologna*
*Via Massarenti, 13*
*40128 Bologna, Italy*

The purpose of this study was to compare transvaginal sonographic scanning of the endometrium with hysteroscopical findings and histology.
 Fleischer[1] showed in 1986 that sonography could demonstrate changes in the thickness and morphology of the endometrium, occurring during the normal ovulatory cycling. It has subsequently been suggested that sonography might be beneficial in determining the presence or absence of myometrial invasion in cases of proved endometrial carcinoma. In addition, many authors, such as Osmers[2] and Goldstein,[3] have reported that transvaginal scanning may be useful in monitoring the endometrium in postmenopausal women.
 A disadvantage of transvaginal ultrasound is the limited field of view, and the absence of reliability in the topography of the lesions.
 Hysteroscopy is the tool that allows us to make not only a diagnosis of endometrial abnormality, but gives us the chance to evaluate where the lesion is situated.[4,5]
 One hundred postmenopausal women were investigated with transvaginal ultrasound, office hysteroscopy and endometrial biopsy. Endometrium thickness was measured from the highly reflective interface of the junction of the endometrium and myometrium.
 Of these one hundred patients, seventy-eight were symptomatic, and had at least 6 months of amenorrhea prior to bleeding; twenty-two were asymptomatic, but were investigated before starting a hormonal replacement treatment.
 In 31 subjects transvaginal ultrasound showed an endometrial thickness greater than 10 millimeters: then hysteroscopy was performed, followed by an endometrial biopsy.
 We used an office 30° forward-oblique Telescope (Storz, Germany) with a 5-mm examination sheath, and $CO_2$ as distending medium. All the examinations were performed without anesthesia, administrating only Atropine (0.5 mg IM) 15–20 minutes before the procedure was started.
 In 10 patients the histological findings were of *endometrial carcinoma* (32.2%), including two atypical hyperplasia, while in 3 patients the specimens showed a *typical hyperplasia* (9.6%); in 18 subjects the specimens were negative (58.1%).

In 28 patients the ultrasound scan showed an endometrial thickness between 5 and 10 millimeters; hysteroscopic view, confirmed by histological assessment, demonstrated that four patients (13.8%) had *carcinoma*, seven patients (24.1%) had typical hyperplasia, while seventeen subjects (60.7%) had an endometrium without abnormalities.

In 3 subjects ultrasound gave an image of an endometrial thickness between 8 and 10 mm, evenly distributed through the whole cavity, and hysteroscopy showed an isolated, unique fibroglandular polyp.

Hysteroscopic views and histological findings were compared: when a completely atrophic condition of the endometrium was observed during hysteroscopic examination (48 subjects), histological assessment confirmed either atrophy or the insufficiency of the material for diagnosis.

During hysteroscopy the evidence was of atypical hyperplasia for 14 patients, with histological findings of endometrial carcinoma for 12 subjects and of atypical hyperplasia for 2 subjects.

In 9 patients hysteroscopy showed typical hyperplasia, confirmed by histology.

In 29 patients the hysteroscopic and histological evidence was the same: active endometrium.

Even if these results show agreement between hysteroscopic view and histology, hysteroscopy may not be used alone, without histology. A very large experience is necessary to detect small differences between similar endometria; besides that, sometimes, inside an apparently regular fibroglandular polyp, small nests of adenocarcinoma are hidden. Hysteroscopy is a technique that allows us not to lose the area where we are meant to perform biopsy, and to evaluate the cavity invasion, in case of endometrial carcinoma.

Other authors (Nasri,[6] Varner[7]) indicate that if ultrasound scanning shows an endometrial thickness less than 5 mm throughout the whole cavity in postmenopausal women, the endometrium will be atrophic or inactive; otherwise, if ultrasound shows an endometrium greater than 5 millimeters, then we think that hysteroscopy should be performed, in order to have a real evaluation of the cavity, and in order to perform a correct endometrial biopsy.

Certainly hysteroscopy may not evaluate the myometrial invasion of an endometrial carcinoma; probably ultrasonography might give some further information,[8] but at this moment there is not enough published data.

Hysteroscopy is currently a necessary methodology for endometrial investigation, despite distortion by myomata or suboptimal uterine attitude.

Hysteroscopy plus ultrasound examination is a good tool for detecting precancerous or cancerous lesions in postmenopausal women, without performing D&C in each symptomatic woman.

## REFERENCES

1. FLEISCHER, A. C., G. C. KALEMERIS, J. E. MACKIN, S. S. ENTMAN & A. E. JAMES. 1986. Sonographic depiction of normal and abnormal endometrium with histopathic correlation. J. Ultrasound Med. **5:** 445–453.
2. OSMERS, R., M. VOLKSEN & A. SCHAUER. 1990. Vaginosonography for early detection of endometrial carcinoma? Lancet **335:** 1569–1571.
3. GOLDSTEIN, S. R., M. NACHTIGALL, J. R. SNYDER & L. NACHTIGALL. 1990. Endometrial assessment by vaginal ultrasonography before endometrial sampling in patients with postmenopausal bleeding. Am. J. Obstet. Gynecol. **163:** 119–123.
4. CRONJE, H. S. 1984. Diagnostic hysteroscopy after postmenopausal uterine bleeding. S. Afr. Med. J. **20:** 773.

5. GOLDRATH, M. H. & A. I. SHERMAN. 1985. Office hysteroscopy and suction curettage: can we eliminate the hospital dilatation and curettage? Am. J. Obstet. Gynecol. **152**(2): 220–227.
6. NASRI, M. N. & G. J. COAST. 1989. Correlation of ultrasound findings and endometrial histopathology in postmenopausal women. Br. J. Obster. Gynaecol. **96:** 1333–1338.
7. VARNER, R. E. & J. M. SPARKS. 1991. Transvaginal sonography of the endometrium in postmenopausal women. Obstet. Gynecol. **78**(2): 195–199.
8. CACCIATORE, B. & L. PENTI. 1989. Preoperative sonographic evaluation of endometrial cancer. Am. J. Obstet. Gynecol. **160**(1): 133–137.

# Can Hysteroscopic Evaluation of Endometrial Carcinoma Influence Therapeutic Treatment?

G. L. TADDEI,[a] D. MONCINI, G. SCARSELLI,[b]
C. TANTINI,[b] AND G. BARGELLI[b]

*Department of Pathology*
*and*
[b]*Department of Gynecology and Obstetrics*
*University of Florence*
*Florence, Italy*

There is much anatomo-clinical data which must be evaluated for a therapeutic choice and which influences the survival rate of endometrial carcinoma patients (stage, histologic subtype, grading, myometrial infiltration, lymphonodal extension, etc.).[1-9] A correct clinical staging of endometrial carcinoma is therefore an indispensable premise. The distinction between stages I and II, according to the model proposed by the International Federation of Gynaecologists and Obstetricians (FIGO, 1991),[10,11] is tied to the neoplasia's extension to the cervical canal. In the past the presence of the endometrial carcinoma's diffusion to the cervical canal was entrusted to the fractioned curretage, but the data obtained were never quite trustworthy. The possibility of visualizing the cervical canal, given by Hamou's hysteroscope, should allow, by means of a guided biopsy, greater certainty during the preoperatory stage.[12-16] The wide angle view of the endometrial cavity allows the evaluation of the tumor's dimensions. The aim of our study is to correlate the tumoral mass, present in the uterine cavity, to the neoplasia's myometrial infiltration and to evaluate the capability of the hysteroscopic test to document the tumor's presence in the cervical canal. A correct preoperatory evaluation of the neoplasia's extension could lead to a personalized therapeutic programming and could intervene positively in survival rates.

## MATERIALS AND METHODS

Out of 12,121 hysteroscopic examinations done at the Department of Gynaecology and Obstetrics of the University of Florence between 1980 and 1992, we collected 235 cases relative to primitive endometrial carcinomas. The examination of the hysteroscopic sheets gave information regarding: stage, obesity, diabetes, hypertension, nulliparity, menopausal period, initial symptomatology, and the neoplasia's intracavital extension. The neoplasia's intracavital extension, evaluated using a hysteroscopic examination, was arbitrarily divided in 1/3, 2/3, and 3/3 according to the cavity's occupied portion. The terms positive, suspect, nega-

---

[a] Address correspondence to: Prof. Gian Luigi Taddei, Istituto di Anatomia Patologica, viale Morgagni 85, 50134 Florence, Italy.

tive and indeterminable were used to indicate the neoplasia's diffusion to the cervical canal. The histological specimens of each case, kept at the Institute of Histopathology of the University of Florence, were examined and, when necessary, new sections were prepared using the customary histological techniques. This allowed us to classify homogeneously: the histologic subtype, the grading, the growth pattern, the myometrial infiltration, and the cervical diffusion. The histological classification adopted is that suggested by the International Society of Gynaecologists and Pathologists with some modifications.[17] As far as the histological grades of differentiation are concerned, we adopted those indicated by FIGO, and for the grade of cytologic atypia we used the Broders method.[18] The growth pattern was evaluated using the model proposed by S. C. Ming[19] for gastric carcinoma, in expansive and infiltrative forms; the diffuse form was added. This last form has a morphological aspect which cannot be referred to in either of the two preceding entities. The expansive or pushing form is recognizable by the regular, compact, semicircular front of the tumor infiltration; the infiltrating aspect is characterized by the myometrium's penetration by single tumoral portions which give rise to very irregular images of the tumoral infiltration. Myometrial diffusion independent of the clinical stage has been evaluated by arbitrarily dividing the myometrium in two parts, $< 50\%$ and $>$ half the myometrium, as proposed by FIGO (1991). The endometrial carcinoma's extension to the cervical canal has been annotated and considered differently in relation to the superficial or deep involvement, since with the hysteroscope one can only evaluate, as is natural, those forms which have a tumoral extension to the cervical canal's mucosa. The 5-year follow-up is known for 199 patients. The most significative data have been evaluated using a statistical method with the chi-square test.

## RESULTS

The average age of our 235 patients was 61 years (range, 37–94). The anatomo-surgical stage subdivision shows a clearly dominant first stage in relation to the following stages (170 cases, 72.3%, were T1; 49 cases, 20.8%, were T2; 13 at T3; only 3 at T4). The distribution per stage as indicated by FIGO in relation to the survival rate is shown in FIGURE 1. Hypertension, obesity and diabetes were

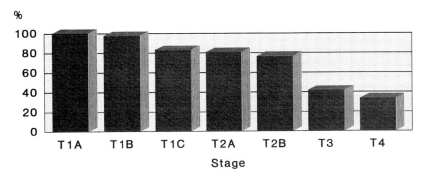

**FIGURE 1.** Five-year survival vs pathologic staging. T1 vs T2, $p = 0.03$; T1b vs T1c, $p = 0.007$.

present in 22.5%; nulliparity in 23.4%; and 35.2% of the women evaluated were in "late" menopause. 9.7% of the patients had no symptoms (abnormal uterine bleeding, AUB) at the moment of diagnosis. In 7 women the cervical canal was not accessible with the hysteroscope examination. The endometrial carcinoma's hysteroscopic positivity in the cervical canal was 19.8% (45/228 patients). The false positives were 9.2% (21/228 patients). The false negatives with the hysteroscope examination were 7.9% (18/228 patients). The intrauterine tumoral extension was focal (1/3) in 97 patients; partial (2/3) in 82 patients; total (3/3) in 47 patients and indeterminable in 9 patients.

The most frequent histologic subtype, comprehensive of some variations (secretory and papillary), is represented by the common adenocarcinoma (65.5%). The clear cell carcinoma (2.5%), the mucinous adenocarcinoma (2.1%) and serous papillary adenocarcinoma (1.7%) were the least frequent histologic subtypes, since in the groups we included only the entities morphologically more characterized. The adenosquamous carcinoma and adenoacanthoma (15.3% and 12.7% respectively) were diagnosed only if they responded to the criteria we had already adopted.[17] The distribution of all the cases in grades of differentiation shows the intermediate grade (41.7%) as slightly prevalent in frequency in relation to the other grades (G1: 34.5%; G3: 23.8%). 90.7% of the women with a tumor having a myometrial infiltration, in conformity with the pushing growth model, are alive after 5 years against 45.4% of the women with diffuse forms independent of the anatomo-surgical stage (FIGURE 2). These data do not change even if we do not evaluate the T3 and T4 cases, as numeric consistency does not substantially modify the percentage.

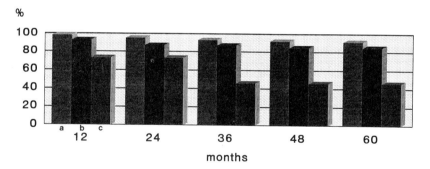

**FIGURE 2.** Five-year survival vs pattern of invasion. (a) Pushing, (b) infiltrative, and (c) diffuse. $p = 0.0001$.

## DISCUSSION

We confirm that the clinical stage is a good prognostic indicator for endometrial carcinoma. The T1a patients are all alive at 5 years; 97.5% of those in T1b and 83.0% in T1c. The survival rate of women in T2a is 80%, which decreases to 76.4% for women in T2b, although the women's numeric consistency in stage III and IV suggests caution in the survival rate's percentage evaluation. Nevertheless, only 41.6% and 33.3%, respectively, of the patients in these stages are alive after

5 years. Statistical comparison between stage I and II, with regard to the survival rate, shows a good significance between the two ($p = 0.003$), but the result is still better if we compare T1b and T1c, both belonging to stage I ($p = 0.007$). This same result does not come through, in our cases, between T2a and T2b, but neither is there a statistical significance if we evaluate the tumor's intrauterine extension in relation to the various clinical stages.

The comparison between histologic subtype, survival rate and myometrial infiltration shows no statistically significant differences which could give the various forms a peculiar anatomoclinical behavior.

A good statistical significance is present between the invasion pattern (pushing and diffuse) and the 5-year survival rate ($p = 0.0001$). The 5-year survival rate is statistically significant when correlated to the myometrial infiltration ($p = 0.003$), while there is no connection ($p = 0.9$) between the neoplasia's intrauterine extension, hysteroscopically ascertained, and the survival rate.

There is no connection between the tumor's intrauterine extension and grading ($p = 0.1$) but there is a high significance between myometrial infiltration and grading ($p = 0.002$). These data are further confirmed when grade and survival rate are compared ($p = 0.001$).

The aim of our study was to verify the possibility of correlating by means of the endometrial cavity's hysteroscopic examination, the endometrial carcinoma's macroscopic aspect to myometrial infiltration and to the cervical canal as recently suggested by some authors.[20,21] The opportunity of a sufficiently large number of cases has allowed us to statistically evaluate these aspects, and it has permitted us to establish that there is no correlation between the endometrial carcinoma's intrauterine extension, myometrial infiltration and survival rate. We instead confirm the close correlation between survival rate, stage, myometrial infiltration, diffusion to the cervical canal and grading, based on nuclear/cytoplasmic abnormalities rather than on morphology alone. Our contribution shows a good correlation between growth type, according to the Ming model and survival rate.

The use of Hamou's hysteroscope, which permits a visual exploration of the cervical canal and of the entire endometrium without anaesthesia, play an important role in the diagnosis of an endometrial carcinoma and allows a quite precise evaluation of the tumor's clinical stage (T1 vs T2), but it is unable to visualize, on the basis of the tumor's intrauterine dimensions, an ulterior subdivision internal to the anatomo-clinical stage I.

## SUMMARY

235 cases of primary endometrial adenocarcinoma (AC) (age range, 37–94; mean age, 61 years) were collected during the period 1980–1992. Hysteroscopic examination of both the endometrial cavity and the cervical canal was performed in every patient prior to hysterectomy, and evaluations of cancer extension in the endometrium (focal: 97 pts; partial: 82 pts; massive: 47 pts; unevaluable: 9 pts) and of endocervical involvement (positive: 45 pts) were compared to the histological findings and survival rates. The $\chi^2$ test was used for statistical analysis, and statistical significance was considered where the $p$ value was <0.05.

Endometrial extension was poorly related to the depth of myometrial invasion (M1 = depth of invasion to <1/2 myometrium, M2 = invasion to >1/2 myometrium): focal AC: M1 57.8%, M2 42.2%; partial AC: M1 40.2%, M2 59.8%; massive AC: M1 51.1%, M2 48.9%; ($p = 0.5$).

Endocervical involvement was unrelated to endometrial extension. No correlation was found between AC histological grade (G1-G3) and entity of endometrial extension, whereas grade showed a significant correlation with myometrial invasion (G1 M1: 69.1%; G3 M1: 41.0%; $p = 0.002$) and survival rates (G1 90.4%, G2 88.5%, G3 69.4%; $p = 0.01$). Five-year survival figures showed no evident correlation with cancer extension (focal AC: 86.5%; partial AC: 87.8%; massive AC: 86.3%; $p = 0.9$) whereas myometrial invasion showed a statistical significance (M1: 91.4%, M2: 79.7%; $p = 0.03$). Three patterns of invasion were defined: pushing (P), infiltrative (I) and diffuse (D) isolated cells. There were significant differences between the various growth patterns and survival rates (P 90.7%; I 84.3%; D 45.4%; $p = 0.0001$). False negative rate of the hysteroscopic diagnosis of cervical involvement was 7.9% (18 cases); however, in 6 of these cases only deep cervical invasion was found.

## REFERENCES

1. KADAR, N., J. H. MALFETANO & H. D. HOMESLEY. 1992. Determinants of survival of surgically staged patients with endometrial carcinoma histologically confined to the uterus: implications for therapy. Obstet. Gynecol. **80:** 655–659.
2. BORONOW, R. C., C. P. MORROW, W. T. CREASMAN, P. J. DiSAIA, S. G. SILVERERG, A. MILLER & J. A. BLESSING. 1984. Surgical staging in endometrial cancer: clinical-pathologic findings of a prospective study. Obstet. Gynecol. **63:** 825–832.
3. HANSON, M. B., J. R. VAN NAGELL, D. E. POWELL, E. S. DONALDSON, H. GALLION, M. MERHIGE & E. J. PAVLIK. 1985. The prognostic significance of lymph-vascular space invasion in stage I endometrial cancer. Cancer **55:** 1753–1757.
4. DiSAIA, P. J., W. T. CREASMAN, R. C. BORONOW & J. A. BLESSING. 1985. Risk factors and recurrent patterns in stage I endometrial cancer. Am. J. Obstet. Gynecol. **151:** 1009–1015.
5. CREASMAN, W. T., C. P. MORROW, B. N. BUNDY, H. D. HOMESLEY, J. E. GRAHAM & P. B. HELLER. 1987. Surgical pathologic spread pattern of endometrial cancer. Cancer **60:** 2035–2041.
6. MORROW, C. P., B. N. BUNDY, R. J. KURMAN, W. T. CREASMAN, P. HELLER, H. D. HOMESLEY & J. E. GRAHAM. 1991. Relationship between surgical-pathological risk factors and outcome in clinical stage I and II carcinoma of the endometrium: a gynecologic oncology group study. Gynecol. Oncol. **40:** 55–65.
7. ABELER, V. M. & K. E. KJORSTAD. 1991. Endometrial adenocarcinoma in Norway. A study of total population. Cancer **67:** 3093–3103.
8. AMBROS, R. A. & R. J. KURMAN. 1992. Combined assessment of vascular and myometrial as a model to predict prognosis in stage I endometrioid adenocarcinoma of the uterine corpus. Cancer **69:** 1424–1431.
9. BURKE, T. W., P. B. HELLER, J. E. WOODWARD, S. A. DAVIDSON, W. J. HOSKINS & R. C. PARK. 1990. Treatment failure in endometrial carcinoma. Obstet. Gynecol. **75:** 96–101.
10. MIKUTA, J. J. 1993. International Federation of Gynecology and Obstetrics staging of endometrial cancer 1988. Cancer 71: 1460–1463.
11. GUSBERG, S. B. 1966. The problem of staging endometrial cancer. Obstet. Gynecol. **28:** 305–308.
12. SAVINO, L., G. SCARSELLI, F. BRANCONI, F. LOCATELLI, M. DI TOMMASO, L. MENCAGLIA & G. TANTINI. 1982. Usefulness of hysteroscopy in endometrial adenocarcinoma staging. Eur. J. Gynaecol. Oncol. **3:** 210–213.
13. SCARSELLI, G., L. MENCAGLIA & J. HAMOU. 1981. Atlante di microcolpoisteroscopia. Cofese. Palermo.
14. HAMOU, J. 1981. Hysteroscopy and microhysteroscopy with a new instrument: the microhysteroscope. Acta Eur. Fertil. **12:** 1.
15. IOSSA, A., L. CIANFERONI, S. CIATTO, S. CECCHINI, C. CAMPATELLI & F. LO STUMBO.

1991. Hysteroscopy and endometrial cancer diagnosis: a review of 2007 consecutive examinations in self-referred patients. Tumori **77:** 479–483.
16. STELMACHOW, J. 1982. The role of hysteroscopy in gynecologic oncology. Gynecol. Oncol. **14:** 392–395.
17. TADDEI, G. L. Carcinoma dell'endometrio. *In* Progressi clinici: ginecologia ed ostetricia. Sezione Anatomia Patologica. Ed. Piccin. Padova. In press.
18. BRODERS, A. C. 1926. Carcinoma: grading and practical application. Arch. Pathol. **2:** 376–380.
19. MING, S. C. 1977. Gastric carcinoma. A pathobiological classification. Cancer **39:** 2475–2485.
20. GUBBINI, G., A. MARABINI, I. LINSALATA, G. MARTINELLI & C. ORLANDI. 1989. Nuova classificazione isteroscopica del carcinoma endometriale al I stadio. Oncol. Ginecol. **8:** 21–24.
21. MARABINI, A., G. GUBBINI, I. LINSALATA, D. SANTINI & C. ORLANDI. 1992. Staging of endometrial cancer. *In* Fifth European Congress on Hysteroscopy and Endoscopic Surgery. June 3–6, Hamburg, Germany. Abstracts. Pg. 4.

# Hysteroscopic Metroplasty

ALBERTO MARABINI, GIAMPIETRO GUBBINI,
ROBERTA STAGNOZZI, MARCO STEFANETTI,
MANUELA FILONI, AND ALESSANDRO BOVICELLI

*Second Department of Obstetrics and Gynecology*
*University of Bologna*
*Via Massarenti, 13*
*40138 Bologna, Italy*

## INTRODUCTION

The reproductive outcome of women with septate uterus is assumed to be poor even if uterine septa may be present in asymptomatic women who conceive and have normal pregnancies and deliveries.

Nonetheless, among symptomatic patients septate uterus is frequently associated with reproductive wastage.[1,4,6,9,10]

Recently several studies demonstrated that hysteroscopic metroplasty is the treatment of choice and may replace abdominal metroplasty.[4,6,10,13,14] The procedure is usually simple, safe and effective and may be performed by several different methods and instruments including scissors,[4,6,8,10,14] laser[2,3] and resectoscope.[5,7,11]

This study reports the surgical outcome and subsequent reproductive outcome in the patients treated in the last four years at the Second Department of Obstetrics and Gynecology of the University of Bologna, Italy.

## MATERIALS AND METHODS

Between February 1990 and June 1993, 40 patients with septate uterus underwent hysteroscopic metroplasty (Class Vb as defined in the Buttram and Gibbons Classification).[1]

The mean age was 33.2 (range, 20–41 years).

Twenty-six patients had previous miscarriages (65%) with a live birth rate of 3.8% and fourteen were infertile (35%) (TABLE 1).

To confirm the diagnosis of septate uterus, laparoscopy was performed in 38 cases and ultrasound in 2 cases.

Preoperative treatment with Danazol (Winthrop Laboratories, New York, NY) was given to 15 patients, 400 mg/daily for 4 weeks, to reduce endometrial thickness. Moreover, 1 g of cefazolin was injected intramuscularly one hour before surgery and twelve hours after surgery.

In twenty-four patients gemeprost, a $PGE_1$ analogue (Seromo Pharmaceutical Company, Japan), was administered vaginally 3 hours before surgery to soften the cervix and to make easier cervical dilatation and resectoscope progression in the cervical canal.

TABLE 1. Reproductive History

|  | No. of Cases |  |
|---|---|---|
| No. of previous miscarriages |  |  |
| 0 | 14 |  |
| 1 | 12 |  |
| 2 | 9 |  |
| >2 | 5 |  |
| Living children |  | 2 |

Under general endotracheal anesthesia the procedure was performed by means of Hamou resectoscope (Storz Endoscopy, Tuttlingen, Germany). The distension of the uterine cavity was obtained by Hamou Hysteromat (Storz) using sorbitol-mannitol solution as distending medium.

After identification of the septum and tubal ostia, the section was started from the septum apex and carried cephalad with progressive horizontal cuts.

The section was considered complete when both tubal ostia were seen simultaneously, and the resectoscope moved freely from one tubal ostium to the other.

The mean operating time was 20 minutes and the mean fluid absorption 400 ml (range, 150–700 ml). No postoperative treatment was administered to the patients and no intrauterine device was inserted.

Forty to sixty days after the operation a diagnostic hysteroscopy was performed in 33 patients (82.5%) to evaluate the repair and the morphology of the uterine cavity.

## RESULTS

Hysteroscopic metroplasty is a safe procedure: no intraoperative and postoperative complications occurred. All patients were discharged within 24 hours. At the follow-up hysteroscopy a wide uterine cavity was observed in all the cases without intrauterine adhesions. A residual portion of the septum in the fundus was present in one case that required a second hysteroscopic operation.

Postoperative reproductive outcome was evaluated in 26 patients with a mean follow-up of 21.1 months (range, 7–43 months). The remaining 14 cases were not considered because three patients were lost to follow-up, four have not tried to conceive since the operation and seven had a short follow-up (less than 6 months). The cumulative pregnancy rate was 73%, live birth 86%, spontaneous abortions 10% (TABLE 2). Eight women delivered vaginally (61%) and five by cesarean section (39%).

Two patients had cesarean sections for fetal distress, one for breech presentation, one for failure to progress in labor and one because her obstetrician believed that hysteroscopic metroplasty was a risk factor for uterine rupture.

In two women cervical cerclage was performed because of cervical incompetence. Gestational age was never less than 38 weeks and fetal weight never less than 2500 g (TABLE 3).

Among the infertile group, five patients underwent additional therapy to achieve pregnancy: one clomiphene citrate, two husband-donor inseminations and two IVF.

Only the patient treated by clomiphene citrate became pregnant.

TABLE 2. Pregnancy Outcome (No. of Cases 26)

|  | Infertility (n = 9) | | Previous Miscarriages (n = 17) | | Total (n = 26) | |
| --- | --- | --- | --- | --- | --- | --- |
|  | No. of Cases | % | No. of Cases | % | No. of Cases | % |
| Abortions | 1 | 25 | 1 | 6 | 2 | 10 |
| Preterm deliveries | 0 | — | 0 | — | 0 | — |
| Vaginal deliveries | 2 | 67 | 6 | 60 | 8 | 61 |
| Cesarean sections | 1 | 33 | 4 | 40 | 5 | 39 |
| Ongoing pregnancies | 0 |  | 4 |  | 4 |  |
| Pregnancy rate |  | 44 |  | 88 |  | 73 |
| Live birth |  | 75 |  | 91 |  | 86 |

In the infertile group pregnancy and live birth rates were much lower than in previous miscarriage group (TABLE 2).

## COMMENT

Hysteroscopic section of uterine septa by Hamou resectoscope is a safe, simple, quick and effective procedure. Compared to scissors the technique is quicker but more expensive.

March[10] suggested that the resectoscope may lead to excessive tissue damage and intrauterine adhesions and does not permit the section of those septa that originate at the internal os.

In our series we observed a complete epithelialization of the uterine cavity without adhesions in all the cases after surgery, and the section was performed in all kinds of septa.

The procedure is generally simple: after the section of the lowermost portion of the septum, the uterine cavity becomes progressively wider. The resectoscope can be introduced in both the horns so that it is possible to cut the septum in the midline from both sides.

Due to the diameter of the Hamou resectoscope, sometimes the dilatation of the cervix to 9.5 mm is difficult. Gemeprost preoperative application reduces cervical traumatism and makes easy cervical dilatation and resectoscope progression into the cervical canal.

TABLE 3. Birth Weight and Gestational Age at Delivery (n = 13)

|  | No. of Cases | % |
| --- | --- | --- |
| Birth weight (g) |  |  |
| <2.500 | 0 | — |
| 2.500 to 3.500 | 11 | 84.6% |
| >3.500 | 2 | 16.6% |
| Gestational age |  |  |
| <38 weeks | 0 | — |
| >=38 weeks | 13 | 100 |

Compared to laser the resectoscope is less expensive and the procedure is quicker.

Fedele[7] did not observe any differences in postoperative intracavitary morphology of the uterus comparing all these three methods.

Bleeding is minimal if the procedure is correct and the section is stopped when the pinkish myometrial color is seen.

Hemostasis was always good, and it was never necessary to insert a Foley catheter.

No injury to surrounding viscera was induced by electrocautery.

We never observed complications due to sorbitol-mannitol distending medium and the quantity of absorbed fluid was always low. On the contrary Vercellini[15] reported one case of hypervolemic pulmonary edema and severe coagulopathy after dextran instillation.

Laparoscopy was used in almost all cases to verify the globular shape of the uterus, to rule out a possible bicornuate configuration, to diagnose associated pelvic diseases and to control accidental perforation during the operation.

Now it is possible to diagnose uterine septum by ultrasound, which can be also used for the monitoring of the hysteroscopic operative procedure.[12]

Laparoscopy is recommended in infertile patients.

The reproductive outcome of our patients was successful and similar to that reported in the literature.[3-8,10,13,14]

The abortion rate was equal to that of the normal population. No case of premature delivery or placenta previa was observed.

In infertile patients pregnancy and live birth rates were lower than in patients with previous miscarriages due to undetectable causes compromising fertility. In two patients IVF was unsuccessful.

Hysteroscopic metroplasty did not seem to improve fertility in these patients but may have prevented subsequent fetal wastage. Therefore, for its minimal morbidity and low cost, hysteroscopic metroplasty is recommended in infertile patients before using different therapeutic strategies.

## SUMMARY

Between February 1990 and June 1993 40 patients underwent hysteroscopic metroplasty for septate uterus. Twenty-six patients had previous miscarriages (65%) and fourteen were infertile (35%).

Hysteroscopic section of uterine septa was performed by means of Hamou resectoscope with sorbitol-mannitol solution as distending medium.

Surgical outcome was excellent without intraoperative and postoperative morbidity. After 40–60 days the uterine cavity was completely epithelialized without intrauterine adhesions in all the cases. One patient had incomplete septum section that required a second procedure. Postoperative reproductive outcome was evaluated in 26 patients: the cumulative pregnancy and birth rate was 73% and 86%, respectively. Five patients delivered by cesarean section (39%). In the infertile group the pregnancy and birth rate was much lower (44% and 75%, respectively) than in previous miscarriage group (88% and 91%, respectively).

Infertile patients do not seem to be cured by hysteroscopic metroplasty; however, in these cases the endoscopic operation should be performed, because it may prevent subsequent miscarriage.

Hysteroscopic metroplasty by means of Hamou resectoscope is a very successful, quick, simple and safe procedure that may replace abdominal metroplasty.

## REFERENCES

1. BUTTRAM, V. C. & W. E. GIBBONS. 1979. Mullerian anomalies: a proposed classification (an analysis of 144 cases). Fertil. Steril. **32:** 40.
2. CANDIANI, G. B., P. VERCELLINI, L. FEDELE, S. GARSIA, D. BRIOSCHI & L. VILLA. 1991. Argon laser versus microscissor for hysteroscopic incision of uterine septa. Am. J. Obstet. Gynecol. **164**(1): 87.
3. CHOE, J. K. & M. S. BAGGISH. 1992. Hysteroscopic treatment of septate uterus with neodymium YAG laser. Fertil. Steril. **57**(1): 81.
4. DALY, C. D., D. MAJER & C. S. ALBROS. 1989. Hysteroscopic metroplasty: six years' experience. Obstet. Gynecol. **73:** 201.
5. DE CHERNEY, A. H., J. B. RUSSEL, R. A. GRAEBE & M. L. POLAN. 1986. Resectoscopic management of mullerian fusion defects. Fertil. Steril. **45:** 726.
6. FAYEZ, J. A. 1986. Comparison between abdominal and hysteroscopic metroplasty. Obstet. Gynecol. **68:** 339.
7. FEDELE, L., L. ARCAINI, F. PARAZZINI, P. VERCELLINI & G. DI NOLA. 1993. Reproductive prognosis after hysteroscopic metroplasty in 102 women: life table analysis. Fertil. Steril. **59**(4): 768.
8. GUARINO, S., S. INCANDELA, M. MANESCHI, G. VEGNA, M. R. D'ANNA, S. LEONE & F. MANESCHI. 1989. Hysteroscopic treatment of uterine septum. Acta Eur. Fertil. **20**(5): 321.
9. JONES, H. W., JR. 1981. Reproductive impairment and the malformed uterus. Fertil. Steril. **36:** 137.
10. MARCH, C. M. & R. ISRAEL. 1987. Hysteroscopic management of recurrent abortion caused by septate uterus. Am. J. Obstet. Gynecol. **156:** 834.
11. MCLUCAS, B. 1991. Intrauterine applications of the resectoscope. Surgery. Obstet. Gynecol. **164**(1): 425.
12. PERINO, A., E. CATINELLA, R. COMPARETTO, R. VENEZIA, P. CANDELA, C. CIMINO & C. ZANGARA. 1987. Hysteroscopic metroplasty: the role of ultrasound in the diagnosis and monitoring of patients with uterine septa. Acta Eur. Fertil. **18**(5): 349.
13. PERINO, A., L. MENCAGLIA, J. HAMOU & E. CITTADINI. 1987. Hysteroscopy for metroplasty of uterine septa: report of 24 cases. Fertil. Steril. **48**(2): 321.
14. VALLE, R. F. & J. J. SCIARRA. 1986. Hysteroscopic treatment of the septate uterus. Obstet. Gynecol. **67**(2): 253.
15. VERCELLINI, P., R. ROSSI, B. PAGNONI & L. FEDELE. 1992. Hypervolemic pulmonary edema and severe coagulopathy after intrauterine dextran instillation. Obstet. Gynecol. **79:** 838.

# Subject Index

**A**ctivin, parturition and, 380
Adenylate cyclase, parathyroid hormone stimulating, 365
Adhesion formation, pathophysiology of, 447
Adhesion molecules
   expression of, during endometrial cycle, 103
   immunological implications of, 43
Adjunctive progestogen, estrogen replacement therapy and, 278
Alkaline phosphatase, 285
Amniochorion, prelabor rupture of fetal membranes and, 430
Amniotic fluid
   activin in, 381
   vasopressin in, 374
Androgens, ovarian, 216
Antiestrogenic effect, 194
Antiprogestins, induction of labor and, 387
Apo E, trophoblast cells and, 94
Appendectomy, 434
Aquadissection, 456
Arteries, uterine, innervation of, 51

**B**enign cystic teratoma, 455
Beta-endorphin, steroid hormones and, 245
Biochemical ligand techniques, 27
Biopsy, hormone replacement therapy and, 263
Bleeding, uterine, role of PAI-1 in, 57
Blood flow, uterine, effects of some peptides on, 52
Bowel resection, 439
Breast cancer, adjuvant therapy for, 310
Bridging ligand, bifunctional, 115
Burch procedure, 436

**C**A125, deeply infiltrating endometriosis and, 334
Calcium channels, antiprogestins and, 398
cAMP
   fibronectin expression regulated by, 133
   parathyroid hormone and, 368
   prolactin induced by, 22
Cancer, endometrial, hormonal production and, 80
Cardiovascular disease, 19-nortestosterone and, 87
Cardiovascular protection, 274
CD44, expression of, in human endometrium, 113

Cell cultures, endometrial, proliferation of, 238
Cell surface, endometrial, implantation and, 103
Cell-mediated immune mechanism, 235
Cellular proliferation, cytokine regulation of, 322
Cervical canal, endometrial carcinoma and, 485
Cervical ripening
   preterm labor and, 415
   RU 486 and, 402
Cervix, antiprogestins and, 399
Circulation, endometrial, 51
Climacteric symptoms, 264
Clomiphene citrate, 193
$CO_2$ laser
   cystectomy and, 456
   deeply infiltrating endometriosis and, 335
Colony-stimulating factor, leukemia inhibitory factor and, 158
Colpotomy, large myomas and, 452
Common terminal pathway of parturition, 414
Complications
   laparoscopy and laparotomy and, 441
   uterine septa resection and, 473
Contraception, hormonal, 257
Contraceptives, oral, 260
Controlled ovarian hyperstimulation cycles, 216
Corticotropin-releasing factor, parturition and, 380
Culdotomy incision, 457
Cystectomy, laparoscopic, 455
Cytokine regulation, endometriosis and, 322
Cytokines
   development of microenvironments in human endometrium and, 1
   uterine cell proliferation and implantation and, 158
   uterine cervix and, 403
Cytotrophoblasts, 166

**D**9B1 epitope, 109
1-Deamino-2-D-(OEt)-4-Thr-8-Orn-oxytocin, 53
Death rates, cancer, 276
Decidua, placental, vasopressin in, 375
Decidual cells, hemostasis and menstruation and, 58
Decidual/membrane activation, preterm labor and, 417

Decidual receptors, 27
Decidualization
  ECM turnover in, 33
  growth factors and, 7
  protease expression during, 33
  stromal cells, 19, 21
Diethylstilbestrol, dual estrogenic and progestagenic activities and, 286
Distal pathology, laparoscopy for, 463
Donor oocyte program, 198
Dual estrogenic and progestagenic activities, compounds with, 293
Dynorphin, steroid hormones and, 245
Dysfunctional uterine bleeding, 80
Dysmenorrhoea, primary, spontaneous blood flow in, 53

Echo pattern, endometrial, 198
Echographic dendometrial patterns, tamoxifen and, 314
Ectopic pregnancy, 435
Egg donation model, 209
Embryo-endometrial interaction, 221
Embryo-epithelial stimulation, MUC-1 and, 116
Endometrial ablation for abnormal uterine bleeding, 469
Endometrial cancer
  estrogen replacement therapy and, 278
  hormonal treatment and, 306
  tamoxifen and, 310
Endometrial carcinoma
  epidermal growth factor receptor and, 300
  hysteroscopic evaluation of, 482
Endometrial contraception, 153
Endometrial differentiation, synthetic steroids and, 237
Endometrial hyperplasia
  estrogen replacement therapy and, 278–279
  hormonal treatment and, 306
Endometrial maturation, embryo's developmental stage and, 221
Endometrial preparation, adequate, 149
Endometrial receptivity, 193
Endometriosis
  bowel, 439
  cytokine regulation of cellular proliferation in, 322
  deeply infiltrating, 333
  endometrioid carcinoma and, 438
  epidemiology and diagnosis of, 352
  peritoneal, 439
    3-D evaluation of, 342
  prevalence of, 354

  recurrence of, 358
  severe, bladder resection for, 435
Endometrium (see also Human endometrium)
  donor oocyte program and, 198
  ectopic, 322
  eutopic, 322
  receptive, 143
  retarded, 180
Endoscopic surgery, medical suppressive therapy prior to, 445
Endoscopy, tubal evaluation and, 462
Epidermal growth factor
  decidual differentiation markers induced by, 8
  expression of, by cytotrophoblasts, 128
  leukemia inhibitory factor and, 158
Epidermal growth factor receptor, endometrial cancer histotypes and, 298
Epithelial cells, cell surface and secretory mucins in, 103
Estradiol, dual estrogenic and progestagenic activities and, 286
Estrogen receptors, decidual, 26, 29
Estrogen replacement therapy
  cardiovascular disease and, 274
  progestins and, 266–267
Estrogenic activities, progestagenic activities and, 285
Estrogens, epidermal growth factor receptor and, 302
Extracellular matrix, decidualization and, 33
Extracellular matrix protein expression, placental, 133

Fetal membranes, 166
  activin in, 381
  vasopressin in, 374
Fibronectin expression, placental, 133
First uterine pass, 212

Gap junctions, antiprogestins and, 395
Gemeprost, 490
Genital atrophy, estrogen replacement therapy and, 272
Giant mitochondria, 174
Glucocorticoids, placental fibronectin expression by, 132
Glycogen vacuole, 170
Glycosylation, MUC-1 and, 107
Gonadotropin-releasing hormone agonist
  deeply infiltrating endometriosis and, 335
  endometriosis recurrence and, 360

# SUBJECT INDEX

hysteroscopic surgery and, 475
medical suppression and, 445
premature luteinization and, 195
tubal obstruction and, 466
vascularization of endometriotic foci and, 345
Gonadotropin-releasing hormone analogs, hyperplastic endometria and, 308
Gonadotropins, cAMP induced by, 21
Granulated lymphocytes, endometrial, 187
Granulated metrial gland cell, 188
Growth factors, decidualization and, 7

Hemostasis, endometrial, 58
Histologic structures, 2-D image analysis program and, 344
Histological assessment, 479
Histological patterns, hormone replacement therapy and, 263
Histology
 endometriosis and, 323
 tamoxifen and, 314
Histones H2A, H2B, H3, H4, 147
Histotype, endometrial carcinoma and, 301
HLA-DR expression of endometrial epithelium, 2
HLA-G, 126
Hormonal and antihormonal activities, *in vitro* bioassays for, 285
Hormonal control, 209
Hormonal treatment, abnormal endometrial growth and, 306
Hormone antagonists, 143
Hormone replacement therapy
 aspects of, 271
 human endometrium and, 263
Human endometrial stromal cells, adhesion molecules on, 43
Human endometrium
 fragments of, *in vitro* bioassays with, 286
 hormone replacement therapy and, 263
 IFN-gamma in, 1
 microenvironments in, 1
 MUC-1 polypeptide in, 104
Human menopausal gonadotropin, 194
Hyperplasia, hormone replacement therapy and, 268
Hyperstimulation, egg donation model and, 209
Hyperstimulation regimen, donor oocyte program and, 198
Hysterectomy, laparoscopic, 436
Hysteroscopic evaluation, endometrial carcinoma and, 482

Hysteroscopic metroplasty, 489
Hysteroscopy, 479
 operative, ten years' experience of, 469
 tamoxifen and, 315

Immunity, altered cellular, 43
Immunocytochemistry, endometriosis and, 323
Immunohistochemical evaluation, primary endometrial carcinoma and, 299
Immunohistochemical methods, 27
Immunohistochemistry
 endometrial and trophoblastic tissues and, 222
 endometrial proteins and, 179
Immunologically mediated abortion, 235
Immunosuppression, 188
Implantation
 donor oocyte program and, 198
 endometrial and embryonic factors in, 221
 endometrial cell surface and, 103
 endometrial hemostasis and, 57
 LDL receptor proteins and, 91
 leukemia inhibitory factor and, 157
Implantation failures, intravenous immunoglobulin in prevention of, 232
*In situ* hybridization, endometriosis and, 324
*In vitro* bioassays, 285
*In vitro* fertilization
 donor oocyte program and, 198
 third factor hypothesis and, 215
 tubal infertility and, 465
*In vitro* influence of growth factors, 240
*In vitro* influence of physiological steroids, 237
*In vitro* studies, 176
Infertility, primary unexplained, 189
Insulin-like growth factor binding protein-1, regulation of, 12, 15
Insulin-like growth factor I and II, proliferation of stromal cells and, 9
Integrin, 125
Integrins, cytotrophoblastic differentiation and, 166
Intercellular adhesion molecule-1, stromal cells and, 43
Interferon gamma
 regulatory roles of, 1
 endometriosis and, 324
Interleukin-1, leukemia inhibitory factor and, 159
Intrauterine fetal death, RU 486 and, 394
Intravenous immunoglobulin, implantation failures and, 232

Ishikawa cells
  dual estrogenic and progestagenic activities in, 285
  secretion of β-endorphin and dynorphins from, 245–246

**K**eratan sulphate, presence of, in human endometrium, 111

**L**abor, antiprogestins in induction of, 387
Lactosaminoglycans, MUC-1 and, 108
Laparoscopy
  advantages of, over laparotomy, 453
  deeply infiltrating endometriosis and, 333
  endometriosis recurrence after, 359
  pelvic endometriosis and, 352
  peritoneal endometriosis and, 342
Laparotomy
  endometriosis recurrence after, 359
  pelvic endometriosis and, 352
Laser densitometric assessment, 150
Lectins, staining patterns for, 172
Lesions
  deeply infiltrating endometriosis and, 334
  endometriotic, in pelvis, 355
  red, 343
  subtle, 342
  typical, 342
  white, 344
Leukemia inhibitory factor
  implantation and, 157
  presence of, in endometrial fluids, 224
Leukocytes, ectopic endometrium and, 329
Ligand binding activities, overlapping, 91
Low density lipoprotein receptor family of proteins, implantation and, 91
Luminal epithelium, 175
Luteal inadequacy, 149
Luteal phase diagnostics, 153
Luteinization, premature, 195
Luteinizing hormone peak, 169
Luteinizing hormone-releasing hormone, β-endorphin secretion and, 250
Lymphocyte function-related antigen-3, stromal cells and, 43

$α_2$-**M**acroglobulin, trophoblast cells and, 99
Macrophages, ectopic endometrium and, 329
Mammals
  lower, induction of parturition studies in, 390
  regulation of implantation in, 157
Management of recurrent endometriosis, 360
Marshall-Marchetti-Krantz procedure, 436

Maternal peripheral venous plasma, 373
Matrigel, 178
Medical suppressive therapy, rationale for use of, 445
Medrogestone, 87
Medroxyprogesterone acetate, estrogenic and progestagenic activities and, 286
Menstrual cycle, endometrial circulation during, 51
Menstruation, role of PAI-1 in, 57
Metalloproteinases, 125
  ECM degradation and, 34
Metroplasty, hysteroscopic, 489
Metroplasty for uterine septa, 469
Metrorrhagia, DUB and, 80
Mice, leukemia inhibitory factor in, 158
Myoma
  intramural, 451
  pedunculated, 451
  submucous, 474
Myomectomy
  hysteroscopic, 471
  laparoscopic, operative procedure for, 450
  laparoscopic and minilaparotomy approach to, 437
Myometrial infiltration, 5-year survival rate and, 485
Myometrial responsiveness, antiprogestins and, 391

**N**atural killer cell, 187–188
Nitric oxide system, antiprogestins and, 396
Noncontraceptive health benefits of oral contraceptives, 260
19-Nortestosterone, cardiovascular disease and, 87
Nuclear channel system, 173
Nucleolar channel systems, 195

**O**nfFN expression in cytotrophoblasts, 133
Oocyte, donor, 198
Oocytes fertilization, steps of, 226
Oophorectomy, laparoscopic, 437, 455
Opioids, endometrial, regulation of, 253
ORG OD14, alkaline phosphatase activity and, 289
Osteoporosis
  estrogen replacement therapy and, 274
  potential risk of, 80
Ovarian cystic endometriosis, deeply infiltrating endometriosis and, 339
Ovarian cysts, other endometriomas differentiated from, 356
Ovarian remnant management, 438
Oxytocin receptors, antiprogestins and, 396

# SUBJECT INDEX

**P**AI-1, trophoblast cells and, 94
Parathyroid hormone-related protein, 365
Parturition
　activin and CRF in, 380
　common terminal pathway of, 414
　vasopressin and, 372
Peptides, effects of, on human uterine blood flow, 52
Peritoneal fluid, deeply infiltrating endometriosis and, 334
Placenta
　activin and, 381
　fibronectin expression in, 133
Placentation, LDL receptor proteins and, 91
Plasma estradiol/progesterone ratio, 212
Plasminogen activator inhibitor type 1, endometrial hemostasis and, 61
Plasminogen activators, ECM degradation and, 34
Polarized cells, 177
Polymorphic mucin MUC-1, 103
Polyps, tamoxifen and, 314
Population explosion control, 259
Pouch of Douglas, 334
　myomectomy and, 452
PP14, deeply infiltrating endometriosis and, 334
Preeclampsia, 126
Pregnancy rate, donor oocyte program and, 198
Prelabor rupture of fetal membranes, 430
Presacral neurectomy, 439
Preterm birth, 430
Preterm labor syndrome, 414
Prevical instrument, 145
Primates, nonhuman, induction of parturition with antiprogestins in, 391
Prodynorphin probe, 249
Progestagenic activities, estrogenic activities and, 285
Progesterone
　donor oocyte program and, 198
　dual estrogenic and progestagenic activities and, 286
　first uterine pass and, 212
　pregnancy maintenance and, 404
　production of, 80
Progesterone antagonists, 144
Progesterone receptors, decidual, 26, 29
Progestins
　endometrial stromal cells and, 23
　estrogen replacement therapy and, 266
Progestogens, addition of, caution against, 87
Prolactin, cAMP and, 22
Prolactin secretion, regulation of, by IGFs, 13, 15
Proliferation, extent of, 2

Proopiomelanocortin probe, 249
Prostaglandin $E_2$, decidualization process and, 24
Prostaglandin synthesis, parturition and, 381
Prostaglandins
　bioavailability of, 418
　uterine, effects of antiprogestins on, 394
　uterine cervix and, 403
Protease expression, 33
Protein patterns, 143
Psychological symptoms, estrogen replacement therapy and, 272

**Q**uality of life, estrogen replacement therapy and, 272

**R**2323 (gestrinone), progestagenic effects of, 293
RAP, trophoblast cells and, 97
Rat uterine explants, MUC-1 and, 108
Recanalization, tubal, 465
Receptivity, endometrial, hormonal control of, 209
Relaxin, decidualization process and, 24
Resection of submucous myomas, 469
Resectoscope, 491
RU 486 (mifepristone), 152
　$\beta$-endorphin secretion and, 250
　cervical ripening with, 402
　chemical structure of, 389
　concentration-dependent antagonistic effects of, 291

**S**acral colpopexy, 440
Second-trimester pregnancy termination, 393
Secretion
　delayed, 144
　human endometrial, 143
Septate uterus, 488
Shared oocyte program, 198
Sialoglycan epitope, D9B1 and, 109
Spontaneous abortion, 190
Squamous metaplasia, 303
Steric hindrance, MUC-1 and, 115
Steroids
　ovarian
　　endometrial circulation during menstrual cycle and, 51
　　protease expression and, 35
　　synthetic, regulation of endometrial differentiation by, 237
Stromal cell cultures
　metalloproteinase expression in, 37
　plasminogen expression in, 36

Stromal cells, parathyroid hormone and, 366
Stromal cells decidualization, mechanism of, 19, 21
Survival, endometrial carcinoma and, 483–484

T cell receptor, 186
T cells, ectopic endometrium and, 329
T lymphocytes, endometrial, 185
T47D cells, dual estrogenic and progestagenic activities in, 285
Tamoxifen
  effect of, on the endometrium, 307
  endometrial cancer and, 310
Thickness, endometrial
  donor oocyte program and, 198
  tamoxifen and, 314
Third factor hypothesis, 216
Three-dimensional architecture of endometriosis, 346
Tissue factor, endometrial hemostasis and, 58
Tissues, endometrial and trophoblastic, 222
Toxicity, tamoxifen, 318
Transcervical tuboscopy, 464
Transcriptional regulation, MUC-1 and, 105
Transfimbria tuboscopy, 464
Transforming growth factor $\beta1$, 222
Transvaginal administration of progesterone, 212
Transvaginal ultrasound, tamoxifen and, 313
Trophectoderm, 117
Trophoblast cells, LDL receptor family and, 94
Tubal infertility, therapeutic strategy in, 460
Two-dimensional image analysis program, 344

Ultrasound, 479
Ultrastructure, 172
UMR-106 cells, parathyroid hormone and, 367
Ureteroureterostomy, 440
Urokinase, trophoblast cells and, 94
Urokinase type-plasminogen activator, seminal fluid samples and, 225
Uterine contractility, 415
Uterine fluid, modulating embryo growth and, 227
Uterine secretion electrophoretic (USE) patterns, assessment of, 149
Uterine secretion proteins, 145
Uterine tissue, ligands for LDL receptor family produced by, 99
Uterus, septate, 488

Vaginal cytodiagnosis, tamoxifen and, 313
Variable number tandem repeat (VNTR) domain, structure of MUC-1 and, 104
Vascularization, morphometric study of, 344
Vasculature, arterial and capillary, of the human uterus, 48
Vasomotor symptoms, 271
Vasopressin, parturition and, 372

ZK 98299 (onapristone)
  chemical structure of, 389
  concentration-dependent antagonistic effects of, 291
Zoladex, suppression of ovarian activity obtained with, 87

# Index of Contributors

Aguzzoli, L., 380–386
Ajossa, S., 352–357
Åkerlund, M., 47–56
Amadori, A., 298–305
Angiolucci, M., 352–357
Aplin, J. D., 103–121
Audibert, F., 460–468

Baracchini, P., 263–270
Bargelli, G., 482–487
Bass, K. E., 122–131
Behzad, F., 103–121
Beier, H. M., 143–156
Beier-Hellwig, K., 143–156
Bell, S. C., 166–168, 430–432
Bergeron, C., 209–220
Bevini, M., 479–481
Bianchi, S., 358–364
Biglia, N., 310–321
Birkenfeld, A., 193–197
Bonn, B., 143–156
Borri, P., 26–32
Bouchard, P., 209–220
Bovicelli, A., 488–492
Branconi, F., 26–32
Bulletti, C., xi, 80–90, 221–231, 235–236
Bulmer, J. N., 185–192
Busacca, M., 43–46, 358–364
Buttram, V. C., Jr., 445–449
Bygdeman, M., 143–156

Caffiero, A., 352–357
Campbell, S., 103–121
Candiani, M., 358–364
Cappiello, F., 232–234
Casanas-Roux, F., 342–351
Casey, M. L., 365–371
Ceccarelli, C., 298–305
Chapron, C., 450–454
Check, J. H., 198–208
Chianchiano, N., 469–478
Chwalisz, K., 387–413
Colacurci, N., 232–234
Coukos, G., 91–102
Coutifaris, C., 91–102
Cristoforoni, P., 263–270, 469–478
Cudemo, V., 33–42

D'Hooghe, T., 333–341
De Cecco, L., 263–270
De Grandis, T., 310–321
De Las Fuentes, L., 7–18
de Micheroux, A. A., 380–386

De Placido, G., 232–234
De Vita, D., 380–386
De Ziegler, D., 209–220
Dey, T. D., 322–332
Di Carlo, C., 380–386
Di Nola, G., 358–364
Donnez, J., 342–351
Dubuisson, J-B., 450–454

Erk, A., 365–371

Fanchin, R., 209–220
Fedele, L., 358–364
Ferraiolo, A., 263–270
Ferrari, A., 380–386
Feygin, N., 33–42
Filoni, M., 488–492
Fisher, S. J., 122–131
Flamigni, C., xi, 80–90, 235–236, 479–481
Florio, P., 380–386
Frydman, R., 209–220

Gabrielli, S., 479–481
Gåfvels, M. E., 91–102
Galasso, M., 414–429
Gallinelli, A., 380–386
Garfield, R. E., 387–413
Gavi, B., 33–42
Gemzell-Danielsson, K., 143–156
Genazzani, A. D., 380–386
Gerbaldo, D., 263–270
Giacomucci, E., 80–90, 235–236
Giai, M., 310–321
Giudice, L. C., 7–18
Gomez, R., 414–429
Graham, R. A., 103–121
Gravanis, A., 245–256
Gubbini, G., 488–492
Guerriero, S., 352–357
Guller, S., 19–25, 132–142
Gurpide, E., xi, 19–25, 285–297

Hausknecht, V., 33–42, 57–79
Hey, N. A., 103–121
Hill, C. J., 169–184
Hilmes, U., 143–156
Holinka, C. F., 257–262, 271–284

Irwin, J. C., 7–18

Jasonni, V. M., 298–305, 479–481

**K**erenyi, T., 57–79
Kiesel, L., 237–244
Klein, N. A., 322–332
Koninckx, P. R., 333–341
Krikun, G., 33–42, 57–79

**L**eibman, M. I., 132–142
Li, T. C., 169–184
Licastro, F., 221–231
Lockwood, C. J., 33–42, 57–79, 132–142
López de la Osa González, E., 306–309

**M**acDonald, P. C., 365–371
Magri, B., 43–46
Mais, V., 352–357
Makrigiannakis, A., 245–256
Malak, T. M., 166–168, 430–432
Mappes, M., 237–244
Marabini, A., 488–492
Margioris, A. N., 245–256
Markiewicz, L., 33–42, 57–79, 285–297
Massonneau, M., 209–220
Matsuo, H., 91–102
Mauri, A., 372–379
Mazor, M., 414–429
Mazzone, S., 479–481
McMaster, M. T., 122–131
Melis, G. B., 352–357
Messeri, G., 26–32
Meuleman, C., 333–341
Mollo, A., 232–234
Moncini, D., 482–487
Montoya, I. A., 322–332
Mulholland, G., 430–432
Munoz, H., 414–429
Muserra, G., 479–481

**N**aldi, S., 298–305, 479–481
Nazzaro, A., 232–234
Nezhat, Camran, 433–444
Nezhat, Ceana, 433–444
Nezhat, F., 433–444
Nisolle, M., 342–351
Noci, I., 26–32
Nutini, L., 26–32

**O**osterlynck, D., 333–341

**P**aglierani, M., 26–32
Palumbo, G., 232–234
Paoletti, A. M., 352–357
Papp, C., 33–42, 57–79
Papp, Z., 33–42, 57–79
Pareschi, A., 479–481

Parmeggiani, R., 221–231
Pérgola, G. M., 322–332
Perino, A., 469–478
Periti, E., 26–32
Petraglia, F., 380–386
Piccione, E., 372–379
Piras, B., 352–357
Polli, V., 80–90, 221–231, 235–236
Possati, G., 479–481
Prefetto, R. A., 80–90
Pulcheri, E., 263–270

**R**emorgida, V., 263–270
Romero, R., 414–429
Rosati, M., 455–459

**S**antini, D., 298–305
Saravelos, H., 169–184
Scarselli, G., 26–32, 482–487
Schatz, F., 33–42, 57–79
Schenken, R. S., 322–332
Seif, M. W., 103–121
Sherer, D. M., 414–429
Sismondi, P., 310–321
Stagnozzi, R., 488–492
Stefanetti, M., 488–492
Sterzik, K., 143–156
Stewart, C. L., 157–165
Stournaras, C., 245–256
Strauss, J. F. III, 91–102
Strickland, D. K., 91–102

**T**abibzadeh, S., 1–6
Taddei, G. L., 26–32, 482–487
Tang, B., 19–25
Tantini, C., 482–487
Tekmal, R. R., 322–332
Ticconi, C., 372–379
Torricelli, F., 26–32
Toth-Pal, E., 33–42, 57–79
Tozzi, P., 26–32

**V**iganò, P., 43–46
Vignali, M., 43–46, 358–364
Volpe, A., 372–379
Volpi, E., 310–321

**W**ang, E-Y., 33–42, 57–79
Warren, M. A., 169–184
Wittmaack, F., 91–102
Wozniak, R., 132–142

**Z**hou, X., 57–79
Zullo, F., 232–234